Essentials of Global Mental Health

Essentials of Global Mental Health

Edited by

Samuel O. Okpaku
Executive Director of the Center for Health, Culture, and Society, Nashville, Tennessee, USA

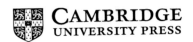

CAMBRIDGE
UNIVERSITY PRESS

CAMBRIDGE
UNIVERSITY PRESS

University Printing House, Cambridge CB2 8BS, United Kingdom

One Liberty Plaza, 20th Floor, New York, NY 10006, USA

477 Williamstown Road, Port Melbourne, VIC 3207, Australia

314-321, 3rd Floor, Plot 3, Splendor Forum, Jasola District Centre, New Delhi - 110025, India

79 Anson Road, #06-04/06, Singapore 079906

Cambridge University Press is part of the University of Cambridge.

It furthers the University's mission by disseminating knowledge in the pursuit of education, learning and research at the highest international levels of excellence.

www.cambridge.org
Information on this title: www.cambridge.org/9781107022324

© Cambridge University Press 2014

First published 2014
Reprinted 2015

A catalogue record for this publication is available from the British Library

Library of Congress Cataloging in Publication data
Essentials of global mental health / [edited by] Samuel O. Okpaku.
        p. ; cm.
Includes bibliographical references.
ISBN 978-1-107-02232-4 (Hardback)
I. Okpaku, Samuel O., editor of compilation.
[DNLM: 1. Mental Health.   2. Developing Countries.
3. Mental Disorders.   4. Mental Health Services.
5. World Health. WM 101]
RA790.55
362.19689–dc23
2013026598

ISBN 978-1-107-02232-4 Hardback

. . . .

To my departed parents, sisters, uncles and aunts, who always had confidence in me and supported my dreams

Contents

Section 1 – History and background of global mental health

Section 2 – Advocacy and reduction of stigma

Section 3 – Systems of development

Section 8 – Research and monitoring the progress of countries

Contributors

Zachary W. Adams, PhD
National Crime Victims Research & Treatment Center, Department of Psychiatry & Behavioral Sciences, Medical University of South Carolina, SC, USA

Margarita Alegría, PhD
Professor, Department of Psychiatry, Harvard Medical School; Director, Center for Multicultural Mental Health Research, Cambridge Health Alliance, Somerville, MA, USA

Atalay Alem, MD
Professor of Psychiatry, Department of Psychiatry, School of Medicine, College of Health Sciences, Addis Ababa University, Ethiopia

Jordi Alonso, MD, PhD
Epidemiology and Public Health Program, IMIM (Institut Hospital del Mar d'Investigacions Mèdiques); Pompeu Fabra University (UPF); CIBER en Epidemiología y Salud Pública (CIBERESP), Barcelona, Spain

Victor Aparicio, MD, PhD
Director of Management, Mental Health Clinic, Asturias Central University Hospital (Hospital Universitario Central de Asturias), Oviedo, Spain

Rifat Atun, MBBS, MBA
Professor of International Health Management, Imperial College, London, UK

Florence Baingana, MBChB, MMed (Psych), MSc (HPPF)
Makerere University School of Public Health, Uganda; Personal Social Services Research Unit, London School of Economics and Political Sciences, London, UK

Emily Baron, BSc, MSc
Perinatal Mental Health Project, Alan J Flisher Centre for Public Mental Health, Department of Psychiatry and Mental Health, University of Cape Town, Cape Town, South Africa

Marco Bertelli, MD
Scientific Director, CREA (Research and Clinical Centre), San Sebastiano Foundation, Florence, Italy

Dinesh Bhugra, PhD, FRCPsych
Professor of Mental Health and Cultural Diversity, Institute of Psychiatry, King's College London, London, UK

Sanchita Biswas, MA, MPhil
Vice-Principal, AL Noor Public School, Aligarh, India

José Miguel Caldas de Almeida, MD, PhD
NOVA Medical School & CEDOC (Chronic Diseases Research Center), NOVA University of Lisbon, Portugal

Edwin Cameron, BA, LLB
Justice of the Constitutional Court of South Africa, Johannesburg, South Africa

Somnath Chatterji, MD
Global Burden Disease Unit, World Health Organization, Geneva, Switzerland

Erminia Colucci, PhD
Centre for International Mental Health, School of Population Health, the University of Melbourne, Melbourne, Vic., Australia

Janice L. Cooper, PhD
Department of Health Policy and Management, Emory University, Atlanta, GA, USA; College of Science and Technology, University of Liberia, Monrovia, Liberia

Carla Kmett Danielson, PhD
Associate Professor of Psychiatry, National Crime Victims Research & Treatment Center, Medical University of South Carolina, Charleston, SC, USA

Diego De Leo, MD, PhD
Professor of Psychiatry; Director, Australian Institute for Suicide Research and Prevention, Griffith University, Mt Gravatt, Qld., Australia

Mary-Jo DelVecchio Good, PhD
Professor of Social Medicine, Department of Global Health and Social Medicine, Harvard Medical School, Harvard University, Boston, MA, USA

Marten W. de Vries, MD, PhD
Professor of Social Psychiatry and Public Mental Health (emeritus), Maastricht University, The Netherlands

Maureen S. Durkin, PhD, DrPH
Waisman Center, University of Wisconsin-Madison, Madison, WI, USA

Xiangming Fang, PhD
Professor of Applied Economics, Director, International Center for Applied Economics and Policy, China Agricultural University, Beijing, China

Julia W. Felton, MD
Assistant Clinical Professor, Department of Psychology, University of Maryland, College Park, MD, USA

Sally Field, BA, MA
Perinatal Mental Health Project, Alan J Flisher Centre for Public Mental Health, Department of Psychiatry and Mental Health, University of Cape Town, Cape Town, South Africa

Andrea Fiorillo, MD, PhD
Department of Psychiatry, University of Naples SUN, Italy

Lance Gable, JD, MPH
Wayne State University Law School, Detroit, MI, USA

Teddy Gafna, BA
Project Officer with Africa Mental Health Foundation

Sandro Galea, MD, DrPH
Gelman Professor and Chair, Department of Epidemiology, Mailman School of Public Health, Columbia University, New York, NY, USA

Patrick Gatonga, MD, MBA
Department of Public Health, University of Nairobi, Kenya

Sofia Halperin-Goldstein
Macalester College, St. Paul, MN, USA

Yanling He, MD
Department of Psychiatric Epidemiology, Shanghai Mental Health Center, Shanghai, China

Grace A. Herbert, BA
Center for Health, Culture, and Society, Nashville, TN, USA

Sabrina Hermosilla, MIA, MPH, MS
Department of Epidemiology, Mailman School of Public Health, Columbia University, New York, NY, USA

Simone Honikman, MD, MPhil
Perinatal Mental Health Project, Alan J Flisher Centre for Public Mental Health, Department of Psychiatry and Mental Health, University of Cape Town, Cape Town, South Africa

Takashi Izutsu, PhD
Department of Forensic Psychiatry, National Institute of Mental Health, National Center of Neurology and Psychiatry, Chiba, Japan

Ruwan M. Jayatunge, MD
Former Medical Officer of Mental Health, Ministry of Health, Sri Lanka

Janis H. Jenkins, PhD
Professor of Anthropology, Adjunct Professor of Psychiatry, University of California at San Diego, CA, USA

Rachel Jenkins, MB BChir, MD
Professor of Epidemiology and International Mental Health Policy, Institute of Psychiatry, King's College London, London, UK

Lynne Jones OBE, MBChB, PhD
Honorary Consultant, South London and Maudsley NHS Trust; Honorary Senior Clinical Fellow, Department of Psychiatry, Cambridge University, UK

Jayanthi Karunaratne, BA, PGDJ
Center for Health, Culture, and Society, Nashville, TN, USA

Ronald C. Kessler, PhD
Department of Health Care Policy, Harvard Medical School, Harvard University, Boston, Massachusetts, USA

Rob Keukens
Department of Community Mental Health Nursing, HAN University of Applied Sciences, Nijmegen, The Netherlands

Lincoln I. Khasakhala, MBChB
Senior Lecturer, Daystar University, Nairobi; Honorary Lecturer, Department of Psychiatry, University of Nairobi, Kenya

Hanna Kienzler, PhD
Department of Social Science, Health & Medicine, King's College London, London, UK

Sarah Kippen Wood, MPH
International Research Manager, BasicNeeds, Bangalore, India

M. Thomas Kishore, PhD
Reader in Health Psychology, University of Hyderabad, India

Robert Kohn, MD, MPhil
Professor, Psychiatry and Human Behavior, The Warren Alpert Medical School of Brown University, The Miriam Hospital, Providence, RI, USA

Natasja Koitzsch Jensen, MPH
Danish Research Centre for Migration, Ethnicity and Health, University of Copenhagen, Copenhagen, Denmark

Sheri Lapatin, MIA
Associate Director, Center for Mulitcultural Mental Health Research, Somerville, MA, USA

Anna Lessios, BA
Center for Mulitcultural Mental Health Research, Somerville, MA, USA

Isabel Louro Bernal, PhD
National School of Public Health (Escuela Nacional de Salud Publica, ENSAP), University of Medical Sciences, Havana, Cuba

Feijun Luo, PhD
National Center on Birth Defects and Developmental Disabilities, Centers for Disease Control and Prevention, Atlanta, GA, USA

Laura MacPherson, PhD
Associate Professor, Department of Psychology, University of Maryland, College Park, MD, USA

Matthew J. Maenner, PhD
Waisman Center, University of Wisconsin-Madison, Madison, WI, USA

Anne W. Mbwayo, PhD
WIMA Africa and United States International University – Africa, Nairobi, Kenya

David McDaid, MSc
Research Fellow in Health Policy and Health Economics, London School of Economics and Political Science, London, UK

Ingrid Meintjes, MSocSc
Perinatal Mental Health Project, Alan J Flisher Centre for Public Mental Health, Department of Psychiatry and Mental Health, University of Cape Town, Cape Town, South Africa

Victoria N. Mutiso, PhD
Clinical Psychologist and Research Director, Africa Mental Health Foundation, Nairobi, Kenya

David M. Ndetei, MD
Professor of Psychiatry, University of Nairobi; Director, Africa Mental Health Foundation, Nairobi, Kenya

Samuel O. Okpaku, MD, PhD
Executive Director of the Center for Health, Culture, and Society, Nashville, TN, USA

Lijing Ouyang, PhD
National Center on Birth Defects and Developmental Disabilities, Centers for Disease Control and Prevention, Atlanta, GA, USA

Ramachandran Padmavati, MD, DPM
Schizophrenia Research Foundation, Tamilnadu, India

Clare Pain, MD, MSc, FRCPC
Associate Professor, Department of Psychiatry, University of Toronto; Director, Psychological Trauma Program, Mount Sinai Hospital, Toronto, Canada

Duncan Pedersen, PhD
Associate Scientific Director, Douglas Mental Health University Institute, McGill University, Montreal, Canada

Jordan Pfau
BasicNeeds, Bangalore, India

Felipe Picon, MD, MSc
Child and Adolescent Psychiatrist, Porto Alegre, Brazil

Rodney D. Presley, MSW
Project Director and Operational Manager, John F. Kennedy Memorial Medical Center/Grant Mental Health Hospital, Monrovia, Liberia

Reima Pryor, BBSci
Director, Research and Evaluation, Drummond Street Services, Carlton, Melbourne, Vic., Australia

Shoba Raja, MA
Director, Policy and Practice, BasicNeeds, Bangalore, India

Thara Rangaswamy, MD, PhD
Director, Schizophrenia Research Foundation, Chennai, India

Jorge Rodriguez, MD, PhD
Senior Advisor, Mental Health, Pan American Health Organization, Washington, DC, USA

Diana Rose, PhD
Reader in User-Led Research, Institute of Psychiatry, King's College London, London, UK

Moosa Salie, BSc, BEd
Former Chair and Co-Chair, World Network of Users and Survivors of Psychiatry

Norman Sartorius, MD, PhD
President, Association for the Improvement of Mental Health Programmes (AMH), Geneva, Switzerland

Ester Shapiro, PhD
Psychology Department, Gaston Institute for Latino Community Development and Public Policy, University of Massachusetts, Boston, MA, USA

Manuela Silva, MD, MSc
Hospital de Santa Maria and Faculty of Medicine, University of Lisbon, Lisbon, Portugal

Daya Somasundaram, MD
Clinical Associate Professor, Discipline of Psychiatry, University of Adelaide; Consultant Psychiatrist, Glenside Mental Health Services, SA, Australia

Katherine Sorsdahl, PhD
Department of Psychiatry and Mental Health, University of Cape Town, Cape Town, South Africa

Dan J. Stein, MD, PhD
Department of Psychiatry and Mental Health, University of Cape Town, Cape Town, South Africa

Deborah M. Stone, ScD, MSW, MPH
National Center for Injury Prevention and Control, Centers for Disease Control and Prevention, Atlanta, GA, USA

Heather Stuart, MA, PhD
Professor and Bell Canada Mental Health and Anti-Stigma Research Chair, Department of Community Health Epidemiology, Queen's University, Kingston, ON, Canada

Athula Sumathipala, MBBS, DFM, MD, PhD
Senior Lecturer, Institute of Psychiatry, King's College London, London, UK; Director, Institute for Research and Development, Battaramulla, Sri Lanka

Hema Tharoor, DPM, DNB, MNAMS
Consultant Psychiatrist, Schizophrenia Research Foundation (SCARF), Chennai, India

Rita Thom, PhD
Department of Psychiatry, University of the Witwatersrand, Johannesburg, South Africa

Lay San Too
Australian Institute for Suicide Research and Prevention, Griffith University, Mt Gravatt, Qld., Australia

Atsuro Tsutsumi, PhD
United Nations University International Institute for Global Health (UNU-IIGH), Kuala Lumpur, Malaysia

Chris Underhill, MBE
Founder Director, BasicNeeds, Leamington Spa, Warwickshire, UK

Anne Valentine, MPH
Center for Multicultural Mental Health Research,
Somerville, MA, USA

Claire van der Westhuizen, MBChB
Department of Psychiatry and Mental Health, Groote
Schuur Hospital, Cape Town, South Africa

Thandi van Heyningen, MA, MA ClinPsych
Perinatal Mental Health Project, Alan
J Flisher Centre for Public Mental Health,
Department of Psychiatry and Mental Health,
University of Cape Town, Cape Town,
South Africa

Robert van Voren, PhD
Chief Executive, Global Initiative on Psychiatry;
Professor of Political Science, Vytautas Magnus
University, Kaunas, Lithuania; Professor of Political
Science, Ilia Chavchavadze State University, Tbilisi,
Georgia

Inka Weissbecker, PhD MPH
Global Mental Health and Psychosocial Advisor,
International Medical Corps

Gail Wyatt, PhD
Professor of Psychology, University of California, Los
Angeles, CA, USA

Preface

Modern globalization refers to a one-world system that has been triggered by a telecommunication revolution, quicker air travel, and mass migration. It implies the presence of some dominant factors which are influential in the field of economics, politics, culture, ideology, and public health. In their article "Global health law: a definition and grand challenges," Gostin and Taylor define globalization thus:

> Globalization can be broadly understood as a process characterized by changes in a range of social spheres including economic, political, technological, cultural and environmental. These processes of global change are restructuring human societies, ushering in new patterns of health and disease and reshaping the broad determinants of health. Indeed, the globalization of trade, travel, communication, migration, information and lifestyles has obscured the traditional distinction between national and global health. Increasingly human activities have profound health consequences for people in all parts of the world, and no country can insulate itself from the effects. Members of the world's community are interdependent and reliant on one another for health security.
>
> (Gostin & Taylor 2008)

No matter the derivation and background, globalization cannot be divorced from issues of international trade, commerce, communication, and politics. Hence, global health cannot be seen in isolation from such considerations, or divorced from such a contextual framework.

The world is a smaller place, and the individual and community relationships in this shrunken place have been significantly affected by radio, television, cell phones, and the internet. These technological innovations bring world events to living rooms and offices worldwide. Evidence the 2010 rescue of 33 miners in Chile who were trapped underground for 64 days. The international collaboration which brought about their rescue along with the worldwide attention paid to the dramatic events is just one example of our new-found interconnectivity. State borders and barriers are shifting. We are witnessing the rise of transnational corporations, and globalization studies are mushrooming in many universities. There are calls for universities to shift their traditional roles and pay greater attention to global issues, community development, and research. Non-governmental organizations (NGOs) such as the Gates Foundation and the Wellcome Trust are playing a significant role in the eradication of poverty and disease. In this respect, discourse on human rights and the eradication of poverty has taken a global perspective. Needless to say, the word *global* has replaced *international*. This world view signifies new dynamic approaches and attitudes which have relevance for global health and global mental health. The World Health Organization (WHO) has a slogan, "There is no health without mental health" (Prince *et al.* 2007). I would go further, and suggest that if we perceive human activities as a hierarchical pyramid, the apex of the pyramid is mental health, followed by physical health, and then other human priorities. An individual's will, motivation, self-esteem, and perceptions are dependent on his or her psychological state and well-being. These then influence physical health, relationships to family and caregivers, workplace functioning, creativity, and productivity. In other words, one's mental health is paramount. From a clinical point of view, depression often affects the natural history and outcome of many physical illnesses.

So what is meant by global health and global mental health? In the preamble to its constitution, the WHO defined health as "a state of complete physical, mental and social well-being and not merely the absence of disease or infirmity" (WHO 1946), and in 2001 the WHO stated that:

> Mental health is as important as physical health to the overall well-being of individuals, societies and countries. Yet only a small minority of the 450 million people suffering from mental or behavioural disorders are

receiving treatment ... like many physical illnesses, mental and behavioural disorders are the result of a complex interaction between biological, physiological and social factors. While there is still much to be learned, we already have the knowledge and power to reduce the burden of mental and behavioural disorders worldwide.

(World Health Organization 2001)

The Global Initiative in Psychiatry group conceptualized the WHO message thus:

Mental health problems are the result of the complex – and still not fully understood – interaction of biological factors such as heredity and birth trauma, physiological factors such as lack of care and love, and social factors such as social exclusion. By contrast, intellectual disability is most commonly present at birth. Both nevertheless place affected individuals and their immediate care-givers in an extremely vulnerable position in terms of their basic human rights, social integration and access to educational and economic opportunities.

(Global Initiative on Psychiatry 2008)

From my perspective, the mere substitution of the term *global mental health* for *international mental health* will be no more than window dressing if there are no innovative strategies for a clarion call for greater attention to the core values of autonomy, equality, empowerment, advocacy, and respect for diversity and human rights. Therefore, global mental health should be seen as a new approach to the ideals of mental health services and research worldwide. It is a movement with both a humanitarian and a philosophical basis. Our experiences from unwanted consequences of the community mental health movement and the increase of mentally ill individuals in prisons, or the rise of homelessness, should alert us to the need for careful articulation, planning, and execution of the movement for global mental health.

Similarly, there is some strenuous criticism of the term *global mental health*. The globalization trend has not gained universal acceptance. We can recall the confrontations which heralded the International Monetary Fund meetings in Seattle and Toronto, and the more recent Occupy Wall Street movement. There are fears of neo-colonialism or neo-liberalism and capitalism, with the potential for the rich to get richer and the poor to get poorer.

New Partnership for Africa's Development (NEPAD), an African Union strategic framework for pan-African socioeconomic development, while addressing the challenges of globalization says,

In the absence of fair and just global rules, globalisation has increased the ability of the strong to advance their interests to the detriment of the weak, especially in the areas of trade, finance and technology. It has limited space for developing countries to control their own development, as the system makes no provision for compensating the weak. The conditions of those marginalized in this process have worsened in real terms. A fissure between inclusion and exclusion has emerged within and among nations.

(NEPAD 2001)

In the same context of challenges of globalization the ex-World Bank President Wolfensohn stated, "We cannot turn back globalisation. Our challenge is to make globalisation an instrument of opportunity and inclusion – not of fear and insecurity. Globalisation must work for all" (Wolfensohn 2001).

The marketplace and capitalism are not perfect. These criticisms should not be dismissed but should be fully confronted. For example, it is true that global activities have now become a way to justify career paths, and to increase research funding and salaries. All this, however, should pale against the moral basis and humanitarian ideals of international cooperation. It is not difficult to make a moral case for global mental health. We are all in this together. There is widespread suffering in many developed and developing countries. In many countries manpower and infrastructure are very limited. There are countries with fewer than 10 psychiatrists. Therefore, global mental health underscores our interconnectivity and interconnectedness. Witness the enthusiasm of young professionals and students who participate in exchange programs, the dedication of aid workers, and the contribution of NGOs.

Nevertheless, there is a cautionary note from D. Summerfield, who argues that Western definitions and solutions cannot be routinely applied to problems in developing countries. He also challenges the claim that, for example, every year up to 30% of the global population will develop some form of mental disorder (Summerfield 2008). His point of view has to be fully addressed. This implies the need for attention to diversity, cultural relevance, and local conditions. There is an urgent need for capacity building and sustainability, as funding tends to occur in cycles. Trust between donors and recipient entities has become a sine qua non.

Furthermore, there is always a need to explore the mutual benefits of international collaboration. No nation can produce enough mental health professionals to meet her needs. Poverty, which is a major cause of illness and depression, is worldwide, even in the United States, as shown by the latest study conducted by the Urban Institute (Nichols 2012). There are slums in New York City, London, Mumbai, Rio de Janeiro, and Lagos. Human suffering is ubiquitous. Knowledge from the low-income and middle-income countries can also contribute to mental health services and research in high-income countries. There is an advantage to a more plural knowledge base in mental health against a background of diversity. Research findings and service delivery systems in low- and middle-income countries can provide alternative models of service delivery in the developed countries.

In 1986, I participated in an international conference in Kenya where some African psychiatrists lamented the lack of opportunities for research in their home countries. From my vantage point as a United States resident I was able to observe the numerous opportunities in African countries to address some fundamental issues in mental health. One good example is the application of traditional approaches to post-conflict reconciliation in Rwanda, the Congo, and their extensions to European and American liturgy. Another example is the relative success of integration of mental health services into primary care in developing countries.

There are many competitive definitions of global health. However, I choose to use the definition by Koplan and colleagues, who defined global health as:

> an area of study, research and practice that places a high priority on improving health and achieving equality in health for all people worldwide. Global health emphasizes transnational health issues, determinants, and solutions; involves many disciplines within and beyond the health sciences and promotes interdisciplinary collaboration; and is a synthesis of population-based prevention with individual-level clinical care.
>
> (Koplan et al. 2009)

Generally, in definitions of global health there are no specific references made to mental health and illnesses. Usually, references are made to such major public health burdens as HIV/AIDS, tuberculosis, maternal and infant mortality. Even the Millennium Fund does not make any specific reference to mental health and illness. This is in spite of the relationship

between behavior and lifestyle and their role in the causation of diseases. In fact, mental illness contributes directly to about 14% of the burden of disease, and indirectly much more so (Prince et al. 2007). This contribution of mental illness to the burden of diseases was underscored by the *World Development Report* (World Bank 1993) and the influential *Global Burden of Disease* report (Murray & Lopez 1996). These reports and the concerns they generated led to additional high-level reports. They mobilized further interest and a call to policy makers to act on this problem. These reports with their recommendations included those from the World Federation for Mental Health, the Institute of Medicine, and the WHO (World Federation for Mental Health 2009). Essentially these reports emphasized the need to pay attention to the well-being of those afflicted by mental disorders. More specifically, they made recommendations to expand and improve the current systems of mental health delivery, provide cost-effective interventions, and provide care in the primary care setting of each country.

Other recommendations included:

- the establishment of linkages with other systems
- strengthening the workforce to provide effective care
- enhancing the human resources
- creating medical centers for research and linking these with institutions in high-income countries
- establishing national health policies, legislation and programs
- encouraging families, communities and users to be involved
- engaging in reduction of stigma and discrimination

The above provides a background to the founding of a global mental health movement. Again, for clarity, I have chosen to adopt Dr. Vikram Patel and his colleagues' definition of global mental health as

> the area of study, research and practice that places a priority on improving mental health and achieving equity in mental health for all people worldwide.
>
> (Patel & Prince 2010)

A major objective of this volume is to define the domain of global mental health and draw the boundaries of the field. The underlying philosophy of this international vision is to make cost-effective, evidence-based treatment services available to those potentially ill individuals worldwide, but more especially to individuals in low- and middle-income countries.

The Movement for Global Mental Health has identified five priorities. These are global advocacy, systems of development, research programs, capacity building, and monitoring progress of countries.

These areas are addressed in the pages that follow, as are the barriers and challenges that stand in the way of achieving these complex tasks. The volume also showcases some best practices that have worldwide applications, and it contains discussions about ethical practices in service delivery and research, including the role of donor countries and NGOs. This volume is therefore targeted at students and trainers in relevant mental health and related disciplines, professionals of these fields, administrators, policy makers, and libraries. It should be a useful foundation book for individuals interested in global mental health.

References

Global Initiative on Psychiatry (2008) Prioritizing mental health Improving psychosocial and mental health care in transitional and developing countries. http://www.gip-global.org/images/24/209.pdf (accessed June 2013).

Gostin LO, Taylor AL (2008) Global health law: a definition and grand challenges. *Public Health Ethics* **1**: 53–63. doi: 10.1093/phe/phn005.

Koplan JP, Bond TC, Merson MH, *et al.* (2009) Towards a common definition of global health. *Lancet* **373**: 1993–5.

Murray CJL, Lopez AD (1996) *The Global Burden of Disease: a Comprehensive Assessment of Mortality and Disability from Diseases, Injuries, and Risk Factors in 1990 and Projected to 2020.* Cambridge, MA: Harvard University Press.

NEPAD (2001) *The New Partnership for Africa's Development (NEPAD).*

Abuja, Nigeria. http://www.un.org/africa/osaa/reports/nepad Engversion.pdf (accessed July 2013).

Nichols A (2012) *Poverty in the United States.* Washington, DC: Urban Institute. http://www.urban.org/publications/412653.html (accessed July 2013).

Patel V, Prince M (2010) Global mental health: a new global health field comes of age. *JAMA* **303**: 1976–7. doi: 10.1001/jama.2010.616.

Prince M, Patel V, Saxena S, *et al.* (2007) No health without mental health. *Lancet* **370**: 859–77.

Summerfield D (2008) How scientifically valid is the knowledge base of global mental health? *BMJ* **336**: 992–4.

Wolfensohn JD (2001) The challenges of globalization: the role of the World Bank. Public Discussion Forum, Berlin, Germany, April 2, 2001. http://web.worldbank.org/WBSITE/EXTERNAL/TOPICS/

EXTARD/0,,contentMDK: 20025027~menuPK:336721~ pagePK:64020865~piPK: 149114~theSitePK:336682,00.html (accessed July 2013).

World Bank (1993) *World Development Report 1993: Investing in Health.* Oxford: Oxford University Press.

World Federation for Mental Health (2009) Mental health in primary care: enhancing treatment and promoting mental health. *World Mental Health Day.*

World Health Organization (1946) *Constitution of the World Health Organization.* New York, NY: International Health Conference.

World Health Organization (2001) *The World Health Report 2001. Mental Health: New Understanding, New Hope.* Geneva: WHO. http://www.who.int/whr/2001/en/whr01_en.pdf (accessed July 2013).

Acknowledgments

There is some inscrutability about the impulses that drive an individual to edit a volume. Nevertheless, upon reflection I seem to have been driven by several influences.

One influence is the unique experience of my career. My interest in culture and society, which made me choose psychiatry over neurosurgery or immunology, seems to have persisted. That interest very often propels me to express an African opinion on issues.

Second influence – as an African who has never had the privilege to work in Africa, I have a diasporic need, indeed an Adlerian need, to contribute something, no matter how small, to scaling up mental health services in Africa and elsewhere in the developing world.

Third influence – as an African, I am forced to empathize with the suffering of the poor and mentally ill in low- and middle-income countries. All that stigmatization of the mentally ill is universal, and it takes on a greater depth in developing countries. Witness the mentally ill and their treatment in Kenya and India, as depicted by CNN in a TV series in 2010.

Lastly, any volume that discusses global themes and issues of necessity has to be highly selective. Otherwise it will require a large canvas and the exercise will be chaotic.

In summary, then, my interest in this area derives from my background as a citizen of Nigeria and the USA. This places me in a unique position to empathize with local, national, and international mental health issues. My goal, therefore, was to select what I consider the most relevant issues in global health and recruit experts in these fields to contribute to the volume. Furthermore, the editor generally is a bandmaster and has to rely very much on the contributors. So I would like to express my intense gratitude to all the contributors to the volume.

I am also deeply indebted to the reviewers who were kind enough to review chapters in their areas and make useful suggestions. For undertaking this task I thank Judith Bass, Fred Kigozi, Birthe Loa Knizek, William Lawson, James A. Mercey, Saggane Musisi, Temisan Okpaku, Uma Rao, Maria Tomasic, and Helen Ullrich.

Another group to whom I wish to extend my gratitude consists of people who when I was formulating my ideas gave me helpful suggestions and comments. These individuals included Lawrence Gostin, Jaswant Guzder, Helen Herrman, Laurence Kirmayer, Peter Martin, Donna Stewart, and Mitchell Weiss.

Also I want to express my thanks and gratitude to my full-time or temporary staff as I preoccupied their minds with my own obsessions about global mental health. These people helped at all stages of preparing the manuscript. They included Chris Hack, Mary Hare, Kristen Jackson, Mary Ozanne, and Carol Watson.

My special thanks go to the staff of Cambridge University Press under Richard Marley. It was a delight to work with them, especially with Jane Seakins, whose help and encouragement was extraordinary.

I am greatly indebted to five individuals who contributed immensely to the volume – my youngest son Temisan Okpaku, who was always a sounding board and gave me valuable editorial assistance; Tony Dreher, who provided technical assistance during the middle phase of editing; and Sanchita Biswas, Grace Herbert, and Jayanthi Karunaratne, who worked many hours to make the volume possible.

Lastly, there are those unnamed individuals who contributed in some way to clarify my thoughts but whose names elude me. To them I say thanks. If I have omitted any other names, it is not by design – the omission can be attributed to the vagaries of time and memory.

Introduction

This volume was conceived in an attempt to give some voice to mental health, as the movement for global health and global health diplomacy mushrooms. In spite of the ubiquity of mental illness and the demand for relief, mental illness continues to be ignored in policy and practice. This is despite the evidence that there are possibilities for the promotion of mental health and the prevention of mental illness. The practice of these disciplines does not require expensive instruments and technology, but rather the training and availability of skilled personnel and adequate public health information.

The volume is divided into eight sections.

Section 1: History and background of global mental health

In this section, the terms *globalization* and *global mental health* are defined. The origin of modern global health diplomacy is traced. The role of the United Nations and its specialized agencies are mentioned. A typology of sponsorships of global health initiatives is undertaken. The worldwide burden of mental illness and the gaps between needs and services are addressed.

Section 2: Advocacy and reduction of stigma

Stigma leads to discrimination, and to the exclusion of individuals with mental illness and their families. This section has two chapters written by service users/survivors. Their perspectives serve to underscore the magnitude of the plague of stigma and demonstrate attempts to deal with it. Their chapters are buttressed by a number of chapters written by mental health professionals, analyzing the issues surrounding stigmatization and exclusion, and describing some initiatives in the area of advocacy on behalf of individuals with mental illness.

Section 3: Systems of development

This section addresses salient features of integrating mental health into the general health systems. The challenges of human resources in low- and middle-income countries is addressed, as is the need to recognize and encourage collaboration between traditional and Western practitioners.

Section 4: Systems of development for special populations

Individuals with special needs tend to be overlooked. These groups include children, individuals with intellectual disability, and adolescents with substance abuse problems. This section addresses the special needs of these groups. The problems of child soldiers and child abuse are discussed. Poverty is a major factor in both adult and child mental health illness. The role of poverty as a social determinant and precursor of mental illness is mentioned. The task of developing interventions in a low-resource context is addressed.

Section 5: Gender and equality

The place and role of women in society have been emphasized by various UN declarations and national policies. Women, by their empowerment, their civic rights, and their influence, contribute immensely to a community's development. Their potentials in education and economic empowerment cannot be overstated. The reduction of violence toward women and girls is addressed.

Section 6: Human resources and capacity building

The delivery of efficient mental health services relies on well-trained personnel, education, and communication. The issues of delivery of service become more critical in special contexts, such as in conflict areas and disaster zones – manmade or natural. This section addresses these issues. Additionally, because of the plethora of stakeholders and the need for efficiency, transparency, and accountability in the delivery of services, the issue of good governance is discussed.

Section 7: Depression, suicide, and violence

There are indications that there is a rise in the prevalence of depression worldwide. An associated phenomenon is the risk of suicide. The twin phenomena of depression and suicide are given a place in view of the increasing recognition of the disability and other consequences of depression. The same consideration applies to violence as a public problem. It appears that the world is witnessing greater violence, with reports of terrorism, mass murders, and gun trafficking. The war on drugs in the USA and Central America has failed. This section deals with the implications of increasing depression, public violence, and failed wars on drugs.

Section 8: Research and monitoring the progress of countries

This section addresses the issues of scaling up the mental health services, entailing education, research, and monitoring the progress made in different countries. The challenge of limited infrastructure, human capacity, and material resources is great in developing countries. Research, education, and monitoring progress can contribute to improving service delivery by evaluative studies and their implication for relevant local best practices.

It is anticipated that this volume will provide a foundational reading for scholars, students, practitioners, and policy makers in understanding the potentials and challenges of global mental health. Readers are encouraged to reflect on the relevance of these chapters to their practice or research settings, and on how they can further contribute to the global alleviation of suffering due to mental health.

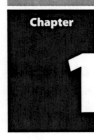

History of global mental health

Samuel O. Okpaku and Sanchita Biswas

Introduction and background

In this chapter, we will attempt to trace the origin and background of modern global mental health and sketch its domain. The history of mental health is punctuated with various movements. These have included the psychoanalytic, the behavioral, the self-help, and the community movements. These movements have been sustained over time and have merged into theory and practice. The less influential movements with shorter half-lives have been eclipsed. In the last decade we have witnessed a surge of activities which have been lumped together and described as *global mental health*. This movement is a relative newcomer to the global health movement.

The history and antecedents of any movement can shed light on the challenges and opportunities associated with it. Social movements are often triggered by some dissatisfaction or a crisis and by the vision of charismatic leaders. Examples are Martin Luther King Jr. and Mahatma Gandhi. Prior to a full discussion of the history of the global mental health movement, some background statements about globalization may be useful.

Globalization

There has been an abundance of definitions of globalization. Each definition highlights one or several themes, but all these definitions tend to emphasize the ascendancy of capitalism and interconnectivity in an ever-shrinking world space. This process has been driven by faster communication, enhanced by the internet and mass communication, faster and more efficient transportation of persons, and quicker and more efficient transfer of information, data, and currency. Perhaps one of the best definitions of globalization is afforded by Giddens (1990), who stated that:

> Globalization can thus be defined as the intensification of worldwide social relations which link distant localities in such a way that local happenings are shaped by events occurring many miles away and vice versa.
>
> (Giddens 1990, p. 64)

Four major dimensions can be distilled from the definitions and descriptions of globalization, which have relevance for global health and mental health. These dimensions are historical, economic, political, and sociocultural. A primary objective of global health and mental health is the eradication of disparities in terms of access to care, quality of life, and well-being worldwide.

- **Historical dimension** – This dimension is very relevant in discussions about global health. Many countries in the developing world have until recently experienced a colonial past. The consequences of this for developing countries are increased suspicion and sensitivity towards the actions of superpowers. "I fear donors when they bring gifts" (Trojan war). In fact, in some quarters, globalization has been described as "neo-colonization" (Akindele *et al.* 2002). In other words, globalization and its attendant processes can be seen as a back-door strategy to continue colonial domination.
- **Economic dimension** – This dimension is a powerful one in a world system where there are now very few dominant financial markets. The powerful nations exercise greater influence while the poorer ones are at risk of greater marginalization. Although the stated vision and goal of the International Monetary Fund and World Bank is the eradication of poverty

Essentials of Global Mental Health, ed. Samuel O. Okpaku. Published by Cambridge University Press. © Cambridge University Press 2014.

worldwide and improved quality of life and well-being for all, there are examples of negative consequences of globalization in low- and middle-income countries (LMICs). There is an exacerbation of poverty in Africa where foreign direct investment (FDI) is falling (UNCTAD 2012).

- **Political dimension** – This domain deals mostly with health, development, and security. In this domain are issues related to the prevention of pandemics and access to affordable pharmaceuticals (e.g. the availability of cheap antiviral medications) (Safreed-Harmon 2008). In this regard, Brazil declared the right to health as a human right. Also, poor health is linked to loss of economic and political viability (United Nations General Assembly 2009).
- **Sociocultural dimension** – The fourth theme in globalization is "a process of cultural mixing and hybridization across locations and identities" (Appadurai 1996). The internet, social media, and mass communications enable individuals to negotiate through different cultures and be subject to different sociocultural forces in real time.

The above themes intersect and are a background to their influences. The resulting opposition to these influences can make understandable the protests against the World Trade Organization (WTO) meetings in Seattle in 1999, Japan in 2003, and Geneva in 2009.

Parenthetically, the same is true of the opposition to the Movement for Global Mental Health and the Grand Challenges of Mental Health. This opposition focused on the lack of attention to local institutions, traditions, and culture as well as that which is intrinsic in capitalism and cultural imperialism. This opposition is to be valued for its watchdog function and for providing the opportunity for reasonable debate. The Movement for Global Mental Health and Grand Challenges of Mental Health are activist programs. Similarly, the opposition to them, especially in the transcultural communities, is also activist. These polar positions are very useful in generating debate in order to protect the poor countries and institutions from further domination from developed countries and their institutions. So the contentious debates are therefore necessary, provided they are held in an honest and disciplined manner.

With that background in mind, what are global health and global mental health?

Global health and global mental health

A frequently used definition of *global health* is that of Koplan and colleagues (2009), who referred to global health as:

> an area for study, research, and practice that places a priority on improving health and achieving equity in health for all people worldwide. Global health emphasizes transnational health issues, determinants, and solutions; involves many disciplines within and beyond the health sciences and promotes interdisciplinary collaboration; and is a synthesis of population-based prevention with individual-level clinical care.
>
> (Koplan *et al.* 2009)

Patel extended this approach to mental health, to come up with a definition of *global mental health* (Patel & Prince 2010).

In this chapter, I would like to suggest a different definition for global mental health, seeing it as a range of activities concerned with mental health that meet five principal criteria:

(1) **Universal and transnational criterion** – The problem/issue should have a universal or transnational aspect. Examples will be the role of poverty in mental illness worldwide and stigma reduction worldwide.
(2) **Public health criterion** – The problem should have a population basis, e.g., violence as a public issue.
(3) **Stakeholders criterion** – The composition of the stakeholders should be international in either bilateral or multilateral arrangements. They could be educational or scientific institutions, government bodies, non-governmental organizations (NGOs), or individuals.
(4) **Problem ownership criterion** – The problem should be owned by the recipient organization, institution, or country.
(5) **Team criterion** – The teams engaged in the project should be multidisciplinary and multi-party.

The above definition enables us to distinguish *global mental health* from *community mental health*, since the two movements have different philosophical backgrounds.

The history of global mental health: three epochs

Global mental health can be traced to a confluence of several influences. One such influence has been the "vision," "imagination," and indefatigability of a set of luminaries – some of whom have suffered the pangs of emotional distress with its attendant humiliation, ostracism, and stigma and others for whom there is less evidence of direct mental illness. For the latter group, their primary motivation appears to be humanitarian. Another major influence was the experience of World War II, which led to extreme barbarism and unbelievable cruelty among men. The third influence has been a resurgence of humanitarianism, a sense of equity bolstered by the Millennium Fund, and a sense that we are all in this together.

The evolution of global mental health is a trajectory that can historically be divided into three epochs. For each epoch, it is possible to identify individuals or agencies that have played a significant role or are currently active in the process. The first epoch was dominated by two Americans, Dorothea Dix and Clifford Beers, who were non-psychiatrists. The second epoch was dominated by prominent social scientists and social psychiatrists, and by the activities of three major organizations, the World Federation for Mental Health (WFMH), the World Health Organization (WHO), and the World Psychiatric Association (WPA). The third epoch is the contemporary era, spearheaded by the Movement for Global Mental Health and the Grand Challenges in Global Mental Health.

The first epoch

As indicated above, Dorothea Dix and Clifford Beers contributed immensely to global mental health and had experiences of mental illness, making their contribution more instructive.

Dorothea Dix (1802–1887)

Dorothea Dix was an individual without any medical training who became very influential in the USA and abroad as an advocate for the humane treatment of mentally ill people. Her father is generally described as an abusive alcoholic. Her grandmother was reputed to be very wealthy, and she contributed to the discipline and training of the young woman. Under her influence Dorothea came into contact with powerful and influential individuals in the Massachusetts area (Tiffany 1890). Dorothea was a Unitarian, and it was reported that she had a call to promote the status of mentally ill individuals and improve their treatment and living conditions. She previously had taught neglected and poor children at home. Meanwhile, she began to visit centers for the custody and treatment of the mentally ill. She was appalled by the conditions she saw. She chronicled her observation of these treatment centers and gave her reports to state legislatures. This resulted in changes in the custody, accommodation, and treatment of mentally ill people. Her activities spread beyond Massachusetts to other states in the United States. This resulted in the creation of large state hospitals. At that time that trend was considered progressive, though that opinion has since changed, especially since de-institutionalization.

Dorothea Dix herself had frequent episodes of mental illness. In attempting to receive respite from one of these episodes, she visited England and met some like-minded individuals interested in reforming the treatment and improving the welfare of those with mental illness. Upon her return to the United States, she continued to investigate the conditions of the mentally ill in state asylums. She worked on a Bill for the benefit of the indigent and the insane. This Bill stipulated that 12 225 000 acres of federal land be set aside for the benefit of such individuals. The Bill passed both houses of Congress, but President Franklin Pierce vetoed it. Disappointed, she returned to the United Kingdom and, reuniting with her co-advocates, conducted surveys of asylums in Scotland and other European countries and chronicled her observations (Tiffany 1890).

With the outbreak of the American Civil War, Dorothea Dix was appointed as the Army's Superintendent of Nurses. Unfortunately, she did not succeed in this capacity and subsequently moved to Morris Plains, New Jersey, where a suite in a state hospital was designated for her private use. She subsequently died and is buried in Cambridge, Massachusetts (Tiffany 1890).

Clifford Beers (1876–1943)

This was the other notable figure to influence advocacy on behalf of mentally ill individuals before World War II. Clifford Beers was born to an upper middle class family. He had four brothers, all of whom suffered from mental illness (Beers 1908). He was able to observe the treatment being meted out to fellow mentally ill individuals. He himself suffered the same humiliations in private and public hospitals in Connecticut.

Beers was a Yale University student and had studied business. He subsequently wrote a book entitled *A Mind That Found Itself* (Beers 1908, Human Spirit Initiative 2009). He became very influential in the field of mental health, and with the support of prominent individuals such as Professor Adolf Meyer of Johns Hopkins Hospital he launched a movement to reform the treatment of mentally ill individuals in Connecticut and subsequently all over the United States.

In 1909 Clifford Beers founded the Connecticut Committee for Mental Hygiene. The following year its national counterpart, the American Mental Health Movement, was founded, and in 1919 followed the International Committee for Mental Hygiene. In 1930, this organization was reorganized as the First International Congress of Mental Hygiene. This was the origin of the World Federation for Mental Health (Brody 2004).

The second epoch

The second epoch is the period of World War II and the years immediately after. The war had caused great devastation and human suffering. This period was the heyday of cultural and social psychiatry. Margaret Mead and Bronislaw Malinowski, two anthropologists, emphasized the cultural influences in the development of personality and human organizations. Mead worked in Samoa and is well known for her book *Coming of Age in Samoa*, and Malinoswki did his research amongst the Trobriand Islanders. It disputed Freud's theory of the Oedipus Complex.

The second epoch was dominated by the activities of certain individuals as well as the activities of three major organizations. These individuals were Drs. George Brock Chisholm, John Rawlings Rees, and Harry Stack Sullivan, all of whom played a significant role in the founding of the WFMH (Brody 2004). The three organizations are the World Federation for Mental Health (WFMH), the World Psychiatric Association (WPA), and the World Health Organization (WHO).

Dr. George Brock Chisholm (1896–1971)

Chisholm, a Canadian and a veteran of World War I, was the first Director-General of the WHO. During World War II, he rose within the ranks of the Canadian military very quickly and was appointed Director-General of Medical Services, becoming the first psychiatrist to head the medical ranks of any army in the world. In 1944, Chisholm was appointed a Deputy Minister of Health in Canada, a post he almost lost because of some of his outspoken pronouncements. He frequently expressed the idea that man's worst enemy was man himself: "The world was sick and the ills from which it was suffering were mainly due to the perversions and his inability to live at peace with himself." He also believed that children should be raised in environments bereft of the moral, political, and religious biases of their parents (Lescouflair 2003).

In 1944, Brock Chisholm also became the Executive Secretary of the Interim Commission of the WHO, and he was one of 16 national experts consulted in drafting the agency's first constitution. It was Chisholm's view that health is a "state of complete physical, mental, and social well-being and not merely the absence of disease or infirmity." He contributed to the founding of the WFMH (Lescouflair 2003).

Dr. John Rawlings Rees (1890–1969)

John Rawlings Rees, like Brock Chisholm and Dorothea Dix, came from a religious background. Dix and Chisholm were Unitarians, and Rees was from a Wesleyan background (Trist & Murray 1989). He was a director of the Tavistock Clinic in London. In 1939, he was invited to take command of British Army psychiatry. He contributed to the British Army in many ways. He assembled a team of psychiatrists, and provided leadership in the screening and placement of inductees and in the education and training of recruits with limited intelligence. He later contributed to the First Mental Health Congress in London in 1948. With his close friend Brock Chisholm, he worked towards the formation of the WFMH, of which he was a director for many years. He also believed in the social roots of mental illness and its treatment (Rees 1966).

Dr. Harry Stack Sullivan (1892–1949)

Harry Stack Sullivan was born in Norwich, New York, to an Irish family. He graduated from Chicago College of Medicine and Surgery (Kimble *et al.* 1991). Early in his career, he was a first lieutenant in the Army Medical Corps and served as US Veterans Bureau Liaison Officer to St. Elizabeth's Hospital in Washington, DC. He believed in the importance of early life experiences and the contribution of interpersonal relationships to the social environment (Rioch 1985). His experience in his role as a consultant at St. Elizabeth's led to important insights in his work with hard-to-reach patients. He died in 1949 in Paris, where he had attended a meeting of the Executive Board of the WFMH (Kimble *et al.* 1991).

World Federation for Mental Health (WFMH)

It was George Chisholm who suggested the creation of the WFMH. Its predecessor was the International Committee for Mental Health. Chisholm's idea was that this would be a non-governmental body that would provide a link between "grassroots" mental health organizations and the United Nations (UN). Another notable contributor to the founding of the WFMH was the anthropologist Margaret Mead. The original Federation began with membership of societies and not of individuals or countries.

Currently, membership in the WFMH is open to individuals, users and survivors, and mental health and disability societies. WFMH remains active in celebrating World Mental Health Day, organizing the biennial World Congress and stimulating advocacy for mental health. The Federation was very active in trying to place mental disorders on the same footing as the non-communicable diseases at the 2011 UN high-level meeting. That goal was not entirely realized, but a mention was made of mental illness. WFMH continues to push and mobilize for prioritizing the needs of the mentally ill (World Federation for Mental Health 2011).

World Health Organization (WHO)

The WHO was founded in 1948 after World War II and the demise of the League of Nations. The WHO, through its division of mental health, has played a vital role in several aspects of mental health worldwide. Its mission is:

> to reduce the burden associated with mental, neurological and substance use diseases, and to promote health world wide
>
> (World Health Organization 1998)

The core functions include:

- Partnership with other organization such as the WPA, WFMH, and other allied professional groups, stakeholders, and NGOs.
- Managing information by providing reliable data, statistics, and information on risk factors, disease burdens, available services, and resources.

- Guidance to interested parties by providing consultation and technical guidelines, training modules, and tools on the development of mental health policies and legislation, and management and policy support (WHO 2004).

At its founding, the overall objective of the WHO was the prevention of infectious diseases. Since then, its activities have broadened. In the 65 years since its founding, the WHO has played a considerable role in promoting mental health all over the world. It has carried out, supported, or publicized major epidemiological studies and promoted international efforts in such areas as the need for each country to have a mental health policy. It also has advocated efforts to reduce stigma. Recently, it has published a Mental Health Gap Action Programme (mhGAP), which is a program to:

- *Tackle priority* conditions – depression, schizophrenia and other psychotic disorders, suicide, epilepsy, dementia, disorders due to use of alcohol and illicit drugs, and mental disorders in children.
- Develop and implement an *essential mental health package* to improve service delivery and reduce inequity.
- *Target countries for intensified support*, i.e., low- and middle-income countries with the maximum burden and a large resource gap.
- Identify and roll out a *strategy to scale up* care (WHO 2008a).

In addition, it also has introduced the Atlas series; each publication in this series presents the latest estimate of global mental health resources available to prevent and treat mental disorders and help protect the human rights of people living with these conditions (WHO 2011a).

The WHO has engaged in efforts to draw attention to mental health as a significant component of health. A primary objective of the Atlas project is to raise public and professional awareness of the inadequacies of existing resources and services and the large inequities in their distribution at national and global level. Hence, "no health without mental health" (Prince *et al.* 2007). This is done in conjunction with WHO regional and country offices. This arrangement helps to assess support and strengthen country systems.

World Psychiatric Association (WPA)

The WPA was founded in 1950 against the background of the period immediately after World War II. There is little doubt that the first-hand experiences of military psychiatrists of the unspeakable devastation wrought by the events of the war led to a desire to understand the inscrutability of war, as well as a desire to help end human suffering. All of this in turn led to the founding of many psychiatric, social welfare, and relief organizations. It is also possible that the dispersion of prominent psychiatrists from the European Continent to other parts of Europe and to the United States fuelled the genesis of psychiatric movements. No matter the impetus, the WPA has grown from it modest origins in 1950 to its current influential role as the world's premier psychiatry organization, with membership societies from 141 countries.

In a way, this was a golden age for psychiatry. There was the rise of psychiatric epidemiology, anthropology, sociology, cultural psychiatry, psychotherapy, and analysis. The field was replete with competitive explanations for mental suffering and treatment.

The predecessor to the WPA was the Association for the Organization of the World Congress of Psychiatry. The first World Congress was held in Paris in 1950, and the second in Zurich in 1957. Its object was to provide educational opportunities for psychiatrists. However, by its formal founding in 1961, the vision had broadened and deepened. The WPA also has contributed to issues of human rights and the political abuse of psychiatry within Russia, Eastern Europe and China. Together with the WFMH and the WHO, the WPA also works to reduce stigma (Patel *et al.* 2010)

In the last two decades, the WPA has increased its efforts in providing educational opportunities, particularly in low- and middle-income countries. Examples include its program on Teaching and Learning about Schizophrenia, the Educational Programme on Depressive Disorders, Social Phobia, the Core Curriculum in Psychiatry for Medical Students, and the Institutional Program on the Core Training Curriculum for Psychiatry (WPA undated)

The third epoch

The third epoch is contemporary, and it has evolved as a result of multiple influences.

The influence of the World Bank and World Health Organization

In 1988, the World Bank supported work that was published as a *Health Sector Priorities Review*. The goal was to have a sense as to "the significance to public health of individual diseases [or related clusters of diseases] and what is now known as the cost and effectiveness of relevant interventions for their control" (Jamison *et al.* 1993). (It is interesting that this work is regarded as being intellectually antedated by work carried out in Ghana, a developing country, by the Ghana Health Assessment Project Team in 1981.) For the *Health Sector Priorities Review* Dr. Christopher Murray introduced the term disability-adjusted life year (DALY). Subsequently Christopher Murray and Alan Lopez edited the *Global Burden of Disease* report. Their work enabled comparisons between different diseases in terms of their contributions to mortality and disability. The measure now incorporates risk factors for different disease groups including mental health and neurological disorders. Mental ill health and neurological conditions contribute about 14% of the burden of disease. Depression contributes about 6% to this burden. It is a matter of concern that suicide has become the highest killer in adolescence in several countries (Murray & Lopez 1996).

In 2003 the WHO commissioned a report on the *Social Determinants of Health*. The report outlined the relative impact of policies, health systems, environmental factors, lifestyle factors, and biology that contribute to well-being and quality of life. These factors are multisectoral and multilevel, hence the need to provide comprehensive approaches to enhance an individual's quality of life and improve the community's health productivity and robustness. The commissioners called for social justice and equality as well as the need to close the health gap in a generation (WHO 2003).

In 2008 WHO published the *Mental Health Gap Action Program* (mhGAP). This volume documents the gap between the service needs and what is available for the treatment of mentally ill people worldwide, especially in low- and middle-income countries. The mhGAP has been followed up by the *mhGAP Intervention Guide* (mhGAP-IG) that provides a grid for the treatment of mentally ill individuals. These interventions are not cast in stone but rather they provide a framework for dealing with disease entities (WHO 2008a, 2010).

The above sequence of events and significant publications illustrates how WHO has systematically shown the need for care and offered suggestions for possible interventions for alleviating suffering and pain worldwide.

Advocacy, humanitarianism, ethics, and mass media

Another major influence in the development of contemporary global mental health is the synergistic relationship of factors such as advocacy, humanitarianism, ethics, and mass media. The mass media has contributed immensely by bringing to individual private rooms, in real time, natural and manmade disasters. Examples of such events are the Asian tsunami of 2004, Hurricane Katrina in 2005, and the rescue of the Chilean miners in 2010. In the last instance the international collaboration was broadcast all over the word. There was collaboration even in the equipment used in the rescue operation. The advocacy factor has been enhanced by the reports of the Commission on the Social Determinants of Health. The report was approved by member states at the 2011 Rio de Janiero Conference (WHO 2011b). Another influential contribution is the role of faith-based organizations. It is likely that this role will expand as the definition of health expands to include matters concerning food and water security and climate change.

Human resources and brain drain, task shifting and sharing

Although no nation can boast of having enough health workers to meet the needs of its citizenry, the problem for developing countries is acute. This problem is made worse by the "brain drain" of health professionals from developing countries to developed countries. It is estimated that 57 countries have a severe shortage of healthcare workers, and 36 of these countries are African (WHO 2008b). This has led to strategies to improve efficiencies in the health systems. Task shifting, which means the delegation of some services to less specialized individuals to free up the highly trained individuals to focus on the more difficult or technical issues, has been derived from experiences in the treatment of HIV/AIDS. More recently some critics are suggesting that a team approach – task sharing, not task shifting – is the way to go. Such critics emphasize that nurses provide a substantial part of the care of HIV/AIDS patients, and that HIV cannot be controlled without the services being provided by nurses (Olson 2012).

The latest epoch of global mental health also was advanced by the publication in 2007 of a series of articles in *The Lancet*. That edition contained a call for action (Lancet Global Mental Health Group 2007). Subsequently, a group of mental health professionals and allied professionals joined to form the Movement for Global Mental Health (MGMH). Since its inauguration, the group has held two biennial conferences, the first in Athens in 2009 and the second in Cape Town in 2011. These meetings were held under the auspices of the WFMH, and at Cape Town a second set of *Lancet* papers was released. The group consists of individuals and institutions with a commitment to improve the plight of mentally ill individuals worldwide, with particular emphasis on low- and middle-income countries. The group emphasizes two major principles, namely, evidence-based approaches and protection of human rights (Lancet Global Mental Health Group 2007). Meanwhile, a project funded by the US National Institute of Mental Health (NIMH) produced a document titled *Grand Challenges in Global Mental Health*. Participants in the project consisted of mental health experts with representation from low- and middle-income countries. Their opinions were sought as to the priorities in scaling up mental health services and research in those countries (Collins *et al.* 2011).

There is no doubt that global health has been greatly influenced by the availability of funds prompted by the availability of the Millennium Development Goals. At the historic summit meeting at the UN headquarters in New York in September 2000, 189 heads of states passed a sweeping resolution designed to eradicate poverty and improve the quality of life worldwide, but especially in the poor low-resource countries (United Nations Development Group 2000). The declaration has eight goals, three of which are specific to health, while the other five have health implications, although not so directly. The goals are financial strategies to be achieved by 2015. The International Monetary Fund (IMF) plays a significant role through various economic and financial strategies which are regarded as more favorable than before by low-income countries. The declaration serves to mobilize public policy agendas for member states (United Nations Development Group 2000).

Commentary and criticism

Quite naturally we do not expect the ideology and the concepts of the MGMH to be accepted universally. There have been strong criticisms of the movement, especially in the transcultural community. Perhaps some of the most vocal criticisms have come from Derek Summerfield, who states "Psychiatry has no answer to the question 'what is a mental disorder?', and instead exalts a way of working it has devised . . . What exactly is 'global mental health'? Can any definition or standard of mental health be definitive universally?" (Summerfield 2012). He has reservations about the term *global mental health*, emphasizing the need for cultural relevance of programs and pointing out that it is unacceptable to apply Western definitions and treatment approaches to non-Western societies.

Suman Fernando stated that "The 'global mental health' movement being pursued by the US NIMH requires considerable modifications if it is to be ethically acceptable in a post-colonial world. Otherwise, the result will be the imposition of Euro-American psychiatry en masse, amounting to cultural imperialism" (Advanced Senior Institute of Transcultural Psychiatry 2012). It is intriguing that considerable energy is being expended in this discussion. We have previously indicated that all psychiatric endeavors are transcultural. So culture is intrinsic in all discussions of mental illness. As an African, but one who has never had the privilege to work in Africa, in my discussions with my colleagues who work in Africa, we seem to come from two worlds. The following is an illustration. In the Western world, there is a standardized protocol for the treatment of alcohol withdrawal, and this is to use benzodiazepines. According to my associates in Africa, the corresponding treatment in Africa is sometimes to encourage the family to purchase more alcohol for the patient to prevent delirium tremens.

An important aspect of global mental health will be the imperative to explore how new and indigenous ways deal with local mental health problems and definitely not attempt to impose Western approaches. Considering examples, especially of places such as the United States, where homelessness is a scourge, or the United Kingdom, where the National Health Service is on the brink of disarray, low- and middle-income countries have to devise their own strategies that take into consideration their local conditions in developing mental health systems. At a recent conference, I was informed by a Ugandan colleague that the success rate for the treatment of depression is higher in Uganda than in the United States. This raises several issues. My opinion is that possibly the profiles of the patients are different in the two countries. Perhaps in Uganda individuals seeking treatments have more serious illness with biological substrates, while in the United States one is dealing with a social problem relative to the social security system. It is not unusual for the American indigent patient to seek continued hospitalization and then to become well at the prospect of his next check, or for individuals to abuse their allotment of annual Medicaid days. Although opposed to the practice of polypharmacy, considering the comorbidities of physical illness and mental illness, in my clinical practice and those of my colleagues, it is not unusual to prescribe for a patient on 10 medications simultaneously. For example, take a male patient who is 65 years old. He has a diagnosis of hypertension, type 2 diabetes, hypercholesterolemia, and major depressive disorder. For his hypertension and diabetes, he is prescribed three medications each, and for his depression two medications (one antidepressant, one antianxiety hypnotic), and for his hypercholesterolemia he is prescribed one medication. His prescription can easily cost between US$1000 and US$1500 per month. This sum would be an enviable income for a family of four in many low- and middle-income countries. Hence new and alternative pathways have to be developed not only for developing countries but also for developed countries where the cost of pharmaceuticals has become exorbitant. So it is incumbent on all stakeholders to explore locally relevant approaches in dealing with problems while being open to outside influences.

The future of global mental health

The future of global health and mental health is likely to be influenced by a variety of driving factors. One of these is activism. This implies a greater role for civil society, patient advocates, and users/survivors as well as their families and communities. WHO agreements, various national policies, and international mental health agencies support this position.

A related driving force is the reduction of stigma and exclusion. Education about mental illness, alongside the rehabilitation and work placement of users/survivors, will continue to be welcome. Related to the above driving factors is the need for self-help and country ownership. Although these concepts have been more prominent in HIV/AIDS treatment and research, it should be anticipated that this trend will spread to other areas.

Another major driving force is the changing perception in the definitions of health and mental health. We have come a long way since the founding of WHO 65 years ago, when the emphasis was on the prevention and management of infectious diseases. Now health and foreign policy of progressive nations make references to quality of life and human dignity. Recently, at least two countries have appointed global health ambassadors. Greater importance is given to the social determinants of health. Poverty, immigration, person trafficking, and modern slavery are highlighted. Mass killings, national and international conflicts and wars draw attention to the role of violence as a risk for mental illness. The current situation is underscored by the spate of mass killings in the USA and the debate over gun ownership. In addition, the mental health consequences of the wars in Iraq and Afghanistan are widespread.

Climate change issues, immigration issues, water shortage, and poverty have their related global mental health consequences. It is anticipated that these issues will continue to hold some presence in foreign policies and international discourse.

An area of promise is the greater implementation and integration of research, policy, and practice. Another level of prominence will come with the increasing integration of mental health services into primary care practices and centers.

Telemedicine and ehealth and other technological advances are likely to shape the future of mental health services in enhancing capacity for service delivery and research, especially in low-resource areas. Related to telemedicine and ehealth is the expansion of task shifting. With the current predictions of increased depression and suicide in the next few decades, the human resources to deal with this demand will have to depend on the availability of community supports.

Lastly, funding remains a major driver in the provision of service delivery and support for research. This is likely to be affected by the contractions and expansions of the economies of the developing countries. It is anticipated that the emerging economies such as the Brazil, Russia, India, China, and South Africa (BRICS) will assume a greater role as donor countries.

Summary

In summary, we have attempted to trace the history of global mental health. We have also described some of the most influential driving factors. There is a clear need to define and operationalize global mental health to improve communication and scholarship. The concerns of global mental health focus largely on the most needy communities, in the low- and middle-income countries, but the vision is worldwide. We must not assume that poverty is restricted to developing countries. Homelessness is worldwide; stigma in people suffering from mental health problems is also worldwide. Human rights abuse of the mentally ill is universal. While we cannot seek a utopia it is nevertheless heartening that the UN and its major health agency the WHO, as well as the related international agencies, the World Bank and IMF play significant roles in contributing to the success of the landmark commitments enshrined in the Millennium Development and Rio de Janeiro treaties. These two treaties affirm a commitment from the UN member states to the eradication of health inequalities and a chance for equitable, dignified, and productive life for all people worldwide irrespective of race, gender, age, or socioeconomic class. We are all in this together.

References

Advanced Senior Institute of Transcultural Psychiatry (2012) *Why Mental Health Matters to Global Health*. Montreal: Advanced Senior Institute of Transcultural Psychiatry.

Akindele ST, Gidado TO, Olaopo OR (2002) Globalisation, its Implications and Consequences for Africa. http://globalization.icaap. org/content/v2.1/01_akindele_etal. html (accessed Juy 2013).

Appadurai A (1996) *Modernity at Large: Cultural Dimensions of Globalization*. Minneapolis, MN: University of Minnesota Press.

Beers C (1908) *A Mind That Found Itself*. Pittsburgh, PA: University of Pittsburgh Press.

Brody, E (2004) The World Federation for Mental Health: its origins and contemporary relevance to WHO and WPA policies. *World Psychiatry.* 3 (1): 54–55.

Collins PY, Patel V, Joestl SS, *et al.* (2011) Grand challenges in global mental health. *Nature* 475: 27–30.

Giddens A (1990) *The Consequences of Modernity*. Cambridge: Polity Press.

Human Spirit Initiative (2009) *Clifford W. Beers: the Founding of Mental Health America 1908–1935: Telling the Story and Showing the Way*. Minneapolis, MN: Human Spirit Initiative.

Jamison DT, Mosley WH, Measham AR, Bobadilla JL, eds. (1993) *Disease Control Priorities in Developing Countries*. New York, NY: Oxford University Press for the World Bank.

Kimble GA, Wertheimer M, White C (1991) *Portraits of Pioneers in Psychology*, Vol. 1. London: Routledge.

Koplan JP, Bond TC, Merson MH, *et al.* (2009). Towards a common definition of global health. *Lancet* **373**: 1993–5.

Lancet Global Mental Health Group (2007) Scale up services for mental disorders: a call for action. *Lancet* **370**: 1241–52.

Lescouflair E (2003) *Brock Chisholm: Director-General, World Health Organization 1896–1971*. Cambridge, MA: Harvard Square Library.

Murray CJL, Lopez AD (1996) *The Global Burden of Disease: a Comprehensive Assessment of Mortality and Disability from Diseases, Injuries, and Risk Factors in 1990 and Projected to 2020*. Cambridge, MA: Harvard University Press.

Olson D (2012) Task sharing not task shifting: team approach is best bet for HIV care. *Global Health Blog*. http://www.intrahealth.org/page/task-sharing-not-task-shifting-team-approach-is-best-bet-for-hiv-care (accessed July 2013).

Patel V, Prince M (2010) Global mental health: a new global health field comes of age. *JAMA* **303**: 1976–7. doi: 10.1001/jama.2010.616.

Patel V, Maj M, Flisher AJ, *et al.* (2010) Reducing the treatment gap for mental disorders: a WPA survey. *World Psychiatry* **9** (3): 169–76.

Prince M, Patel V, Saxena S, *et al.* (2007) No health without mental health. *Lancet* **370**: 859–77.

Rees JR (1966) *Reflections: a Personal History and An Account of the Growth of the World Federation for Mental Health*. New York, NY: WFMH.

Rioch DM (1985) Recollections of Harry Stack Sullivan and of the development of his interpersonal psychiatry. *Psychiatry* **48** (2): 141–58.

Safreed-Harmon K (2008) Human rights and HIV/AIDS in Brazil. *GMHC Treatment Issues*. http://www.gmhc.org/files/editor/file/ti_poz_0408.pdf (accessed July 2013).

Summerfield D (2012). Afterword: against "global mental health". *Transcultural Psychiatry* **49** (3) 1–12.

Tiffany F (1890) *The Life of Dorothea Lynde Dix*. Boston, MA: Houghton, Mifflin.

Trist E, Murray H (1989) The foundation and development of the Tavistock Institute to 1989. http://www.moderntimesworkplace.com/archives/ericsess/tavis1/tavis1.html (accessed July 2013).

United Nations Conference on Trade and Development (UNCTAD) (2012) Global flows of foreign direct investment exceeding pre-crisis level in 2011, despite turmoil in the global economy. *Global Investment Trends Monitor* (8).

United Nations Development Group (2000) *Millennium Declaration*. New York, NY: Millennium Development Goals Summit.

United Nations General Assembly (2009) Global health and foreign policy: strategic opportunities and challenges. Note by the Secretary-General. (A/64/365). New York, NY: UN.

World Federation for Mental Health (2011) World Federation for Mental Health Activities at the United Nations for 2010–2011. Conference on advocacy for the inclusion of mental health among Non-Communicable Diseases.

World Health Organization (1998) *Primary Prevention of Mental, Neurological and Psychosocial Disorders*. Geneva: WHO.

World Health Organization (2003) *Social Determinants of Health: the Solid Facts*. Based on the World Conference on Social Determinants of Health. Geneva: WHO.

World Health Organization (2004) *Prevention of Mental Disorders: Effective Interventions and Policy Options*. Geneva: WHO.

World Health Organization (2008a) *mhGAP: Mental Health Gap Action Programme. Scaling up Care for Mental, Neurological, and Substance Use Disorders*. Geneva: WHO.

World Health Organization (2008b) *Task Shifting: Rational Redistribution of Tasks Among Health Workforce Teams: Global Recommendations and Guidelines*. First Global Conference on Task Shifting Addis Ababa, Ethiopia. Geneva: WHO.

World Health Organization (2010) *mhGAP Intervention Guide for Mental, Neurological and Substance Use Disorders in Non-Specialized Health Settings*. Geneva: WHO.

World Health Organization (2011a) *Mental Health Atlas 2011*. Geneva: WHO.

World Health Organization (2011b) Rio Political Declaration on Social Determinants of Health, Rio de Janeiro, Brazil, 21 October 2011. World Conference on Social Determinants of Health.

World Psychiatric Association (undated) WPA Educational Programs *Core Training Curriculum for Psychiatry* Retrieved from http://www.wpanet.org.

Chapter

2

Burden of illness

Jordi Alonso, Somnath Chatterji, Yanling He, and Ronald C. Kessler

Introduction

The concept of global burden of disease was first publicized in a landmark report commissioned by the World Bank (1993). The measure developed in that report to operationalize the definition of disease burden combined the years lost due to premature mortality with those years "lost" due to living with disabling non-fatal conditions into a single measure of the impact of health conditions. This measure was designed to assess the population's health gap, taking into account not only mortality but also non-fatal decrements in health that result from health conditions. As a continuation of that work, the World Health Organization (WHO) and Harvard University published *The Global Burden of Disease* (GBD) study (Murray & Lopez 1996) as a systematic effort to estimate the leading causes of death globally and to combine these estimates with the leading causes of disability. The GBD study provided comprehensive estimates of the disability-adjusted life years (DALYs) due to more than 100 diseases and 19 risk factors. The first publication of the GBD study showed that in 1990 unipolar major depression was the fourth leading cause of DALYs worldwide (3.7%), exceeded only by respiratory infections (8.2%), diarrheal diseases (7.2%), and perinatal conditions (6.7%). Projections estimated that unipolar major depression would be the leading cause of total disability worldwide by the year 2030 (World Health Organization 2008).

A subsequent systematic review of epidemiological studies of mental disorders examined estimates of frequency (one-year prevalence), risk of mortality, and disability associated with 10 mental disorders (Eaton *et al.* 2007). In that review, one-year prevalence of major depressive disorders (median of 42 studies) was 5.3% of the adult population, with a median excess risk of mortality of 70% (OR = 1.7) and a disability weight between 0.35 (0 worst, 1 best) and a Sheehan Disability Score of 58 (0 worst, 100 best). As a consequence of their high frequency and associated significant disability, the costs of mental disorders in Western countries were estimated in this review to be huge. In Europe it was estimated that mental disorders had a total cost, in 2011, of 461 billion euros (approaching 1000 euros per inhabitant) (Gustavsson *et al.* 2011). Of those costs, 39% corresponded to direct medical costs (due to utilization of professional services, medical interventions, and use of medication), 13% to other direct non-medical services, and almost half (48%) to indirect costs (those incurred due to sick leave, early retirement, and premature death) (Gustavsson *et al.* 2011). Affective disorders, and especially unipolar depression alone, accounted for more than half of the indirect costs, indicating a very important toll on European social productivity.

Initiated a decade after the GBD study, the WHO World Mental Health (WMH) surveys, with over 150 000 respondents surveyed across 28 different countries, is the largest ongoing cross-national series of community epidemiological surveys of mental disorders ever carried out (Kessler & Ustun 2008). The WMH surveys represent an important contribution to knowledge about the global burden of mental disorders. WMH estimates the prevalence of mental disorders using the most updated instrument for use in community surveys, the WHO Composite International Diagnostic Interview (CIDI version 3.0) (Kessler & Ustun 2004). WMH also evaluates the disability associated with mental (and non-mental) disorders in the general population samples collected in the 28 countries studied.

Essentials of Global Mental Health, ed. Samuel O. Okpaku. Published by Cambridge University Press. © Cambridge University Press 2014.

In this chapter we describe and discuss the results of the WMH surveys regarding the burden of mental disorders. We pay particular attention to the frequency of mental disorders, and to their associations with important outcomes over the life course (such as education, marriage, occupation, and income), productivity (role function), and general health (perceived health status). These data, which are so extensive that they are only presented in summary fashion in this chapter, are described more fully in a volume in the WHO World Mental Health Survey series on the burdens of mental disorders (Alonso *et al.* 2013).

The World Mental Health (WMH) surveys initiative

Study samples

The data presented in this chapter come from 25 WMH surveys carried out in 24 countries. These results, based on the most complete subset of the growing number of WMH surveys continuing to be carried out throughout the world, are grouped according to the World Bank country income categories. These countries include six that are classified by the World Bank as low/lower-middle-income countries (Colombia, the Indian region of Pondicherry, Iraq, Nigeria, the People's Republic of China metropolitan areas of Beijing and Shanghai, and Ukraine), six others classified as upper-middle-income countries (the Brazilian metropolitan area of São Paulo, Bulgaria, Lebanon, Mexico, Romania, and South Africa), and 12 classified as high-income countries (Belgium, France, Germany, Israel, Italy, Japan, Netherlands, New Zealand, Northern Ireland, Portugal, Spain, and the United States).

All surveys were based on probability samples of the adult household population of the participating countries. The samples were selected either to be nationally representative (in the majority of countries), representative of all urbanized areas in the country (Colombia and Mexico), or representative of particular regions of the country (Brazil, India, Japan, Nigeria, and China). More details of sampling methods are provided elsewhere (Heeringa *et al.* 2008). The total sample size of respondents aged 18 and older was 121 902, with individual country samples ranging from 2357 in Romania to 12 790 in New Zealand. The weighted (by sample size) average response rate across surveys was 72.0%, ranging from

45.9% in France to 98.8% in Pondicherry, India. In all surveys, the CIDI 3.0, described below, was used to assess mental disorders. Interviews were administered face-to-face by trained lay interviewers using training and field quality control procedures described elsewhere (Pennell *et al.* 2008). Informed consent was obtained before beginning interviews, using procedures approved by the institutional review board of the organization coordinating the survey in each country.

Other than in Romania, Israel, Iraq, and South Africa, where all respondents were administered the full WMH interview, subsampling was used to reduce respondent burden by dividing the interview into two parts. Part I included core diagnostic assessment and was completed by all respondents. All Part I respondents who met criteria for any core mental disorder, plus a probability subsample of other Part I respondents, were administered Part II, which assessed correlates and disorders of secondary interest to the study. Weights were used to adjust for differential probabilities of selection within households as well as for residual discrepancies between sample and population distributions on a range of sociodemographic and geographic variables. Part II data were additionally weighted to adjust for the undersampling of Part II non-cases, thus making the weighted Part II sample representative of the full Part I sample. WMH weighting procedures are discussed in more detail elsewhere (Heeringa *et al.* 2008).

The Part II sample included 62 971 respondents in all countries (16 051 from low/lower-middle-income countries, 14 811 from upper-middle-income countries, and 32 109 from high-income countries). Because physical conditions, marital status records, and some mental disorders were only asked about in the Part II sample, the present analyses are limited to this group of respondents.

Diagnostic assessment
Mental disorders

As noted above, mental disorders were assessed with the CIDI, a fully structured lay-administered interview designed to generate research diagnoses of commonly occurring mental disorders according to the definitions and criteria of both the *Diagnostic and Statistical Manual of Mental Disorders* (DSM-IV) and *International Classification of Diseases* (ICD-10) Diagnostic Criteria for Research (DCR) diagnostic systems (Kessler & Ustun 2004). The disorders considered in this report were based on DSM-IV criteria and included anxiety disorders (panic disorder, agoraphobia without panic, specific phobia, social phobia, generalized anxiety disorder (GAD), post-traumatic stress disorder (PTSD), separation anxiety disorder), mood disorders (major depression, dysthymia, bipolar disorder I or II), impulse control disorders (oppositional defiant disorder, conduct disorder, attention-deficit/hyperactivity disorder, intermittent explosive disorder), and substance use disorders (alcohol and drug abuse/dependence). Blind clinical re-interviews using the Structured Clinical Interview for DSM-IV (SCID) (2011) with a probability subsample of WMH survey respondents found generally good concordance between CIDI diagnoses and SCID diagnoses (Haro *et al.* 2006).

The CIDI included retrospective disorder age-of-onset (AOO) reports based on a special question sequence that has been shown experimentally to improve recall accuracy (Knauper *et al.* 1999). Premarital onset of any mental disorder was defined as having a disorder with AOO less than age at first marriage. Either lifetime disorders, together with AOO of the disorder, or disorders present in the 12 months before interview were considered, depending on the research question.

Chronic physical conditions

Physical conditions were assessed with a standard chronic conditions checklist. Checklists of this sort have been shown to yield more complete and accurate reports of condition prevalence than estimates derived from responses to open-ended question (Centers for Disease Control and Prevention 2004). Reports based on such checklists have also been shown in previous methodological studies to have moderate to good concordance with medical records (Knight *et al.* 2001). The 10 conditions considered here are: arthritis, cancer, cardiovascular disorders (heart attack, heart disease, hypertension, stroke), chronic pain conditions (chronic back or neck pain, other chronic pain), diabetes, migraines or other frequent or severe headaches, insomnia, neurological disorders (multiple sclerosis, Parkinson's disease, epilepsy or seizures), digestive disorders (stomach or intestinal ulcers, irritable bowel disorder), and respiratory disorders (seasonal allergies, asthma, COPD, emphysema). The symptom-based disorders in this set (arthritis, pain disorders, heart attack, and stroke) were assessed with respondent reports as to

whether or not they ever experienced the condition, while the remaining conditions were assessed with respondent reports of whether or not a doctor or other health professional ever told them they had the condition. Questions were asked about AOO of all conditions, while questions about persistence were asked about conditions that can remit. The focus in this report is on conditions present in the 12 months before interview.

Outcome variables of burden of disease in the WMH surveys
Educational attainment

Respondents were asked how many years of education they had completed. Since countries varied by the age of starting school and the duration of each stage of schooling, we standardized the stage of education within country by years of education. We assumed an orderly academic progression and defined four educational milestones as follows: finishing primary education after eight years of education, finishing secondary education after 12 years of education, entry to tertiary education after 13 years of education, and graduation from tertiary education (such as university or other higher levels of education after secondary education) after a total of 16 years of education. The standardization of these educational stages was carried out for all the countries studied (higher, middle, and lower income levels) with the help of researchers from the participating countries.

Marriage and divorce

We assessed the impact of early mental disorders on timing of marriage (*early marriage* = marriage prior to age 18, *on-time marriage* = between age 18 and the country-specific 75th percentile of age at marriage, and *late marriage* = above the country-specific 75th percentile of age at marriage). Data on history of marriage was sought in 19 of the 24 countries (not assessed in South Africa, Iraq, Israel, North Ireland, and Portugal). Twelve of these countries also collected information on whether this first marriage ended in divorce or separation, and the age at which that occurred. The countries lacking data on divorce were all high-income countries (Belgium, France, Germany, Italy, Netherlands, Spain, and New Zealand). In addition, for a subsample of married study participants, their partners were randomly recruited. Both members of the couple were assessed concerning physical violence in their current marriage using questions based on the modified Conflict Tactics Scale (Straus *et al.* 1996). The couples' samples were assessed in 11 of the WMH countries.

Household income and personal earnings

This was assessed in the Part II sample and focused on income in the past 12 months. Respondents were asked if they were employed or self-employed at any time in that period. Those who responded positively were asked about *personal earnings*, which were defined as including only wages and other stipends from employment, excluding pensions, investments, financial assistance, and other sources of income. We also assessed spouse earnings and separately assessed all "other" household income. Income-earnings reports were divided by median within-country values to pool across countries but retain information about between-countries differences in income-earnings variation.

Days out of role

A modified version of the WHO Disability Assessment Schedule (WHODAS II) (Von Korff *et al.* 2008) was used to ask respondents the number of days in the 30 days before interview (i.e., beginning the day before the interview and going back 30 days) that they were *totally unable* to work or carry out their normal activities because of problems with either physical health or mental health, or because of the use of alcohol or drugs. In addition, questions on *partial disability* asked about the number of days on which respondents (a) had to cut down on what they did, (b) had to cut back on the quality of what they did, or (c) had extreme effort to perform as usual. Partial disability was expressed in full day equivalents to allow for the variation in the number of disability hours per day. Good concordance of these reports has been documented both with payroll records of employed people (Kessler *et al.* 2003) and with prospective daily diary reports (Gureje 2009).

Perceived overall health

After all physical and mental conditions had been assessed, respondents were asked to rate their own overall physical and mental health in the 30 days prior to the interview, using a 0–100 visual analog scale (VAS) where 0 represents the worst possible health a person can have and 100 represents perfect health,

taking into consideration all the physical and mental conditions reviewed in the survey.

Statistical analyses

In addition to standard descriptive and association analyses, several innovative statistical approaches were used in the WMH surveys to assess the burdens of mental disorders. Among these innovative analyses were discrete-time survival analysis and generalized linear modeling. *Discrete-time survival analysis* was applied to consider the AOO of mental disorders and the time elapsed until the outcome considered (for instance, termination of education, first marriage, first divorce). In these analyses, disorders were treated as time-varying predictors of the functional outcomes using a retrospective follow-back analysis logic. *Generalized linear modeling* (GLM) was used to assess the effects of mental disorders on continuous outcome variables with skewed distributions, such as a 0–100 visual analog scale of perceived health and a measure of the number of days the respondent was totally unable to carry out normal activities in the month before the interview. We also used simulation procedures to estimate the impact of mental and physical disorders at the individual level (*individual effects*) and at the level of the whole adult population (*societal effects*). The effects of the complex survey design (i.e., the use of weighting and clustering) in the WMH data were taken into account in all these analyses using design-based methods of significance testing. The statistical note in the appendix to this chapter provides more detailed information about the statistical methods used in the analyses.

Prevalence of mental disorders and age of onset in the WMH surveys

Lifetime prevalence

The WMH surveys that have been completed so far (which are only a subset of the 28 so far in the initiative) show clearly that the mental disorders assessed in the CIDI are quite common in all the countries studied. The interquartile range (IQR; 25th–75th percentiles across countries) of lifetime prevalence estimates of any DSM-V/CIDI disorder is 18.1–36.1% in this set of surveys. A lifetime DSM/CIDI diagnosis was found among more than one-third of respondents in five countries (Colombia, France, New Zealand, Ukraine, United States),

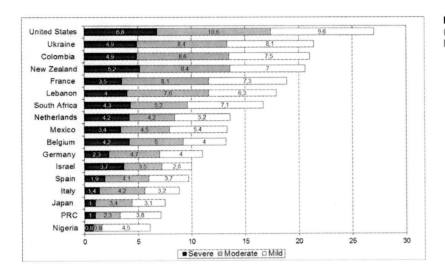

Figure 2.1 Twelve-month prevalence (%) of any mental disorder by country, by level of severity. WMH surveys.

more than one-fourth in six (Belgium, Germany, Lebanon, Mexico, Netherlands, South Africa), and more than one-sixth in four (Israel, Italy, Japan, Spain). The remaining two countries, China (13.2%) and Nigeria (12.0%), had considerably lower prevalence estimates, which are likely to be downwardly biased (Gureje *et al.* 2006). When coupled with the fact that our clinical reappraisal studies showed prevalence estimates in developed countries to be accurate (Haro *et al.* 2006, Ghimire *et al.* 2013) and with the possibility that prevalence in less developed countries is underestimated, these results argue persuasively that mental disorders have great public health importance throughout the world.

Twelve-month prevalence

A more convenient indicator of the frequency of mental disorders refers to those that have occurred sometime during a given year. This is a particularly common period to assess the frequency of disorders for health policy analyses, where the access to care is linked with the presence of disease. Figure 2.1 shows the 12-month prevalence of mental disorders, ordered by frequency. The joint 12-month prevalence of any of the mental disorders considered in the WMH surveys varied considerably, from just above 6% (Nigeria) to more than 30% of the population (Metropolitan São Paulo, Brazil, and the United States). The figure also shows the distribution of severity

within each survey. Contrary to the suggestion that larger prevalence of mental disorders would be driven by mild cases (Regier *et al.* 1998), it can be seen that surveys with the highest overall prevalence of mental disorders tended to show the highest proportion of severe cases (as in the São Paulo metropolitan area of Brazil, the USA, Northern Ireland, and New Zealand). Conversely, countries with very low overall prevalence showed a clear predominance of mild cases.

Age of onset (AOO)

The WMH retrospectively assessed when the disorder first occurred among people with a lifetime history of a disorder. The WMH surveys contain the most comprehensive AOO data for mental disorders ever published. These data are remarkably consistent across countries, as well as consistent with the AOO data reported in previous studies. Median AOO (i.e., the 50th percentile on the AOO distribution) of lifetime disorders, which was assessed retrospectively, was estimated to be earlier for anxiety disorders (age 11) and behavior disorders (age 11) than for substance use disorders (age 20) or mood disorders (age 30) (Kessler *et al.* 2007). AOO was also found to be concentrated in a very narrow age range for most disorders, with the interquartile range (IQR; the number of years between the 25th and 75th percentiles of the AOO distributions) only eight years (ages 7–15) for behavior disorders, nine years (ages 18–27) for substance use disorders, and 15 years (ages 6–21) for anxiety disorders. The AOO IQR was wider, however, for mood disorders (25 years, ages 18–43). These AOO results are quite similar to those found in comparable surveys in other countries. A note of caution is needed in interpreting these results, as they are based on retrospective lifetime recall and thus are subject to bias. Indeed, somewhat earlier AOO estimates are generally found in prospective longitudinal studies than in the analysis of retrospective AOO reports (Wittchen *et al.* 1999, 2011). Nonetheless, these prospective data are generally quite consistent with the AOO distributions seen in the retrospective WMH data.

Early mental disorders and key life-course outcomes in the WMH surveys
Premature termination of education

Education is a basic asset for individuals to realize a productive and healthy life. Premature termination of education puts individuals at clear risk of lower productivity, health, and self-realization in their adulthood (Lee *et al.* 2009). WMH data show that early mental disorders (i.e., mental disorders with AOO before the termination of education) were associated with a premature termination of education. In higher-income countries, prior substance use disorders were associated with termination of education at all stages (OR ranging from 1.4 to 12.8). Prior anxiety disorders (OR = 1.3), prior mood disorders (OR = 1.5), and prior impulse control disorders (OR = 1.8) were associated with termination of secondary education. In the other countries the association of early-onset mental disorder and premature termination of education was less consistent, with only prior impulse control disorders and prior substance use disorders associated with termination of secondary education.

The expected risks of failure in educational attainment of the population in the presence or absence of any prior mental disorders are presented in Table 2.1. Comparison of these estimates shows the change in the probability of failing to complete a particular stage of education attributable to all mental disorders, assuming the observed associations were causal. For example, in the USA, the probability of people failing to complete secondary education would be increased by 11.4% in the presence of any mental disorder. The overall pattern shows that the percentage change of people failing at educational milestones attributable to prior mental disorders was generally larger in developed countries than in developing countries. Among all educational milestones, the change in probability between those with mental disorder and those without was largest for the stage of completing secondary education, in both developed and developing countries.

Early marriage, divorce, and marital violence

A broad range of evidence shows that marriage is associated with a wide variety of positive life outcomes, including health, longevity, and well-being (Breslau *et al.* 2011). Conversely, divorce has negative effects in terms of distress, loss of income, and lower child well-being. In the WMH surveys only a few associations were found for prior mental disorders and timing of marriage: major depressive disorder, bipolar disorder, and alcohol abuse were significantly associated with lower likelihood of both on-time and late marriage. Prior impulse control disorders tended to be associated with a higher chance of early marriage (i.e., before age 18). Contrary to the scarce associations found between early mental disorders and marriage, there is evidence of an association between specific disorders and divorce, as they were associated with a higher likelihood of divorce in most of the countries, irrespective of their income level. As shown in Figure 2.2, prior major depressive episode (MDE), alcohol abuse (AA), and drug abuse (DA) were associated with the highest likelihood of divorce.

By computing population attributable risk proportions (PARPs), which combine information on the prevalence and strength of association with the outcome for each disorder into a single term that can be compared across individual disorders, we assessed the impact of mental disorders on marital life: they explain a 3.9% increase in the prevalence of early marriage, a 3.3% reduction in on-time marriage, a 12.3% reduction in late marriage, and a 12% increase in the prevalence of divorce. Social phobia has the largest effects, followed by major depressive episode.

Marital violence was assessed in 1281 married couples from 11 countries. Any physical violence was reported by one or both spouses in 20%, and it was associated with husbands' externalizing disorders (OR = 1.2–2.3) (Miller *et al.* 2011). About 1 in 6 cases

Table 2.1 Early mental disorders and educational achievement

Country	Failure in completing primary school			Failure in completing secondary education			Failure in entering tertiary education			Failure in completing tertiary education		
	Without disorder	With disorder	% change	Without disorder	With disorder	% change	Without disorder	With disorder	% change	Without disorder	With disorder	% change
Developed												
Belgium	0.0597	0.0597	0	0.2973	0.3015	1.41	0.5181	0.5361	3.47	0.7531	0.7641	1.46
Germany	0.0049	0.0053	8.16	0.3660	0.3662	0.05	0.5816	0.5826	0.17	0.9649	0.9649	0
Israel	0.0069	0.0069	0	0.2596	0.2611	0.58	0.5420	0.5427	0.13	0.7533	0.7537	0.05
Italy	0.2954	0.2960	0.20	0.6133	0.6147	0.23	0.8096	0.8092	−0.05	0.8750	0.8767	0.19
Japan	0.0125	0.0125	0	0.2961	0.2961	0	0.6227	0.6227	0	0.8070	0.8107	0.46
Netherlands	0.0518	0.0518	0	0.3013	0.3097	2.79	0.4110	0.4195	2.07	0.6530	0.6618	1.35
New Zealand	0.0084	0.0090	7.14	0.3836	0.4026	4.95	0.6476	0.6753	4.28	0.7946	0.8147	2.53
Spain	0.2654	0.2663	0.34	0.5870	0.5901	0.53	0.6401	0.6427	0.41	0.7998	0.8079	1.01
USA	0.0275	0.0286	4	0.1521	0.1694	11.37	0.4687	0.4905	4.65	0.7417	0.7613	2.64
Developing												
Colombia	0.1674	0.1674	0	0.5367	0.5436	1.29	0.7488	0.7519	0.41	0.8889	0.8903	0.16
Lebanon	0.2523	0.2541	0.71	0.6008	0.6077	1.15	0.7172	0.7220	0.67	0.8108	0.8136	0.35
Mexico	0.1749	0.1754	0.29	0.6959	0.6996	0.53	0.8136	0.8157	0.26	0.8661	0.8692	0.36
Nigeria	0.2188	0.2188	0	0.6476	0.6477	0.02	0.8183	0.8184	0.01	0.9234	0.9246	0.13
PR China	0.0684	0.0684	0	0.4577	0.4577	0	0.6960	0.6960	0	0.9696	0.9698	0.02
South Africa	0.1978	0.1978	0	0.6187	0.6194	0.11	0.8454	0.8472	0.22	0.9670	0.9682	0.12
Ukraine	0.0638	0.0638	0	0.1789	0.1844	3.07	0.3208	0.3277	2.15	0.6421	0.6454	0.51

From Lee *et al.* (2009), *British Journal of Psychiatry* **194**: 411–17.

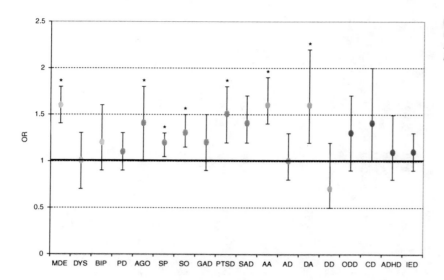

Figure 2.2 Association of premarital mental disorders and age of first divorce. Adapted from Breslau *et al.* (2011), *Acta Psychiatrica Scandinavica* **124**: 474–86.

of marital violence can be attributed to premarital mental disorders (Miller *et al.* 2011).

Household income and personal earnings losses

Mental disorders are associated with lower earnings (Levinson *et al.* 2010). This might be due to a number of causes: mental disorders can lead to low educational attainment, which in turn will lower earnings and/or reduce motivation or ability to work, or lead to difficulties in work performance, impairments in interpersonal functioning, or discrimination, all of which are likely to reduce occupational advancement and increase disability (Kawakami *et al.* 2012). In the WMH surveys, respondents with mental disorders as of the age of completing education had reduced household income, personal earnings, and spouse earnings, as well as greater disability and a lower probability of employment, marriage, and having an employed spouse (Table 2.2). The number of mental disorders explained 1% reduction of total household income. Disability to work, unemployment, and personal earnings among men, and disability to work and not having an employed spouse among women most explained the association. Among these mental disorders, specific phobia and agoraphobia without panic were significantly and negatively associated with total household income. The number of mental disorders was also associated with decreased household income: slightly for 1 or 2 disorders, moderately

for 3 disorders, and highly for 4 or 5+ disorders. About a 16% reduction in total household income is estimated for those who had 4 or 5+ disorders compared to those who had no disorder. The overall association of mental disorders with personal earnings was also significant among those employed and those with other household income. Major depressive disorder or dysthymia, and agoraphobia without panic, were significantly and negatively associated with personal earnings among those employed. Specific phobia was significantly and negatively associated with spouse earnings among those married with an employed spouse. Alcohol abuse was significantly and negatively associated with other household income, while major depressive disorder or dysthymia and oppositional defiant disorder were significantly and positively associated with other household income.

Impact of common mental disorders and physical conditions
Productivity loss

Studies have estimated that there are 3.6 billion annual health-related days out of role in the USA (Kawakami *et al.* 2012), and that the annual human capital costs of health-related days out of role in Europe exceed 136 billion euros (Gustavsson *et al.* 2011). In fact, a good portion of the costs of mental disorders is driven by the so-called indirect costs,

Table 2.2 Household income and personal earnings (regressions of total family income and continuous income component measures on type and number of early-onset mental disorders among WMH respondents who were 18–64 years old at the time of interview)

	Total household income		Personal earnings among the employed	
	Estimate	**(SE)**	**Estimate**	**(SE)**
I. Mental disorders				
Mood disorders				
Major depression or dysthymia	–0.02	(0.02)	–0.06*	(0.02)
Broad spectrum bipolar disorder	–0.08	(0.05)	–0.02	(0.06)
Anxiety disorders				
Panic disorder	–0.02	(0.05)	–0.07	(0.07)
Generalized anxiety disorder	–0.04	(0.05)	–0.02	(0.05)
Social phobia	–0.02	(0.02)	–0.01	(0.03)
Specific phobia	–0.04*	(0.02)	–0.05	(0.03)
Agoraphobia without panic	–0.17*	(0.06)	–0.25*	(0.06)
Post-traumatic stress disorder	–0.07	(0.04)	0.00	(0.05)
Separation anxiety disorder	–0.03	(0.03)	–0.02	(0.04)
Disruptive behavior disorders				
Oppositional defiant disorder	0.05	(0.03)	0.04	(0.05)
Conduct disorder	–0.02	(0.04)	–0.03	(0.04)
Attention-deficit/hyperactivity disorder	0.03	(0.03)	0.03	(0.04)
Intermittent explosive disorder	0.04	(0.03)	0.05	(0.03)
Substance disorders				
Alcohol abuse	–0.04	(0.03)	0.01	(0.04)
Alcohol abuse with dependence	–0.08	(0.06)	–0.08	(0.06)
Drug abuse	–0.03	(0.04)	–0.08	(0.05)
Drug abuse with dependence	0.01	(0.07)	0.01	(0.08)
χ^2_{17}	60.5*		67.4*	
χ^2_{16}	29.6*		44.4*	
II. Number of disorders				
Exactly 1 disorder	–0.02	(0.02)	–0.02	(0.02)
Exactly 2 disorders	–0.02	(0.02)	–0.01	(0.03)
Exactly 3 disorders	0.08*	(0.03)	–0.10*	(0.03)
Exactly 4 disorders	–0.18*	(0.04)	–0.09	(0.06)
5+ disorders	–0.18*	(0.04)	–0.17*	(0.05)
χ^2_5	40.0*		22.4*	
(n)	(37 741)		(25 460)	

* Significant at the 0.05 level, two-sided test.
From Kawakami et al. (2012), *Biological Psychiatry* **72**: 228–37.

A. Mean annual number of days totally out of role

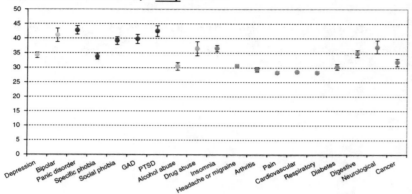

Figure 2.3 Productivity loss associated with mental disorders and physical conditions. (A) Mean additional annual number of days totally out of role; adapted from Alonso *et al.* (2011a), *Molecular Psychiatry* **16**: 1234–46. (B) Proportion of partial disability attributable to mental and physical disorders; from Bruffaerts *et al.* (2012), *British Journal of Psychiatry* **200**: 454–61.

B. Proportion(%) of partial disability attributable to mental and physical disorders

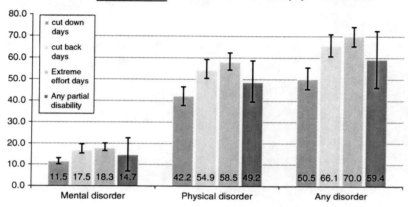

which account for the productivity loss (including work absenteeism and presenteeism, and early retirement).

Figure 2.3A shows the additional days totally out of role in a year among respondents of the WMH surveys with a disorder (individual-level effect). These estimates were adjusted by age, gender, marital status, and employment, as well as the number and type of comorbid disorders. Mental disorders were associated with a higher level of disability measured by the additional days totally out of role (more than 40 for panic disorder, PTSD, and bipolar disorders). Rank correlations of individual effects of the conditions were low across country type (from 0.12 to 0.26). Interactions were found to be subadditive for most disorders in all three income groups: i.e., the incremental increase in days out of role is smaller when a disorder occurs comorbidly compared to when the same disorder occurs in isolation. This may imply that for preventing

disability more effectively, as many as possible of the coexisting disorders should be addressed together. Addressing only one disorder will result in a less effective outcome (Alonso *et al.* 2011a).

In addition to those days totally out of role due to their health, respondents had days where their health partially affected their functioning. The number of additional disability days varied considerably by type of disorder, but was in the 2.30–4.19 range for physical disorders (median = 3.09 days) and in the 2.32–5.26 range for mental disorders (median = 4.04 days). Respondents with PTSD (5.26 days), GAD (4.52 days), and bipolar disorder (4.22 days) reported the highest number of partial disability days. Generally, respondents with mental disorders systematically reported 15–28% more partial disability days than respondents with physical disorders. Partial disability was higher in high-income countries (median impact range = 3.58–4.37), compared to middle-income countries

A

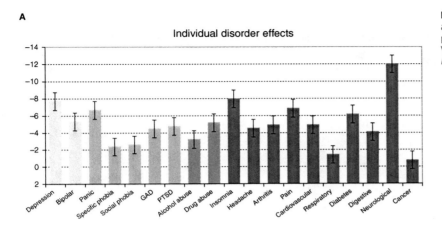

Figure 2.4 Impact of mental disorders and physical conditions on overall perceived health (visual analog scale, VAS). From Alonso *et al.* (2011b), *Psychological Medicine* **41**: 873–86.

B

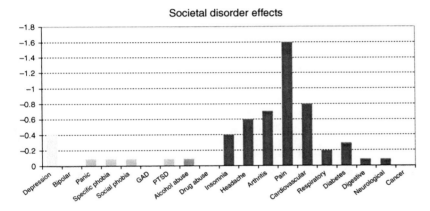

(median impact range = 2.50–3.59) or low-income countries (median impact range = 2.77–3.43).

Mental disorders (especially PTSD, depression, and bipolar disorder) yielded higher individual-level effects than physical disorders on partial disability days. At the societal level, all disorders analyzed accounted for about 59% of all partial disability days (last column in Figure 2.3B)

Physical disorders were responsible for the majority of these days at the societal level, accounting for 49% of the reported disability, compared to 15% accounted for by mental disorders (Bruffaerts *et al.* 2012).

Decreased perceived health status

Table 2.3 shows the individual effect of physical conditions and mental disorders on overall perceived health status (bivariate and multivariate estimations). It can be seen that all coefficients are negative (i.e., they lower the overall perception of health). With the exception of neurological disorders and insomnia, bivariate impacts were higher for mental disorders (range −7.3 to −17.8). In the table, we can also observe that multivariate estimates tend to be more similar for physical and mental conditions. A likely explanation of this is that, with few exceptions, individuals with mental disorders, on average, tend to suffer from a higher number of additional conditions (last column in Table 2.3). Multivariate estimates of impact are also depicted in Figure 2.3A.

Conversely, Figure 2.3B shows the population attributable risk proportion (PARP) estimates of the same conditions, what we have called in this chapter the societal-level impact of disorders.

Table 2.3 Individual-level condition-specific estimates on overall perceived health (VAS)

	Bivariate (Bib)[a]		Multivariate (Multib)		Multib/Bib[b]	Mean comorbidity[c]
	Estimate	(SE)	Estimate	(SE)	Estimate	#
I. Chronic physical conditions						
Arthritis	−9.5	(0.5)	−4.9	(0.4)	0.51	2.0
Cancer	−2.6	(1.1)	−0.8	0.9	0.31	2.1
Cardiovascular disorders	−8.4	(0.4)	−4.9	(0.4)	0.59	1.8
Chronic pain conditions	−10.9	(0.4)	−6.8	(0.4)	0.63	1.8
Diabetes	−8.8	(1.0)	−6.1	(0.8)	0.70	2.0
Digestive disorders	−9.9	(0.9)	−4.1	(0.8)	0.41	2.3
Headaches or migraines	−9.9	(0.4)	−4.5	(0.4)	0.45	2.0
Insomnia	−16.0	(0.7)	−7.9	(0.7)	0.50	2.9
Neurological disorders	−17.8	(1.7)	−12.0	(1.4)	0.67	2.6
Respiratory disorders	−4.3	(0.4)	−1.4	(0.4)	0.31	1.6
II. Mental conditions						
Alcohol abuse	−7.3	(1.1)	−3.2	(1.1)	0.44	1.8
Bipolar disorder	−17.8	(1.4)	−5.3	(1.5)	0.30	3.9
Drug abuse	−12.4	(1.8)	−5.2	(1.7)	0.42	2.6
Generalized anxiety disorder	−13.4	(1.1)	−4.5	(1.1)	0.34	3.0
Major depressive episode	−14.8	(0.5)	−7.6	(0.5)	0.52	2.5
Panic disorder	−16.6	(1.0)	−6.7	(1.0)	0.40	3.4
PTSD	−15.3	(1.1)	−4.7	(0.9)	0.31	3.5
Social phobia	−11.2	(0.8)	−2.6	(0.9)	0.24	2.9
Specific phobia	−8.1	(0.6)	−2.3	(0.6)	0.29	2.2

[a] 19 models with one condition at a time adjusted by demographic controls.
[b] The ratio of the estimate based on the best-fitting model to the estimate based on the bivariate model.
[c] Mean comorbidity = the mean number of other conditions reported by respondents with the condition in the row.
From Alonso et al. (2011b), Psychological Medicine **41**: 873–86.

PARPs are a joint function of prevalence and severity. As can be seen in the figure, the rank ordering of disorders is different for societal impact, where physical pain disorders (such as back and neck pain), cardiovascular disorders, and arthritis are the most burdensome disorders. Among mental disorders, depression is the one with the highest societal burden on overall perceived health. The top five conditions in the rank ordering of societal burden are the same across different income-level countries.

Conclusions

The WMH surveys paint a very detailed and textured picture of the impact of mental disorders. As compared to the GBD, which is focused on health decrements alone, the WMH surveys examine impacts at various levels such as impact on work and income, burden on the family, and changes in the life course due to mental disorders. This describes the wide impact of mental disorders beyond just decrements in health. The following is a short list of conclusions from our work:

- *Burden of mental disorders* – Mental disorders are a very important cause of disease burden in many countries throughout the world. These disorders have a clear and pervasive impact on relevant life-cycle outcomes such as educational achievement, marriage, and divorce, as well as on day-to-day role functioning. Our results are very consistent with prospective studies and call for more efforts to prevent the appearance of mental disorders at an early age. Efforts should be made in different sectors (health, educational, social services).

- *Mental disorders and physical conditions* – Mental disorders are important causes of productivity loss and low perceived health. They are among the most important disorders at both individual and societal levels, although more important at the individual level due to differences in prevalence compared to some of the most common physical disorders. Clearly, both mental and physical disorders must be addressed to increase personal and societal productivity.

- *International variation* – The WMH surveys document considerable international variation in the prevalence of common mental disorders. By using strictly comparable methods and paying considerable attention to cultural issues, the WMH surveys suggest that variation in the prevalence of mental disorders is much more closely associated to contextual variables in the participating countries (such as education level or inequalities) than to methodological issues (such as survey methods or response rates). Whether international variation in the prevalence of mental disorders is due to cultural and other factors that question the equivalence and/or relevance of current definitions of mental disorders should be disentangled. Nevertheless, more worrisome are differences found in access to health services among those with mental disorders. Lower-income countries are at a clear disadvantage (Wang *et al.* 2007). In sharp contrast to the abovementioned variation, the association of mental disorders with life-course disadvantages, disability, and low perceived health is remarkably similar across countries of different economic development levels.

- *Research challenges* – The WMH Consortium has stimulated the active interaction of a large

community of researchers worldwide. Some research projects have been developed as a fruit of this interaction. Studies focusing on adolescents have been carried out in some countries. In other sites DNA samples have been collected at the time of the interview, and these will subsequently be analyzed to try to contribute to the study of genome variation and mental disorders, as well as of gene-by-environment interactions. Methodological studies for refining instruments that can be used in different settings, such as the general population and the health services, are being planned. No doubt the WMH surveys will continue to contribute to improving our knowledge of the burden of mental disorders worldwide. But there are still many research challenges that need to be addressed, if we are to gauge the scale of this important problem.

Appendix: statistical note
Discrete-time survival

Discrete-time survival models (Kalbfleisch & Prentice 1980) were specified to estimate covariate adjusted associations between mental disorders pre-existing to the outcome of interest, specifically early education termination, age of first marriage in the entire sample, and age of first divorce in the subsample of respondents with at least one marriage. In these models, each year a respondent is at risk, up to their age at the occurrence of the outcome or their age at interview, is represented by a separate observation. The resulting person-year datasets are analyzed using logistic regression models with dummy-variable covariates specifying the year of life that each observation represents. Chronological age was used as the time scale. Models allow control for variables of interest (e.g., sex, age, educational attainment, and country in the analysis of age at first marriage; while for models for divorce, statistical controls were included for sex, age, educational attainment, years since marriage, months dating prior to marriage, and country). Pre-existing mental disorders were added as time-varying covariates, i.e. as present in the year of onset and subsequent person-years. Model coefficients are presented as odds ratios, which indicate the relative odds of the outcome in a person who had onset of a disorder prior to the outcome compared with someone without the disorder at the time of the outcome.

GLM modeling

Multiple regression analysis was used to examine multivariate associations of the physical and mental disorders assessed in the survey with perceived health status (VAS) and with reported days out of role in the past 30 days. Statistical controls were included for age, gender, and country (VAS), and additional controls were included for employment in the case of days out of role. As substantial comorbidity was found among the disorders, we included terms to capture the effects of comorbidity in the regression models. Given that the number of possible combinations of comorbid disorders in the data far exceeds the number of respondents, it was necessary to impose some structure on the terms used to capture the effects of comorbidity. This was done by including terms for total number of comorbid disorders and separate interaction terms for the extent to which the regression coefficient of each separate disorder changed as a function of number of comorbid disorders. In days out of role models, the interaction terms were obtained taking into account the size of the coefficients associated with the comorbid disorders. Nonlinear regression methods requiring iterative estimation procedures (Seber & Wild 1989) were used for this purpose.

As both outcome variables (i.e., the 0–30 measure of number of days out of role and the 0–100 VAS measure of perceived health status) were highly skewed, we investigated a number of different model specifications that included an ordinary least squares (OLS) regression model and six generalized linear models (GLMs) that considered the conjunction of two link functions (logarithmic or square root) and three error structures (constant, error variance proportional to the mean, and error variance proportional to the mean squared). In order to choose the model specification that provided the best-fitting results, the following procedures were conducted: (a) the means of predicted values according to each model were plotted against means of observed values, by deciles of the predicted values; the actual decile means form a 45° line, and points above and below the line indicate either underestimation or overestimation; (b) the means of the predicted values were compared with the means of the observed values for different groups of interest; (c) the mean square error (MSE) and the mean absolute predict error (MAPE) were calculated for each of the models. Standard diagnostic procedures to compare model fit (Buntin & Zaslavsky 2004) showed that the OLS model was the best-fitting model when the VAS

perceived health was modeled. For the days out of role variable, the GLM with a log link function was the model that provided the best results in terms of fit.

Estimation of burden: individual and societal effects

As the prediction equation includes interaction terms, the predictive effect of each disorder is distributed across a number of different coefficients. Simulation was used to produce a single term that summarizes all these component effects. This was done by estimating the predicted value of the outcome for each respondent from the coefficients in the final model (the base estimate) and then repeating this exercise in modified form 19 different times, each time assuming that one of the 19 disorders no longer existed.

Individual effects – The difference between the predicted mean of the outcome generated by the simulated estimate and the base estimate was divided by the number of respondents with the disorder in question to obtain the estimated individual-level effect of the disorder on the outcomes. The same procedure was used to calculate total effects of any physical disorder, any mental disorder, and any disorder.

Societal effects – In the models to study perceived health, the estimated societal-level effect of the disorder was then obtained by multiplying the individual-level estimate by the prevalence of the disorder. For days out of role, the proportions of the attributable risk in the population (PARPs) were calculated as societal effects. To obtain them, the two estimates of predicted days out of role described above were used. We then averaged both estimates across the entire population, and computed percentage difference between them.

Complex sampling design

The fact that the WMH survey data are geographically clustered and weighted implied that design-based methods were needed to obtain accurate estimates of standard errors and statistical significance. The Taylor series linearization method implemented in SAS 9.1 (SAS Institute Inc. 2002) was used to do this for the basic model. The more computationally intensive method of Jackknife Repeated Replications (Wolter 1985) implemented in a SAS macro that we wrote for this purpose was used to obtain standard errors of the simulated estimates of individual-level and societal-level disorder effects. Significance tests were consistently evaluated using 0.05-level, two-sided design-based tests.

References

Alonso J, Petukhova M, Vilagut G, et al. (2011a) Days out of role due to common physical and mental conditions: results from the WHO World Mental Health surveys. *Molecular Psychiatry* 16: 1234–46.

Alonso J, Vilagut G, Chatterji S, et al. (2011b) Including information about co-morbidity in estimates of disease burden: results from the World Health Organization World Mental Health Surveys. *Psychological Medicine* 41: 873–86.

Alonso J, Chatterji S, He Y (2013) *The Burden of Mental Disorders: from the WHO World Mental Health Surveys.* Cambridge: Cambridge University Press.

Breslau J, Miller E, Jin R, et al. (2011) A multinational study of mental disorders, marriage, and divorce. *Acta Psychiatrica Scandinavica* 124: 474–86.

Bruffaerts R, Vilagut G, Demyttenaere K, et al. (2012) Role of common mental and physical disorders in partial disability around the world. *British Journal of Psychiatry* 200: 454–61.

Buntin MB, Zaslavsky AM (2004) Too much ado about two-part models and transformation? Comparing methods of modeling Medicare expenditures. *Journal of Health Economics* 23: 525–42.

Centers for Disease Control and Prevention (2004) Health United States. www.cdc.gov (accessed November 2012).

Eaton WW, Martins SS, Nestadt G, et al. (2008) The burden of mental disorders. *Epidemiologic Reviews* 30: 1–14.

Ghimire D, Chardoul S, Kessler RC, Axinn WG, Adhikari BP (2013) Modifying and validating the Composite International Diagnostic Interview (CIDI) for use in Nepal. *International Journal of Methods in Psychiatric Research* 22: 71–81.

Gureje O (2009) The pattern and nature of mental-physical comorbidity: specific or general? In MR Von Korff, KM Scott, O Gureje, eds., *Global perspectives on mental-physical comorbidity in the WHO World Mental Health Surveys.* Cambridge: Cambridge University Press; pp. 51–83.

Gureje O, Lasebikan VO, Kola L, Makanjuola VA (2006) Lifetime and 12-month prevalence of mental disorders in the Nigerian Survey of Mental Health and Well-Being. *British Journal of Psychiatry* 188: 465–71.

Gustavsson A, Svensson M, Jacobi F, et al. (2011) Cost of disorders of the brain in Europe 2010. *European of Neuropsychopharmacology* 21: 718–79.

Haro JM, Arbabzadeh-Bouchez S, Brugha TS, et al. (2006) Concordance of the Composite International Diagnostic Interview Version 3.0 (CIDI 3.0) with standardized clinical assessments in the WHO World Mental Health surveys. *International Journal of Methods in Psychiatric Research* 15: 167–80.

Heeringa S, Wells JE, Hubbard F, et al. (2008) Sample designs and sampling procedures. In RC Kessler, TB Ustun, eds., *The WHO World Mental Health Surveys: Global Perspectives on the Epidemiology of Mental Disorders.* New York, NY: Cambridge University Press; pp. 14–32.

Kalbfleisch JD, Prentice RL (1980) *The Statistical Analysis of Failure Time Data.* New York, NY: Wiley.

Kawakami N, Abdulghani EA, Alonso J, et al. (2012) Early-life mental disorders and adult household income in the World Mental Health Surveys. *Biological Psychiatry* 72: 228–37.

Kessler RC, Ustun TB (2004) The World Mental Health (WMH) survey initiative version of the World Health Organization (WHO) Composite International Diagnostic Interview (CIDI). *International Journal of Methods in Psychiatric Research* 13: 93–121.

Kessler RC, Ustun TB (2008) *The WHO World Mental Health Surveys: Global Perspectives on the Epidemiology of Mental Disorders.* New York, NY: Cambridge University Press.

Kessler RC, Ormel J, Demler O, Stang PE (2003) Comorbid mental disorders account for the role impairment of commonly occurring chronic physical disorders: results from the National Comorbidity Survey. *Journal of Occupational Environmental Medicine* 45: 1257–66.

Kessler RC, Amminger GP, Aguilar-Gaxiola S, et al. (2007) Age of onset of mental disorders: a review of recent literature. *Current Opinion in Psychiatry* 20: 359–64.

Knauper B, Cannell CF, Schwarz N, Bruce ML, Kessler RC (1999) Improving accuracy of major depression age-of-onset reports in the US National Comorbidity Survey. *International Journal of Methods in Psychiatric Research* 8: 39–48.

Knight M, Stewart-Brown S, Fletcher L (2001) Estimating health needs: the impact of a checklist of conditions and quality of life measurement on health information derived from community surveys. *Journal of Public Health Medicine* 23: 179–86.

Lee S, Tsang A, Breslau J, et al. (2009) Mental disorders and termination of education in high-income and low- and middle-income countries: epidemiological study. *British Journal of Psychiatry* 194: 411–17.

Levinson D, Lakoma MD, Petukhova M, et al. (2010) Associations of serious mental illness with earnings: results from the WHO World Mental Health surveys *British Journal of Psychiatry* 197: 114–21.

Miller E, Breslau J, Petukhova M, et al. (2011) Premarital mental disorders and physical violence in marriage: cross-national study of married couples. *British Journal of Psychiatry* **199**: 330–7.

Murray CJ, Lopez AD (1996) Evidence-based health policy: lessons from the Global Burden of Disease Study. *Science* **274**: 740–3.

Pennell BE, Mneimneh ZN, Bowers A, *et al.* (2008) Implementation of the World Mental Health Surveys. Chapter 3. Part I. Methods. In CK Ronald, ed., *The WHO World Mental Health Surveys: Global Perspectives on the Epidemiology of Mental Disorders.* New York, NY: Cambridge University Press; pp. 33–57.

Regier DA, Kaelber CT, Rae DS, *et al.* (1998) Limitations of diagnostic criteria and assessment instruments for mental disorders: implications for research and policy. *Archives of General Psychiatry* **55**: 109–15.

SAS Institute inc. (2002) *SAS/STAT® software, version 9.1 for Windows.* Cary, NC: SAS Institute Inc.

Seber GAF, Wild CL (1989) *Nonlinear Regression.* New York, NY: Wiley.

Shen YC, Zhang MY, Huang YQ, *et al.* (2006) Twelve-month prevalence, severity, and unmet need for treatment of mental disorders in metropolitan China. *Psychological Medicine* **36**: 257–67.

Straus MA, Hamby SL, Boney-McCoy S, Sugarman DB. (1996) The revised conflict tactics scales (CTS2). *Journal of Family Issues* **17**: 283–316.

Structured Clinical Interview for DSM disorders (SCID) (2011) www.scid4.org/ (accessed January 2013).

Von Korff M, Crane PK, Alonso J, *et al.* (2008) Modified WHODAS-II provides valid measure of global disability but filter items increased skewness. *Journal of Clinical Epidemiology* **61**: 1132–43.

Wang PS, Aguilar-Gaxiola S, Alonso J, *et al.* (2007) Use of mental health services for anxiety, mood, and substance disorders in 17 countries in the WHO world mental health surveys. *Lancet* **370**: 841–50.

Wittchen HU, Lieb R, Schuster P, Oldehinkel T (1999) When is onset? Investigations into early developmental stages of anxiety and depressive disorders. In JL Rapoport, ed., *Childhood Onset of "Adult" Psychopathology: Clinical and Research Advances.* Washington, DC: American Psychiatric Press; pp. 259–302.

Wittchen HU, Jacobi F, Rehm J, *et al.* (2011) The size and burden of mental disorders and other disorders of the brain in Europe 2010. *European Neuropsychopharmacology* **21**: 655–79.

World Bank (1993) *World Development Report 1993: Investing in Health.* Oxford: Oxford University Press.

World Health Organization (2008) *The Global Burden of Disease: 2004 Update.* Geneva: WHO.

Wolter KM (1985) *Introduction to Variance Estimation.* New York, NY: Springer-Verlag.

Chapter

3

Trends, gaps, and disparities in mental health

Robert Kohn

Introduction

The prevention, care, and rehabilitation of mental disorders is a growing public health problem globally. Addressing the increasing public health burden of mental disorders worldwide requires an understanding of the prevalence, associated disability, and treatment gap associated with these disorders. Community-based psychiatric epidemiological studies provide insights into the magnitude of the burden.

Estimates of the prevalence of specific mental disorders in numerous countries globally have been established using either structured or semi-structured interview schedules linked to current diagnostic criteria that have improved the reliability and validity of psychiatric diagnoses. The World Mental Health (WMH) surveys (Kessler *et al.* 2009) and the International Consortium of Psychiatric Epidemiology (Andrade *et al.* 2003) are cross-national initiatives that have demonstrated that mental disorders are highly prevalent throughout the world; lifetime prevalences range from 12.0% to 47.4% (median 26%) in the WMH surveys. In addition to these important international collaborations, there are numerous other nationally representative studies (e.g., from Australia, Canada, Ethiopia, and the United Kingdom) that have highlighted the high prevalence of mental disorders throughout different societies (Henderson *et al.* 2000, Paykel *et al.* 2003, Gravel *et al.* 2005, Kebede *et al.* 2005).

The increasing burden of illness of neuropsychiatric disorders is due not only to the high prevalence of mental disorders, but also to the early age of onset of these disorders. About half of all lifetime mental disorders start by the mid-teens, and three-quarters by the mid-twenties (Kessler *et al.* 2007).

The burden of neuropsychiatric disorders

Neuropsychiatric conditions account for a disproportionate amount of burden of disease, although they result in few direct deaths. To assess burden of disease two time-based metrics are used: years of life lost because of premature mortality (YLL) and years of healthy life lost as a result of disability (YLD). YLD is weighted by the severity of disability. The sum of these two components results in a measure of years expected to be lived in full health lost as a result of the incidence of specific diseases and injury, or disability-adjusted life years (DALY). The DALY, as defined by Murray and Lopez (1996), is a health gap measure that extends the concept of potential years of life lost due to premature death to include equivalent years of healthy life lost by virtue of individuals being in states of poor health or disability. One DALY can be thought of as one lost year of healthy life. The DALY is also a measure of the gap between current status and an ideal situation where everyone lives into old age free from disease and disability.

Neuropsychiatric conditions in 2010 were estimated to account for 10.4% of the DALY across all age groups, and 16.6% for those between the ages of 15 and 59, the age range at highest risk for mental disorders (Global Burden of Disease Study 2010 2012). The amount of YLD attributable to neuropsychiatric disorders was even more dramatic, 28.2%, and for those between the ages of 30 and 59 it was 34.1%. The burden of neuropsychiatric disorders varies across regions of the world: DALY and YLD are highest in high-income countries and lowest in low-income countries (Table 3.1).

Table 3.1 Percentage of DALYs and YLDs attributed to neuropsychiatric conditions by region (2010)

Region	DALYs (%)	YLDs (%)
World	10.4	28.2
High-income Asia Pacific	14.8	32.8
Western Europe	19.0	29.3
Australasia	6.8	25.3
High-income North America	12.5	32.9
Central Europe	13.1	28.0
Southern Latin America	14.7	34.0
Eastern Europe	4.3	23.7
East Asia	11.5	27.3
Tropical Latin America	11.7	30.1
Central Latin America	5.9	24.2
Southeast Asia	13.7	25.6
Central Asia	18.7	32.5
Andean Latin America	14.2	30.9
North Africa and Middle East	7.6	26.2
Caribbean	9.4	27.0
South Asia	11.5	30.5
Oceania	16.2	33.5
Southern sub-Saharan Africa	6.7	25.1
Eastern sub-Saharan Africa	15.6	34.1
Central sub-Saharan Africa	17.0	27.8
Western sub-Saharan Africa	4.8	22.2

Unipolar depressive disorders accounted for 9.5% of YLD, and among adults at highest risk, age 15–59, they accounted for 11.4% of the YLD. Among 15–59-year-old females, unipolar depressive disorders accounted for 13.5% of the YLD. Unipolar depressive disorder across all age groups accounted for 3.0% of all DALYs. Among adults at highest risk, age 15–59, 5.0% of DALYs were due to unipolar depressive disorders; and for females in that age group 6.9%. Of all disorders, unipolar depressive disorder ranks seventh across all age groups, behind ischemic heart disease, low back pain, malaria, preterm birth complications, chronic obstructive pulmonary disease, and cirrhosis of the liver secondary to alcohol use, as one of the leading causes of DALY globally, and it is the second

leading cause of YLD. Figures 3.1 and 3.2 illustrate the distribution of DALY and YLD attributable to neuropsychiatric conditions in relation to other medical disorders.

In part, the excess disability due to neuropsychiatric disorders is a result of the early age of onset, compared to other chronic conditions, and the high prevalence of mental disorders. In addition, the increased disability associated with mental disorders may be due to failure to receive treatment; the proportion of individuals who receive treatment in the specialized mental health system or the general healthcare system is small in comparison to those who require treatment (Alegría *et al.* 2000). In addition, those who receive treatment often delay treatment for years (Wang *et al.* 2007a); in other words, there is a treatment lag. Reasons for the delay in treatment include failing to seek help because the problem is not acknowledged, perceiving that treatment is not effective, believing that the problem will go away by itself, and desiring to deal with the problem without outside help. In addition, a lack of knowledge about mental disorders and stigma remain major barriers to care. Factors that are direct barriers to care also preclude treatment, including financial considerations and issues of accessibility, as well as limited availability or lack of availability of services in many countries or for some populations (Kohn *et al.* 2004, Saldivia *et al.* 2004). The burden of psychiatric disorders is increasing, and this may be a result of the epidemiological transition from infectious diseases to chronic illness, or of an increased focus on emergent disorders such as violence and HIV/AIDS, as well as due to a changing population structure away from a very young population to a relatively older population at increased risk for mental disorders.

The treatment gap

If disability is to be reduced, the "treatment gap" must be bridged. The treatment gap represents the absolute difference between the true prevalence of a disorder and the treated proportion of individuals affected by the disorder (Kohn *et al.* 2004). The treatment gap may be expressed as the percentage of individuals who require care but do not receive treatment. Estimating the treatment gap depends on the prevalence period of the disorder, the time frame of the examination of service utilization, and the demographic representativeness of the study sample with reference to

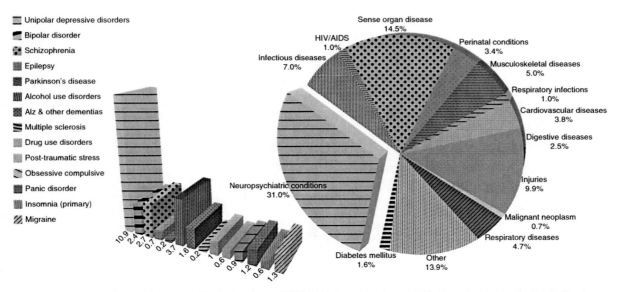

Figure 3.1 The contribution of neuropsychiatric disorders to DALY, 2010 (based on data available from the Institute for Health Metrics and Evaluation).

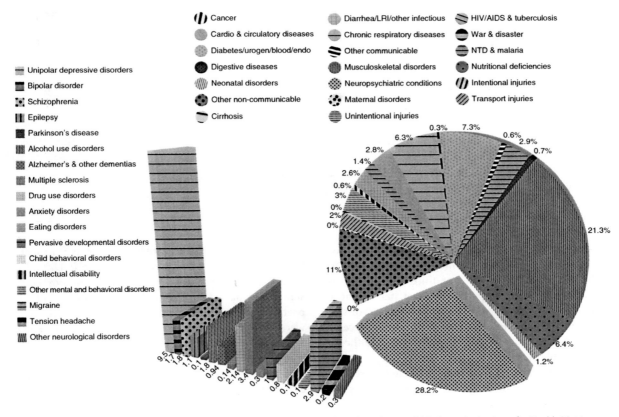

Figure 3.2 The contribution of neuropsychiatric disorders to YLD, 2010 (based on data available from the Institute for Health Metrics and Evaluation).

29

Table 3.2 Median treatment gap, 1980–2002, by region (%)

Diagnosis	Global	AFR	AMR	EMR	EUR	SEAR	WPR
Non-affective psychosis	32.2	–	56.8	–	17.8	28.7	35.9
Major depression	56.3	67.0	56.9	70.2	45.4	–	48.1
Dysthymia	56.0	–	48.6	–	43.9	–	50.0
Bipolar disorder	50.2	–	60.2	–	39.9	–	52.6
Generalized anxiety disorder	57.5	–	55.4	–	47.2	–	66.7
Panic disorder	55.9	–	49.6	–	62.3	–	55.6
Obsessive compulsive disorder	59.5	–	82.0	–	24.6	–	62.7
Alcohol abuse/dependence	78.1	–	72.6	–	92.4	–	71.6

AFR, Africa; AMR, Americas; EMR, Eastern Mediterranean; EUR, Europe; SEAR, South East Asia; WPR, Western Pacific.
Adapted from Kohn *et al.* (2004), *Bulletin of the World Health Organization* **82**: 858–66.

the target population. Kohn and colleagues (2004) formally defined calculation of the treatment gap as

$$G = \frac{\sum [(1 - S_c) R_c P_c]}{\sum [R_c P_c]}$$

Regional treatment gap (*G*) calculations take into account the service utilization rate (S_c), the prevalence rate (R_c), and the population size (P_c) of each of the countries.

In 2004 Kohn *et al.* estimated the treatment gap worldwide, based on studies published between 1980 and 2002 (Table 3.2). The median treatment gap across all studies for schizophrenia, including other non-affective psychosis, was 32.2%; major depression, 56.3%; dysthymia, 56.0%; bipolar disorder, 50.2%; panic disorder, 55.9%; generalized anxiety disorder, 57.5%; and obsessive compulsive disorder, 59.5%. Alcohol abuse and dependence had the largest treatment gap, 78.1%.

More recently, estimates of the treatment gap for Latin America and the Caribbean were published (Kohn & Levav 2009). Over one-third of the individuals with non-affective psychosis, over half of those with an anxiety disorder, and some three-quarters of those with an alcohol use disorder did not receive mental health care from the formal healthcare system (Table 3.3).

The WMH surveys have published data on service utilization in most of the participating countries for anxiety disorders, mood disorders, and substance use disorders. The treatment gap for mood disorders ranges from 43.6% in the USA to 88.5% in Nigeria.

Table 3.3 Mean and median treatment gap for mental disorders in Latin America and the Caribbean, based on published studies from 1980 to the present

Disorder	Treatment gap	
	Mean	Median
Non-affective psychosis	37.4	44.4
Major depression	58.9	57.9
Dysthymia	58.8	58.0
Bipolar disorder	64.0	62.2
Generalized anxiety disorder	63.1	58.2
Panic disorder	52.9	58.9
Obsessive–compulsive disorder	59.9	59.9
Alcohol abuse/dependence	71.4	76.0

Adapted from Kohn & Levav (2009), in *Epidemiología de los Trastornos Mentales en América Latina y el Caribe*, pp. 300–15.

For anxiety disorders the treatment gap is lowest in the USA (57.8%) and highest in Lebanon (93.5%). In some countries almost no one seeks help for substance use disorders (Table 3.4). A summary of 17 participating countries based on whether disorders were severe, moderate, or mild found a wide range of service utilization, whether from the formal healthcare system or from complementary and alternative medicine, between countries (Wang *et al.* 2007b). For example, among those with severe mental disorders in Nigeria, 78.7% did not receive any form of treatment, while in Belgium, the country with the highest service utilization, 39.1% of those with severe disorders had

Table 3.4 Treatment gap for mood, anxiety, and substance use disorders in selected World Mental Health (WMH) survey countries

Country	Mood	Anxiety	Substance use	Reference
Nigeria	88.5	89.6	~100	Gureje & Lasebikan 2006
Ukraine[a]	83.4	78.9	91.6	Bromet *et al.* 2005
Colombia	82.4	84.8	92.5	Posada-Villa *et al.* 2004
South Africa	81.2	73.4	66.4	Seedat *et al.* 2009
Lebanon	80.7	93.5	~100	Karam *et al.* 2006
Mexico	77.8	86.8	82.9	Borges *et al.* 2006
ESEMeD[b]	69.1	73.8	66.8	ESEMeD 2004
Japan	67.0	78.5	80.0	Naganuma *et al.* 2006
New Zealand	44.9	60.6	70.1	Oakley Browne *et al.* 2006
USA	43.6	57.8	61.9	Wang *et al.* 2005

[a] Lifetime service utilization rates
[b] ESEMeD: Belgium, France, Germany, Italy, the Netherlands, and Spain

not utilized any form of mental health services in the past year (Table 3.5).

The World Health Organization Assessment Instrument for Mental Health Systems (WHO-AIMS) was used to assess the treatment gap for schizophrenic disorders, in order to update the estimates published in the 2004 report (Lora *et al.* 2012). The treatment gap measurement was based on the number of cases treated per 100 000 persons with schizophrenic disorders, and it was compared with subregional estimates based on the GBD 2004 update report. Roughly two-thirds (69%) of the people with schizophrenic disorders were not receiving treatment. The treatment gap for schizophrenic disorders was found to be larger in lower-income countries (89%) than in lower-middle-income (69%) and upper-middle-income countries (63%). The treatment gap for schizophrenic disorders was found to be considerably larger than the earlier 2004 estimates. The size of the treatment gap showed a significant negative association with the prevalence of schizophrenic disorders in the general population, gross national income, the number of mental hospital beds per 100 000 population, the number of psychiatrists per 100 000 population, and the number of nurses in mental health facilities per 100 000 population.

A limited number of studies provide data on service utilization in children and adolescents. An analysis of the WHO-AIMS in 42 low- and middle-income countries confirmed that mental health services for children and adolescents are extremely scarce and access to appropriate care is greatly limited (Morris *et al.* 2011). In Chile, for example, 59.4% of children and adolescents who have a psychiatric disorder with significant impairment do not receive treatment, whether from the formal healthcare system or from their school (Vicente *et al.* 2012). Similarly, in an Israel-based study 66% of adolescents with mental disorders had unmet needs based on self-report and 60% based on maternal reports (Mansbach-Kleinfeld *et al.* 2010). In the USA the 2001–2004 NHANES study reported an increase in service utilization among children, age 8–15, in comparison to past studies, but the treatment gap remained greater than 50% (Merikangas *et al.* 2010). The NHANES study reported a range for the treatment gap from 67.8% for generalized anxiety disorder and panic disorder to 52.3% for attention-deficit/hyperactivity disorder. Studies from low-income countries are non-existent.

Resources for mental health in low-income countries

Clearly, the worldwide treatment gap is underestimated, based on studies available, as few studies from low/lower-middle-income countries exist, and of those not all are nationally representative, but limited to large population centers where treatment is more readily available. An illustration of how much greater the treatment gap may be in a low-income country

Table 3.5 Treatment gap and severity of disorders in World Mental Health (WMH) survey countries

Country	Severe	Moderate	Mild
Low income			
Nigeria	78.7	86.2	90.0
Lower-middle income			
China	89.0	76.5	98.3
Colombia	72.2	89.7	92.2
South Africa	73.8	73.4	76.9
Ukraine	74.3	78.8	92.4
Upper-middle income			
Lebanon	79.9	88.4	96.0
Mexico	74.2	82.1	88.1
High income			
Belgium	39.1	63.5	86.1
France	52.0	70.6	78.9
Israel	46.9	67.7	85.6
Germany	60.0	76.1	79.7
Italy	49.0	74.1	82.7
Japan	75.8	75.8	87.2
Netherlands	49.6	68.7	83.9
New Zealand	43.4	60.2	77.8
Spain	41.3	62.6	82.7
USA	40.3	60.1	73.8

Adapted from Wang *et al.* (2007b), *Lancet* **270**: 841–50.

was a treatment prevalence study conducted in Belize based on a review of medical records of all healthcare providers who treated mental illness. It was found that about 63% of individuals with schizophrenia were untreated; this was also true for 89% of those with affective disorders, and for 99% of those with anxiety disorders (Bonander *et al.* 2000). More recently, the prevalence study in Nigeria, the only low-income country represented in the WMH survey, revealed a treatment gap ranging from 78.9% to 90.0% depending on severity (Gureje & Lasebikan 2006). Lora *et al.* (2012) found a treatment gap for schizophrenia alone of 89% in low-income countries.

Additional evidence of the shortfall in mental health services based on income distribution of countries is available from the WHO *Mental Health Atlas* (2011). There are marked disparities between low- and high-income countries in the resources available, in terms of legislation on mental health, health budget allocation for mental health, and number of treatment facilities and human resources committed to the care of the mentally ill (Table 3.6). A review for the *Lancet* series on mental health concluded that this shortage of resources is likely to worsen unless substantial investments are made to train a wider range of mental health workers in much higher numbers (Kakuma *et al.* 2011). In addition, it was suggested that task shifting seems to be an effective and feasible approach, but would also entail substantial investment, innovative thinking, and effective leadership.

Recommendations to reduce the treatment gap

If countries are to successfully reduce the disability associated with inadequate care provision, much more emphasis needs to be placed on addressing both the direct and indirect barriers that continue to persist. The WHO (2001) outlined 10 recommendations for developing countries to implement at both national and community levels in order to reduce the treatment gap in mental health: make mental health treatment accessible in primary care; make psychotropic drugs readily available; shift care away from institutions toward community care; educate the public; involve family, communities, and consumers; establish national mental health programs; increase and improve training of mental health professionals; increase links with other governmental and non-governmental institutions; provide monitoring of the mental health system with quality indicators; and support more research.

More recently, the *Lancet* series on global mental health made recommendations for overcoming barriers to mental health care (Table 3.7) (Saraceno *et al.* 2007). The study group concluded that there were four basic lessons to be learned in overcoming barriers to mental health reform and reducing the treatment gap: political will; advocacy for people with mental illness; development of secondary care-level community mental health services; and more effective use of available formal and informal resources.

To close the treatment gap in mental health, the National Institute of Mental Health, using an

Table 3.6 Mental health resources according to World Bank income level of countries

	Country income level				
	Low	Lower-middle	Upper-middle	High	World
Percent of countries with mental health plan	61.5	72.5	65.1	87.5	72.4
Percent of countries with mental health legislation	38.5	47.1	76.7	77.1	60.2
Median percent of health budget	0.53	1.90	2.38	5.10	2.82
Mental health outpatient facilities per 100 000 population	0.04	0.29	1.05	2.32	0.61
Annual rate treated in mental health outpatient facilities per 100 000 population	48	271	861	1829	110
Day treatment facilities per 100 000 population	0.006	0.010	0.075	0.517	0.046
Psychiatric beds per 100 000 population	0.6	0.4	2.7	13.6	1.4
Psychiatrists per 100 000 population	0.01	0.04	0.08	0.30	0.04
Psychologists per 100 000 population	0.02	0.03	0.15	2.15	0.09
Social workers per 100 000 population	0.01	0.00	0.00	4.10	0.01
Nurses per 100 000 patients in the mental health sector	0.42	2.93	9.72	29.15	4.95

Data from *Mental Health Atlas 2011* (WHO 2011).

Table 3.7 Barriers to improvement of mental health services and challenges to overcoming them

Barriers	Challenges to overcoming barriers
Insufficient funding for mental health services	Inconsistent and unclear advocacy Perception that mental health indicators are weak People with mental disorders are currently not a sufficiently powerful lobby Social stigma Incorrect belief that care is not cost-effective
Mental health resources centralized in and near big cities and in large institutions	Historical reliance on mental hospitals Division of mental health responsibilities between government departments Differences between central and provincial government priorities Vested interests of mental health professionals and workers in continuity of large hospitals Political risk associated with trade union protests Need for transitional funding to shift to community-based services
Complexities of integrating mental health care effectively in primary care services	Primary care workers already overburdened Lack of supervision and specialist support after training Lack of continuous supply of psychotropics in primary care
Low numbers and limited types of health workers trained and supervised in mental health care	Poor working conditions in public mental health services Lack of incentives to work in rural areas Professional establishment opposes expanded role for non-specialists in mental health workforces

Table 3.7 (*cont.*)

Barriers	Challenges to overcoming barriers
	Medical students and psychiatric residents trained only in mental hospitals Inadequate training of general health workforce Mental health specialists spend time providing care rather than training and supervising others Lack of infrastructure to enable community-based supervision
Mental health leaders often deficient in public health skills and experiences	Those who rise to leadership positions often only trained in clinical management Public health training does not include mental health Resistance of psychiatrists to accept others as leaders Lack of training courses in public mental health Leaders overburdened by clinical and management responsibilities and private practice

Adapted from Saraceno *et al.* (2007), *Lancet* **370**: 1164–74.

international Delphi panel, identified 25 "grand challenges" as research priorities for the next 10 years (Collins *et al.* 2011, National Institute of Mental Health 2011):

Goal A – identify root causes, risk and protective factors

- identify modifiable social and biological risk factors across the life course
- understand the impact of poverty, violence, war, migration, and disaster
- identify biomarkers

Goal B – advance prevention and implementation of early interventions

- support community environments that promote physical and mental well-being throughout life
- reduce the duration of untreated illness by developing culturally sensitive early interventions across settings
- develop interventions to reduce the long-term negative impact of low childhood socioeconomic status on cognitive ability and mental health
- develop an evidence-based set of primary prevention interventions for a range of mental disorders
- develop locally appropriate strategies to eliminate childhood abuse and enhance child protection

Goal C – improve treatments to expand access to care

- integrate screening and core packages of services into routine primary health care
- reduce cost and improve the supply of effective medications
- develop effective treatments for use by non-specialists, including lay health workers with minimal training
- incorporate functional impairment and disability into assessment
- provide effective and affordable community-based care and rehabilitation
- improve children's access to evidence-based care by trained health providers in low- and middle-income countries
- develop mobile and IT technologies to increase access to evidence-based care

Goal D – raise awareness of the global burden

- develop culturally informed methods to eliminate stigma, discrimination, and social exclusion of patients and families across cultural settings
- establish cross-national evidence on cultural, socioeconomic, and services factors underlying disparities in incidence, diagnosis, treatment, and outcomes
- develop valid and reliable definitions, models, and measurement tools for quantitative assessment at the individual

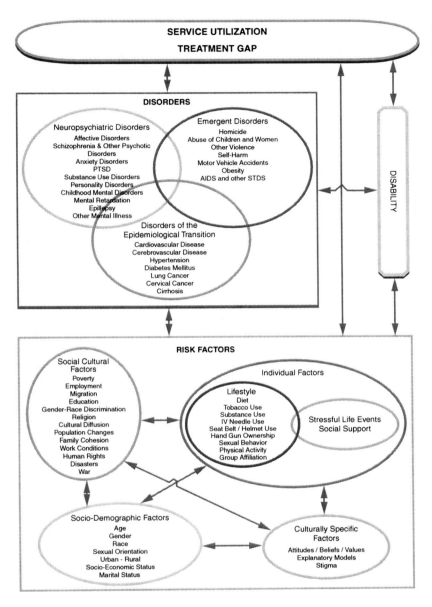

Figure 3.3 Treatment gap and disability, and transitions in the role of mental health.

and population levels for use across cultural settings

- establish shared, standardized global data systems for collecting surveillance data on the prevalence, treatment patterns, and availability of human resources and services

Goal E – build human resource capacity

- increase capacity in low- and middle-income countries by creating regional centers for

mental health research, education, training, and practice that incorporate the views and needs of local people

- develop sustainable models to train and increase the number of culturally diverse lay and specialist providers to deliver evidence-based services
- strengthen the mental health component in the training of all healthcare personnel

Goal F – transform health-system and policy responses

- establish and implement minimum healthcare standards for mental disorders around the world
- redesign health systems to integrate mental disorders with other chronic disease care, and create parity between mental and physical illness in investment into research, training, treatment, and prevention
- incorporate a mental health component into international aid and development programs

The *Lancet* mental health series has called for a "scaling up" of mental health care, including coverage, the range of services offered, services based on scientific evidence base, and strengthening the healthcare system (Eaton *et al.* 2011). Scaling up also includes mobilization of political will, human resource development, an increase in the availability of essential medicines, and monitoring and evaluation (Mangham & Hanson 2010).

Conclusions

Mental disorders are highly prevalent, and the burden of mental disorders is growing in most low- and middle-income countries. The population's mental health burden is not just a reflection of the rate of psychopathology, but is also an aggregate of conditions and problems in which behavior plays a dominant role.

Historically, mental health care has concerned itself only with psychiatric disorders and with disorders that may fall under the broader categorization of neuropsychiatric. Depending on such factors as the resources available and the prevailing planning tradition, some countries limit mental health programs to severe mental illnesses. Such a narrow perspective of mental health care will not suffice, given the changing population structures. The mental health field will be asked to play an increasingly important role in the prevention and treatment of chronic diseases and emergent disorders that have behavioral components (Figure 3.3). A shift toward a larger role for mental health care has begun in industrialized nations, with an emphasis on primary care detection, behavioral medicine programs, and the health of the elderly.

Recommendations on reducing the treatment gap set forth by the *Lancet* mental health series, the National Institute of Mental Health, and the World Health Organization need to be broadly accepted and implemented. Even established market economies or high-income countries have unacceptable treatment gap rates, resulting in an extremely high global burden of disease for mental illness. If this were the pattern for any other category of chronic illness a call for action would have long been heeded, as failure to address such a public health burden would not have been an option. As appropriately stated in the *Lancet* mental health series, "there is no health without mental health" (Prince *et al.* 2007).

References

Alegría M, Kessler RC, Bijl R, *et al.* (2000) Comparing data on mental health service use between countries. In G Andrews, S Henderson, eds., *Unmet Need in Psychiatry.* New York, NY: Cambridge University Press; pp. 97–118.

Andrade L, Caraveo-Anduaga JJ, Berglund P, *et al.* (2003) The epidemiology of major depressive episodes: results from the International Consortium of Psychiatric Epidemiology (ICPE) surveys. *International Journal of Methods in Psychiatric Research* 12: 3–21.

Bonander J, Kohn R, Arana B, *et al.* (2000) An anthropological and epidemiological overview of mental health in Belize. *Transcultural Psychiatry* 37: 57–72.

Borges G, Medina-Mora ME, Wang PS, *et al.* (2006) Treatment and adequacy of treatment of mental disorders among respondents to the Mexico National Comorbidity Survey. *American Journal of Psychiatry* 163: 1371–8.

Bromet EJ, Gluzman SF, Paniotto VI, *et al.* (2005) Epidemiology of psychiatric and alcohol disorders in Ukraine: findings from the Ukraine World Mental Health survey. *Social Psychiatry and Psychiatric Epidemiology* 40: 681–90.

Collins PY, Patel V, Joestl SS, *et al.* (2011) Grand challenges in global mental health. *Nature* 475: 27–30.

Eaton J, McCay L, Semrau M, *et al.* (2011) Scale up of services for mental health in low-income and middle-income countries. *Lancet* 278: 1592–603.

ESEMeD / MHEDEA 2000 investigators (2004) Use of mental health services in Europe: results from the European Study of the Epidemiology of Mental Disorders (ESEMeD) project. *Acta Psychiatrica Scandinavica* 109 (Suppl. 420): 47–54.

Global Burden of Disease Study 2010 (GBD 2010) (2012) *Global Burden of Disease Study 2010: Results by Cause 1990–2010.* Seattle, WA: Institute for Health Metrics and Evaluation (IHME).

Gravel R, Béland Y (2005) The Canadian community health survey: mental health and well-being. *Canadian Journal of Psychiatry* **50**: 573–9.

Gureje O, Lasebikan VO (2006) Use of mental health services in a developing country: results from the Nigerian survey of mental health and well-being. *Social Psychiatry and Psychiatric Epidemiology* **41**: 44–9.

Henderson S, Andrews G, Hall W (2000) Australia's mental health: an overview of the general population survey. *Australia and New Zealand Journal of Psychiatry* **34**: 197–205.

Kakuma R, Minas H, van Ginneken N, *et al.* (2011) Human resources for mental health care: current situation and strategies for action. *Lancet* **378**: 1654–63.

Karam EG, Mneimneh ZN, Karam AN, *et al.* (2006) Prevalence and treatment of mental disorders in Lebanon: a national epidemiological survey. *Lancet* **367**: 1000–6.

Kebede D, Alem A, Shibre T, *et al.* (2005) Short-term symptomatic and functional outcomes of schizophrenia in Butajira, Ethiopia. *Schizophrenia Research* **78**: 171–85.

Kessler RC, Amminger GP, Aguilar-Gaxiola S, *et al.* (2007) Age of onset of mental disorders: a review of recent literature. *Current Opinion in Psychiatry* **20**: 359–64.

Kessler RC, Aguilar-Gaxiola S, Alonso J, *et al.* (2009) The global burden of mental disorders: an update from the WHO World Mental Health (WMH) surveys. *Epidemiologia e Psichiatria Sociale* **18**: 23–33.

Kohn R, Levav I (2009) La utilización de los servicios de salud mental y la brecha de tratamiento en América Latina y el Caribe. In J Rodríguez, R Kohn, S Aguilar-Gaxiola, eds., *Epidemiología de los Trastornos Mentales en América Latina y el Caribe*. Washington DC: Pan American Health Organization; pp. 300–15.

Kohn R, Saxena S, Levav I, *et al.* (2004) The treatment gap in mental health care. *Bulletin of the World Health Organization* **82**: 858–66.

Lora A, Kohn R, Levav I, *et al.* (2012) Service availability and utilization and treatment gap for schizophrenic disorders: a survey in 50 low- and middle-income countries. *Bulletin of the World Health Organization* **90**: 47–54B.

Mangham LJ, Hanson K (2010) Scaling up in international health: what are the key issues? *Health Policy Planning* **25**: 85–96.

Mansbach-Kleinfeld I, Palti H, Farbstein I, *et al.* (2010) Service use for mental disorders and unmet need: results from the Israel Survey on Mental Health Among Adolescents. *Psychiatric Services* **61**: 241–9.

Merikangas KR, He JP, Brody D, *et al.* (2010) Prevalence and treatment of mental disorders among US children in the 2001–2004 NHANES. *Pediatrics* **125**: 75–81.

Morris J, Belfer M, Daniels A, *et al.* (2011) Treated prevalence of and mental health services received by children and adolescents in 42 low- and middle-income countries *Journal of Child Psychology and Psychiatry* **52**: 1239–46.

Murray CJL, Lopez AD (1996) *The Global Burden of Disease: a Comprehensive Assessment of Mortality and Disability from Diseases, Injuries, and Risk Factors in 1990 and Projected to 2020*. Cambridge, MA: Harvard University Press.

Naganuma Y, Tachimori H, Kawakami N, *et al.* (2006) Twelve-month use of mental health services in four areas in Japan: findings from the World Mental Health Japan Survey 2002–2003. *Psychiatry and Clinical Neurosciences* **60**: 240–8.

National Institute of Mental Health (2011) Grand Challenges in Global Mental Health. http:// grandchallengesgmh.nimh.nih.gov (accessed June 2013).

Oakley Browne MA, Wells JE, McGee MA, *et al.* (2006) Twelve-month and lifetime health service use in Te Rau Hinengaro: the New Zealand Mental Health Survey. *Australian and New Zealand Journal of Psychiatry* **40**: 855–64.

Paykel E, Abbott R, Jenkins R, *et al.* (2003) Urban–rural mental health differences in Great Britain: findings from the National Morbidity Survey. *International Review of Psychiatry* **15**: 97–107.

Posada-Villa JA, Aguilar-Gaxiola SA, Magaña CG, *et al.* (2004) Prevalencia de trastornos mentales y uso de servicios: resultados preliminares del Estudio nacional de salud mental. Colombia 2003. *Revista Colombiana Psiquiatria* **33**: 241–62.

Prince M, Patel V, Saxena S, *et al.* (2007) No health without mental health. *Lancet* **370**: 859–77.

Saldivia S, Vicente B, Kohn R, *et al.* (2004) Use of mental health services in Chile. *Psychiatric Services* **55**: 71–6.

Saraceno B, van Ommeren M, Batniji R, *et al.* (2007) Barriers to improvement of mental health services in low-income and middle-income countries. *Lancet* **370**: 1164–74.

Seedat S, William DR, Herman AA (2009) Mental health service use among South Africans for mood, anxiety and substance use disorders. *South African Medical Journal* **99**: 346–52.

Vicente B, Saldivia S, de la Barra F, *et al.* (2012) Prevalence of child and adolescent mental disorders in Chile: a community epidemiological study. *Journal of Child Psychology and Psychiatry* **53**: 1026–53.

Wang PS, Lane M, Olfson M, *et al.* (2005) Twelve-month use of mental health services in the United States: results from the National Comorbidity Survey Replication. *Archives of General Psychiatry* **62**: 629–40.

Wang PS, Angermeyer M, Borges G, *et al.* (2007a) Delay and failure in treatment seeking after first onset of mental disorders in the World Health Organization's World Mental Health Survey Initiative. *World Psychiatry* **6**: 177–85.

Wang PS, Aguilar-Gaxiola S, Alonso J, *et al.* (2007b) Use of mental health services for anxiety, mood, and substance disorders in 17 countries in the WHO world mental health surveys. *Lancet* **270**: 841–50.

World Health Organization (2001) *The World Health Report 2001. Mental Health: New Understanding, New Hope.* Geneva: WHO.

World Health Organization (2008) *The Global Burden of Disease: 2004 Update.* Geneva: WHO.

World Health Organization (2011) *Mental Health Atlas 2011.* Geneva: WHO.

Global health and mental health as diplomacy

Samuel O. Okpaku

Introduction and background

The last few decades have witnessed considerable discussions and activities in global health diplomacy. The relationship between physical health and mental health is an intricate one. Therefore it would be artificial to consider global mental health in the absence of physical health. For pragmatic reasons we will discuss global health and global mental health diplomacy jointly, but when global mental health diplomacy has any ascendancy or priority, it will be emphasized.

In this chapter we will establish some academic definitions of global health policy. Then we will explore heuristic instances where global health drives foreign policy and vice versa, bearing in mind that these two processes frequently overlap and sometimes intersect. A chronology of significant milestones in the modern history of global health diplomacy is undertaken, using a typology of sponsorship/initiatives. This is followed by a review of predictions for the future of global health (Fidler 2003). The chapter concludes with a discussion and summary.

In considering global health as diplomacy, some preliminary statements are in order:

(1) This is not a new phenomenon. As early as 1851 there were treaties to regulate human movement and trade in order to protect nation states from infectious diseases such as cholera. However, modern global health has become a complex set of processes.

(2) Because of modern interconnectivity, the international system has to be seen as an open and single system which is porous and allows of outside influences.

(3) The players and stakeholders are individuals and organizations with different backgrounds funding practices and objectives.

(4) There has been an apparent shift in strategy, with powerful nations tending to use soft and smart diplomacy instead of big-stick diplomacy to gain influence, trust, and authority.

Definitions of global health diplomacy

Several authors have explored definitions of global health diplomacy and have attempted various analyses using different reference points. The following are some definitions of global health diplomacy:

> Winning hearts and minds of people in poor countries by exporting medical care, expertise and personnel to help those who need it most.
>
> (Fauci 2007)

> The cultivation of trust and negotiation of mutual benefit in the context of global health goals.
>
> (Aldis 2008)

> Health diplomacy is the chosen method of interaction between stakeholders engaged in public health and politics for the purpose of representation, cooperation, resolving disputes, improving health systems, and securing the right to health for vulnerable populations.
>
> (Health Diplomats undated)

Labonté (2008) examined the different frames that have been employed by different governments to support placing health in their foreign policies. The frames he selected were security development, global public goods, trade, human rights, and ethical/moral reasoning. He was interested in two issues in particular:

(1) What reasons have governments stated for positioning health in their foreign policy objectives?

(2) What is the potential of this framing to advance global health equity?

Essentials of Global Mental Health, ed. Samuel O. Okpaku. Published by Cambridge University Press. © Cambridge University Press 2014.

Labonté and Gagnon (2010) reviewed major English-language health and foreign policy documents from 2000 to 2009. Their findings include the fact that security and development were the most often cited frames. The British government is an example of a government that has positioned health security and development as a major consideration. In making reference to the work of Fidler, Labonté and Gagnon identified their position with Fidler's conceptualization of remediation. Fidler had conceptualized the insertion of health considerations into foreign policy as:

(1) revolution
(2) remediation
(3) regression

According to Fidler, revolution, as a concept, referred to the transformative nature of health in relation to foreign policy. Remediation referred to the traditional role of foreign policy in understanding another issue, this time health. His conceptualization of regression indicates deterioration and a failure of public health efforts in an attempt to "stay the course" (Fidler 2005).

Lee and Smith (2011) contributed to this definition to distinguish between traditional and new diplomacy. New diplomacy occurs within a global context, the stakeholders are diverse, and the processes involved are innovative. Lee and Smith suggested that a more precise definition of global health diplomacy is helpful for greater scholarship in this area.

Beyond these academic definitions, diplomacy can be parsimoniously stated simply as skilled negotiations in international relations. In other words, global health can be operationalized as skilled negotiations that relate to foreign policy. With this definition we can now explore opportunities for global health and global mental health.

Global health and foreign policies

As previously indicated, global health and foreign policy frequently overlap and intersect. Global health can drive foreign policy and vice versa. We will now explore these two sets of driving forces.

Global health driving foreign policy

Examples for this category are immigration and refugee issues, natural and manmade disasters, and violence as a public health issue.

Immigration and refugees

It is reported that the total number of immigrants worldwide has increased over the last 10 years, with an estimated 214 million international migrants at present (UN Department of Economic and Social Affairs 2009). Some have migrated for economic reasons. A proportion has left their homelands because of conflict and civil wars. Their settlement frequently requires diplomatic consultations and compromises. Issues in human rights are also frequently involved. Sometimes these immigrants have children. Deservingness and citizenship rights become issues. Should these individuals have access to education and health care? What of the health implications for undocumented and illegal immigrants who may seek medical care and are excluded from medical care? What are some of the humanitarian issues? A good example of the diplomatic underpinnings of immigration is the recent debate about immigration into the United States. In the past, the US government has had restrictions on sick indivudals coming into the United States, but more recently it has eased the health criteria for individuals with HIV/AIDS to enter the USA. Many countries now have global health centers to help detect immigrants whose entry may pose a threat to the recipient countries. In addition, their universities and research centers are devoted to the care of immigrants and their families.

Any discussion of immigration driving foreign policy will be incomplete without a mention of the "brain drain" of medical professionals from developing countries to developed nations. An example is the case of Sri Lanka, where recent figures show 106 Sri Lankan-trained psychiatrists working in the USA while only 38 remain in Sri Lanka. The corresponding figures for Nigeria and India are 167 in the USA and 114 remaining in Nigeria, 3293 in the USA and 2162 remaining in India (Jenkins *et al.* 2010). As a result, mental health services in these countries are suffering, with a shortage of qualified psychiatrists as well as fewer opportunities for specialist training programs. This is an ethical question without any easy solution, as it touches on individual rights, state rights, and public good. Different countries have dealt with this in diverse ways. In the United Kingdom in the early 1970s there was a practice to encourage Commonwealth-born physicians to return to their homelands. Further research on this matter and effective policy agreements are necessary for more equitable health care.

Disasters

Several chapters in this volume refer to the global implications of natural disasters and manmade disasters. Major disasters in the last two decades include Hurricane Katrina, the Chilean mine disaster, the Chilean earthquake, the Haitian earthquake, the Indonesian tsunami, the Japanese tsunami, and its threat of nuclear disaster. These disasters were graphically captured in the world news and on television. The Chilean mine disaster was especially poignant as the world watched the result of a collaborative and elaborate rescue, with even the rescue equipment coming from different countries. The Haitian rescue was similar, and the cooperation of the United Nations (UN) agencies, non-governmental organizations (NGOs), and individual aid workers emphasized the need for diplomatic action.

Violence as a public health issue

Through public health measures and advances in medicine the world was starting to see a reduction in death by infectious diseases towards the middle of the twentieth century. At that time, homicide and suicide were becoming leading causes of deaths. Public health professionals and organizations began focusing on behavioral challenges and social problems (Dahlberg & Mercy 2009). Dr. Gro Harlem Brundtland, a former Director-General of the World Health Organization (WHO), is credited with drawing attention to violence as a public health issue in a global context. In a 1996 resolution, the World Health Assembly called on the WHO to develop a typology of violence. Since then, the UN's efforts to end violence and prevent violence have grown (WHO 1996). The current UN Secretary-General, Ban Ki-moon, initiated the UNiTE campaign to end violence against women and girls. Through the mechanism of UNiTE the UN agencies collaborate with member states, civil societies, and NGOs to work towards ending violence to women and girls in its various forms. These include intimate partner violence as well as sex trafficking (UN Secretary-General 2008).

The activities in these areas are a matter for diplomatic collaboration. For example, the British government in its action plan stipulated that one of its actions should be partnership with the New York police, the World Bank, and the Council of Europe, in reducing violence against women and girls (HM Government 2011). The partnership with the New York police is to learn about that department's successful proactive strategies in reducing violence against women. Another objective is to support the poorest countries in their efforts to reduce domestic violence against women and girls by providing expertise, knowledge, and technology. In that document, the UK government affirms the belief that violence and lack of security can undermine the ability of women and girls to achieve their highest potential. This belief is likely to hinder one of the attainments of the Millennium Goals. The UK government, as a signatory to the convention on the elimination of all forms of discrimination, is therefore active in the domestic, European, and international arenas, as well as providing support to the European Union's action plan on gender equality and women's empowerment and development (European Commission 2010a).

Foreign policy driving global health

The following are examples of foreign policies of a number of states that have implications for health, security, and development. Although these policies have much in common, there are some variations in their philosophical priorities and agenda.

British foreign policy

The British government in its document *Health is Global* stated the following five policies for action (HM Government 2008):
(1) better global health security
(2) stronger, fairer, and safer systems to deliver health
(3) more effective international health organizations
(4) stronger, freer, and fairer trade for better health
(5) strengthening the way we develop and use
     evidence to improve policy and practice

US foreign policy

For the USA, global health is a crucial aspect of national security. This policy strives to establish alliances with foreign partners in the interest of security and peace. For example, the US government has spent considerable sums of money in the fight against AIDS.

In 2002 the Bush Administration commissioned the National Intelligence Council to report on HIV/AIDS in Nigeria, Ethiopia, Russia, India, and China, and on potential consequences of the excess mortality on US national security interests. A total of US$15 billion was committed to the fight against HIV for 2003–08. That amount constitutes one of the highest contributions by one state to another state in the fight against a disease entity. This massive funding was renewed as the Tom Lantis and Henry J. Hyde United States Global Leadership against HIV/AIDS, and Tuberculosis Reauthorization Act of 2008 (US Congress 2008).

The US Centers for Disease Control and Prevention (CDC) aims to achieve the following goals (CDC 2012):

Goal 1. Health impact: improve the health and well-being of people around the world.

Goal 2. Health security: improve capabilities to prepare for and respond to infectious disease, other emerging health threats, and public health emergencies.

Goal 3. Health capacity: build country public health capacity.

Goal 4. Organizational capacity: maximize the potential of CDC's global programs to achieve impact.

Swiss foreign policy

The Swiss government prides itself as the first country to adopt an interministerial agreement on health. Swiss foreign policy objectives place emphasis on increasing stakeholder participation, and the policy is buttressed by the Swiss values of the rule of the law, human rights, and its strength as a health capital. The policy also broadens the definition of "developed" to imply living a life of dignity (FDFA & FDHA 2006).

Swedish foreign policy: shared responsibility

In May 2003 the Swedish government's Bill Shared Responsibility was presented to parliament. The Bill promoted an overall policy for global development with a common objective for all policy areas. Thus the main theme of the Bill is policy coherence built on a multisetorial system. A major objective of this policy is to contribute to an equitable and sustainable development globally. The policy is to be driven by a human rights perspective that derives from international human rights conventions as well as by "perspectives of the poor." The policy therefore focuses on poor people and poor countries, and it proposes equity and sustainability in all policy sectors including trade, agriculture, migration, and security (Swedish Ministry of Foreign Affairs 2003).

Norwegian foreign policy

The cornerstone of Norwegian policy is to promote and respect fundamental human rights. The principle of equal access to health services based on comprehensive, robust health systems serves as a guideline (Norwegian Ministry of Foreign Affairs 2012).

Norway's Policy Coherence Commission reported:

> The aim here is not fighting poverty through increasing aid or loans to poor people or countries, but framework conditions that can make it easier for these countries to create long-term economic growth and reduce poverty themselves . . . Aid can be a crucial and necessary catalyst for contributing to development, but it is far from adequate as a tool to make this sustainable.
> (Policy Coherence Commission 2008)

As Norway's foreign minister, Jonas Gahr Støre, noted in tacit acknowledgement of where global power lies (markets, and those who dominate them):

> We need to find new ways of portraying health expenditures as more than costs, but also as an investment. We need to . . . get to the core of the economic dimension and speak a language that people with power really understand.
> (Støre 2008)

The overall objectives of Norway towards global health (Norwegian Ministry of Foreign Affairs 2012) are to:

(1) fight poverty by helping to achieve the UN Millennium Development Goals

(2) support and promote the right to health services

(3) help to reduce the great social inequalities in the world

(4) help to reduce the burden of disease

(5) promote women's rights and gender equality

Milestones in modern global health diplomacy

It might be useful to examine global mental health from a typology of the sponsorships of the diplomatic initiatives:

(1) UN and universal initiatives

(2) multinational initiatives

(3) regional initiatives

(4) bilateral initiatives

(5) NGOs, including foundations, civil societies of users, survivors, and advocacy groups

UN and universal initiatives

Under the auspices of the UN and WHO, the following examples chronologically demonstrate the evolution of global health diplomacy.

The Alma Ata Declaration of 1978

At an international conference on primary care, the Alma Ata Declaration was adopted. There are essentially five major prongs to this declaration (WHO 1978):

(1) It defined health as not merely the absence of disease or infirmity.
(2) It affirmed the inequality between the developing countries and the developed world, between the haves and have-nots. It framed this inequity as socially, politically, and economically unacceptable.
(3) It declared health as a socioeconomic matter and as a human right.
(4) It underlined the role of the state in providing appropriate social and health programs. A by-product of this was the concept of "health for all."
(5) The goals were to be obtained through the mechanism of primary health care.

All stakeholders – governments, international organizations, civil societies, health workers, and development communities – were to dedicate themselves to the above ideals. WHO worked together with major UN agencies towards "intersectoral action for health" in order to implement comprehensive "health for all" primary health care (WHO 1986). These sentiments were reaffirmed during the 20th anniversary of the Alma Ata Declaration in 1998 (WHO 1998).

The UN General Assembly of 1991

In 1991 the UN produced a document listing 25 principles geared to protect mentally ill individuals from discrimination and exclusion, promoting access to humane treatment and establishing other fundamental rights such as counsel, independent authority, mental health care, mental health facility, mental health practitioners, and opportunity for due process (UN General Assembly 1991).

The UN Declaration on the Elimination of Violence against Women, 1993

The Declaration on the Elimination of Violence against Women was adopted by the UN General Assembly in 1993. This document defined gender-based abuse and emphasized the role of governments. The General Assembly has since dealt with various forms of violence including all forms of violence against women (UN General Assembly 1993):

(1) trafficking in women and girls
(2) crimes committed in the name of honor
(3) violence against women migrant workers
(4) traditional or customary practices affecting the health of women and girls
(5) domestic violence

Since 1999, November 25 has been designated as the International Day for the Elimination of Violence against Women (UN General Assembly 1999).

The World Report on Violence and Health, 1994

This humanitarian and human rights approach to health is likely to gain momentum as the consequences of health-related effects of world hunger and poverty, climate change, and violence become more apparent. At the International Conference on Population and Development held in Cairo under the auspices of the UN, the action plan included the request to countries to consider population factors in their development plans as well as to take action to reduce violence against women. Some of this violence may be due to traditional beliefs and practices, including femicide and female genital mutilation (UN 1994).

In 1996, Resolution WHA 49.25 was adopted by the 49th World Health Assembly. The resolution declared violence as a major public health problem globally (WHO 1996).

World Health Report 2001

This report, titled *New Understanding, New Hope*, focuses on the fact that mental health is crucial to the overall well-being of individuals, societies, and countries. The report advocates policies that are urgently needed to ensure that stigma and discrimination are broken down and that effective prevention and treatment are put in place (WHO 2001).

In 2002, a major report was published by WHO. The foreword was written by Nelson Mandela, who reflected on his own personal experience in South Africa (Krug *et al.* 2002).

WHO Mental Health Policy Project and Human Rights Day, 2005

This project provided guiding tools for all the stakeholders, governments, and non-governmental agencies to collaborate with WHO to address the behavioral health needs of society. Several papers were published, in particular *WHO Mental Health Policy and Service Guidance Package, WHO Resource Book on Mental Health, Human Rights, and Legislation*, and *Mental Health Promotion*. The documents linked the protection of human rights to improving the quality of life for people with mental disorders (WHO undated). Furthermore, these documents supported the initiative to decrease the international burden of mental illness and promoted "the importance of mental health to the overall health of individuals, communities, cities, and even entire nations." (WHO 2005a).

Millennium Development Goals Achievement Fund, 2007

As outlined by the UN General Assembly in the Millennium Declaration of 2000, 80 heads of state committed themselves to "a collective responsibility to uphold the principles of human dignity, equality, and equity at the global level" (UN General Assembly 2000). This resolution was expanded into a set of priorities and challenges, known as the Millennium Development Goals (MDGs), with eight specific objectives to be achieved by 2015. The eight goals are as follows (WHO 2005b):

(1) end poverty and hunger
(2) provide access to universal education
(3) promote gender equality
(4) improve child health
(5) improve maternal health
(6) combat HIV/AIDS
(7) promote environmental sustainability
(8) promote global partnerships

The commitment by the heads of state is to include adequate appropriation of funds in order to accomplish the above goals. In 2007 the Millennium Development Goals Achievement Fund (MDG-F) was set up by the government of Spain and the UN system. The availability or the prospect of funds has led to a mushrooming of services and activities to make the MDGs a reality (MDG Achievement Fund undated).

It should be noted that mental health is not specifically mentioned in the MDGs. However, it is indisputable that issues related to poverty and hunger, gender equality, child health, and maternal health are central to individuals and states searching for better equity and quality of life for all.

It is also important to mention the fact that some nations have not committed adequate funding to the MDG-F. This jeopardizes the acceleration in achievement of the MDGs. The performance of many African countries is lagging behind. Overall, the agreement on the goals to be achieved by the MDG-F was a major victory for UN Secretary-General Kofi Annan as a consensus had to be driven among states that differ politically, ideologically, and religiously. Examples are the discussions over the role of women, and family planning practices.

The First Global Conference on Healthy Lifestyles and Non-Communicable Disease Control, 2011

This conference was sponsored by the Russian Federation and WHO. It was a major milestone in the international effort to reduce the disease burden of four non-communicable diseases (NCDs): cancers, cardiovascular diseases, diabetes, and chronic lung diseases (WHO 2011a). Prior to the meeting, Ms. Zsuzsanna Jakab, WHO Regional Director for Europe, stated that NCDs constitute "a global problem that needs national solutions." She called on health ministries to involve foreign ministries and other sectors in their search for solutions (WHO Regional Office for Europe 2011).

UN High Level General Assembly Meeting on Non-Communicable Diseases, 2011

This was the second time in the history of the UN General Assembly that a health issue was placed on the agenda. The heads of state declared that the four NCDs resulted in a major burden and a major obstacle to twenty-first-century development, thereby recognizing the primary role of governments in the control and prevention of these conditions. Mental health disorders were not part of the resolution but had a mention (UN General Assembly 2011).

The World Conference on Social Determinants of Health Declaration, 2011

Appointed by WHO in 2005, the Commission on Social Determinants of Health set forth the inequities of health and in their report called to action a team to explore the major social determinants of health outcomes (WHO 2008). In 2011 at Rio de Janeiro, Brazil, the World Conference on Social Determinants of Health adopted a declaration affirming the commitment of member states for an "all for equity" global action plan.. These recommendations were as follows (WHO 2011b):

(1) adopt improved governance for health and development
(2) promote participation in policy meetings and implementation
(3) further orient the health sector towards promoting health and reducing health inequities
(4) strengthen global governance and collaboration
(5) monitor programs and increase accountability

The document was very important, as it challenges the hegemony of biomedical explanations of health and emphasizes the economic, social, and environmental lifestyle factors that determine health outcomes.

The Sixty-fifth World Health Assembly, 2012

The 65th World Health Assembly recognized the disease burden of mental health, cited the lack of investment in mental health prevention and control, and called for mental health action (WHO 2012).

Multinational initiatives

In addition to the above agreements and instruments of the UN, sometimes a group of member states may come together to support and adopt some initiatives. Some examples are listed below.

The Helsinki Accord: Declaration on Human Rights, 1975

The Helsinki Accord emphasized "Respect for human rights and fundamental freedoms – including the freedom of thought, conscience, religion, or belief." This was an agreement signed by 35 states including the defunct USSR, the USA, and 33 European states. The civil rights section is perhaps the most relevant. This has implications for fundamental human rights including the treatment of the mentally ill and dissidents (Conference on Security and Co-operation in Europe 1975)

Paris Declaration and aid effectiveness principles, 2005

This declaration was developed at a forum in March 2005 in Paris organized by the Organisation for Economic Co-operation and Development (OECD). The declaration aimed at the accountability of developed and developing countries for delivering

and managing aid in terms of five principles (OECD 2005):

(1) **ownership** – partner countries exercise effective leadership over their development policies and strategies, and coordinate development actions
(2) **alignment** – donors base their overall support on partner countries' national development strategies, institutions, and procedures
(3) **harmonization** – donor's actions are more harmonized, transparent, and collectively effective
(4) **managing for results** – managing resources and improving decision making for results
(5) **mutual accountability** – donors and partners are accountable for development results

Oslo Ministerial Declaration on Global Health, 2007

In March 2007, foreign ministers from Brazil, France, Indonesia, Senegal, South Africa, and Thailand under their initiative on global health and foreign policy declared:

> In today's era of globalization and interdependence there is an urgent need to broaden the scope of foreign policy. We believe that health as a foreign policy issue needs a stronger strategic focus on the international agenda. We have therefore agreed to make impact on health a point of departure and a defining lens that each of our countries will use to examine key elements of foreign policy and development strategies, and to engage in a dialogue on how to deal with policy options from this perspective.
>
> (Oslo Ministerial Declaration 2007)

That meeting and declaration has been pivotal. First, the ministerial group consisted of the cooperation of foreign ministers, not health ministers. In addition, they came from different parts of the world with different economic statuses and cultures. Thus their action brings diversity to the discussion of global health diplomacy in a new arrangement, in contrast to the previous North–South or South–South configuration.

Brazil, Russia, India, China, and South Africa (BRICS) Beijing Declaration, 2011

The BRICS states consist of Brazil, Russia, India, China, and South Africa. The group first came together as BRIC in 2006, and the first formal annual summit was held in Russia in June 2009. In 2010 South Africa was added to the BRIC club, whence the name BRICS. These countries have expanding economies, and as funding from the USA and Europe shrinks the potential contribution of the BRICS becomes more important. In addition, it is believed that these countries still will have considerable proportions of their respective populations under the poverty line, and the models they develop are likely to have implications for low- and middle-income countries (LMICs). At their health ministerial meeting in 2011 they declared a collaboration on common health challenges as well as support to other countries for the sake of "health for all" (BRICS Health Ministers 2011).

Regional initiatives

In some instances neighboring states may find that they have a common interest in health security.

WHO European Ministerial Conference on Mental Health, Helsinki, 2005

In January 2005 the WHO European Region organized a conference on mental health. Present at this conference were health ministers from 52 countries of the WHO European Region, the European Union, and the Council of Europe. This conference dealt with the epidemic of psychosocial distress and mental health impacts on the well-being of Europeans. The result was a Mental Health Declaration for Europe and an Action Plan. The group committed itself to action in 12 areas to improve the quality of life of all citizens and to reduce stigma and exclusion (WHO 2005c).

Lisbon Treaty, 2007–2009

The Lisbon Treaty was built on two previous treaties, namely the Treaty on European Union (TEU, the Maastricht Treaty) and the Treaty Establishing the European Community (TEC, Treaty of Rome), which has been renamed the Treaty on the Functioning of the European Union (TFEU). The articles of the Lisbon Treaty have to do with cross-border health issues, fundamental human rights in health decisions, promotion of well-being in the citizenry, high standards of health systems, and citizen engagements in health policies (European Commission 2010b). With these core responsibilities in mind, the commission presented its health strategy *Together for Health: a Strategic Approach to the EU 2008–2013*. This incorporates the "health in all policies" framework, highlighting the integrated political nature of public health (European Commission 2007).

Merida Initiative, 2007–2008

The initiative was announced in October 2007 and signed into law in June 2008. This is a treaty signed between USA, Mexico, and the countries of Central America. It pledges to combat drug trafficking, transnational organized crime, and money laundering. Part of the Merida strategy aims to provide alternatives to drug trafficking and consumption by providing development assistance (Seelke & Finklea 2013).

The Association of South East Asian Nations (ASEAN)

This group consists of 10 countries, namely Indonesia, Malaysia, the Phillipines, Singapore, Thailand, Brunei, Myanmar, Cambodia, Laos, and Vietnam. Together the group ranks as the eighth largest economy in the world. In addition to peace, security, and economic growth, another focus of this group is the advancement of global health (Foreign and Commonwealth Office 2013). An example of one of their inititives is the Global Healh Program, which brings together health professionals and diplomats from ASEAN countries.

Bilateral inititiaves

State bilateral collaborations may exist between two countries in the area of global health and diplomacy. In the Cold War era many countries offered medical training scholarships to African countries. Other examples are as follows:

- In the early 1990s, Nigeria sent medical personnel to Gambia, a small country highly limited in medical personnel.
- Cuba has considerable experience in providing aid and medical services to its neighbors in South America as well as in Africa. Between 1999 and 2004, Cuban doctors made 36.7 million visits to low-income communities and taught 900 000 medical education courses to local health professionals.
- There are instances of China attempting to emulate Cuba, but its contribution does not represent the full potential that it has. In addition, there is some discontent, especially amongst Africans, concerning the approaches by China either in terms of their demand for resources or in the failure of the Chinese representatives to acclimatize or adapt to local conditions (Kerry *et al.* 2010).

Non-governmental organizations: foundations, civil societies, users, survivors, and advocacy groups

Foundations such as the Wellcome Trust, the Bill & Melinda Gates Foundation, and Oxfam are some of the major players in global health diplomacy. In fact the name of Bill Gates is sometimes mentioned in the same breath as the UN and the WHO. In other words, the wealth of some foundations has made them very powerful stakeholders. Another important component in the global activities of the NGOs and foundations are the members of various religious groups, university students, and faculty members of universities who engage in global activities. The young ambassadors with their dedication and enthusiasm contribute to these global efforts.

Sometimes there are different permutations and combinations of these actors and stakeholders. Also the above typology can be useful for epistemological and heuristic reasons. In fact, there is the emergence of a new discipline, which attempts to explore the role of multilateral proto-institutions in global health. For example, Gómez and Atun (2013) compared the coalition formation processes of state and non-state actors with two well-established multilateral donors. The first group, called proto-institutions, was represented by the Global Fund to Fight AIDS, Tuberculosis and Malaria and the GAVI Alliance (Global Alliance for Vaccines and Immunisation). The second group consisted of the World Bank and the Asian Development Bank. They found that the former, the proto-institutions groups, were "more adaptive in strengthening their governance processes" (Gómez & Atun 2013).

Predicting future directions in global health and diplomacy

The future of global health and mental health depends at least to some extent on the fate of globalization. Bearing in mind that political and economic serendipities can occur at any time, it is hazardous to predict the future with a great deal of confidence. For example, a single unanticipated event, such as 9/11 or a banking failure, can be disruptive of national or international trajectories. Hence, only a few economists are willing to predict the future of globalization.

Hirst and Thompson (1995) explored the question as to whether nation states will continue as the major loci for governance in an increasingly complex globalized world. They concluded that nation states will continue to mediate between international agencies and subnational entities, and that national economic processes remain pivotal. In other words, the nation states will continue to protect their citizens. Khan and Najam (2009) took a different slant. They identified the key drivers that are likely to affect the future of globalization: (1) information and communications technology (ICT), (2) markets, (3) mobility, and (4) policy orientation. They applied these drivers to the following dominant areas: exclusion and inequality, human insecurity, health, cultural and social, environmental, institutions and governance. They then proceeded to apply a scenario analysis, which according to United Nations Environmental Program (UNEP) is the most suitable method for making future predictions in complex and indeterminate systems such as the planetary systems or social systems. According to UNEP, in such systems there are significant elements of "surprise, ignorance, and volition" (UNEP 2004). Adapting this work, Khan and Najam (2009) arrived at three possible scenarios, "the Global Marketplace, the Managed Planet, and the Fortress World." They then used the dominant characteristics of each scenario to see how the various drivers of globalization will impact the domains enumerated above.

The Global Marketplace is characterized by a supreme free-market economy and political thinking. The Managed Planet is characterized by dominant policy institutions and value systems. The Fortress World represents a break from current policy institutions and value systems. The first two scenarios are continuities from the present. The Fortress World shows a discontinuity. Increasing marginalization and poverty is predicted in this scenario, alongside increased authoritarianism. Khan and Najam (2009) concluded that a combination of the first two scenarios would be the most desirable, and they made some recommendations to humanitarian relief agencies. They suggested that the international relief agencies have to be strategic in choosing the drivers that meet their needs and how best to achieve their goals. They suggested that relief agencies can (1) participate in creating dominant belief systems, (2) become policy actors and entrepreneurs, (3) utilize ICT advances, and (4) influence advances in ICT developments. Of the six impact areas Khan and Najam (2009) recommended great watchfulness in the domain of exclusion and inequality, as its consequences may be very decisive.

Discussion

In a recent presentation in Washington, John Sopko, the US Special Inspector-General for Afghanistan Reconstruction, suggested a template of seven questions that are critical in the planning and evaluative phase in the reconstruction project (Sopko 2013). Although he spoke specifically about Afghanistan, consideration of these questions may apply to other foreign aid projects as well. These questions can be paraphrased as follows:

(1) Does the project or program make a clear and identified contribution to national interests or strategic objectives of donor countries?
(2) Does the recipient country want or need the project?
(3) Has the project been coordinated with other donor implementing agencies, the recipient government, and other international donors?
(4) Are security conditions favorable to effective implementations oversight?
(5) Are there adequate safeguards to detect, deter, and mitigate corruption?
(6) Does the recipient nation have the financial resources, technical capacity, and political will to sustain the program?
(7) Have the various stakeholders established meaningful and measurable metrics for determining success?

In other words, the issues of country ownership, transparency, corruption, sustainability, and measurement of effective outcomes are central to the initial planning and execution of foreign aid projects. A major concern for donors and donor countries is pervasive corruption in recipient countries. There will be an increasing need to deal with this and come up with measurable effectiveness and outcome strategies. This implies greater engagement between donors and recipients during the planning and other stages of the project. The musician activist Bono, in a recent lecture to Georgetown University students, was optimistic about the corruption issue. He expressed the view that the internet and its capability will help to provide

a paper trail for identifying corruption amongst senior politicians and civil servants (Bono 2012).

It is envisaged that the current push to reform the structures and functions of the UN and its agencies, particularly the WHO, will place emphasis on inclusion, transparency, accountability, and greater sensitivity to the needs of the LMICs. We will anticipate more stakeholders wishing for voting and observer statuses. We hope that the policies of the World Bank and the International Monetary Fund (IMF) will positively impact the economies and development of LMICs. The policy of structural adjustments should be more supportive of country ownership.

Related to the above issues are the issues of advocacy and humanitarianism. These two driving factors are likely to increase in our contemporary society. Lancaster (2010) has made reference to how internal politics may affect external foreign aid policies. This differs from nation to nation. In the USA, Lancaster has cited the example of the growing roles of Evangelical churches, even if conservative. These churches are likely to play a bigger role in issues concerning human civil rights, poverty, and climate change worldwide. She also cites the role of the green parties in Europe emphasizing foreign aid policies as they negotiate their coalitions. In the last two decades, many institutions and organizations (intergovernmental and non-governmental) have invested considerable energy and funding in global health (Lancaster 2010).

So global health and its interconnectivity are likely to stay. There is likely to be more discussion on a level playing field as the teams become more diversified. Groups such as BRICS with its emerging markets will play a more important role and answer the call from the USA to contribute more to foreign aid (parenthetically, in spite of popular sentiments the USA contributes less than 1% of its GDP in foreign aid: Eischen 2012). Similarly, it is anticipated that donor and recipient countries will heed a call for host countries to own their problems and reduce foreign-aid dependency.

However, there are influences other than economic and financial factors that contribute to the globalization. These factors are humanitarianism and equity. These influences, especially through religious groups, socially responsible NGOs, and transnational cooperations, are likely to continue their contributions and efforts. The humanitarian factors are likely to persist, as modern communications and technologies bring the impact of natural and man-made disasters into the living rooms of ordinary citizens.

Similarly, as previously discussed, the broadened portfolio of global mental health now involves the mental health effects of poverty, climate change, and food shortages. Events in these areas are likely to continue humanitarian responses from NGOs. Also the issues of equity will continue to be a concern for governments and transnational organizations that have framed health as a component in their social and foreign policy.

In addition, immigration and human mobility with their consequent brain drain may continue to be a significant factor. Individuals in their various diaspora spaces will continue to show interest in the welfare of their homelands. The remittances sent to the homelands can sometimes play a significant role in the revenue and economy of some countries. Another factor that is likely to continue the ideal of globalization is the activity of a constituency of young

ambassadors – university students and volunteers – who have participated in overseas programs and have had a practical experience in global health. The future is theirs.

Summary

In this chapter we have reviewed some definitions of global health and mental health diplomacy. We have traced the evolution and suggested a typology of sponsoring agencies and institutions. We have also reviewed some predictions for the future in global health and global mental health diplomacy. It is to be anticipated that with an expanded portfolio for health, global mental health will have a more important positioning in foreign policies. Also, it is anticipated that for more cost-effective international interventions, increased governance is a sine qua non. Lastly, there is a need for reciprocal relationships and a new partnership to discourage an aid-dependency culture.

References

Aldis W (2008) Health security as a public health concept: a critical analysis. *Health Policy Plan* 23: 369–375

Bono (2012) Webcast: U2's Bono speaks at GU global social enterprise event. Washington, DC: Georgetown University. http://www.georgetown.edu/webcast/bono-social-enterprise.html (accessed July 2013).

BRICS Health Minsters (2011) Beijing Declaration. BRICS Health Ministers' Meeting, Beijing, China.

Centers for Disease Control and Prevention (2012) *CDC Global Health Strategy 2012–2015*. Atlanta, GA: CDC. http://www.cdc.gov/globalhealth/strategy/pdf/CDC-GlobalHealthStrategy.pdf (accessed July 2013).

Conference on Security and Co-operation in Europe (1975) The Final Act of the Conference on Security and Cooperation in Europe, Aug. 1, 1975, 14 I.L.M. 1292 (Helsinki Declaration).

Dahlberg LL, Mercy JA (2009) History of violence as a public health issue. *Virtual Mentor* 11: 167–72.

Eischen F (2012) Foreign aid spending and the US budget [Newsgroup post, August 5, 2012]. Independent Voter Network website: http://ivn.us/2012/08/05/united-states-foreign-aid-and-budget (accessed July 2013).

European Commission (2007) *Together for Health: a Strategic Approach to the EU 2008–2013*. White Paper. Brussels: European Union.

European Commission (2010a). *EU Plan of Action on Gender Equality and Women's Empowerment in Development 2010–2015*. Brussels: EU Commission.

European Commission (2010b) Consolidated versions of the Treaty on European Union and the Treaty on the Functioning of the European Union. [The Treaty of Lisbon.] *Official Journal of the European Union*. 53 (C83).

Fauci AS (2007) The expanding global health agenda: a welcome development. *Nature Medicine* 33: 1169–71.

Federal Department of Foreign Affairs, Federal Department of Home Affairs (2006). *Swiss Health Foreign Policy: Agreement on Health Foreign Policy Objectives*. Bern: Swiss Government.

Fidler DP (2003) Emerging trends in international law concerning global infectious disease control. *Emerging Infectious Diseases* 9: 285–90.

Fidler DP (2005) Health and foreign policy: a conceptual overview. Lecture at a conference on "Health in Foreign Policy Forum," sponsored by Academy Health, February 4, 2005, Washington, DC.

Foreign and Commonwealth Office (2013) *ASEAN Economic Bulletin*, May 2013.

Gómez EJ, Atun R (2013) Emergence of multilateral proto-institutions in global health and new approaches to governance: analysis using path dependency and institutional theory. *Globalization and Health* 9 (18).

Health Diplomats (undated) Health diplomacy. http://www.healthdiplomats.com/index.php?page=31_health_overview (accessed January 10, 2013).

Hirst P, Thompson G (1995) Globalization and the future of the nation state. *Economy and Society* **24**: 408–42.

HM Government (2008) *Health is Global: a UK Government Strategy 2008–2013*. London: Department of Health.

HM Government (2011) *Call to End Violence Against Women and Girls: Action Plan*. London: Cabinet Office.

Jenkins R, Kydd R, Mullen P, *et al.* (2010) International migration of doctors, and its impact on availability of psychiatrists in low and middle income countries. *PLoS ONE* **5** (2): e9049.

Kerry VB, Auld SA, Farmer P (2010) An international service corps for health: an unconventional prescription for diplomacy. *New England Journal of Medicine* **363**: 1199–201.

Khan S, Najam A (2009) *The Future of Globalization and its Humanitarian Impacts*. Humanitarian Futures Programme. http://www.humanitarianfutures.org/wp-content/uploads/2013/06/The-Future-of-Globalisation-and-its-Humanitarian-Impacts.pdf (accessed July 2013).

Krug EG, Dahlberg LL, Mercy JA, Zwi AB, Lozano R, eds. (2002) *World Report on Violence and Health*. Geneva: World Health Organization.

Labonté R (2008) Global health in public policy: finding the right frame? *Critical Public Health* **18**:4, 467–482

Labonté R, Gagnon ML (2010) Framing health and foreign policy: lessons for global health diplomacy. *Globalization and Health* **6** (14): 1–19.

Lancaster C (2010) Redesigning foreign aid. *Foreign Affairs* **79** (5): 74–88.

Lee K, Smith R (2011) "Global health diplomacy"? A conceptual review. *Global Health Governance* **5** (1).

MDG Achievement Fund (undated) MDG Achievement Fund: About us. http://mdgfund.org/aboutus (accessed July 2013).

Norwegian Ministry of Foreign Affairs (2012) *Global Health in Foreign Policy and Development*. Meld. St. 11 (2011–2012). Report to the Storting [White Paper].

OECD (2005) *The Paris Declaration on Aid Effectiveness*. http://www.oecd.org/development/effectiveness/34428351.pdf (accessed July 2013).

Oslo Ministerial Declaration (2007) Oslo Ministerial Declaration – global health: a pressing foreign policy issue of our time. *Lancet* **369**: 1373–8.

Policy Coherence Commission (2008) *Coherent for Development? How Coherent Norwegian Policies Can Assist Development in Poor Countries*. Official Norwegian Reports 2008: 14.

Seelke CR, Finklea KM (2013) *U.S.–Mexican Security Cooperation: the Mérida Initiative and Beyond*. CRS Report for Congress 7-5700 R41349. Washington, DC: Congressional Research Service. http://www.fas.org/sgp/crs/row/R41349.pdf (accessed July 2013).

Sopko J (2013) U.S. reconstruction effort in Afghanistan. Q & A segment presented at Simpson Center, Washington, DC, January 10, 2013. C-SPAN Video Library. http://www.c-spanvideo.org/program/310312-1 (accessed July 2013).

Støre JG (2008) Global health and the foreign policy agenda. Speech given at the State of the Planet Conference, New York, NY, March 27, 2008.

Swedish Ministry of Foreign Affairs (2003) *Shared Responsibility: Sweden's Policy for Global Development*. Stockholm: Government Bill (2002/03) 122.

United Nations (1994) *The Report of the International Conference on Population and Development (A/CONF.171/13/Rev.1)*. Cairo, Egypt.

United Nations Department of Economic and Social Affairs (2009) *Trends in International Migrant Stock: the 2008 Revision*. United Nations Database (POP/DB/MIG/STOCK/REV.2008).

United Nations Environment Program (2004) *Global Environment Outlook Scenario Framework: Background Paper for UNEP's Third Global Environment Outlook Report (GEO-3)*. Nairobi: Division of Early Warning and Assessment (DEWA).

United Nations General Assembly (1991) *The Protection of Persons with Mental Illness and the Improvement of Mental Health Care (A/RES/46/119)*. New York, NY: UN.

United Nations General Assembly (1993) *Declaration on the Elimination of Violence against Women (A/RES/48/104)*. New York, NY: UN.

United Nations General Assembly (1999) *International Day for the Elimination of Violence against Women (A/RES/54/134)*. New York, NY: UN.

United Nations General Assembly (2000) *United Nations Millennium Declaration (A/RES/55/2)*. New York, NY: UN.

United Nations General Assembly (2011) *Political Declaration of the High-level Meeting of the General Assembly on the Prevention and Control of Non-communicable Disease (A/66/L.1)*. New York, NY: UN.

United Nations Secretary-General (2008) UNiTE to end violence against women: about UNiTE. http://www.un.org/en/women/endviolence/about.shtml (accessed July 2013).

United States Congress (2008) *Tom Lantos and Henry J. Hyde United*

States Global Leadership Against HIV/AIDS, Tuberculosis, and Malaria Reauthorization Act of 2008. US Congress Public Law 110(293).

World Health Organization (1978) *Declaration of Alma-Ata.* International Conference on Primary Health Care, Alma-Ata, USSR, 6-12 September 1978.

World Health Organization (1986) *Intersectoral Action for Health: the Role of Intersectoral Cooperation in National Strategies for Health for All.* Geneva: WHO.

World Health Organization (1996) Prevention of violence: a public health priority. 49th World Health Assembly, Geneva (Resolution 49.25). Geneva: WHO.

World Health Organization (1998) *Primary Health Care 21: "Everybody's Business".* An International Meeting to Celebrate 20 years after Alma-Ata: Almaty, Kazakhstan. Geneva: WHO.

World Health Organization (2001) *The World Health Report 2001. Mental Health: New Understanding, New Hope.* Geneva: WHO.

World Health Organization (2005a) *Promoting Mental Health: Concepts, Emerging Evidence, Practice.* A Report of the World Health Organization, Department of Mental Health and Substance Abuse in collaboration with the Victorian Health Promotion Foundation. Geneva: WHO.

World Health Organization (2005b) *Health and the Millennium Development Goals.* Geneva: WHO.

World Health Organization (2005c) *Mental Health: Facing the Challenges, Building Solutions. WHO European Ministerial Conference.* Geneva: WHO.

World Health Organization (2008) *Closing the Gap in a Generation: Health Equity Through Action on the Social Determinants of Health.* Final Report of the Commission on Social Determinants of Health. Geneva: WHO.

World Health Organization (2011a) Prevention and control of NCDs: priorities for investment. First Global Ministerial Conference on Healthy Lifestyles and Noncommunicable Disease Control (Moscow, April 28–29, 2011).

Discussion paper. http://www.who.int/nmh/publications/who_bestbuys_to_prevent_ncds.pdf (accessed July 2013).

World Health Organization (2011b) Rio Political Declaration on Social Determinants of Health, Rio de Janeiro, Brazil, 21 October 2011. World Conference on Social Determinants of Health.

World Health Organization (2012) Resolutions and Decisions Annexes, 65th World Health Assembly (65/2012/REC/1). Geneva: WHO.

World Health Organization (undated) Addressing Needs, Improving Services. WHO Mental Health Policy Project (MHPP). Geneva: WHO.

World Health Organization Regional Office for Europe (2011) Noncommunicable diseases on global health agenda. http://www.euro.who.int/en/what-we-do/health-topics/disease-prevention/sections/news/2011/05/noncommunicable-diseases-on-global-health-agenda (accessed July 2013).

5

Global mental health and the United Nations

Takashi Izutsu and Atsuro Tsutsumi

Introduction

In the area of global mental health, the role played by the United Nations (UN) has not been widely discussed, despite its critical impact. This chapter looks into the basics of the UN, and its work related to mental health and psychological well-being, so that the mental health community can strengthen partnership with the UN as a key stakeholder in global mental health.

The UN is an international organization founded in 1945 committed to maintaining international peace and security, promoting economic, social and cultural development, and responding to humanitarian crises, based on a principle of protecting and promoting the human rights of all people.

In the UN, based on resolutions adopted by Member States in its *principal organs* such as the UN General Assembly, *subsidiary organs*, particularly implementing entities called *funds and programmes*, execute activities through their country offices worldwide. The term *United Nations* usually represents the principal and the subsidiary organs.

In addition to the UN itself, there are a number of UN *specialized agencies*, which are autonomous but have collaborative relationships with the UN. Specialized agencies include the World Health Organization (WHO), the United Nations Educational, Scientific and Cultural Organization (UNESCO), and the World Bank, among others.

The UN, including its principal and subsidiary organs together with the specialized agencies, can be said to make up the "United Nations system."

The United Nations system

Principal organs

The UN principal organs include the UN General Assembly, the Security Council, the Economic and Social Council (ECOSOC), the Trusteeship Council (currently inactive), the International Court of Justice, and the UN Secretariat.

The UN General Assembly is composed of all 193 UN member states, and meets in regular yearly sessions. Each member state has one vote. The General Assembly may discuss any issues within the scope of the mandate of the UN.

The Security Council consists of 15 members of the UN. In addition to five permanent members of the Council (China, France, Russian Federation, United Kingdom, United States), 10 non-permanent members are elected for a term of two years. The Security Council discusses matters related to the maintenance of international peace and security.

ECOSOC consists of 54 members elected by the General Assembly. Each member state is elected for a term of three years. ECOSOC makes and initiates studies and reports with respect to international economic, social, cultural, educational, health, and related matters, and may make recommendations to the General Assembly, the members of the UN, and the specialized agencies concerned.

Lastly, the UN Secretariat is composed of the Secretary-General, assisted by international civil servants. It services other principal organs of the UN and administers the programs and policies as laid down by them.

Essentials of Global Mental Health, ed. Samuel O. Okpaku. Published by Cambridge University Press. © Cambridge University Press 2014.

Subsidiary organs

The UN General Assembly and the Security Council can establish subsidiary organs as they deem necessary for the performance of their functions.

Among them, funds and programs such as the United Nations Development Programme (UNDP), the United Nations Population Fund (UNFPA), the United Nations Children's Fund (Unicef), and others play key roles as implementing entities of the decisions (such as resolutions) made by the UN principal organs. Guided by each organization's strategic plan, these funds and programs implement capacity building of governments, in-country policy and program development, and implementation support, for more than 150 countries through their country offices.

Specialized agencies

When funds and programs of the UN implement their programs, technical guidance is provided by the specialized agencies. The role of the specialized agencies is mainly to provide state-of-the-art technical guidance and tools which have been developed in collaboration with external experts such as academia and non-governmental organizations (NGOs). Global implementation often needs to be executed by funds and programs or other stakeholders, since specialized agencies tend to have limited human and financial resources on the ground.

UN country teams

In each program country, the UN system forms a UN Country Team (UNCT). Each UNCT coordinates among all the UN entities in the country in order to promote efficiency and prevent duplication.

Each UNCT develops a United Nations Development Assistance Framework (UNDAF), which is a joint mid-term plan developed with its host government. All the UN entities participate in this process together by implementing joint assessment, discussing priorities and goals, and developing plans of activities and budget. For a mental health program to be realized, it is important that it is integrated into the UNDAF.

Global mental health and the United Nations

Definition of health and the right to health made by the United Nations

Mental health has been an important and major component of health and the right to health as defined by the UN from its early days.

First, "health" is defined in the Preamble to the Constitution of the WHO as "a state of complete physical, *mental* and social *well-being* and not merely the absence of disease or infirmity" (World Health Organization 1946; emphasis added).

The "right to health" referred to in the International Covenant on Economic, Social and Cultural Rights (ICESCR) is "the right of everyone to the enjoyment of the highest attainable standard of physical and mental health" (United Nations 1966, Article 12). The ICESCR is part of the International Bill of Human Rights and constitutes one of the most fundamental principles of the UN's activities.

Thus, when the term "health" is used in the UN context, it always includes mental health.

Key UN human rights conventions and mental health

Conventions are legally binding tools for the member states that have ratified them. After ratification, "states parties" are required to change their laws and policies in compliance with the conventions.

Convention on the Rights of Persons with Disabilities (CRPD) (United Nations 2006)

In 2006, the UN General Assembly adopted the Convention on the Rights of Persons with Disabilities (CRPD) by consensus. Article 1 states that "Persons with disabilities include those who have long-term physical, *mental*, intellectual, or sensory impairments which in interaction with various barriers may hinder their full and effective participation in society on an equal basis with others."

Article 17 recognizes that every person with disabilities has a right to respect for his or her *mental integrity* on an equal basis with others. CRPD also states that states parties need to take measures to enable persons with disabilities to attain and maintain maximum *mental ability*. To that end, states parties need to organize, strengthen, and extend comprehensive habilitation and rehabilitation services and programs (Article 26.1). In relation to education, it specifies that states parties shall ensure an inclusive education system and lifelong learning directed to the development of persons with disabilities' *mental ability* to their fullest potential (24.1).

Article 16.4 states that states parties need to promote cognitive and *psychological recovery*, rehabilitation and social integration of persons with disabilities who become victims of exploitation, violence, and abuse.

Convention on the Rights of the Child (CRC) (United Nations 1989)

The Convention on the Rights of the Child (CRC) recognizes the rights of children with regard to mental health. The convention states that every child must have a standard of living adequate for the child's physical, *mental*, spiritual, moral, and social *development* (Article 27.1). It also mentions that children need to be directed to ensure the development of the child's *mental* and physical *abilities* to their fullest potential (29.1). In addition, the convention recognizes the importance of the mass media and that the child has access to information and material which aims to promote his or her physical and *mental health* (17).

CRC states that children need to be protected from economic exploitation and from any work that is harmful to the child's health or *mental development* (32.1). The convention also calls for all appropriate measures to protect the child from all forms of physical or *mental violence* (19) and the illicit use of narcotic drugs and *psychotropic* substances (33). Article 39 says that all appropriate measures must be taken to promote the *psychological recovery* of child victims of any form of neglect, exploitation, abuse, or torture among other cruel, inhuman, or degrading treatments or punishments, including armed conflicts.

In Article 23.1 and 23.4, the rights of children *with mental or physical disabilities* are recognized, and promotion of the international exchange of appropriate information in the field of preventive health care and of medical, *psychological*, and functional *treatment* of children with disabilities is encouraged. Also, states parties shall recognize the right to periodic review of treatment provided to children who are placed in institutions because of their physical or *mental health* (25).

CRC has two optional protocols. The Optional Protocol to the CRC on the Involvement of Children in Armed Conflict (OP-CRC-AC) (United Nations 2000) reiterates the needs of *psychosocial rehabilitation* of children who are victims of armed conflict (Preamble), and assistance for their *psychological recovery* (6.3). The Optional Protocol to the Convention on the Rights of the Child on the Sale of Children, Child Prostitution and Child Pornography (OP-CRC-SC) (United Nations 2000) reiterates the right of the child to be protected from economic exploitation and from performing any work that is likely to be harmful to the child's *mental development*. Article 8.4 outlines measures to ensure appropriate *psychological training* for the persons who work with victims of the offences mentioned in this optional protocol. For the victims of such offences, the optional protocol calls for all feasible measures with the aim of ensuring all appropriate assistance including their full *psychological recovery* (9.3). Article 10.2 states that states parties shall promote international cooperation to assist child victims in their *psychological recovery*.

Convention against Torture and Other Cruel, Inhuman or Degrading Treatment or Punishment (CAT) (United Nations 1984)

This convention is also relevant to the mental health. Article 1 defines torture as "any act by which severe pain or suffering, whether physical or *mental*, is intentionally inflicted on a person for such purposes as obtaining from him or a third person information or a confession, punishing him for an act he or a third person has committed or is suspected of having committed, or intimidating or coercing him or a third person, or for any reason based on discrimination of any kind, when such pain or suffering is inflicted by or at the instigation of or with the consent or acquiescence of a public official or other person acting in an official capacity."

Major UN global conferences: outcome documents

World Conference on Disaster Reduction (Hyogo): Hyogo Declaration and Hyogo Framework for Action 2005–2015: Building the Resilience of Nations and Communities to Disasters (United Nations 2005)

Enhancing recovery schemes including *psychosocial training programs* in order to mitigate the *psychological damage* of vulnerable populations, particularly children, in the aftermath of disasters is included as part of the priority for action (Para. 19).

World Summit on Sustainable Development (Johannesburg): Plan of Implementation of the World Summit on Sustainable Development (United Nations 2002)

The plan of implementation includes developing or strengthening, where applicable, preventive, promotive, and curative programs to address noncommunicable diseases and conditions which include *mental health disorders* and associated risk factors, including alcohol and tobacco (Article 54 (o)).

United Nations Conference on Human Settlement (HABITAT II) (Istanbul): the Habitat Agenda (United Nations 1996)

Para. 36 of Goals and Principles states that human health and quality of life are at the center of the effort to develop sustainable human settlements, and the goals of universal and equal access to the highest attainable standard of physical and *mental health* need to be promoted and attained.

Its Global Plan of Action: Strategies for Implementation includes provision of special living facilities and shelter solutions for persons with *mental disabilities* (Para. 97), and promotion of crime prevention by addressing lack of *mental health services* (123).

The Fourth World Conference on Women: Platform for Action (Beijing) (United Nations 1995)

The Platform for Action (PFA) reaffirms that women have the right to enjoy the highest attainable standard of physical and *mental health*. In addition, it states that women's health involves their *emotional*, social and physical *well-being* (Para. 89). It clearly states that "*mental disorders* related to marginalization, powerlessness and poverty, along with overwork and stress and the growing incidence of domestic violence as well as *substance abuse*, are among other health issues of growing concern to women" (100).

It pays special attention to sexual and gender-based violence, including physical and *psychological abuse*, trafficking in women and girls, sexual exploitation, and states that women are at high risk of physical and *mental trauma* due to these types of abuse (99). In its description of violence against women, the document specifically includes *psychological abuse* (112).

In Para. 113, the term "violence against women" is defined as any act of gender-based violence that results in, or is likely to result in, physical, sexual, or *psychological harm* or suffering to women, which encompasses but is not limited to physical, sexual, and *psychological violence* occurring in the family and the community. PFA stresses that adolescent girls are both biologically and *psychosocially* more vulnerable than boys to sexual abuse, violence, and prostitution, and to the consequences of unprotected and premature sexual relations (93). It states that governments and other stakeholders need to provide well-funded shelters and relief support for girls and women subjected to violence, including *psychological and other counseling services*. It also states that governments of countries of origin, transit, and destination, as well as regional and international organizations, need to allocate resources to provide comprehensive programs designed to heal and rehabilitate into society the victims of trafficking, including *psychological care* (130).

As to women and armed conflict, Para. 135 recognizes the *psychologically traumatic consequences* of armed conflict, foreign occupation, and alien domination. With regard to the systematic practice of rape and other forms of inhuman and degrading treatment of women as a deliberate instrument of war and ethnic cleansing, PFA urges that steps are taken to ensure that full assistance is provided to the victims of such abuse for their physical and *mental rehabilitation* (145). To promote a culture of peace, Para. 146 states that governments, international and regional institutions, and NGOS shall develop and disseminate research on the physical, *psychological*, and other *effects* of armed conflicts on women (146).

Concerning the girl child, PFA mentions that they have less access to *mental health care* (39), and the existing discrimination in their access to *mental health services* endangers their health (266). Therefore, it states that all barriers must be eliminated to enable girls to develop their full potential and skills through equal access to physical and *mental health care and related information* (272). In particular, there is a call for governments to protect the girl child from economic exploitation and from performing any work that is harmful to the child's health or *mental development* (282.a). In addition, it calls for action by governments and partners to "take appropriate legislative, administrative, social and educational measures to protect the girl child, in the household and in society, from all forms of physical or *mental violence*, injury or abuse, neglect or negligent treatment" (283.b) and develop age-appropriate safe and confidential *psychological support services* to assist girls who are subjected to violence (283.d).

PFA states a need to develop information, programs, and services, to assist women in understanding and adapting to changes associated with aging, paying particular attention to those who are physically or *psychologically dependent* (106.n).

With recognizing the lack of necessary *psychological support* in current health systems (91), PFA calls for action by governments and relevant stakeholders to "reaffirm the right to the enjoyment of the highest attainable standards of physical and *mental health*," and "incorporate it in national legislation" (106.b.) and "integrate *mental health services* into primary healthcare systems or other appropriate levels, develop supportive programs and train primary health workers to recognize and care for girls and women of all ages who have experienced any form of violence" (106.q.). PFA reiterates the definition of reproductive health set by the International Conference on Population and Development to include *mental well-being* (94). Furthermore, governments are urged to take steps to ensure that full assistance is provided to the victims of systematic rape and other forms of inhuman and degrading treatment of women as a deliberate instrument of war and ethnic cleansing for their physical and *mental rehabilitation* (144.c). It also calls for action by governments and relevant stakeholders to place special focus on programs to educate women and men, especially parents, on the importance of girls' physical and *mental health and well-being* (277.d) and to strengthen and reorientate health education and health services, particularly primary healthcare programs that meet the physical and *mental needs* of girls and women (281.c).

PFA also calls for action by governments, the UN system, health professions, research institutions, NGOs, donors, pharmaceutical industries, and the mass media as appropriate, to conduct research to understand and better address the determinants and consequences of unsafe abortion, including its effects on health conditions including *mental health* (109.i).

International Conference on Population and Development (Cairo): Programme of Action (United Nations 1994a)

The International Conference on Population Development (ICPD) Programme of Action (PoA) reiterates in its principles that "everyone has the right to the enjoyment of the highest attainable standard of physical and *mental health*. States should take all appropriate measures to ensure, on a basis of gender equality, universal access to healthcare services, including those related to reproductive health care, which includes family planning and sexual health" (Principle 8). Principle 11 stresses children's rights in this regard, and states that it is the responsibility of all states to protect by appropriate legislative, administrative, social, and educational measures from all forms of physical or *mental violence*.

The ICPD PoA defines reproductive health as a state of complete physical, *mental* and social *well-being* and not merely the absence of disease or infirmity, in all matters relating to the reproductive system and to its functions and processes (7.2).

The ICPD PoA calls for actions by countries regarding *mental rehabilitation* for victims of the systematic practice of rape and other forms of inhuman and degrading treatment of women as a deliberate instrument of war and ethnic cleansing (4.10), enforcement of laws against *mental abuse* of children (6.10), providing parents with information and education about childcare, including the use of *mental stimulation* (8.17), *emotional support* for breastfeeding mothers (8.18), devising special programs to provide emotional support to people affected by AIDS, including their families (8.34), and research on the determinants and consequences of induced abortion, including its effects on subsequent *mental health* (12.17).

World Conference on Human Rights (Vienna): Vienna Declaration and Programme of Action (United Nations 1993)

The World Conference on Human Rights recognizes the importance of the enjoyment of the highest standard of physical and *mental health* by women throughout their lifespan (Para. 41).

The Vienna Declaration and Programme of Action stresses the importance of further concrete action in providing assistance to victims of torture and to ensure more effective remedies for their *psychological rehabilitation*, and it states that providing the necessary resources for this purpose should be given high priority (59).

World Summit for Children (New York): Plan of Action for Implementing the World Declaration on the Survival, Protection and Development of Children in the 1990s (United Nations 1990)

As part of the specific actions for child survival, protection, and development, the outcome document calls for concerted action by governments and inter-governmental agencies to combat illicit production, supply, demand, trafficking, and distribution of narcotic drugs and *psychotropic substances*, and tobacco and *alcohol abuse*.

UN General Assembly resolutions related to mental health

More than 100 UN General Assembly resolutions mention mental health or psychological well-being. A compendium of these resolutions will be published by the United Nations University (UNU) International Institute for Global Health (IIGH) in collaboration with the UN Secretariat and other partners in the near future. Among them are two key mental disability-related resolutions.

Declaration on the Rights of Mentally Retarded Persons (A/RES/2856(XXVI)) (United Nations 1971)

The declaration was adopted by the General Assembly on December 20, 1971, and represented a significant step in terms of raising awareness of the human rights of persons with intellectual disabilities.

The declaration states the right of persons with intellectual disabilities to: (1) proper medical care, physical therapy, education, training, rehabilitation, and guidance to develop their ability and maximum potential; (2) economic security and decent standards of living, to perform productive work and engage in any meaningful occupation; (3) live with their own families or foster care, and to participate in community life; (4) a qualified guardian when required to protect their personal well-being and interest; and (5) protection from exploitation, abuse, degrading treatment, with due process of law.

Over time, some of its expressions and concepts became outdated – notably, the charity models of disability, which serve to reinforce paternalistic attitudes to the lives of persons with disabilities. It is also outdated in its qualifying the scope of rights of persons with intellectual disabilities both in providing that "the mentally retarded person has, to the maximum degree of feasibility, the same rights as other human beings" and in terms of its goal for societies, which is to promote "their integration as far as possible in normal life." These provisions were problematic because they appeared to suggest that the rights to which persons with intellectual disabilities were entitled were somehow more restricted than those of other groups of people. The former Special Rapporteur on Disability, Mr. Bengt Lindqvist, noted that in so far as "its inappropriate terminology shows, the Declaration is in many ways outdated. It reflects an approach to disability commonly referred to as the 'medical model,' in which persons with disabilities are primarily seen as individuals with medical problems, dependent on social security and welfare and in need of separate services and institutions" (United Nations 2003).

Principles for the Protection of Persons with Mental Illness and the Improvement of Mental Health Care (A/RES/46/119) (United Nations 1991)

After years of deliberations on the rights of persons admitted to or detained in mental health institutions, the General Assembly adopted the Principles in December of 1991.

The 25 principles address: the fundamental freedoms and basic rights; protection of minors; life in the community; determination of mental illness; medical examination; confidentiality; role of community and culture; standards of care; treatment; medication; consent to treatment; notice of rights; rights and conditions in mental health facilities; resources for mental health facilities; admission principles; involuntary admission; review body, procedural safeguards; access to information; criminal offenders; complaints; monitoring and remedies; implementation; scope of principles relating to mental health facilities; and saving of existing rights.

Over time, some of the terminologies and concepts in this tool are also outdated, since the Principles employed the "medical model" and limited the rights of persons with mental disabilities.

International Days

The General Assembly declared April 2 as World Autism Awareness Day (A/RES/62/139), March 21 as World Down Syndrome Day (A/RES/66/149),

June 26 as the International Day against Drug Abuse and Illicit Trafficking (A/RES/42/112). In addition, December 3 is declared as the International Day of Persons with Disabilities (A/RES/47/3).

The UN also commemorates Mental Health Day (October 10) and World Suicide Prevention Day (September 10).

UN humanitarian response and mental health

One of the areas where mental health is most integrated into the UN activities is in its humanitarian response. Based on WHO's leadership, the following key guidelines have been published.

IASC Guidelines for Mental Health and Psychosocial Support in Emergency Settings (Inter-Agency Standing Committee 2006)

In 2006, the Inter-Agency Standing Committee (IASC) published the *IASC Guidelines for Mental Health and Psychosocial Support in Emergency Settings* (MHPSS) as an outcome of collaboration among the broad range of the UN and non-UN humanitarian organizations: the UN Secretariat, Unicef, the Office of the UN High Commissioner for Refugees (UNHCR), UNFPA, World Food Programme (WFP), WHO, International Organization for Migration (IOM), Action Contre la Faim (AFC), Inter Action, Inter-Agency Network for Education in Emergencies (INEE), International Council of Voluntary Agencies (ICVA), and International Federation of Red Cross and Red Crescent Societies (IFRC), among others.

The purpose of the guidelines is to enable humanitarian actors and communities to plan, establish, and coordinate a set of minimum multisectoral responses to protect and improve people's mental health and psychosocial well-being in the midst of an emergency, with special attention paid to the do-no-harm principle.

The guidelines have been used in a variety of emergency settings as the gold standard by global, national, and community stakeholders. Whenever a severe emergency occurs, the IASC Reference Group coordinates their activities across UN entities and NGOs through teleconference and field coordination. These have been instrumental in making mental health and psychosocial aspects integral to relevant policies and activities within different sectors. The IASC MHPSS activities by different stakeholders are described concisely in a special issue of the journal *Intervention* (2008).

The IASC Reference Group on MHPSS has also published *IASC Guidelines on Mental Health and Psychosocial Support in Emergency Settings: Checklist for Field Use* (2008).

WHO Psychological First Aid: Guide for Field Workers (WHO 2011)

The WHO, the War Trauma Foundation, and World Vision International in collaboration with the UN Secretariat, UNHCR, Unicef, OHCHR, and others published *Psychological First Aid: Guide for Field Workers* in 2011. This guide was developed in order to have widely agreed-upon psychological first aid materials available to enable humane, supportive, and practical help among fellow human beings suffering serious crisis events.

Others

In addition to these tools, an increased number of guidelines have started to integrate mental health and psychological well-being as a key priority humanitarian response. These include:

- UNFPA, Save the Children USA (2009). *Adolescent Sexual and Reproductive Health Toolkit for Humanitarian Settings: a Companion to the Inter-Agency Field Manual on Reproductive Health in Humanitarian Settings.*
- IOM, London School for Hygiene and Tropical Medicine, United Nations Global Initiative to Fight Trafficking in Persons (UN.GIFT) (2009). *Caring for Trafficked Persons: Guidance for Health Providers.*

UN development efforts and mental health

Integration of mental health and psychological well-being into UN development efforts had been limited. For example, the UN Millennium Development Goals (MDGs) do not mention mental health or psychological well-being at all. However, collaboration between UNFPA and WHO led to some remarkable achievements in this area. Recently, the UN Department of Economic and Social Affairs (DESA) and the UNU together with WHO started to play key roles in integrating mental health as a mainstream element of development.

UNFPA Strategic Plan 2008–2013 (UNFPA 2007)

As one of the first initiatives to mainstream mental health and psychological aspects into organizational priorities among the funds and programs, UNFPA has integrated mental health and psychological well-being into its mandate of universal access to reproductive health, particularly as it relates to the achievement of MDG 5 on promoting maternal health in its strategic plan, which is the most important organizational medium-term policy. In addition, UNFPA held expert meetings on mental health and reproductive health with WHO and issued publications including Executive Director's statements on integrating mental health into sexual and reproductive, maternal, newborn, and child health.

UNFPA–WHO Maternal Mental Health and Child Survival, Health and Development in Resource-Constrained Settings: Essential for Achieving the Millennium Development Goals (Hanoi Expert Statement) (UNFPA, WHO 2007)

In June 2007 UNFPA, WHO, the Key Center for Women's Health in Society, and the Research and Training Center for Community Development, Vietnam, convened the International Expert Meeting on Maternal Mental Health and Child Health and Development in Resource-Constrained Settings. It aimed to appraise the evidence on the nature, prevalence, and risks for common perinatal mental disorders in women, the consequences of these for child health, and development and ameliorative strategies in these contexts.

The meeting outcome is the Hanoi Expert Statement. It argues that the MDGs to improve maternal health, reduce child mortality, promote gender equality and empower women, achieve universal primary education and eradicate extreme poverty and hunger cannot be attained without a specific focus on women's mental health. It was co-signed by the international expert group, UNFPA, and WHO.

United Nations–WHO Policy Analysis: Mental Health and Development: Integrating Mental Health into All Development Efforts including MDGs (UN, WHO 2010)

In September 2010, UN DESA and WHO held a panel discussion, An Emerging Development Issue: Integrating Mental Health into Efforts to Realize MDGs and Beyond. Panelists included the Assistant Secretary-General, DESA, UN; the Assistant Director-General in Non-Communicable Disease and Mental Health, WHO; the Director of the Technical Division, UNFPA; the Deputy Permanent Representative of Finland to the UN; and civil society organizations including self-advocates for persons with mental disabilities.

The policy analysis states that "mental health represents a critical indicator of human development, serves as a key determinant of well-being, quality of life, and hope, has an impact on a range of development outcomes, and is a basis for social stability." It also points out that "poor mental health is both a cause and a consequence of poverty, compromised education, gender inequality, ill-health, violence and other global challenges. It impedes the individual's capacity to work productively, realize their potential and make a contribution to their community. On the other hand, positive mental health is linked to a range of development outcomes, including enhanced productivity and earnings, better employment, higher educational achievement, improved human rights protection and promotion, better health status and improved quality of life."

Others

Currently, Unicef, WHO, and other partners including the UN Secretariat are preparing an outcome document on mental health and young people out of the Round Table on Bridging the Mental Health Gap: Reaching the World's Adolescents, which was organized by Unicef, WHO, and the Center for Global Health, George Washington University, in Washington DC in April 2011.

Further, UNU-IIGH in collaboration with the UN Secretariat, WHO, UNAIDS, and other partners is developing an outcome document on HIV and mental health based on the International Seminar on Socio-economic and Mental Health Burden of HIV/AIDS in Developing Countries, held in Kuala Lumpur in November 2011.

Peace and security and mental health

Mental health and psychological well-being aspects of peace and security is an emerging area.

Among the UN Security Council resolutions, mental health and psychological well-being are drawing attention as part of mandates of international/special tribunals related to peace and security

(S/RES/955 on establishment of International Tribunal for Rwanda and adoption of the Statute of the Tribunal, and S/RES/1757 on the establishment of a Special Tribunal for Lebanon) (United Nations 1994b, 2007).

In addition, psychosocial aspects of sexual violence are discussed (S/RES/1888 and S/RES/1960 on sexual violence against women and children in situations of armed conflict) (United Nations 2009, 2010).

The UNESCO Constitution (1945) states that "since wars begin in the minds of men, it is in the minds of men that the defenses of peace must be constructed." In this context, it is more and more important to integrate mental health and psychological perspectives into the discussion, policy, programs, and activities related to peace and security.

The way forward

Mental health and psychological aspects have been defined as a key aspect of various areas of UN work. Many of them are listed as action points in the conventions and key UN resolutions. This means that the UN and the international community have an obligation to integrate mental health and psychlogical aspects into their activities, and to realize mental health and psychological well-being on the ground.

In order to accomplish this, it is very important to understand the implications of these UN tools, and to utilize them strategically. In addition, analysis of these tools and efforts to fill gaps are also an urgent priority. One of the limitations the global mental health communities have suffered from is the lack of attention paid to the UN tools, including the resolutions. The efforts to develop a compendium of key UN documents related to mental health and psychological well-being by the UNU and the UN will give a useful foundation for this work.

It is also very important to understand the division of labour, the different mandates, and the comparative advantages of each actor in the UN system. In particular, among the most prominent priorities is linking WHO's technical expertise with funds and programs for implementation. This would address the current gap between theory and practice, evident in the lack of implementation of existing tools. In addition, linking WHO's expertise with the normative functions of the UN principal organs is critical for the development of global frameworks and other

tools. For example, WHO (2010) published the *mhGAP Intervention Guide for Mental, Neurological and Substance Use Disorders in Non-Specialized Health Settings* (mhGAP-IG). Finally, the international community has a key "solution package" for mental health problems. Currently, the post-MDG framework and other important mechanisms are under discussion at the UN. Now is the time to integrate mental health and psychological well-being as a key determinant and consequence, indicator and priority, into global priorities.

In order to systematize these tasks, developing the Secretary-General Report system and some General Assembly Resolutions on mental health and psychological well-being could be very useful. In addition, an interagency mechanism on mental health and psychosocial well-being should be established to support integration of mental health into existing and emerging priorities of the UN policies and programs.

As the international communities are shifting to "human" development and a human rights-based approach vis-à-vis economic or materialistic development, human emotional aspects of peace and security, humanitarian response, development, and human rights protection and promotion are receiving increased attention. This is natural, since humans are emotional beings, and our emotions determine our thoughts and behaviors. Additionally, there are relevant and encouraging new developments such as the adoption of the Convention on the Rights of Persons with Disabilities (United Nations 2006) and the new General Assembly Resolution on Happiness (United Nations 2012).

As the international community evolves, it might also be useful to start discussing a possible new terminology which strategically and comprehensively represents human mental, psychological, and emotional well-being.

It is impossible to attain peace and security, humanitarian response, development, or human rights protection and promotion, without the mental health and psychological perspective, given that human beings are the target. At the same time, global mental health cannot be achieved without linking the UN-related international priorities. Further integration of mental health and psychological well-being into the UN policies and programs is critical in order to realize mental and psychological well-being for all.

References

Inter-Agency Standing Committee (2006) *IASC Guidelines on Mental Health and Psychosocial Support in Emergency Settings*. Geneva: IASC.

Inter-Agency Standing Committee (2008) *Mental Health and Psychosocial Support: Checklist for Field Use*. Geneva: IASC.

Intervention (2008) Special issue: the IASC Guidelines on Mental Health and Psychosocial Support in Emergency Settings. *Intervention* 6 (3/4): 193–360.

IOM, London School for Hygiene and Tropical Medicine, United Nations Global Initiative to Fight Trafficking in Persons (UN.GIFT) (2009) *Caring for Trafficked Persons: Guidance for Health Providers*. Geneva: International Organization for Migration.

UNESCO (1945) *Constitution of the United Nations Educational, Scientific and Cultural Organization*. London: United Nations.

UNFPA (2007) *UNFPA Strategic Plan 2008–2011: Accelerating Progress and National Ownership of the ICPD Programme of Action*. New York, NY: UNFPA.

UNFPA, Save the Children USA (2009) *Adolescent Sexual and Reproductive Health Toolkit for Humanitarian Settings: A Companion to the Inter-Agency Field Manual on Reproductive Health in Humanitarian Settings*. New York, NY: UNFPA.

UNFPA, World Health Organization (2007) *UNFPA-WHO Maternal Mental Health and Child Survival, Health and Development in Resource-Constrained Settings: Essential for Achieving the Millennium Development Goals*. Geneva: WHO.

United Nations (1966) *International Covenant on Economic, Social and Cultural Rights, International Covenant on Civil and Political Rights and Optional Protocol to the International Covenant on Civil and Political Rights (A/RES/21/2200 (XXI))*. New York, NY: UN.

United Nations (1971) *Declaration on the Rights of Mentally Retarded Persons (A/RES/2856(XXVI))*. New York, NY: UN.

United Nations (1984) *Convention against Torture and Other Cruel, Inhuman or Degrading Treatment or Punishment (A/RES/39/46)*. New York, NY: UN.

United Nations (1989) *Convention on the Rights of the Child (A/RES/44/25)*. New York, NY: UN.

United Nations (1990) *Plan of Action for Implementing the World Declaration on the Survival, Protection and Development of Children in the 1990s*. New York, NY: UN.

United Nations (1991) *The Protection of Persons with Mental Illness and the Improvement of Mental Health Care (A/RES/46/119)*. New York, NY: UN.

United Nations (1993) *Vienna Declaration and Programme of Action (A/CONF.157/23)*. New York, NY: UN.

United Nations (1994a) *Report of the International Conference on Population and Development (A/CONF.171/13)*. New York, NY: UN.

Untied Nations (1994b) *Resolution 955 Adopted by the Security Council: Establishment of International Tribunal for Rwanda and adoption of the Statute of the Tribunal*. New York, NY: UN.

United Nations (1995) *Report of the Fourth World Conference on Women (A/CONF.177/20)*. New York, NY: UN.

United Nations (1996) *Report of the United Nations Conference on Human Settlements (HABITAT II) (A/CONF.165/14)*. New York, NY: UN.

United Nations (2000) *Optional Protocols to the Convention on the Rights of the Child on the Involvement of Children in Armed Conflict and on the Sale of Children, Child Prostitution and Child Pornography*. New York, NY: UN.

United Nations (2002) *Report of the World Summit on Sustainable Development (A/CONF.199/20)*. New York, NY: UN.

United Nations (2003) *Progress of efforts to ensure the full recognition and enjoyment of the human rights of persons with disabilities: Report of the Secretary-General (A/58/181)*. New York, NY: UN.

United Nations (2005) *Report of the World Conference on Disaster Reduction (A/CONF.206/6)*. New York, NY: UN.

United Nations (2006) *Convention on the Rights of Persons with Disabilities (A/RES/61/106)*. New York, NY: UN.

United Nations (2007) *Resolution 1757 Adopted by the Security Council: Establishment of a Special Tribunal for Lebanon*. New York, NY: UN.

United Nations (2009) *Resolution 1888 Adopted by the Security Council: Sexual Violence against Women and Children in Situations of Armed Conflict*. New York, NY: UN.

United Nations (2010) *Resolution 1960 Adopted by the Security Council: Sexual Violence against Women and Children in Situations of Armed Conflict*. New York, NY: UN.

United Nations (2012) *Happiness: Towards a Holistic Approach to Development (A/RES/65/309)*. New York, NY: UN.

United Nations, World Health Organization (2010) *United Nations (DESA)-WHO Policy Analysis: Mental Health and Development: Integrating Mental Health into All Development Efforts including MDGs*. New York, NY: UN.

World Health Organization (1946) *Constitution of the World Health Organization*. New York, NY: International Health Conference.

World Health Organization (2010) *mhGAP Intervention Guide for Mental, Neurological and Substance Use Disorders in Non-Specialized Health Settings*. Geneva: WHO.

World Health Organization (2011) *Psychological First Aid: Guide for Field Workers*. Geneva: WHO.

Chapter

6

The voice of the user/survivor

Moosa Salie

Introduction

The life experiences of the "mentally ill" have always been difficult. Throughout history, in every society, it has been the practice that "the mad" were denied the right to fully experience life like everyone else, because of the fears, ignorance, intolerance, and lack of patience and understanding of mainstream society. When organized psychiatry arose during the last few hundred years, treatments for the "mentally ill" still continued to go hand in hand with violations of the human rights of those regarded as afflicted with "mental illness."

The user/survivor movement emerged in the early 1970s and became formalized in 2001 when it was launched at its founding conference in Vancouver, Canada. The participants at that conference adopted the statement drafted by Paolo del Vecchio, one of the co-chairs of the organisation known as the World Federation of Psychiatric Users, in 1994. In it the urgent need for the self-organising of "mental patients," who later referred to themselves as "users and survivors of psychiatry," was emphasized. The original statement of del Vecchio from 1994 was amended and reaffirmed in 2001 by the participants at the launch of the World Network of Users and Survivors of Psychiatry (WNUSP) in Vancouver:

> We have taken it upon ourselves to become vocal and active participants in changing how we are treated in order to better meet our needs and to strive towards dignity and independence.
>
> (WNUSP 2001a)

The desire to become active agents with respect to our own lives and treatment decisions was thus the starting point of organizing the "mentally ill."

This set us on the path to becoming active holders of rights rather than passive recipients of care. It was a recognition of the emerging voice of users/survivors and an awareness that "we are not useless" and that "we have a value." This was at the same time an expression of the need to have our human dignity and independence respected, especially at times of crisis, when we very often found that the psychiatric help we received in fact resulted in our retraumatization or, as it was stated in the vision statement of the Icarus Project, a network of people living with and/or affected by experiences that are often diagnosed and labeled as psychiatric conditions:

> Together, we seek new space and freedom for extreme states of consciousness. We support alternatives to the medical model and acknowledge the traumatic legacy of psychiatric abuse. We recognize that we all live in a crazy world, and believe that sensitivities, visions, and inspirations are not necessarily symptoms of illness . . . We call for more options in understanding and treating emotional distress.
>
> (Icarus Project undated)

The desire to be regarded as fully human, especially in times of crisis and amidst the pain and suffering caused by our condition, emerged in many places simultaneously, and the purpose of this chapter is to look at how these voices, calling out for respect for our dignity and independence, became more and more organized, and how they consistently articulated the same message, which became more and more framed within human rights law and eventually enabled us to give our inputs into the groundbreaking first human rights treaty of the twenty-first century, the Convention on the Rights of Persons with Disabilities (CRPD) (United Nations 2006).

Essentials of Global Mental Health, ed. Samuel O. Okpaku. Published by Cambridge University Press. © Cambridge University Press 2014.

An overview of self-organizing of users/survivors of psychiatry

This voice of the "mentally ill" was first organized as the World Federation of Psychiatric Users (WFPU) in the early 1990s, to reflect the change from being regarded as objects of psychiatric treatment to being endowed with the right to make key decisions involving our treatment and thus becoming partners in the process of our recovery journeys.

In this chapter I will draw upon significant milestones in this discourse from within the user/survivor movement, starting with the paper written in 1999 by Mary O'Hagan, the founder and one of the first co-chairs of the WFPU, called "A call to open the door" (O'Hagan 1999), which was a plain-language parable on human rights for people with "psychiatric disabilities." The WFPU in 1997 became the World Network of Users and Survivors of Psychiatry (WNUSP). This name change reflected the experience of some of our peers who sought help from psychiatry but received involuntary treatment and found that experience to be extremely traumatic to the point of even endangering their lives in many cases. It is important to note that this name does not imply that users and survivors of psychiatry see psychiatrists as their "enemies," but it is a reflection of the pain and suffering that was caused, through psychiatry, for many of us.

The human rights statement drafted by Paolo del Vecchio in 1994 was later adapted to become the "Human Rights Position Paper of the World Network of Users and Survivors of Psychiatry" adopted by the assembly at the launch of the WNUSP in Vancouver in 2001 (WNUSP 2001a). At the General Assembly of the WNUSP in 2004, in Vejle, Denmark, the assembly adopted the Vejle Declaration (ENUSP & WNUSP 2004), which further articulated the aspirations of the global user/survivor movement for the respecting of their dignity and independence.

This was also a key juncture in the history of the user/survivor movement, as it was at this point that members of the movement coalesced into a coherent lobby with members from all continents who came together at the United Nations Ad Hoc Committee (AHC) tasked with drafting the CRPD. Throughout the period of the drafting of the CRPD, the team of the WNUSP, led by Tina Minkowitz, made significant input into the final text, and played a leading role in the International Disability Caucus (IDC), which was a broad coalition of non-governmental organizations

(NGOs) and disabled people's organizations (DPOs) that acted as a united civil society voice during the negotiations. In fact, this was the first UN treaty in which civil society played such a big role in the course of negotiating the document.

Other WNUSP participants who were present at many meetings of the AHC include Gabor Gombos, Maths Jesperson, Chris Hansen, Judi Chamberlin, Karl Bach Jensen, Alpha Boubacar Diop, Daniel Iga, Janet Amegathcher, Celia Brown, Myra Kovary, Sylvia Caras, John McCarthy, Amita Dhanda, amongst other users/survivors from the USA and the rest of the world. The attention of the rest of the movement was focused on the deliberations at the UN, and they actively provided input from their lived experiences into the text through their participation in the email list of the WNUSP.

Soon after the CRPD came into force, the WNUSP held its third general assembly in Uganda under the theme *Making our Rights a Reality – Human Rights in the Age of the CRPD*. The global membership of the WNUSP all agreed upon the Kampala Declaration (WNUSP 2009), which further articulated the evolving human rights concerns of users/survivors, especially then in the light of the recently signed CRPD, which was at that point being ratified by more and more countries.

In March 2011 the WNUSP released its position paper on the implications of the CRPD on forced treatment, which has been endorsed by many individuals and organizations from all around the world. This is a very significant period as, at both the national and international level, critical mass has been developing which is pushing states parties to the CRPD as well as international agencies such as the WHO to come out with regulations, guidelines, and policy changes which would ensure that they are in line and compliant with the CRPD.

The early period

This period starts in the early 1970s when the pioneering leaders of user/survivor movement started their activism. One of the first was Judi Chamberlin, who in 1978 published the book, *On Our Own: Patient-Controlled Alternatives to the Mental Health System* (Chamberlin 1978), in which she speaks about her personal experiences receiving treatment in locked facilities and her eventually becoming involved in user/survivor organizing. At the core of the book she talks about the emerging consensus amongst users/survivors on how we would like to be treated, which was the first time that human rights principles that all agreed upon were articulated.

The writings of Paolo del Vecchio and Mary O'Hagan emerged as the first clear human rights documents from the movement during the 1990s. In her paper "A call to open the door," O'Hagan, from New Zealand, was the first from within the movement to look at human rights for users/survivors in a complete way. She spells out the concerns and dreams of users/survivors or, as she refers to us, people with psychiatric disabilities.

She eloquently talks about how the stories told by users/survivors all share common threads. Apart from talking "of their suffering during episodes of mental distress," they talk about their "shame and rejection" by others; "being locked up in institutions and being subjected to forced treatment, physical and sexual abuse, and neglect"; being "trapped in institutions for years with no legal processes to help get them out"; suffering "serious harm from psychiatric treatments," such as tardive dyskinesia; "not being able to use community mental health services when they need them"; living "in degrading institutions, houses or hostels where they have no say, in dilapidated boarding houses, in prisons or on the street"; never finding "employment on the open market, being subjected to sheltered workshops where they do repetitive work for a pittance"; and spending "their lives in living rooms and day centres without any opportunity to contribute to their communities" (O'Hagan 1999).

O'Hagan then continues to talk about the "locked door," which in her parable explains how users/survivors have been kept outside of mainstream society. The author also sees this "locked door" as an apt metaphor for all of those who are locked away and in this way remain "outside" of society. O'Hagan goes on to explain why "the conception of mental illness and disability is too narrow and doesn't facilitate recovery." She clearly emphasizes the connection between the prevailing concept of mental health/illness and service delivery, and warns of the prejudicial nature of some service providers' attitudes and beliefs in the predeterminism of "psychiatric labels":

A society's underlying conceptualizations about mental illness and disability will profoundly influence the way services are delivered and whether the door to our communities is open or shut to us.

Disability and mental illness are judgments, not facts.

Disability and mental illness have no real meaning outside the context of our social relationships and how we understand things like productivity, communication, attractiveness, independence and status.

Disability would merely indicate the different requirements of certain minorities to live a fulfilling life, rather than all the baggage and labels that say we are helpless, useless, unattractive and needy.

When disability and mental illness are viewed as inherent facts about individuals, it places these concepts beyond questioning.

(O'Hagan 1999)

In these words she announces the social and human rights model of disability that was later firmly introduced by the CRPD, which clearly sees disability as a part of human diversity to be celebrated, and not a label to demean one's human dignity. Apart from the underfunding for services, she also very importantly notes that the state discriminates against us by allowing coercive treatments by mental health services.

Discrimination by mental health services thus mainly happens because of coercion and paternalistic practices. We are forced to accept services where we are mostly not allowed to have a say in decisions regarding treatment, rehabilitation and vocational services; and, most importantly, services are provided which violate our human rights because they are delivered without informed consent. Her biggest complaint against community level discrimination is that they "passively discriminate against people with psychiatric disabilities by abdicating too much responsibility for our lives, often to the state" (O'Hagan 1999).

At the same time she is well aware of a broader picture, and recognizes that the problems users/survivors face cannot be addressed within psychiatry alone since they involve the whole society and communities: "Communities don't always demonstrate they have the will to see to the ordinary needs of all citizens for housing, income, work and family life." She concludes by saying that "the sad reality is that no specialist service can cater for these ordinary universal needs as well as willing friends, peers, families, clubs, community groups, neighborhoods or business communities."

The rest of O'Hagan's paper talks about what the quality of the services should be that will be suitable to us, which would not violate our human rights and keep us locked out and excluded from experiencing full lives like everyone else. She closes with this wish for the kind of "care" we would want, and which the writer believes is still not being delivered to users/survivors in most places:

> "care" must be concerned with standing alongside people with disabilities to assist us, on our terms, to open the door to freedom, inclusion and a valued place in our communities.
>
> (O'Hagan 1999)

First human rights position paper

The paper first drafted by Paolo del Vecchio in 1994, adapted and adopted by the first assembly of WNUSP at its launch in 2001, represents the first time that users/survivors collectively expressed their expectations on human rights. The paper is entitled *Human Rights Position Paper of the World Network of Users and Survivors of Psychiatry* (WNUSP 2001a).

The paper is composed of two parts, the first part expressing the values of the WNUSP and the second part the principles which will ensure that the goals and values are adhered to. The statement of principles in fact reads like a manifesto of demands on society, governments, the community at large, and especially on mental health service providers. The WNUSP position paper is a strong human rights document, and its values became entrenched in the CRPD. Among the principles stated in the WNUSP position paper, I wish particularly to highlight those pertaining to the kind of treatment that would be in compliance with human rights standards:

Every user/survivor shall be:
- free from any and all human rights abuses
- free from any and all forms of discrimination
- granted self-determination and the ability to make informed choices
- granted full political, legal, and civil rights
- fully integrated as any and all citizens within any community

Every user/survivor shall:
- have the opportunity to organize collectively
- have the right to refuse any and all "treatments or procedures"
- have the right to representation on his/her behalf
- have the right to handle one's personal affairs

- have the right to be paid at equitable pay for any work performed
- have the right to confidentiality and access to any records or documents concerning one's self

The following principles outline in more detail what respect of human rights in a hospital setting entails:

Every user/survivor within a hospital or mental health setting shall in addition to these principles have the following rights:
- unrestricted and private communication including receiving and sending unopened letters and to have outgoing letters stamped and mailed, to have access to telephones, to receive visitors of one's own choice, and to make grievances and have those grievances heard and adjudicated promptly with appeals processes in place
- to keep, use and sell personal possessions
- to participate in the development and review of one's "treatment" plan, and
- to be discharged or released upon one's wishes

No user/survivor shall be forced to work or be paid beneath equitable rate scales for equitable work.

Every user/survivor shall be notified of their rights and these principles.

The following paragraphs show how the voices and real-life experiences of users and survivors of psychiatry expressed in these principles were translated into a legally binding international human rights treaty, the UN Convention on the Rights of Persons with Disabilities (CRPD).

The negotiation of the CRPD

The Convention on the Rights of Persons with Disabilities and its Optional Protocol (United Nations 2006) was adopted on December 13, 2006, at the UN Headquarters in New York, and was opened for signature on March 30, 2007. There were 82 signatories to the Convention, 44 signatories to the Optional Protocol, and one ratification of the Convention. This is the highest number of signatories in history to a UN Convention on its opening day. It is the first comprehensive human rights treaty of the twenty-first century, and the first human rights convention to be open for signature by regional integration organizations. The Convention entered into force on 3 May 2008.

The CRPD was the fastest ever negotiated UN treaty. As mentioned earlier, it was the first time that representatives of the states parties negotiating an international human rights treaty worked with the representatives of persons whose lives would be directly influenced by the document. This practice reflected the motto of the international disability movement, *Nothing about us without us*, which recognized the importance and value of inputs by experiential experts on an equal footing with experts by learning.

As was mentioned in the introduction, thanks to the efforts and presence of key leaders of the movement, persons who experience and have experienced mental distress, i.e., users and survivors of psychiatry, at the negotiations, we had a chance to have our concerns voiced as well as an opportunity to suggest and negotiate ways of redress with representatives of states parties. The results of these efforts were then presented in the 50 articles of the CRPD.

The CRPD's "non-definition" of disability

Persons with disabilities include those who have long-term physical, mental, intellectual or sensory impairments which in interaction with various barriers may hinder their full and effective participation in society on an equal basis with others.

The "definition" clearly states that persons with mental or psychosocial disability are entitled to the same level of protection offered by the CRPD as other disability groups.

The CRPD recognizes disability rights as human rights. Unlike previous human rights documents (e.g., the UN Declaration on the Rights of Disabled Persons: United Nations 1975), which saw disability as a natural impediment to exercising human rights, the CRPD imposes an obligation on the state to provide reasonable accommodation in the environment and support so that any "impairments" a person has would not result in their exclusion from the society. The crucial paradigm shift introduced by the CRPD is that it recognized that it is societal barriers which turn an impairment into a disability, preventing the individual from realizing his/her full human potential.

This is the very reason why the CRPD intentionally does not define disability per se. In fact, this omission or non-definition is intentional, and it clearly illustrates the fact that disability is not an internal flaw in the individual, but is socially constructed when society is not inclusive enough to facilitate the accessibility needs of all people.

Forced treatment is a violation of human rights

Going into the negotiations, the WNUSP team already had a clear mandate from the membership to engage at the UN on our concerns, which in most cases reflected the experiences of all disability groups. What has always been a core issue of the user/survivor movement was the consensus position amongst all that forced treatment is a violation of our human rights. The Vejle Declaration (ENUSP & WNUSP 2004) reiterates the consensus from within the movement against discrimination and for an approach to mental health services which would be based on equality and not on unilateralism.

Very early in the process of the Ad Hoc Committee (AHC) drafting the treaty at the UN, the mandate by the membership was renewed to have the WNUSP team engage at the UN in order to ensure that we would arrive at a treaty which would fulfill our aspiration on how we like to be treated. Our core advocacy concern has been to end forced or coercive treatments, that is, treatments against the will of the person.

Many different terminologies have been used to explain what forced treatment is. It has been called involuntary hospitalization, compulsory treatment orders, sectioning, certification, etc. Mostly it means that people in a serious mental or emotional crisis could be deemed a "danger to themselves and others," and forcibly treated against their will, through losing their liberty when being locked up in a mental hospital or institution, and forcibly administered psychotropic drugs, placed into seclusion or isolation cells, or when they are, without consent, administered potentially harmful "treatments" such as electroshock therapy or insulin shock therapy.

The WNUSP assembly of 2001 made a very important statement in this regard in responding to the UN *Principles for the Protection of Persons with Mental Illness and for the Improvement of Mental Health Care* adopted by the General Assembly in its resolution 46/119 of December 17, 1991, commonly referred to as the MI Principles (United Nations 1991, WNUSP 2001b). Once again the movement clearly articulated its disagreement with the MI Principles in that it "endorses involuntary detention and treatment." Long before international human rights law as encapsulated by the CRPD forbade involuntary psychiatric detention and treatment without free and informed consent, many members of the user/survivor movement adopted the fight against forced treatment, as so many of us have experienced, and continue to experience, the horrors and traumatizing effects of coercion. In fact one of the slogans which emerged out of the movement very early on has been, *If it is not voluntary, then it is not treatment.*

User/survivor principles embedded in the UN Convention on the Rights of Persons with Disabilities

There are quite a few places where the CRPD directly addresses the WNUSP statement of principles, which is a proof of Team WNUSP's success at the AHC and in mobilizing support from and showing leadership in the International Disability Caucus (IDC), which was the single civil society voice representing DPOs and NGOs.

The key articles for users/survivors in the CRPD are Articles 12, 13, 14, 15, 16, 17, 19, 22, 23, 25, 27, 29. Table 6.1 shows the correlation between the pre-CRPD principles and the CRPD.

The 2009 Kampala Declaration, which expressed the wishes of the global assembly of users/survivors at the third assembly and world conference, reiterates the same concerns and once again highlights the articles mentioned above and how we expect them to be understood and implemented (WNUSP 2009). The declaration reflects our intentions as a collective to proceed with love, hope, and dignity.

The global north/south division in the treatment of persons with psychosocial disability

While countries of the so-called global north have an elaborate system of care, often based on hospitals and institutions, for the long-term placement of persons the system has failed to rehabilitate, the global south lacks that kind of infrastructure. In line with the paradigm shift introduced by the CRPD, which recognizes that people are better off in their communities even when they lack sophisticated care provided by institutionalized lives, the global south might make a leapfrog and simply avoid developing a system of institutions, focusing instead on the provision of services in the community where people live.

Yet another issue is the issue of mental health legislation, which in most countries merely serves to legalize coercion, i.e., forced hospitalization and medicating. These are now recognized by international human rights law to be high-risk situations for severe violations of basic human rights, while in many countries of the global south these matters are not legally regulated, and most human rights violations occur outside of the framework of mainstream mental health services. Chaining and locking away relatives who have "mental illnesses" in backrooms and sheds, as well is in prayer camps, churches, mosques and temples takes place in many parts of the world.

Conclusion

Some key international agencies, the World Health Organization in particular, have not yet come out with clear guidelines to governments on how to make everyday practice comply with the CRPD. However, I applaud the WHO for its recent *QualityRights Tool Kit* (World Health Organization 2012), which I feel is a big step in the right direction towards having CRPD principles apply in mental health services, and putting an end to coercive or forced interventions. Much work has to be done also around mental health legislation, regulations, and policies. In countries where mental health legislation has traditionally been used to enforce involuntary treatment, the feeling from this movement has been to call for the abolition of these laws, as they will not be able to be amended to be CRPD-compliant.

In many developing countries very few laws and regulations exist which have a bearing on mental health service provision. Here the challenge is whether to attempt to draft CRPD-compliant mental health laws, or to have one health or disability law which is fully CRPD-compliant. These are not just challenges for governments, which have obligations under international human rights law, but remain a challenge for most of humanity, be it communities, families, or society at large – as Mary O'Hagan pointed out back in 1999.

We would like to see a world where people who experience emotional distress, altered states, madness, or spiritual illnesses receive the appropriate care they need, which will not demean them or reduce them to dependent beings, but empower them to exist in this world on the same basis as

Table 6.1 A comparison of the Articles of the CRPD and pre-CRPD principles as formulated by the WNUSP

CRPD Article	WNUSP pre-CRPD principle
Article 12: right to enjoy legal capacity	Every user/survivor shall be granted self-determination and the ability to make informed choices – no user/survivor shall be denied the opportunity to make educated decisions affecting their lives.
Article 13: access to justice	Every user/survivor shall have the right to representation on his/her behalf – no user/survivor shall be denied the opportunity to have an advocate or attorney to ensure the protection of one's rights.
Article 14: liberty and security of the person on an equal basis with others, ensuring that disability cannot justify a deprivation of liberty	Every user/survivor within a hospital or mental health setting shall be discharged or released upon one's wishes.
Article 15: prohibition of torture and cruel, inhuman, or degrading treatment or punishment	Every user/survivor shall have the right to refuse any and all "treatments or procedures" – no user/survivor shall be subjected to coerced or forced psychosurgery, sterilization, over-medication, psychiatric drugging, chemical restraints, physical restraints, insulin shock, electroshock, or inpatient or outpatient commitment.
Article 16: freedom from exploitation, violence, and abuse	Every user/survivor shall be free from any and all human rights abuses – no user/survivor shall be subject to physical, sexual, or emotional abuse.
Article 17: protecting the integrity of the person	Every user/survivor shall be treated with the basic respect and dignity afforded to all persons.
Article 19: the right to live in the community with choices equal to those of others	Every user/survivor shall be as fully integrated as any and all citizens within any community – no user/survivor shall be segregated and relegated in separate housing or separate areas of communities.
Article 22: respect for privacy	Every user/survivor shall have the right to confidentiality and access to any records or documents concerning one's self – no user/survivor shall have their privacy rights violated. Every user/survivor within a hospital or mental health setting shall have unrestricted and private communication including receiving and sending unopened letters, and the right to have outgoing letters stamped and mailed, and access to telephones.
Article 23: respect for home and the family	Every user/survivor shall have the right to handle one's personal affairs – no user/survivor shall be denied the opportunity for holding a driver's license or professional license, engaging in personal intimate relationships of one's choice, marrying, obtaining a divorce, etc.
Article 25: equality in health care and services, including the requirement of free and informed consent	Every user/survivor shall have the right to refuse any and all "treatments or procedures" Every user/survivor within a hospital or mental health setting shall: • participate in the development and review of one's "treatment" plan, and • be discharged or released upon one's wishes.

Table 6.1 (*cont.*)

CRPD Article	WNUSP pre-CRPD principle
Article 27: work and employment	Every user/survivor shall have the right to be paid at equitable pay for any work performed – no user/survivor shall be forced to work or be paid beneath equitable rate scales for equitable work.
Article 29: participation in political and public life	Every user/survivor shall be: • granted self-determination and the ability to make informed choices – no user/survivor shall be denied the opportunity to make educated decisions affecting their lives including full informed participation and informed consent in all mental health "treatment" matters; additionally, users/survivors shall have the opportunity to fully participate in the planning, policy development, delivery, evaluation, and research of mental health services. • granted full political, legal, and civil rights – no user/survivor shall be denied the right to participate fully in society including the right to participate in political processes, practice one's religion and free speech, and to petition their governments. Every user/survivor shall: • have the opportunity to organize collectively – no user/survivor shall be denied the opportunity to assemble for mutual support and political action. • have the opportunity to become informed of the user/survivor movement.

everyone else, having the autonomy to make their own decisions, marry and form families, participate in the civil and political arena, and to be free from stigma, exclusion, and other abuses of their human rights.

We ask a simple thing: to be fully human in this world and to live our lives with the same opportunities and outcomes as everyone else, with all the reasonable accommodations required for everyone's particular needs.

References

Chamberlin J (1978) *On Our Own: Patient-Controlled Alternatives to the Mental Health System.* New York, NY: Hawthorn Books.

Icarus Project (undated) The Icarus Project. http://theicarusproject.net (accessed July 2013).

ENUSP, WNUSP (2004) Vejle Declaration, approved by the General Assemblies of ENUSP & WNUSP July 20, 2004. http://www.wnusp.net/index.php/vejle-declaration.html (accessed July 2013).

O'Hagan M (1999) A call to open the door: a psychiatric disability perspective on "rethinking care." http://www.dinf.ne.jp/doc/english/resource/acallto_eng.html (accessed July 2013).

United Nations (1975) *Declaration on the Rights of Disabled Persons.* New York, NY: UN.

United Nations (1991) The protection of persons with mental illness and the improvement of mental health care. A/RES/46/119. New York, NY: UN.http://www.un.org/documents/ga/res/46/a46r119.htm (accessed July 2013).

United Nations (2006) *Convention on the Rights of Persons with Disabilities (A/RES/61/106).* New York, NY: UN.

WNUSP (2001a) Human rights position paper of the World Network of Users and Survivors of Psychiatry. http://www.wnusp.net/index.php/human-rights-position-paper-of-the-world-network-of-users-and-survivors-of-psychiatry.html (accessed July 2013).

WNUSP (2001b) Minutes: Initial Congress of WNUSP, 20th and 21st July 2001 in Vancouver. http://www.wnusp.net/documents/

GeneralAssembly2001.pdf (accessed July 2013).

WNUSP (2009) Kampala Declaration. http://www.wnusp.net/documents/ WNUSP_KampalaDeclaration2009. pdf (accessed July 2013).

WNUSP (2011) Position paper on the implications of the CRPD. *WNUSP Newsletter*, March 2011. http://wnusp.rafus.dk/ newsletters (accessed July 2013).

World Health Organization (2012) *WHO QualityRights Tool Kit: Assessing and improving quality and human rights in mental health and social care facilities*. Geneva: WHO.

Chapter

7

Internalized stigma

Edwin Cameron

Introduction

One of the most perplexing and elusive phenomena in the HIV epidemic is the concept of internalized stigma.

HIV was first reported in the *Morbidity and Mortality Weekly Reports* (MMWR) of the US Centers for Disease Control in May 1981, over 32 years ago (Gottlieb 1981). From its inception the chief feature of the political, social, and medical response to the disease has been stigma. President Ronald Reagan, who held office in the USA as the epidemic became a deathly nightmare in the gay male communities of the east and west coasts, refused even to mention the word "AIDS" until 1987 (Salyer 2004). His silence was seen as a judgment – one condemning the gay men, who were falling sick and dying in their tens of thousands, because they deserved it.

In my own country, the stigma has also stalked the political management of the disease. President Nelson Mandela – though for reasons very different from those of President Reagan – also remained mute about the disease, as its toll rose under his presidency (Quist-Arcton 2003). He first mentioned the word "AIDS" in February 1997, nearly three years after he had taken office. And he did so in a speech outside South Africa – at the World Economic Forum in Davos, Switzerland (Mandela 1997). His successor, President Thabo Mbeki, refused to accept that AIDS was a disease caused by a virus that was sexually transmitted (Murphy 2003). He castigated Western medical scientists, doctors, and epidemiologists for propounding that a mass heterosexually transmitted epidemic of AIDS had manifested only on the African continent (Mbeki 2005). But President Mbeki's disastrous and tragic misconceptions themselves rested on

stigma – the idea that it was shameful to have a disease with sexual vectors in Africa. He even told opposition leader Tony Leon in July 2000 that the assertion that AIDS originated in Africa was "insulting" (Mbeki 2000).

The phenomenon of stigma and AIDS

The phenomenon of stigma is well understood and lavishly described in the AIDS literature (Mahajan *et al.* 2008). Classically, stigma is a mark of disgrace placed upon a member of society because of an unacceptable feature or trait or behavior. Stigma is disapproval, condemnation, judgment, rejection, ostracism, and abandonment. It is an attitude of devaluation that manifests in a social process and is exacerbated by class, gender, sexual, and racial differences (Parker & Aggleton 2002). In its enacted manifestation, stigma is discrimination and ostracism (Roura *et al.* 2009). Its external manifestations are widely documented. This is because their effect is so real – they can be easily perceived and easily described (Greeff *et al.* 2008)

In addition, enacted or external stigma can be socially countered. One can enact laws and pass resolutions and adopt policies against discrimination and ostracism. What is far more insidious, and much more difficult to describe, is the internalized dimension of stigma. In all the vast literature that has arisen in the AIDS epidemic, relatively little attention is given to internal stigma, and some of that attention exhibits basic misunderstanding of its nature and operation (Malcolm *et al.* 1998). The result is a gaping omission – internalized stigma forms virtually no part of individual, professional, or programmatic responses to AIDS.

Essentials of Global Mental Health, ed. Samuel O. Okpaku. Published by Cambridge University Press. © Cambridge University Press 2014.

What is internal stigma?

Internal stigma is the individual's internal appropriation of the fear, rejection, and condemnation with which many react to AIDS. In some of the literature, it is wrongly grouped together, or confused with, perceived, experienced, anticipated, or "felt" stigma (Greeff *et al.* 2008). Internal stigma is not the same as apprehended stigma. It is not the fear of others' condemnation – but the appropriation, internalization, and self-enactment of that condemnation (Cameron 2008). It is therefore more revealing of the motive dynamic of internal stigma to speak of "internalized" stigma.

Internalized stigma consists of self-disabling inner feelings of contamination, shame, self-rejection, and self-loathing experienced by people with HIV, and those who fear they have HIV, *even when there is no objective reason to fear rejection or discrimination, and even when there is good objective reason to believe that they will receive external support, protection, treatment, and acceptance.*

Internalized stigma has its most pernicious operation when the subject knows, cognitively, that he or she will receive support and acceptance (Cameron 2008). It is not merely external, or enacted, stigma that constitutes an impediment to the effective management of the AIDS epidemic. It is also internalized stigma. Many people with HIV, or at risk of it, feel overwhelming dread at discovering that they are infected with a socially reviled virus. This dread is often stronger than a cognitive appreciation that friends, family, and colleagues will support and accept them. It is stronger than the knowledge that life-saving treatment is now available. And it may even be stronger than the individual's capacity to make life-saving choices.

Internalized stigma is a dread of HIV that may have its origin externally – but it is located not in others, but within the self. It is the most intractable part of stigma. It is more insidious, and more destructive, than external stigma, for it eludes the direct, politically conscious confrontation with which we rightly respond to overt discrimination.

In my memoir, *Witness to AIDS*, I try to grapple with this internal dimension of stigma. I speak of my own horror and dismay when in 1986 I discovered I had HIV (Cameron 2005). Although working at a human rights public-interest law center, surrounded by rights-defending comrades, so deep was my sense

of self-revulsion that I felt entirely incapable of accessing their solidarity and support. It was impossible to say a word to them – or to anyone else.

I write of how the external stigma of AIDS – the fear of others' often-real adverse reactions – all too often finds an ally within: an ally that rejects health-affirming choices in favor of paralysed inaction, postponement, delay, denial, and death. I suggest that we fail to understand stigma fully if we concentrate solely on its external manifestations and causes, and neglect the inner dimension that may be altogether more deadly.

I write, also, of a man from Zimbabwe who worked for me as a gardener: a quiet, gentle man, who knew full well that I had HIV, and that I had survived AIDS because antiretroviral treatment had saved me – and who knew, also, that if he had HIV I would secure treatment for him. Despite this knowledge, my gardener, while visibly wasting away from what everyone 'knew' was AIDS, repeatedly denied that he had HIV or that he was sick with anything more than tuberculosis. He ultimately returned to Zimbabwe to die what must have been a lonely and medically untended death.

The story in my book is told in self-reproach. The point I make is that I should have been more proactive in helping my gardener ascertain his HIV status; that I should not have left him to the isolation and loneliness of his own fears. I should have done more to insist that he be tested and diagnosed and treated. I should, through my external actions, have created a bridge for him to cross over the perilous rapids within that were preventing him from accessing medical diagnosis, care, and treatment.

But the point of the story is broader. It is that our failure to grapple with and understand the internalization of stigma is impeding our understanding of the epidemic. It is costing us lives. We are now in what epidemiologists call "a mature epidemic" (Hearst & Mandel 1997). This means an epidemic in which everyone knows someone who has died of HIV. The consequence is that stigma generally abates. Despite this, the story of my gardener is still being replicated today.

Although South Africa has the world's biggest publicly provided antiretroviral treatment program, Statistics SA estimates that there were still more than 281 404 AIDS deaths in 2010 (this is down from the UNAIDS estimate of 310 000 AIDS-related deaths in 2009) (Statistics of South Africa 2010). Some of these deaths would have been due to inaccessibility of medical care or the unavailability of treatment (Statistics of South Africa 2010).

But too many of them are also due to fear. Fear not outside – but fear appropriated and enacted inside. Fear, propelled from within, that avoids diagnosis, testing, disclosure, and treatment. Fear that eludes loving and supportive colleagues, friends, neighbors, and family. Fear unto death.

The puzzle of internalized stigma

The non-description, or mis-description, of internalized stigma in the literature of AIDS is the more puzzling because the phenomenon is well-known in other settings. The "self-hating Jew" and the "self-loathing gay man" are readily recognizable constructs of the psychological and other literature (e.g., Lessing 1930)

In South Africa's vile past of racial hatred, Steven Bantu Biko recognized that the stigma of racial subordination had an internal impact that had to be eradicated first, if notions of white superiority and black subordination were to be effectively overcome (Biko 1977). Indeed, the founding analysis of stigma, that by Erving Goffman in 1963, itself recognizes that "the social label of deviance compels stigmatized individuals *to view themselves* ... as discredited or undesirable" (Goffman 1963).

Why has internalized stigma been so hard to see and to understand in the AIDS epidemic – when its effects are so profound? I think there are a number of reasons.

First, it is easy to condemn the condemner, the discriminator, the excluder. With external stigma we have a perpetrator and we have a victim. The villain is easy to see. By contrast, with internalized stigma, we have only a victim. A search for a perpetrator seems, unsettlingly, to lead to blaming the victim (Hasan *et al.* 2012). And, indeed, blaming the victim of internalized stigma would replicate the very experience of self-condemnation, self-disentitlement, and self-disablement that are its operational effects.

A second reason may be that it is harder to discern. The operation of internalized stigma consists in self-disablement, and therefore in inaction or omission (avoidance of testing, care, treatment). Hence it is harder to detect. It is an internal phenomenon and deeply elusive.

A third reason may be that we shy away from internalized stigma because we wouldn't know what to do with it when we found it. It is so intractably difficult to address that we run away from it.

How internalized stigma operates

Internalized stigma is deadly because it incapacitates health-seeking choices. Even when diagnosis, care, and treatment are available, they become not only unattractive but unpalatable, because they require an embrace, by the self, of a condition that is internally reviled. What is the practical significance of all of this? I think it is threefold.

First, we need to speak up for internalized stigma. It has been a poor, neglected, and shabbily treated player in the drama of AIDS. We need to accept that it exists if we are to understand its psychological operation and to appreciate its impact on volition.

Second, understanding internal stigma has a dramatic impact on the management of the individual patient–health-carer relationship. To understand this, we must understand the history of the AIDS epidemic and the inextricable role of stigma in it. Because AIDS affected largely the vulnerable, the marginalized and the dispossessed (gay men, sex-workers, the poor of Africa), and because those with HIV in these groups were blamed for their own condition (Turan *et al.* 2012), it became imperative for the effective public management of the disease to introduce special measures (Bayer 1991). These included special anti-discrimination measures for those with HIV. They also included special measures inhibiting ordinary physician–patient protocols and procedures.

Thus, it became unacceptable to test a patient for HIV without obtaining consent that had to be both express and specific. It became impossible to recount to others that someone had HIV because the stigmatizing fallout was almost invariably so high. The necessity for human rights protections for those with and at risk of HIV was called "the AIDS paradox" (Kirby 1995) – the recognition that protecting the rights of those with the disease was not inimical, but complementary to, effectively containing the epidemic. Coercive measures were recognized as not just needlessly punitive; they put the very public they were designed to protect at unnecessary risk of further infection by driving those with HIV away from diagnosis, counseling, and behavior change. But this paradox led to a further paradox. The protections in the healthcare setting for those with or at risk of HIV began to imperil those they were designed to protect.

They were designed for a world in which there was only temporary palliation for AIDS, and in which nothing could be done to halt inevitable decline and death (Richter *et al.* 2010). This pre-dated treatment.

But that has all changed. Treatment is now available. And it works. It is relatively easy to administer, side effects are being minimized, and the number of tablets and the frequency with which they have to be taken are being reduced.

My own life has given me joyous opportunity to celebrate this. Sixteen years ago, in September 1997, 11 years after my diagnosis with HIV, I was dying of AIDS. I would, had treatment not been available, surely have been dead by mid-2000. Instead, I started on antiretroviral treatment in November 1997. Within weeks I knew that the medication was working. My energy, my life force, and my vitality returned. My appetite became ravenous. My will to work and to exercise were resurgent. I have not looked back. The last time I had a detectable viral load was in October 2000. For more than a decade, no instrument of science or medicine has been able to detect the virus itself in my body. All this while I feel privileged to lead a bountifully full, energetic, and productive life.

Now, rather than protecting the patient against inevitable stigma and discrimination, inhibitions on diagnosis and treatment have the opposite effect. They can only increase suffering and hasten death. It is for this reason that I have become convinced that, in the southern African epidemic conditions, the medical community must step far outside the traditional boundaries of HIV testing. It must be actively *directive, interventive, and prescriptive* (Gillon 1987) in urging patients to test for HIV and to obtain treatment (Richter *et al.* 2012).

In the setting of our epidemic, it has become the physician's duty to assert his or her hierarchical power and authoritative command in exercise of the duty of beneficence. This is because without direct external intervention, all too many people with or at risk of HIV are too scared to be tested and diagnosed. The physician in these circumstances becomes duty-bound to help overcome the patient's internalization of self-disabling condemnation and stigma. This has two implications – one for the patient and one for the physician. For the patient, it implies an invocation of and reliance upon medical beneficence when diagnosis is overwhelmingly likely to lead to life-saving treatment. For the physician, it implies a caring

conquering of his or her own fears, misconceptions, and condemnations in relation to HIV and AIDS. It means that health carers must actively recognize, address, and overcome their own stigmatizing conceptions of HIV and AIDS in dealing with their patients.

At present, a collusive resonance all too often arises between the patient's internalized condemnatory fear of diagnosis, and the physician's partly stigmatizing fear of overcoming it and thus encountering HIV (Crisp 1987, Gillon 1987). For the doctor–patient management of the epidemic, recognizing and understanding internalized stigma therefore entails a revolution. It has been one that some of my human rights comrades have been slow to embrace (Brazier & Lobjoit 1990). Too many have clung to outmoded and inappropriate inhibition on physician-initiated or -encouraged testing. Too many have fought against medical technology, such as rapid tests, or self-testing kits, that would help disseminate HIV diagnosis rapidly and widely – and emporeringly – in the hands of patients themselves (Richter *et al.* 2012).

But, third, and lastly, recognizing internalized stigma should entail also a revolution in the public management of the disease. It is not enough for the public management of the epidemic to recognize and seek to counter external manifestations of stigma. The self-disabling internal workings of it must also be recognized and countered. This means that public messaging should address the fact that people blame themselves for HIV and incapacitate themselves from seeking help and health. This task can partly be undertaken by diminishing the external sources of stigma that are the source of internalized stigma. There has been significant progress in addressing the external manifestations of stigma by way of training, advocacy, and community outreach programs.

In addition, the fact that we are in what I called earlier a "mature" epidemic, together with the widespread availability of treatment, and the increasing knowledge that it works, have helped diminish stigma. But still the effects of internalized stigma operate. A fellow lawyer who is a close friend recently told me the tragic story of his sister who died of AIDS in a remote village in KwaZulu-Natal, even though he encouraged her to seek and take treatment, and offered her unqualified love and support in doing so. Hence the reduction of external stigma is not enough. The public management of the disease must recognize that, uniquely, AIDS inflicts an internal burden that is costing lives and causing immense suffering.

The public message should be, not only that you can live healthily with HIV, but that those with and at risk of HIV are not alone; that their internal fears are real and can operate brutally; but also that they can be overcome.

I do not pretend that this is an easy message to proliferate – or even to articulate. One of the difficulties is that the perils of *blame* and *exceptionalism* do not lie far from our good intent. However, the correct articulation of the phenomenon the patient faces, *in conjunction* with the reassurance that this is a common and understandable feeling, which can be addressed and treated, is of urgent significance.

The message, "You are not alone" is pivotal, because the patient feels a self-disabling assortment of feelings – "loneliness," "shame," "isolation," and "stigmatization." But we must beware of a risk – the risk that to articulate those notions to the patient could serve to augment and intensify those very emotions. To tell the person with or at risk of HIV "you feel isolated" or "you feel ashamed" may only give external definition to a tacit internal turmoil. The message should therefore not overdramatize the feelings the patient experiences, but must seek to reassure and counsel against those feelings. Learned members of the medical profession should give medical and academic credence to the particularities of internal stigma.

Conclusion

The story of stigma in AIDS is a story of human fear and fallibility. And the role of stigma in that story is the same as with any form of irrational blame, rejection, or condemnation. It can be fearsome and intractable. It was stigma that led to the gas chambers of Auschwitz, and to the Rwandan genocide of 1994. But ignorance, fear, and prejudice are conditions of the mind. And all conditions of the mind can be made subject to change – immediately. Internalized stigma is more difficult to address not only because it is less visible but because its object, and therefore its victim, is the self. We do ourselves a disservice, however, when we fail, in addressing any of the complex social burdens we carry that are exacerbated by externally or internally directed fear or hatred, to recognize them and to tackle them. The profession of psychiatry concerns itself with agonies of the mind, and psychiatrists probably see more human anguish and suffering than lawyers. Medication and prescription drugs have an important role to play in relieving human distress. But understanding the complexity of our own external and internalized thought processes is an indispensable part of the remedy.

References

Bayer R (1991) Sounding board: an end to HIV exceptionalism? *New England Journal of Medicine* **324**: 1500–4.

Biko S (1977) [Statement attributed to Biko]. *Boston Globe*, 25 October 1977.

Brazier M, Lobjoit M (1990) AIDS, ethics and the respiratory physician. *Thorax* **45** (4): 283–6.

Cameron E (2005) *Witness to AIDS*. London: I. B. Tauris.

Cameron E (2008) Moving from promises to actions. *XVII International AIDS Conference*, August 6, 2008.

Crisp R (1989) Autonomy, welfare and the treatment of AIDS. *Journal of Medical Ethics* **15**: 68–73.

Gillon R (1989) Refusal to treat AIDS and HIV positive patients. *British Medical Journal* **294**: 1332–3.

Goffman E (1963) *Stigma: Notes on the Management of Spoiled Identity*. Englewood Cliffs, NJ: Prentice Hall.

Gottlieb MS, Schanker HM, Fan PT, Saxon A, Weisman JD (1981) Pneumocystis Pneumonia: Los Angeles. *Morbidity and Mortality Weekly Report* **30** (21): 1–3.

Greeff M, Uys LR, Holzemer WL, *et al.* (2008) Experiences of HIV/AIDS stigma of persons living with HIV/AIDS and nurses involved in their care from five African countries. *African Journal of Nursing and Midwifery* **10**: 78–108.

Hasan MT, Nath SR, Khan NS, *et al.* (2012) Internalized HIV/AIDS-related stigma in a sample of HIV-positive people in Bangladesh. *Journal of Health, Population, and Nutrition* 2012; **30** (1): 22–30.

Hearst N, Mandel JS (1997) A research agenda for AIDS prevention in the developing world. *AIDS* **11** (Suppl 1): S1–4.

Kirby M (1995) Law and HIV: a paradoxical relationship of mutual interest. Law and Justice Foundation of New South Wales, IUDVT World STD/AIDS Congress, 22 March 1995.

Lessing T (1930) *Der Jüdische Selbsthaß*. Berlin: Jüdischer Verlag.

Mahajan AP, Sayles JN, Patel VA, *et al.* (2008) Stigma in the HIV/AIDS epidemic: a review of the literature and recommendations for the way forward. *AIDS (London, England)* **22** (Suppl 2): S67–79.

Malcolm A, Aggleton P, Bronfman M, *et al.* (1998) HIV-related stigmatization and discrimination: its form and context. *Critical Public Health* **8**: 347–70.

Mandela N (1997) Address at the World Economic Forum Session on AIDS, Davos, Switzerland, February 3, 1997.

Mbeki T (2000) Letter to Tony Leon dated 1 July 2000. http://www. virusmyth.com/aids/news/letmbeki. htm (accessed July 2013).

Mbeki T (2005) Lies have short legs. *ANC Today*, May/June 2005.

Murphy V (2003) Mbeki stirs up AIDS controversy. *BBC News Online*, September 23, 2003.

Parker R, Aggleton P (2002) *HIV/ AIDS-Related Stigma and*

Discrimination: a Conceptual Framework and an Agenda for Action. Population Council (Horizons Project). http://www. popcouncil.org/pdfs/horizons/ sdcncptlfrmwrk.pdf (accessed 9 July 2013).

Quist-Arcton O (2003) South Africa: Mandela deluged with tributes as he turns 85. *AllAfrica*, July 19, 2003.

Richter M, Venter WD, Gray A (2010) Home self-testing for HIV: AIDS exceptionalism gone wrong. *South African Medical Journal* 2010; **100** (10): 636–42.

Richter M, Venter WD, Gray A (2012) Enabling HIV self-testing in South Africa: a rapid overview. *South African Journal of HIV Medicine* **13**: 186–7.

Roura M, Wringe A, Busza J, *et al.* (2009) "Just like fever": a qualitative

study on the impact of antiretroviral provision on the normalisation of HIV in rural Tanzania and its implications for prevention. *BMC International Health and Human Rights* **9**: 22. http://www. biomedcentral.com/1472-698X/9/22 (accessed July 2013).

Salyer D (2004) Ronald Reagan and AIDS. *AIDS Survival Project.* http://www.thebody.com/content/ art32196.html (accessed July 2012).

Statistics South Africa (2010) Mid-year population estimates 2010. Statistical Release PO302, released 20th July 2010.

Turan JM, Hatcher AH, Medema-Wijnveen J, *et al.* (2012) The role of HIV-related stigma in utilization of skilled childbirth services in rural Kenya: a prospective mixed-methods study. *PloS Medicine* **9** (8): e1001295.

Chapter

8

Definition and process of stigma

Heather Stuart

Introduction

This chapter reviews the origins and nature of stigma. Placing it within evolving disability discourse, it traces a shift from considering stigma from the perspective of those stigmatized – viewing them as indelibly marked – to a broader social determinants framework that considers stigma from the perspective of the stigmatizing groups – as a form of social oppression. Theoretical thinking on the topic is described, and evidence describing the effects of stigma on people who have a mental illness, on their family members, and on mental health system delivery is reviewed. It closes with a review of promising approaches that can be used to fight stigma.

Though there is a rich theoretical literature on social reactions to mental illnesses dating from the mid-twentieth century, clinical and public health communities have only recently recognized the importance of social inclusion for people with a disability. For example, signatories to the United Nations Convention on the Rights of Persons with Disabilities have agreed to eliminate discrimination on the basis of a disability and promote the full and effective participation of people with a physical or mental disability. This includes raising awareness about rights, fostering respect and dignity, combating stereotypes, prejudices, and harmful practices, and promoting awareness of the capabilities and contributions of people with a disability (United Nations 2006). Raising awareness of the global burden of mental, neurological, and substance abuse disorders and eliminating social stigma, discrimination, and social exclusion of patients and families has been identified as one of the grand challenges in global mental health that must be addressed in order to make an impact on the lives of people living with mental disorders (Collins *et al.* 2011).

Origins and nature of stigma

The origin of the term stigma is often traced to early Greece, where a sharp stick, or *stig*, was used to tattoo or brand marks on slaves, criminals, and other social undesirables to signify their ownership or their inferior social position. Though there is no evidence that the early Greeks branded people with a mental illness in this way, mental illness was associated with deep shame and guilt, as evidenced from early Greek literature linking mental illnesses with murderous madness, shame, loss of face, humiliation, and social banishment. In the Christian tradition, stigmata were the marks of grace – physical marks that resembled the crucifixion wounds of Christ. Another important use of the term was to refer to a mark of service where a tattoo or mark signified that the bearer was dedicated to a particular god. The more negative connotation, signifying a mark of shame or degradation, appeared later and was well established by the late sixteenth and early seventeenth centuries (Simon 1992). This most likely occurred when mental illnesses were linked with sin (Anderson 1970).

By the early nineteenth century, most mental illnesses were explained by heredity and understood as the result of a degenerative taint in the family. Clinicians of the day thought that people who were mentally ill displayed morphological stigmata such as pointed ears, stunted growth, or cranial abnormalities (Shortt 1986). Patients' symptoms, signs, behavior, body configuration, skull measurements, and detailed descriptions of their face, ears, and other characteristics were made. Kraepelin is generally credited with creating the clearest and most meaningful categorization of stigmata. The denigration of people with a mental illness was further explicated by Lombroso, who identified stigmata of degeneration as a means of

Essentials of Global Mental Health, ed. Samuel O. Okpaku. Published by Cambridge University Press. © Cambridge University Press 2014.

marking criminality. Important textbooks of the day began to include photographs and line drawings which portrayed the mentally ill as bizarre, comic, vulgar, and extreme. In this era, mental illnesses were considered to be so bizarre, comic, or disgusting that they could only occur in grossly abnormal creatures (Leigh 1957). Indeed, this thinking was a driving force behind the eugenics movement. Though normally associated with Nazi Germany, the eugenics movement had blossomed throughout the early 1900s in much of the United States, Canada, Britain, Scandinavia, elsewhere in Europe, and parts of Latin America and Asia. In Canada and the United States, eugenics laws permitting the sterilization of mentally disabled people reached only as far as public institutions for the mentally ill and mentally handicapped, and did not touch people in private care or in the care of their families (Kevles 1999).

Degeneracy thinking remains evident even today. Research shows that genetic and biological explanations of mental illnesses are linked to prejudicial attitudes. In a review of studies conducted between 1970 and 2000, Haslem, Sayce, and Davies (2006) found that biological explanations were widely linked to stereotypes of dangerousness and unpredictability, and that studies that had challenged biological theories reported reductions in stereotyping and social distance. The association of genetics and biology to mental illness increases beliefs about lack of control over behaviors, an inability to recover (because the brain structure is damaged), and fears of dangerousness and unpredictability (Pescosolido *et al.* 2010).

Theoretical perspectives

Significant contributions to the field of stigma research have been made by sociologists, social psychologists, geographers, psychiatrists, and more recently epidemiologists and public health professionals. A unifying theory does not exist, and stigma has been variously defined and redefined depending on whether the focus is on the psychological scaffolding that underlies prejudicial thinking (Corrigan *et al.* 2003) or on the discriminatory behavioral and social responses to people with a mental illness as a marginalized group (Link & Phelan 2001). Building on these perspectives, public health models have highlighted the process of stigmatization as a series of vicious cycles that involve interactions between individual-level factors (such as self-perceptions, feelings of

shame, or guilt), interpersonal or group factors (such as social cognitions, attributions, stereotypes, or behaviors) and social structural factors (such as laws, policies, institutional practices, power imbalances, and social norms). These interact at various levels to create and maintain social inequities that are based on one's diagnostic or treatment status, even in the absence of visible signs or symptoms (Sartorius & Schulze 2005).

In response to growing criticism from advocates, the term *stigma* is becoming less useful in the context of current disability discourse, as it is thought to place undue emphasis on the characteristics that mark the individual as different, and insufficient emphasis on the underlying social oppression that excludes individuals from the group (Everett 2004). This has led several advocacy groups to call for the retirement of the term stigma. In light of this discourse, it may be more useful to refer to the "process of stigmatization," rather than stigma per se. For it is through the process of stigmatization that people with a mental illness are marginalized, disenfranchised, socially excluded, and denied their human rights and social entitlements.

Social psychologists make a distinction between pre-judgments, which may be based on inaccurate overgeneralizations, and prejudice, a negative evaluation of others based on a characteristic or group membership. Pre-judgments are receptive to new information and can be corrected in the light of new facts. Pre-judgments become prejudices when they are not reversible when exposed to new data. There is an emotional undertone to prejudice, which may become activated when the prejudice is threatened or contradicted. One cannot rectify a prejudice without considerable emotional resistance. Thus, a prejudice is an emotional antipathy that is rooted in inflexible and incorrect generalizations. Prejudices may be directed toward an entire group, or an individual within the group, based on that person's group membership (Stangor 2000).

This helps to explain why a growing body of evidence is showing that good mental health literacy (defined as knowledge about symptoms and treatments) coexists with high levels of social intolerance. Comparing the attitudes of the American public between 1950 and 1996, Phelan and colleagues (2000) found that conceptions of mental illness had broadened significantly to include more non-psychotic disorders, so more closely approached professional definitions. At the same time, stereotypes of violence and other frightening characteristics linked to mental illnesses had increased. Comparing changes in knowledge about the causes of mental illnesses and public stereotypes between 1996 and 2006, Pescoso-lido *et al.* (2010) found increases in the proportion of the public that embraced neurobiological explan-ations for disorders such as schizophrenia or depres-sion, and in the proportion that endorsed medical treatments. Despite improvements in mental health literacy and knowledge, levels of social intolerance remained high and unchanged. In 2006, the majority of respondents continued to report high social dis-tance, expressed as an unwillingness to work or social-ize with a person described in a study vignette. Holding a neurobiological explanation was unrelated to stigma, or it increased the odds of a stigmatizing reaction. These results highlight the fact that know-ledge (or lack of knowledge) is not the central modi-fiable characteristic underlying the stigmatization of mental illnesses.

Sociologists such as Link and Phelan (2001) have reminded us that only powerful social groups can stigmatize. Thus, the process of stigmatization is rooted in power differentials that make it possible for a dominant group to disenfranchise and margin-alize another, less powerful group. In their reconcep-tualization of stigma, Link and Phelan highlight several interrelated elements, beginning with the labeling of a difference by the dominant social group, followed by cultural beliefs that link the label and the labeled individual to negative stereotypes that are used to create clear social distinctions. Once labeled and separated, stigmatized groups experience status loss and discrimination. In this model, stigmatization is entirely contingent on structures that allow unequal access to the social, economic, and political power necessary to the process of stigmatization. When powerful groups are motivated to stigmatize, there are many ways in which discrimination can be per-petuated, ranging from overt discrimination to more covert and sophisticated forms, if the overt becomes ideologically difficult to sustain.

Stigma will exist to the extent that members of the dominant group control access to major life domains (education, employment, housing, health care). As long as stigma is embedded in power differentials and the dominant group sustains its stigmatized view, decreasing the use of one mechanism will give rise to another. Successful anti-stigma interventions will be those that bring about fundamental changes in the

attitudes, beliefs, and behaviors of powerful groups, or those that limit the power of these groups to act on their attitudes and beliefs (Link & Phelan 2001). Corrigan, Roe, and Tsang have argued that stopping discrimination is not enough. Affirming actions, which promote full and effective social inclusion, are also required. This might include legal and policy changes that require deliberate efforts to reach out to people with a mental illness, such as through edu-cational programs, hiring programs, and outreach activities by social and religious groups (Corrigan *et al.* 2011).

Effects of stigma: personal, family, and system

Self-stigma is a form of self-fulfilling prophesy. It occurs when members of a stigmatized group intern-alize negative stereotypes and adopt a stigmatized illness identity. Self-stigma has its origins in cultural conceptions of mental illness that begin in childhood and become crystalized throughout adulthood. Through various modes of cultural transmission, including news and entertainment media, people become aware of the negative cultural stereotypes pertaining to mental illnesses and the mentally ill. Whenever individuals with a mental illness believe that the culturally internalized stereotypes apply to them, self-esteem and self-efficacy suffer. They may avoid social situations in which stigma is expected, and delay treatment seeking in order not to receive s stigmatizing label (Corrigan *et al.* 2006).

Research has shown that self-stigma is inversely associated with hope, self-efficacy, social functioning, and recovery (Corrigan *et al.* 2011). Ritsher and Phe-lan (2004) studied 82 outpatients with severe mental illness. A third of the sample had an internalized stigma score that was over the midpoint of the scale. Half reported that they believed others routinely dis-criminated against them, and 40% reported social withdrawal. High levels of internalized stigma at base-line were associated with low levels of morale at a four-month follow-up. Those with high scores on an alienation subscale reported the most distress at follow-up, suggesting that programs that promote interpersonal engagement may reduce self-stigma and promote recovery.

It is important to note that not everyone is victim-ized by self-stigma. Those who have a sense of personal power over their illness and control over their lives are less likely to experience the negative psychosocial effects of stigma. Consequently, personal empowerment strategies have been offered as an important antidote to self-stigma. These include self-help and mutual aid programs that offer peer supports from people who are in recovery from a mental illness (Corrigan *et al.* 2011) as well as mental health systems that are reoriented to foster personal choice, self-determination, and hope (Amering & Schmolke 2009).

Goffman (1963) used the term *courtesy stigma* to refer to the social blemish that is bestowed on individuals who have courtesy membership in the stigmatized group – those who, by virtue of their close association with the stigmatized, know most about them. Historically, families have borne the brunt of stigma-by-association because they were often viewed as blameworthy by causing the mental illness in the first place (through a genetic taint or poor parenting), or for harboring a dangerous and unpredictable criminal in their midst.

Since deinstitutionalization, people with a mental illness have become more visibly relocated within families, who now provide the bulk of community care and support (Falk 2001). Stigma interferes with family functioning and quality of life. In a study designed to develop an inventory to measure family experiences of stigma, 53% of the family members participating indicated that their experiences with stigma had affected their family's quality of life, 43% indicated that stigma had affected their ability to interact with other relatives, 28% reported that stigma had affected their family's ability to make or keep friends, and 20% indicated that they had personally felt stigmatized because of their relative's mental illness (Stuart *et al.* 2008). To avoid the stigma, family members will often conceal the fact that they have a relative with a mental illness. For example, in a sample of 156 parents and spouses of people who experienced their first admission to a psychiatric hospital, half reported some degree of concealment (Phelan *et al.* 1998). The shame and worry experienced by family members is stress-producing, and in some cases it can produce burn-out and depleted social support. Family members are less able to support their ill relative, and in extreme cases family ties may be severed completely. Reduced social support can exacerbate symptoms and promote a relapse. This is portrayed as a vicious cycle of shame, increased stress, reduced supports, and increased disability (Sartorius & Schulze 2005).

Stigma-by-association also diminishes the quality of care that is provided to people with a mental illness, both within and outside of the mental health system. Despite international protections, the majority of the world's population still has little or no access to even the most basic mental health services or treatments (World Health Organization 2005). Furthermore, community surveys show that 35–50% of people living in developed countries, and 76–85% of those living in developing countries, do not receive treatment even though they meet the criteria for a treatable mental illness (WHO Mental Health Survey Consortium 2004). Inequities in the availability of mental health services and supports and high levels of unmet need reflect a process of structural stigmatization that results from discriminatory policies, practices, and organizational structures. Structural stigmatization gives low priority to mental health programs and reduces the quantity and quality of care available for people who have a mental illness. In turn, this makes it difficult to attract high-quality personnel and contributes to the overall negative perception of mental health services and clients (Sartorius & Schulze 2005).

Approaches to stigma reduction

At least six different approaches to stigma reduction can be identified in the literature, though none has been sufficiently researched to warrant the distinction of being a "best practice" (Arboleda-Flórez & Stuart 2012). At the structural level, legislative reforms that prohibit discrimination on any grounds have offered important protections for the human and civil rights of people with a mental illness. The UN Convention on the Rights of Persons with Disabilities (United Nations 2006) has provided an important rallying point for legislative and social reform. It requires signatories to guard against coercion and forced treatments (termed negative or first-generation rights), and places a duty on them to provide economic, social, and health supports designed to promote full and effective social inclusion (termed positive or second-generation rights). Second-generation protections include employment equity legislation (requiring employers to make reasonable accommodations for people with a mental illness), laws that allow people with a mental illness equal access to training and education, as well as zoning by-laws that make it impossible for neighborhoods to exclude supported residential and housing facilities (Callard *et al.* 2011).

However, legislation alone is insufficient. Advocacy is required to ensure that people with a mental illness actually enjoy the rights and freedoms that legislation guarantees, and offers avenues for redress when policies and procedures violate civil or human rights or entitlements. Advocacy is defined by the World Health Organization as activities that are aimed at raising awareness of the importance of mental health issues and ensuring that these issues are placed on the agendas of governments and decision makers. It can include education, dissemination of information, training, mutual help, counseling, mediating, defending, and denouncing (World Health Organization 2003).

Considerable research now supports the "contact hypothesis," which suggests that positive social contact between group members challenges negative attributions, breaks down cultural stereotypes, and reduces the salience of group divisions (Hewstone 2000). For example, school-based programs use contact-based education and active discussion to break down stereotypes, and these have been a central approach to stigma reduction in many countries (Sartorius & Schulze 2005). In Hong Kong, for example, Chan et al. (2009) compared the effects of traditional education (delivered in a lecture format) with traditional education enhanced with a video of people with a mental illness (contact-based education). The video showed four people (two males and two females) who had been diagnosed with schizophrenia during their early adulthood. They had made a good recovery and were living independently with jobs and a good quality of life. They shared their experiences with symptoms, talked about stigma, and how they overcame it to regain a fulfilling life. Only the students who received the traditional education followed by the contact-based video demonstrated improved attitudes and social tolerance, an effect that remained evident in a one-month follow-up. Similar results have been reported elsewhere (Stuart 2006). The importance of positive portrayals is highlighted in a study that used a video to portray homeless people living on the streets in Toronto, Canada. Students who received the video showed more negative attitudes, reported stronger feelings of danger, and endorsed more restrictions (Tolomiczenko et al. 2001).

Stigma management – which encourages people with a mental illness to overcome their illness

identities to find new personal meanings and valued social roles – is emerging as another promising approach. Removing prejudices and changing the way in which individuals and organizations behave is a long-term task – one that will take generations. In the meantime, stigmatized individuals must find a way to rise above these conditions and lead healthy and productive lives. In order to achieve this, they must understand stigma and learn how to mitigate its negative personal and social consequences. There is a growing literature that suggests that becoming empowered and learning how to overcome stigma and its debilitating effects is fundamental to personal recovery (Shih 2004).

While few modern mental health services would not claim to be "recovery-oriented," the extent to which they are is debatable, given a lack of operational criteria, fidelity measures, and service monitoring data. Current mental health systems remain uncoordinated, lacking in many of the supports that would promote full and effective participation, and continue to be experienced as stigma-promoting (Cobigo & Stuart 2010). In their focus group study, Schulze and Angermeyer (2003) reported that the stigma associated with the delivery of mental health care accounted for one-quarter of the stigmatizing experiences reported by patients and their family members. In a survey of health providers' views of the prognosis and long-term outcomes of depression and schizophrenia, Caldwell and Jorm (2001) found that mental health providers were more negative about whether someone with schizophrenia, even with professional help, would make a full recovery compared to the general public. Two percent of psychiatrists, 3% of psychologists, and 9% of mental health nurses agreed, compared to 30% of the general public. Lauber and colleagues (2006) found psychiatrists were more likely to consider people with a mental illness as dangerous, less skilled, and more socially disturbing than other professional groups.

Finally, two approaches that have been more equivocal have been traditional education and protest. Traditional education attempts to correct misinformation about mental illnesses and replace myths with facts. While these approaches have been demonstrated to improve mental health knowledge (or literacy) and promote help-seeking, evidence supporting their effectiveness in reducing stigma and improving social inclusion for people with a mental illness is lacking. In some cases, greater medical knowledge (particularly etiological theories that are genetically or biologically based) has been associated with greater stigma (Haslam *et al.* 2006). Protest attempts to suppress negative and offensive representations or behaviors by opening objections to them. Although they have been used profitably in some situations to remove offensive media depictions or marketing strategies, the psychological impact of protest campaigns is less certain (Corrigan *et al.* 2001), as there is always a risk that it will polarize perspectives and deepen divisions.

Conclusion

The stigmatization of people who have a mental illness has a long historical tradition and is deeply rooted in our social fabric, through both cultural and religious conceptions of mental illnesses. It denigrates and marginalizes people who have a mental illness. It creates serious inequities in the quality and availability of treatments, reduces the possibility of recovery, undermines the quality of life of people with a mental illness and their family members, and promotes infringements in human and civil rights and entitlements.

References

Amering M, Schmolke M (2009) *Recovery in Mental Health*. Oxford: Wiley.

Anderson R (1970) The history of witchcraft: a review with some psychiatric comments. *American Journal of Psychiatry*, **126**: 69–77.

Arboleda-Flórez J, Stuart H (2012) From sin to science: fighting the stigmatization of mental illness. *Canadian Journal of Psychiatry* **57**: 457–63.

Caldwell T, Jorm A (2001) Mental health nurses' beliefs about likley outcomes for people with schizophrenia or depression: a comparison with the public and other healthcare professionals. *Australian and New Zealand Journal of Mental Health Nursing* **10**: 42–54.

Callard, F, Sartorius N, Arboleda-Flórez J, *et al.* (2011) *Mental Illness, Discrimination and the Law: Fighting for Social Justice*. London: Wiley-Blackwell.

Chan J, Mak W, Law L (2009) Combining education and video-based contact to reduce stigma of mental illness: "The Same or Not the Same" anti-stigma program for secondary schools in Hong Kong. *Social Science and Medicine* **68**: 1521–6.

Cobigo V, Stuart H (2010) Social inclusion and mental health.

Current Opinion in Psychiatry **23**: 453–7.

Collins PY, Patel V, Joestl SS, *et al.* (2011) Grand challenges in global mental health. *Nature* **475**: 27–30.

Corrigan P, Markowitz FE, Watson A, Rowan D, Kubiak MA (2003) An attribution model of public discrimination towards persons with mental illness. *Journal of Health and Social Behavior* **44**: 162–79.

Corrigan P, Watson A, Barr L (2006) The self-stigma of mental illness: implications for self-esteem and self-efficacy. *Journal of Social and Clinical Psychology* **25**: 875–84.

Corrigan PW, River LP, Lundin RK, *et al.* (2001) Three strategies for changing attributions about severe mental illness. *Schizophrenia Bulletin* **27**: 187–95.

Corrigan PW, Roe D, Tsang, H (2011) *Challenging the Stigma of Mental Illness: Lessons for Therapists and Advocates*. Chichester: Wiley-Blackwell.

Everett B (2004) Best practices in workplace mental health: an area for expanded research. *HealthcarePapers* **5**: 114–16.

Falk G (2001) *Stigma: How We Treat Outsiders*. Amherst, NY: Prometheus Books.

Goffman E (1963) *Stigma: Notes on the Management of Spoiled Identity*. Englewood Cliffs, NJ: Prentice Hall.

Haslam R, Sayce N, Davies E (2006) Prejudice and schizophrenia: a review of the "mental illness is an illness like any other" approach. *Acta Psychiatrica Scandinavica* **114**: 303–18.

Hewstone M (2000) Contact and categorization: social psychological interventions to change intergroup relations. In C Stangor, ed., *Stereotypes and Prejudice*. Ann Arbor, MI: Taylor & Francis; pp. 394–418.

Kevles D (1999) Eugenics and human rights. *BMJ* **319**: 435–8.

Lauber C, Nordt C, Braunschweig C, Rossler W (2006) Do mental health proessionals stigmatize their patients? *Acta Psychiatrica Scandinavica*, **113** (Suppl. 429): 51–9.

Leigh D (1957) Recurrent themes in the history of psychiatry. *Medical History* **1** (3): 237–48.

Link BG, Phelan JC (2001) Conceptualizing stigma. *Annual Review of Sociology* **27**: 363–85.

Pescosolido BA, Martin JK, Long JS, *et al.* (2010) "A disease like any other"? A decade of change in public reactions to schizophrenia, depression, and alcohol dependence. *American Journal of Psychiatry* **157**: 1321–30.

Phelan J, Bromet E, Link B (1998) Psychiatric illness and family stigma. *Schizophrenia Bulletin* **24**: 115–26.

Phelan JC, Link BG, Stueve A, Pescosolido BA (2000) Public conceptions of mental illness in 1950 and 1996: what is mental illness and is it to be feared? *Journal of Health and Social Behavior* **41**: 188–207.

Ritsher J, Phelan R (2004) Internalized stigma predicts erosion of morale among psychiatric outpatients. *Psychiatry Research* **129**: 257–65.

Sartorius N, Schulze H (2005) *Reducing the Stigma of Mental Illness.* Cambridge: Cambridge University Press.

Schulze B, Angermeyer MC (2003) Subjective experiences of stigma: a focus group study of schizophrenic patients, their relatives and mental health professionals. *Social Science and Medicine* **56**: 299–312.

Shih M (2004) Positive stigma: examining resilience and empowerment in overcoming stigma. *Annals of the American Academy of Political and Social Science* **591**: 175–85.

Shortt S (1986) *Victorian Lunacy.* Cambridge: Cambridge University Press.

Simon B (1992) Shame, stigma, and mental illness in ancient Greece. In P Fink, A Tasman, eds., *Stigma and Mental Illness.* Washington, DC: American Psychiatric Press.

Stangor C, ed. (2000) *Stereotypes and Prejudice.* Ann Arbour, MI: Taylor & Francis.

Stuart H (2006) Reaching out to high school youth: the effectiveness of a video-based antistigma program. *Canadian Journal of Psychiatry* **51**: 647–53.

Stuart H, Koller M, Milev R (2008) Inventories to measure the scope and impact of stigma experiences from the perspective of those who are stigmatized: consumer and family versions. In J Arboleda-Flórez, N Sartorius, eds., *Understanding the Stigma of Mental Illness: Theory and Interventions.* London: Wiley; pp. 193–204.

Tolomiczenko G, Goering P, Durbin J (2001) Educating the public about mental illness and homelessness: a cautionary note. *Canadian Journal of Psychiatry* **46**: 253–7.

United Nations (2006) *Convention on the Rights of Persons with Disabilities (A/RES/61/106).* New York, NY: UN.

WHO Mental Health Survey Consortium (2004) Prevalence, severity, and unmet need for treatment of mental disorders in the world health organization world mental health surveys. *JAMA* **291**: 2581–90.

World Health Organization (2003) *Advocacy for Mental Health.* Geneva: WHO.

World Health Organization (2005) *Mental Health Atlas 2005.* Geneva: WHO.

Chapter

9

Stigmatization and exclusion

Ramachandran Padmavati

> The stigma attached to mental illness is the greatest obstacle to the improvement of the lives of people with mental illness and their families.
> *(Kadri & Sartorius 2005)*

Introduction

Stigma has been described by Goffman (1963) as an attribute of people who are stigmatized – "an attribute that is deeply discrediting." Stigma is a reflection of the way people relate to one another or the way society relates to a person or group of people. Social exclusion is a multidimensional process of progressive social rupture, detaching groups and individuals from social relations and institutions and preventing them from full participation in the normal, normatively prescribed activities of the society in which they live. Exclusion implies that discrimination occurs through individual (or group) prejudice or institutionally mediated processes. According to Jacobsson (2002), the negative stigmatization process that finally results in discrimination and exclusion of persons with mental illness is the outcome of a more or less conscious continuous evaluation of persons who are perceived as "different."

While cultural differences determine the ways in which stigma manifests, there are certain common universal effects seen. The practical result of discrimination is the everyday avoidance of people with mental illness. They experience social exclusion in a multiplicity of domains, including high rates of unemployment, lower educational achievement, persistent poverty, the loss of friendships, kinship, denial of housing, and rejection by their neighbors. Self-stigma occurs when persons with mental illness internalize stigma and experience diminished self-esteem and self-efficacy

(Watson *et al.* 2007). This results in people not pursuing opportunities, advocating for entitlements, or accessing mainstream activities. Social isolation, loss of family supports, and unemployment all contribute to a worsening in mental health and increase an already high risk for suicide. There is a lack choice and limited access to community, rehabilitation, and treatment supports. People with mental health issues are more likely to have their human rights violated through the use of seclusion, restraints, involuntary admissions, and forced treatments, along with experiencing losses of personal and parental rights. Many people with mental illness are so accustomed to these rejections that they have stopped making the effort to meet new people. But a lack of adequate social networks for themselves can increase the chances of relapse and reduce overall recovery. Thus, stigma can be seen as a culturally induced barrier to recovery.

An exhaustive literature on the subject of stigma over the years has demonstrated the pervasive negative attitudes and discriminatory treatment towards people with mental illness. This chapter focuses on the relationship to stigma from a cultural perspective across the globe. It is not intended as a complete review of all cultural research on stigma, but aims to provide some insights into the processes, with special focus on low- and middle-income countries (LMICs). Issues pertaining to marriage, divorce, work, and media are covered, and the stigma associated with mental health professionals is briefly touched upon. The role of laws and policies is not dealt with in this chapter, as it warrants an entire section.

As one of the most chronic and disabling conditions, schizophrenia has been a "difficult-to-understand" mental disorder since ancient times. Throughout history, and in practically every culture,

---

Essentials of Global Mental Health, ed. Samuel O. Okpaku. Published by Cambridge University Press. © Cambridge University Press 2014.

groups of persons with schizophrenia, including mental patients, have been stigmatized. The reasons for this remain obscure. People with this illness suffer with a loss of individual potential and personal anguish, resulting in significant psychological and social consequences. The latter signifies stigmatization in a crucial way. Fernando (2006) aptly puts it as follows: "To designate someone as a 'schizophrenic' or 'psychotic' invalidates everything they do or say – designates them as 'alien' to society, not to be trusted, not to be taken seriously."

Descriptions through history

Several features in people with mental disorders evoke these negative emotions and reactions. It is obvious that a psychotic, badly dressed, bad-smelling, aggressive, and disturbing person evokes feelings of disgust as well as fear and runs the risk of discrimination and exclusion. These descriptions have been noted over centuries; the stigma of mental illness is probably as old as the civilization itself.

In the ancient texts of Ayurveda, there are detailed descriptions of mental disorders known as *unmada*, and schizophrenia can be correlated with many of the types of *unmada*. Ayurvedic physicians describe schizophrenia as a disorder of the mind caused by the doshas (vata, kapha, and vata) moving in the wrong paths due to increased toxicity. According to the classical Ayurvedic texts, the *Charaka Samhita*, insanity is defined as "the perversion of the mind, intellect, consciousness, knowledge, memory, desire, manners, behavior, and conduct." It is denominated as insanity (*unmada*) because it is madness (*mada*) of the mind caused by a deviation (*unmada*) of the humors (Swami Sadashiva Tirtha 1998). The important thing to note, however, is that insanity is not being specifically discriminated but is considered a kind of disability and mentioned along with other physical disabilities and socially or religiously disapproved behavior (Wig 1997).

Contrarily, there are references to insanity from biblical times that are now recognized as stigmatizing. King Nebuchadnezzar was "punished by God for his vanity, cast out from among men," and on his return to society declared "my reason was restored to me." Similarly, in the fourth century BC, Plato likened injustice to madness, and sickness of the psyche was equated to vice. The historical roots to our thinking that mental disorders reflect moral failings, religious corruptions, or a threat to social cohesion have been described extensively (quoted in Thornicroft 2006)

Stigma across cultures

Psychiatric stigma is reported to occur in most societies. Difficulties arise in understanding how and to what extent this occurs in various cultural settings (Fabrega 1991). For example, since most non-Western cultural traditions handle illness in an integrated way without differentiating it along psychiatric versus non-psychiatric lines (as in the West), the matter of stigma attached to psychiatric illness is difficult to evaluate. Murthy (2002) notes that stigmatization of mental illness probably exists everywhere, even though the form and nature of it may differ across cultures

Direct discrimination against individuals with schizophrenia

Although stigma is generally conceptualized as an attribute of a person, a group of people, or a "thing" such as an illness, Goffman (1963) makes the point that "a language of relationships, not attributes, is really needed" in understanding stigma. In other words, "the process of stigmatization revolves around exclusion of particular individuals from certain types of social interactions" (Kurzban & Leary 2001). Social psychological models highlight that direct discrimination from individuals is the most readily observable mechanism in the stigma process (Crocker 1998, Major & O'Brien 2005). Sources of direct discrimination are diverse; discrimination can stem from community members, employers, mental health caregivers, family members, and friends (Wahl 1999, Dickerson *et al.* 2002).

Research from Western societies strongly corroborates that people with schizophrenia *experience direct discrimination from others* on the individual level. Such discrimination may impact health outcomes as overtly as denying equal access to medical care (Druss *et al.* 2000). Yet people with schizophrenia also suffer psychologically from other forms of interpersonal rejection and discrimination. An American outpatient survey of patients with a schizophrenia spectrum disorder reported being treated as less competent by others or being shunned and avoided (Dickerson *et al.* 2002). This type of directly experienced stigma has been shown to negatively impact both positive and negative self-esteem by affecting perceptions of mastery among a sample of schizophrenic outpatients (Wright *et al.* 2000).

It has been suggested that mental illness may be less stigmatized in developing countries, but there are no convincing data on this point. On the contrary, several research studies point to the fact that mentally ill people in developing countries do experience stigma and discrimination.

In the outpatient services operated by a non-governmental organization (NGO), the Schizophrenia Research Foundation in Chennai, South India, fear of rejection by neighbors and the need to hide the facts from others were some of the more stigmatizing aspects (Thara & Srinivasan 2000). In the same facility, one woman, who was under treatment for schizophrenia, reported that "My husband does not take me for any weddings or family functions. He tells me not to go to my daughter's school also. He says that because I am mentally ill, I cannot talk properly to outsiders." The stigma of accessing the outpatient services was sadly noted in the case of this Hindu woman, who would walk into the clinic clad in a *burkha*, an enveloping outer garment worn by women in some Islamic traditions to cover their bodies in public places, so that they cannot be identified.

In a study on outpatients with schizophrenia in Hong Kong, 59.7% of respondents anticipated that their partner would break up with him/her if he or she were to reveal the illness (Lee *et al.* 2005). In their study of 72 schizophrenic outpatients in Singapore, Lai *et al.* (2001) found that 51% thought that neighbors and colleagues would avoid them if they were aware of their illness.

There is widespread stigmatization of mental illness in the Nigerian community (Gureje *et al.* 2005). Negative attitudes to mental illness may be fueled by notions of causation that suggest that affected people are in some way responsible for their illness, and by fear. As many as 96.5% believed that people with mental illness are dangerous because of their violent behavior. Most would not tolerate even basic social contacts with a mentally ill person.

In Sri Lanka, social and cultural perspectives of stigma attached to mental disorders in both Sinhalese and Tamil communities contribute significantly to the problem. A cross-sectional study carried out among the academic and non-academic staff of the Faculty of Medicine, University of Kelaniya, Ragama, showed

that though prejudice and misconceptions toward completely recovered mentally ill patients were less, the social acceptance of incompletely recovered patients was low. This was seen more markedly with psychotic illnesses than with neurosis. In the same country, in certain rural communities, it may be more culturally acceptable to say that one was possessed by a supernatural power than to admit to being psychiatrically ill (Kuruppuarachchi & Lawrence 2005).

In a retrospective cross-sectional study of patients admitted to a psychiatry ward in Nepal, patients were assessed using a self-report questionnaire that focused on beliefs about discrimination against mental illness, rejection experiences, and ways of coping with stigma (Adhikari *et al.* 2008). Most of the patients were aware of the stigma associated with mental illness. There were experiences of rejection by family members, colleagues, and healthcare professionals. There were strong perceptions of stigmatization felt by patients in different social circumstances. Despite experiencing stigma, patients were generally treated fairly by other people.

Stigma and the caregivers of persons with mental illness

Stigma is also seen to affect the families of persons with mental illness. In a comparative study, it was found that 36% of caregivers in India, compared to 30% in Malaysia, felt that their relative's illness prevented them from having satisfying relationship with friends. One of the reasons for this could be due to stigma associated with mental illness (Talwar & Matheiken 2010). In a study of how patients and families experience direct discrimination from others, a substantial proportion of a sample of 1491 family members of schizophrenic patients in mainland China reported a "moderate" or "severe" effect of stigma on the patient and the family (Phillips *et al.* 2002). Similarly, a significant percentage of 320 schizophrenic outpatients in Hong Kong reported that they had been laid off after revealing their mental condition (44.5%) and that their family members had been treated unfairly due to their illness (41.1%) (Lee *et al.* 2005). These rates of direct discrimination, particularly toward family members (which suggest that relatives suffer severe "social contamination" due to their familial link to patients), are as high as or higher than rates reported in Western studies (Phelan *et al.* 1998, Wahl 1999).

In a study in Ethiopia, 178 relatives of individuals who were diagnosed as suffering from schizophrenia or major affective disorders in a community-based survey were interviewed using the Family Interview Schedule (Shibre *et al.* 2001). About 75% of the respondents perceived that they were stigmatized or had experienced some sort of stigma due to the presence of mental illness in the family, 42% were worried about being treated differently, and 37% wanted to conceal the fact that a relative was ill.

These results imply that the ethnocentric social beliefs in China (Yang 2007), India (Jadhav *et al.* 2007), or Ethiopia (Shibre *et al.* 2001) shape discrimination against the mentally ill at the individual and familial level.

Concealing to protect from exclusion

One common behavioral response by persons with schizophrenia, as well as their families, is to conceal the presence of a "mental" illness. The labeled individual, in addition to using cognitive coping strategies, responds *behaviorally* to anticipated social rejection through actions such as concealing one's treatment from others, or withdrawing from social contact, according to the "modified labeling theory" (Link *et al.* 1989). This leads the mentally ill to endorse secrecy as a predominant coping strategy over other forms (e.g., educating others that mental illness is like any other physical illness).

In a study of perceptions of and reactions to stigma among 156 parents and spouses of a sample of first-admission psychiatric patients, at least half the family members reported concealing the hospitalization at least to some degree, although the majority did not perceive themselves as being avoided by others because of their relative's hospitalization. Family members were more likely to conceal the mental illness if they did not live with their ill relative, if the relative was female, and if the relative had less severe positive symptoms (Phelan *et al.* 1998). Further examples of concealment are dealt with in relation to issues pertaining to marriage and employment.

Marriage and divorce

For persons with mental illnesses, social contexts such as marriage, divorce, or relationships are perhaps the most affected by stigma. Being mentally ill carries a connotation of shame and weakness of character, a shameful condition that causes the person or the family to lose face. This is particularly seen with reference to the issue of marriage.

A study of people with a diagnosis of mental illness, in five different European countries, found that two-thirds were effectively single and only 17% married, thereby concluding that having a diagnosis of mental illness could reduce a person's chances of marrying or staying married (Thornicroft *et al.* 2004). In contrast, Indian families believe marriage to be a cure for mental illnesses, and therefore a history of mental illness is concealed. A study in southern India found that 70% of young adults with a diagnosis of schizophrenia went on to marry in the following 10 years (Thara & Srinivasan 1997).

In many cultures, to have a mentally ill relative could damage the possibilities of advancement of the other members of the family, and might even harm the marriage prospects of other family members. The Vellore study on public attitudes found 65.3% of respondents objected to marital alliance the household of a mental patient (Verghese & Beig 1974). A study on attitudes of psychiatric patients themselves found that three-quarters in India were opposed to marital alliance (Malhotra *et al.* 1981).

Chinese views on the cause of mental illness are multifaceted. It may be regarded as moral transgressions towards ancestors or social norms whereby the family is also held responsible. Alternatively, it can be attributed to hereditary or even ancestral inheritance of misconduct, so that sufferers, and sometimes even their siblings, are traditionally excluded from marriage (Ng 1997).

Divorce and patterns of separation show striking cultural patterns

The social, psychological, and cultural concomitance of being mentally ill and divorced/separated is particularly severe in the Indian culture (Nambi 2005). In addition to the stress of mental illness, hostility from family members, and rejection from society in general, women in particular are ridiculed and ostracized for their divorced/separated status. Interviews with women with a diagnosis of schizophrenia in southern India found that despite no longer living in the marital home, many of them were not legally separated, nor were they receiving maintenance from their husbands. The stigma attached to separation was as distressing as that of being mentally ill, if not more so. Even several years after separation, these women still harbored the hope that they would eventually reunite with their husbands (Thara *et al.* 2003a). Furthermore, for the families (primarily aging parents), the emotional, financial, and physical burden of caring for a severely mentally ill woman is extremely high (Thara *et al.* 2003b).

In the 1980s, people with schizophrenia in China experienced divorce rates nearly 10 times the population norm (Phillips 1993). In Hong Kong about a third reported that their partner broke up with them because of their mental illness or attributed their divorce to their illness (Lee *et al.* 2005). The researchers reported the following anecdotal evidence to describe the severance of a marital relationship: "A 50-year-old participant reported having been abandoned: his wife and his daughter did not visit him in hospital, and a few months later he received a letter demanding a divorce. He never saw them again."

Friendships and intimate relationships in persons with mental illnesses have aroused very little research interest (Thornicroft 2006, p. 27). Key findings include small social networks, more dependent rather than interdependent relationships, social contacts consisting of other users or staff at mental health facilities (Beels 1984, Dunn 1990), or parents having negative views about partners (Desapriya & Nobutada 2002).

Stigma at work

Work is a major determinant of mental health and a socially integrating force. To be excluded from the workforce creates material deprivation, erodes self-confidence, creates a sense of isolation and marginalization, and is a key risk factor for mental disability. Stigmatizing views held by employers make it difficult for people with mental disabilities to enter the competitive workforce.

Discrimination in the workplace drives the low employment rate among people with severe mental illness (Stuart 2006, Latimer 2008). People with mental health problems both have a lower rate of employment than other disabled groups and are more likely than other groups to want to be in employment (Grove 1999).

Finding work as well as keeping work are seen as areas where stigma and discrimination can be a major barrier. People with mental disorders identify employment discrimination as one of their most frequent stigma experiences (Gaebel *et al.* 2005). Compared with individuals with physical disabilities, twice as many people with mental disabilities (the majority)

expect to experience employment-related stigma (Roeloffs *et al.* 2003). One in three mental health consumers in the United States report being turned down for a job once their psychiatric status became known, and in some cases job offers were rescinded when a psychiatric history was revealed (Wahl 1999).

Fear of stigma and rejection by prospective employers may undermine confidence and result in a poorer showing on job interviews. Concealment of mental illness is far more common in efforts at finding jobs or in keeping jobs. In a study of 320 schizophrenic outpatients in Hong Kong, 69.7% of respondents agreed that their chance of being promoted at work would be affected by revealing their mental illness (Lee *et al.* 2005). Chinese immigrants who enter the USA illegally are offered no such protection and thus rely heavily upon secrecy to maintain employment (Chou 2004). In India too, it is not uncommon for persons with schizophrenia to hide their illness status when applying for a job. Loganathan and Murthy (2011) noted that men with schizophrenia reported hiding their illness in job applications, and from others. Patients taking treatment at the Schizophrenia Research Foundation frequently reported being unable to get jobs if mental illness was disclosed. The job placement services at the vocational training center in the same organization faced difficulties in placing patients. Prospective employers wished to hide the problem of mental illness from other employees. They expressed concerns about how others would respond both to behavioral problems in the patient and to their relatively lesser productivity. Over time, people with mental disorders may come to view themselves as unemployable and stop seeking work altogether (Wahl 1999).

Stigma and the media

The news media and the entertainment industry have a critical role to play in informing public opinion. Together and separately, they can either perpetuate the stigma and misunderstanding surrounding mental illness or work to reduce it. Deep-rooted prejudice toward mental illness is entrenched in society, a prominent stereotype being that persons with mental illness are dangerous or unpredictable. Reinforcement of these popular myths through the media perpetuates the stigma surrounding mental illness, precipitating shame, self-blame, and secrecy, all of which discourage affected individuals from seeking treatment (Benbow 2007). Wig (1997) wrote of the "unfortunate role which media in India like cinema, TV, or press, has played in perpetuating the prejudice against mental disorders. Mental illness is always shown as something to ridicule, something to laugh at, or something which is bizarre, disgusting."

Media coverage of mental health can be technically accurate yet misleading, over-reporting negative stories about people with mental illness, or leaving out important data, thus skewing public understanding in the implied link between mental illness and violence. In cinema and television, mental illness is the substrate for comedy, more usually laughing *at* than laughing *with* the characters (Byrne 1997). Indian films are noted to portray mental disorders in the form of crude comedy, showing the victim of mental illness as an object of derision (Pandve & Banerjee 2007).

Further, media gets its information from experts such as psychiatrists, psychologists, or policy makers. The virtual exclusion of the voices of mental health consumers in the press gives the public the misleading impression that the mentally ill are too disturbed and dysfunctional to speak for themselves.

Society is ingrained with prejudice toward mental illness, and sufferers are often widely perceived to be dangerous or unpredictable. The rare person with schizophrenia who acts violently and gets arrested is far more likely to find himself on the front page of a local newspaper than a drunken man who gets into brawl in the middle of the street.

Stigma and the mental health professional

The stigma surrounding mental illness is seen to affect mental health professionals as well. Stanley (2004), as a first-year resident, described the "constant challenge to overcome the stigma associated with becoming a psychiatrist, not just from colleagues, but from family and friends as well."

The attitudes and experiences of mental health professionals have been sparingly studied. In a simple survey at Catawba Hospital in Virginia, USA, 50 clinical staff, including psychiatrists, psychologists, social workers, adjunctive therapists, and nursing staff, were asked to complete a written questionnaire with a yes/no response. "If you were to be diagnosed with schizophrenia, would you be uncomfortable talking about it to a nonprofessional (such as friends or acquaintances)?" "If you answered 'Yes,' is it

because of stigma?" The responses were obtained anonymously. Thirty respondents (60%) said that they would be uncomfortable talking about it to friends and acquaintances. Seventeen (34%) said that it was because of stigma. This brief survey highlighted the feelings of discomfort even professionals experience with a psychiatric diagnosis such as schizophrenia. It is interesting that a third of the respondents perceived stigma. The researchers opined that mental health professionals may be practicing a double standard – expecting consumers and the public to cast off their stigmatizing beliefs but harboring those beliefs themselves (Sriram & Jabbapour 2005).

Similar findings were seen in another survey. In a postal survey of doctors' attitudes to becoming mentally ill in Birmingham, nearly three-quarters (73%) of doctors said they would not seek professional help for mental health problems for fear of damaging their career (33%) or their professional reputation (30%), and because of the perceived stigma of having a mental health problem (20%) (Hassan *et al.* 2009).

In personal conversations, psychiatrists working with the Schizophrenia Research Foundation in Chennai, South India, reported stigma manifested in various ways. Other medical fraternity often had disparaging views of psychiatry and psychiatrists in general, while paradoxically approaching the psychiatrist for personal help in "secrecy." One psychiatrist reported on the comments of a former classmate who is now a surgeon, "You psychiatrists only sedate people." Invitations to social functions from patients and their families were often post-fixed with "Oh, we know you will be too busy to come, doc!" Concealing one's own profession as a psychiatrist in social settings was reported, the reason being the "fear of being scoffed at." The myth that "psychiatrists themselves will become psychiatrically ill in the long run" was common. One colleague, a clinical psychologist, reported difficulties in marriage alliances for siblings.

Conclusion

Stigma is perhaps the major barrier explaining why persons with serious mental illnesses and their carers, especially in LMIC countries, are not able to lead the lives they want to, to hold jobs in keeping with their skills, to socialize, to enjoy their rights as citizens. Stigma is the basis of social exclusion and alienation. Social and cultural dimensions need to be addressed, in addition to policy changes, in order to undo the impact of stigma.

References

Adhikari SR, Pradhan SN, Sharma SC (2008) Experiencing stigma: Nepalese perspectives. *Kathmandu University Medical Journal* **6**: 458–65.

Beels CC, Gutwirth L, Berkeley J, Struening E (1984) Measurements of social support in schizophrenia. *Schizophrenia Bulletin* **10**: 399–411.

Benbow A (2007) Mental illness, stigma and the media. *Journal of Clinical Psychiatry* 2007; **68** (Suppl 2): 31–5.

Byrne P (1997) Psychiatric stigma: past, passing and to come. *Journal of the Royal Society of Medicine* **90**: 618–20.

Chou YW (2004) How stigma manifests in the clinical encounter: case examples among immigrant Chinese-Americans. *Symposium presented at the Asian-American Psychological Association. Honolulu, HI, 2004. In LH Yang, ed., Application of mental illness stigma theory to Chinese societies: synthesis and new directions Singapore Medical Journal* **48**: 977–85.

Crocker J, Major B, Steele C (1998) Social stigma. In D Gilbert, S Fiske, G Lindze, eds., *Handbook of Social Psychology*, 4th edn. Boston, MA: McGraw-Hill; pp. 504–53.

Desapriya EB, Nobutada I (2002) Stigma of mental illness in Japan. *Lancet* **359**: 1866.

Dickerson FB, Sommerville J, Origoni AE, Ringel NB, Parente F (2002) Experiences of stigma among outpatients with schizophrenia. *Schizophrenia Bulletin* **28**: 143–55.

Dunn M, O'Driscoll C, Dayson D, Wills W, Leff J (1990) The TAPS project, 4: An observational study of the social lives of long stay patients. *British Journal of Psychiatry* **157**: 842–8, 852.

Druss BG, Marcus SC, Rosenheck RA, *et al.* (2000) Understanding disability in mental and general medical conditions. *American Journal of Psychiatry* **157**: 1485–91.

Fabrega H (1991) Psychiatric stigma in non-western societies. *Comprehensive Psychiatry* **32**: 534–51.

Fernando S (2006) Stigma, racism and power. *Aotearoa Ethnic Network Journal* **1** (1): 24–8.

Fink PJ, Tasman A (1992) *Stigma and Mental Illness*. Washington, DC: American Psychiatric Press.

Gaebel W, Bauman AE, Zäske H (2005) Intervening in a multilevel network: progress of the German Open the Doors projects. *World Psychiatry* **4** (Suppl 1): 16–20.

Goffman E (1963) *Stigma: Notes on the Management of Spoiled Identity*. Englewood Cliffs, NJ: Prentice Hall.

Grove B (1999) Mental health and employment: shaping a new agenda. *Journal of Mental Health* **8**: 131–40.

Gureje O, Lasebikan VO, Ephraim-Oluwanuga O, Olley BO, Kola L (2005) Community study of knowledge of and attitude to mental illness in Nigeria. *British Journal of Psychiatry* **186**: 436–41.

Hassan TM, Ahmed SO, White AC, *et al.* (2009). A postal survey of doctors' attitudes to becoming mentally ill. *Clinical Medicine* **9**: 327–32.

Jacobsson L (2002) The roots of stigmatization. *World Psychiatry* **1** (1): 25.

Jadhav S, Littlewood R, Ryder AG, *et al.* (2007) Stigmatization of severe mental illness in India: Against the simple industrialization hypothesis. *Indian Journal of Psychiatry* **49**: 189–94.

Kadri N, Sartorius N (2005) The global fight against the stigma of schizophrenia. *PLoS Medicine* **2** (7): e136.

Kuruppuarachchi LA, Lawrence TS (2005) Stigma in developing countries: Sri Lanka. *British Journal of Psychiatry*. http://bjp.rcpsych.org/content/186/5/436/reply (accessed January 2012).

Kurzban R, Leary MR (2001) Evolutionary origins of stigmatization: the functions of social exclusion. *Psychological Bulletin* **127** (2): 187–208.

Lai YM, Hong CP, Chee CY (2001) Stigma of mental illness. *Singapore Medical Journal* **42**: 111–14.

Latimer EA (2008) Individual placement and support programme increases rates of obtaining employment in people with severe mental illness. *Evidence-Based Mental Health* **11**: 52.

Lee S, Lee MT, Chiu MY, Kleinman A (2005) Experience of social stigma by people with schizophrenia in Hong Kong. *British Journal of Psychiatry* **186**: 153–7.

Link BG, Cullen FT, Struening E, Shrout PE, Dohrenwend BP (1989) A modified labeling theory approach to mental disorders: an empirical assessment. *American Sociological Review* 1989; **54**: 400–23.

Loganathan S, Murthy RS (2011) Living with schizophrenia in India: gender perspectives. *Transcultural Psychiatry* **48**: 569–84.

Major B, O'Brien LT (2005) The social psychology of stigma. *Annual Review of Psychology* **56**: 393–421.

Malhotra HK, Inam AS, Chopra HD (1981) Do the psychiatric patients reject themselves? *Indian Journal of Psychiatry* **23**: 44–8.

Murthy RS (2002) Stigma is universal but experiences are local. *World Psychiatry* **1**: 28.

Nambi S (2005) Marriage, mental health and the Indian legislation. *Indian Journal of Psychiatry* **47** (1): 3–14.

Ng CH (1997) The stigma of mental illness in Asian cultures. *Australian and New Zealand Journal of Psychiatry* **31**: 382–90.

Pandve H, Bannerjee A (2007) Do popular media such as movies aggravate the stigma of mental disorders? *Indian Journal of Psychiatry* **49**: 144.

Phelan CJ, Brome EJ, Link BQ (1998) Psychiatric illness and family stigma. *Schizophrenia Bulletin* **24**: 115–26.

Phillips MR (1993) Strategies used by Chinese families in coping with schizophrenia. In D Davis, S Harrell, eds., *Chinese Families in the 1980s*. Berkeley & Los Angeles, CA: University of California Press.

Phillips MR, Pearson V, Li F, Xu M, Yang L (2002) Stigma and expressed emotion: a study of people with schizophrenia and their family members in China. *British Journal of Psychiatry* **181**: 488–93.

Roeloffs CC, Sherbourne J, Unützer A, *et al*. (2003) Stigma and depression among primary care patients. *General Hospital Psychiatry* **25**: 311–15.

Shibre T, Negash A, Kullgren G, *et al*. (2001) Perception of stigma among family members of individuals with schizophrenia and major affective disorders in rural Ethiopia. *Social Psychiatry and Psychiatric Epidemiology* **36** (6): 299–303.

Sriram TG, Jabbarpour YM (2005) Are mental health professionals immune to stigmatizing beliefs? *Psychiatric Services* **56**: 610.

Stanley C (2004) Overcoming psychiatry's stigma: taking pride in healing the mind. *The New Physician* **53** (8).

Stuart H (2006) Mental illness and employment discrimination. *Current Opinion in Psychiatry* **19**: 522–6.

Swami Sadashiva Tirtha (1998) *The Ayurveda Encyclopedia: Natural Secrets to Healing, Prevention, & Longevity*. Bayville, NY: Ayurveda Holistic Center Press.

Talwar P, Matheiken ST (2010) Caregivers in schizophrenia: a cross-cultural perspective. *Indian Journal of Psychological Medicine* **32**: 29–33.

Thara R, Srinivasan TN (1997) Outcome of marriage in schizophrenia. *Social Psychiatry and Psychiatric Epidemiology* **32** (7): 416–20.

Thara R, Srinivasan TN (2000) How stigmatising is schizophrenia in India? *International Journal of Social Psychiatry* **46** (2): **135**–41.

Thara R, Kamath S, Kumar S (2003a) Women with schizophrenia and broken marriages: doubly disadvantaged? Part I: Patient perspective. *International Journal of Social Psychiatry* **49** (3): 225–32.

Thara R, Kamath S, Kumar S (2003b) Women with schizophrenia and broken marriages: doubly disadvantaged? Part II: Family perspective. *International Journal of Social Psychiatry* **49** (3): 233–40.

Thornicroft G, Tansella M, Becker T, *et al*. (2004) The personal impact of schizophrenia in Europe. *Schizophrenia Research* **69** (2–3): 125–32.

Thornicroft G (2006) *Shunned: Discrimination Against People with Mental Illness*. Oxford: Oxford University Press.

Verghese A, Beig A (1974) Public attitudes towards mental illness: the Vellore study. *Indian Journal of Psychiatry* **16**: 8–18.

Wahl OF (1999) Mental health consumers' experience of stigma. *Schizophrenia Bulletin* **25**: 467–78.

Watson AC, Corrigan P, Larsson JE, Sells M (2007) Self stigma in people with mental illness. *Schizophrenia Bulletin* **33**: 1312–18.

Wig NN (1997) Stigma against mental illness. *Indian Journal of Psychiatry* **39** (3): 187–9.

Wright ER, Gronfein WP, Owens TJ (2000) Deinstitutionalization, social rejection, and the self-esteem of former mental patients. *Journal of Health and Social Behavior* **41**: 68–90.

Yang LH (2007) Application of mental illness stigma theory to Chinese societies: synthesis and new directions. *Singapore Medical Journal* **48**: 977–85.

Chapter

10

Grassroots movements in mental health

Chris Underhill, Sarah Kippen Wood, Jordan Pfau, and Shoba Raja

Introduction

A grassroots movement is one driven by the creation of a community in a natural and spontaneous way. Behind many of the greatest advances to the human condition lie powerful grassroots movements. These movements begin as people with a shared interest or identity come together, rejecting traditional stereotypes and realizing that their marginalized status is a consequence of the system's failures, rather than their own personal failures (Klein 1984). Throughout history, such movements have influenced key shifts in thinking toward some of the most vulnerable members of society. From women's rights to African-American civil rights to disability rights, grassroots movements developed as dynamic leaders emerged from within historically disempowered groups, leading others to recognize their own rights and act. While some grassroots movements have resulted in immediate, dramatic changes, the global mental health movement perhaps exemplifies a slow-burning persistent approach to change.

Mental health movements

People with mental illness represent one of the most marginalized groups in society, often isolated and deprived of basic rights (Kleinman 2009). In many countries, the focus for delivering mental health care has traditionally been centralized in large-scale residential institutions, where gross human rights abuses have historically been very common. Outside of institutions, individuals still face stigma and discrimination (World Health Organization 2007). This furthers their descent into poverty and reduces their chances of receiving care. Therefore, deinstitutionalization has been a focus of mental health advocates for

many years. In the 1950s, appalling conditions in hospitals began to be exposed. As people shared their stories, the media caught on and the movement grew.

Some of the most prominent international groups of affected individuals have perceptions about mental health reform that differ considerably from those held by practitioner groups such as the World Health Organization (WHO) and the Pan American Health Organization (PAHO). They feel that people with mental illness should be involved in the decision making, and oppose the power practitioners hold over peoples' lives (Desai 2005). The World Network of Users and Survivors of Psychiatry (WNUSP) has led a movement which has been very critical of psychiatric practice in many countries. They have strongly advocated against involuntary hospitalization and certain forms of treatment that they consider unconscionable. MindFreedom International was created to form an international coalition of grassroots psychiatric survivor groups (MindFreedom International 2012). Likewise, the International Disability Alliance (IDA) works to ensure that practitioners comply with the UN Convention on the Rights of Persons with Disabilities (International Disability Alliance 2012).

The International League Against Epilepsy (ILAE), established with 16 participant countries, seeks to raise awareness, promote research, and improve services for patients in the diagnosis and prevention of epilepsy. In 1997, ILAE partnered with the WHO and the International Bureau for Epilepsy to launch a global awareness campaign (International League Against Epilepsy 2010). Despite these varied perspectives, each has aimed to strengthen the rights of individuals with mental illness and epilepsy. Figure 10.1 shows a timeline of key mental health movement events over the last 50 years.

Essentials of Global Mental Health, ed. Samuel O. Okpaku. Published by Cambridge University Press. © Cambridge University Press 2014.

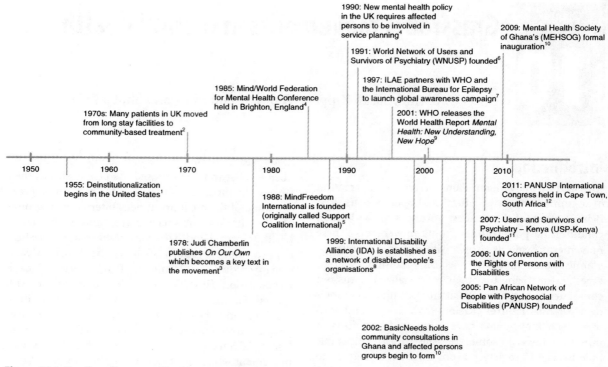

Figure 10.1 Timeline of key mental health movement events since 1950.

References

1. Torrey EF (1997) *Out of the Shadows: Confronting America's Mental Illness Crisis*. New York, NY: Wiley.

2. Mind (2012) The history of mental health and community care: key dates. www.mind.org.uk/help/research_and_policy/ the_history_of_mental_health_and_community_care-key_dates.

3. Shapiro J (2010) Advocate for people with mental illness dies. *National Public Radio*, January 19, 2010. http://www.npr.org/templates/ story/story.php?storyId=122706192.

4. Wallcraft J, Bryant M (2003) The mental health service user movement in England. The Sainsbury Centre for Mental Health. http://www. centreformentalhealth.org.uk/pdfs/policy_paper2_service_user_movement.pdf.

5. MindFreedom International (2012) About David W. Oaks, MindFreedom International Executive Director. http://www.mindfreedom.org/ about-us/david-w-oaks.

6. Amegatcher J (2007) The UN Convention on the Rights of Persons With Disabilities: a rights-based approach to development. *WNUSP News*, June 2007. http://www.enusp.org/wnusp-newsletter-2007-3.pdf.

7. International League Against Epilepsy (2010) *2010 Annual Report*. http://www.ilae.org/Visitors/Documents/ILAEAnnual- Report2010Final_000.pdf.

8. International Disability Alliance (2012) About us. http://www.internationaldisabilityalliance.org/en/about-us.

9. World Health Organization (2001) *The World Health Report 2001. Mental Health: New Understanding, New Hope*. Geneva: WHO

10. Yaro, P. and Menil, V. (2005). Lessons from the African User Movement: The Case of Ghana. In Community Mental Health Care in Low- Income Countries: A Way Forward, eds. Barbato, A. and Vallarino, M. Italy: Press Milan.

11. Keter SC. Interviewed by J. Pfau (February 2, 2012).

12. Pan African Network of People with Psychosocial Disabilities (2011) Announcement 27 October. http://www.panusp.org/wp-content/ uploads/2011/10/2_1_Announcement%20_October_2011.pdf.

National and regional mental health movements

If a group is inspired, motivated and encouraged it will analyse its own problems and after reflection, act!

(Underhill 1996)

Despite the often uphill human rights battle that lies before individuals with mental illness, pioneering individuals and groups have been inspired to act, organizing grassroots movements of affected individuals in a wide variety of contexts. This chapter follows two dynamic country movements in the UK and Ghana, as well as the Pan African Network of People with Psychosocial Disabilities (PANUSP) regional movement, highlighting some of the challenges experienced and critical successes achieved.

United Kingdom

I felt that I couldn't speak about my experience because nobody wanted to listen. But as I started re-evaluating, I realized that wasn't right. I wanted to find others and start talking.

(Dr. Jan Wallcraft – service user/researcher, University of Birmingham, interviewed by Jordan Pfau, February 2012)

Mental health services in the United Kingdom over the past 200 years have fallen short, and major concerns about human rights violations in psychiatric hospitals provided grounds for a grassroots movement (Hervey 1986). Activists were addressing the human rights violations in the system as early as the 1800s. Involuntary confinement was a common practice at the time, and people faced solitary confinement, cold baths, and other inhumane treatment. In the 1840s, former patients of psychiatric hospitals came together as the Alleged Lunatics' Friend Society to publicize the treatment they had received (Hervey 1986). Over 100 years later, in the 1970s, the government enacted several policies that shifted mental health care away from long-stay facilities and placed more focus on the community. This, however, was not the end to human rights abuses for those with mental illness. Stigma, lack of social support, and disregard for patient input in their treatment were ever present.

As people were moved into community-based settings, conversations began to occur at local levels in places such as day centers and hospitals. It was here that many groups critical of the current mental health situation in the country began to form. At this time, other grassroots movements, such as the feminist movement, the gay and lesbian movement, and the disability movement, were developing around the UK. Adding mental health to the conversation was a natural thing. The groups that began to form were various – there were groups for women in mental health, manic depression/bipolar groups, groups for people coming off tranquilizers, groups for carers, and more. These groups provided not only a support system, but also a place to advocate for change (J. Wallcraft, interviewed February 2012).

Growth of the movement

As the movement developed, it increasingly used the media to spread the message of discontent with the psychiatric system. Television programs, newspapers, newsletters, and other media were used, and people stepped forward to share personal experiences (Wallcraft & Bryant 2003). In 1978, after being involuntarily confined in a mental institution in the United States of America, Judi Chamberlin published *On Our Own*, which became a sort of manifesto for the movement both in the USA and abroad (Shapiro 2010). In the UK, the book helped spur other newsletters and publications in which people shared their own experiences. The services available in the country came into the spotlight and were critically examined. Four mental health service networks comprising affected individuals emerged across the groups to create a unified voice for change. The 1985 Mind/World Federation for Mental Health Conference further stimulated the movement, as grassroots groups from the USA and the Netherlands met with those in the UK to discuss their shared goals (Wallcraft and Bryant 2003).

Achievements and challenges

In 1990, there were several changes in mental health policy as a result of the movement's work. The first was the National Health Service and Community Care Act, which established a requirement that people with mental illness be involved in service planning. This was an important step in the right direction and represents a shift in the government's thinking about mental illness and the involvement of those with mental illness. Three subsequent policies were enacted at the end of the 1990s to map out mental health service delivery over the next 10 years. They emphasized the role of people with mental illness as key stakeholders expressing their needs (Wallcraft & Bryant 2003).

In 2008, the mental health charity called Mind launched a large awareness campaign, attempting to involve 10 000 people in advocating for mental health. The campaign was supported by celebrities (Mind 2008). The National Survivor User Network (NSUN) also received funding. With a national network now in place, participants in the movement are in better contact with each other and there is improved oversight and organization (J. Wallcraft, interviewed February 2012). While conditions of care have improved with the closing of institutions, those with mental illness are focused on their entire well-being. This includes reducing stigma and increasing employment opportunities, access to benefits, and full inclusion in society (Wallcraft & Bryant 2003).

The mental health movement in England has provided a voice for those with mental illness, but still faces many challenges. Some recent government policies are putting more restrictions on rights, including forcing people to work, changes to welfare benefits, and other policies that are affecting all disabled people. The Mental Health Act of 2007 allows psychiatrists to make decisions on behalf of adults who they feel lack the capacity to make decisions for themselves. This may include forcing people to take medications or receive treatments against their will, and people may be forced into hospitals if they refuse to do so. The Mental Capacity Act of 2005 in theory gives people the right to refuse treatment and allows them to designate someone to make decisions for them if they become incapacitated, but the new Mental Health Act of 2007 allows psychiatrists to override that provision (J. Wallcraft, interviewed February 2012). These changes are frustrating for the movement, which is trying to fight for rights but is now seeing more rights taken away.

There are also challenges within the movement, where certain minority groups and women are often under-represented, and differing viewpoints can cause tensions. Some groups accept funding from a range of donors including pharmaceutical companies, while others prefer to remain independent. There are differing viewpoints about psychiatry, with some groups feeling that the care they receive is satisfactory, and others feeling that their needs are not being respected or addressed. The movement continues to evolve, yet the core message of promoting human rights, social inclusion, and allowing people to have a voice for themselves remains at the center of its activities. As Jan Wallcraft, a service user and movement researcher, explains:

> Human rights are still not doing very well at the moment. We need to make more noise. There's no way the government will make the changes we want unless we demand it. Everybody deserves the right to an advocate to help them speak up when they need to negotiate services and get support. This is the primary right that we are pushing for.
>
> (J. Wallcraft, interviewed February 2012)

Ghana

> Living in a poor district with very poor health care services, the movement [MEHSOG] advocates regular community-based treatment for its members. It also seeks to promote access to opportunities to engage in income generation activities for its members, and I have personally benefited from this.
>
> (Alhassan Yakubu, Secretary at Ti Bi Gangso Mental
>
> Association, Zabzugu District, interviewed by D. A. Yahaya, February 2012)

The mental health movement in Ghana is more recent, but has grown dramatically from its inception at the grassroots level, to the creation of a national body, providing an interesting case for the affected individual-led movements. The mental health care available in the country has not been able to meet the needs of the population, and most of the services are focused in the capital city in the south. Few people want to receive training to work in mental health because of the stigma that exists. Community psychiatric nurses (CPNs) have been trained by the government and posted to various regions, but they are not able to diagnose patients and are unable to meet all of the mental health needs (Yaro et al. 2005). To add to this, 60% of the 20 CPNs in the north are almost near retiring age, which will leave many without any care at all (Yaro & Menil 2005).

Because of the lack of services available, particularly in the north, BasicNeeds, an international mental health non-governmental organization (NGO), set up its field program here in 2002, and held several community consultation meetings to get feedback on the mental health needs. It was during these consultations that individuals with mental illness and epilepsy first met one another. From these introductions, self-help groups began to form (Peter Yaro, interviewed by Jordan Pfau, November 2011).

Growth of the movement

These groups gained momentum as members identified and reached out to other potential members. Members informed others in the community of the mental health services and outreach clinics available by speaking at community centers, churches, and mosques, and utilizing local media channels. The network of people participating began to spread as they encouraged more people to participate (Yaro & Menil 2005).

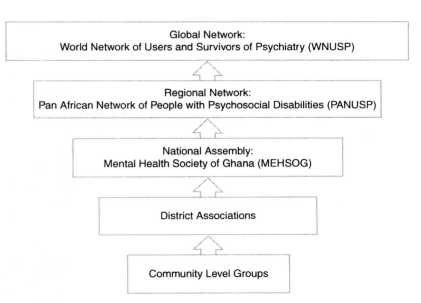

Global Network:
World Network of Users and Survivors of Psychiatry (WNUSP)

Regional Network:
Pan African Network of People with Psychosocial Disabilities (PANUSP)

National Assembly:
Mental Health Society of Ghana (MEHSOG)

District Associations

Community Level Groups

Figure 10.2 Mental health self-help groups in Ghana: structure and links.

As the community groups grew in number, district-level groups were formed to interact with District Assemblies and local authorities, allowing for a more unified stance and increased advocacy on issues relating to mental health. The district groups grew into a more formal structure known as the District Association of Self Help Groups. Members of the District Association are elected representatives of the community groups. Among other things, they conduct community outreach education programs, assist groups with funding and registration, and liaise with the Departments of Community Development and Social Welfare to represent the community-level mental health self-help groups (Yaro & Menil 2005). Figure 10.2 shows the structure of the groups in Ghana and their links beyond Ghana.

Eventually, as members realized that their rights could not be fully enjoyed until they were recognized at the highest levels of government, the Mental Health Society of Ghana (MEHSOG) was formed with support from BasicNeeds. A national steering committee was constituted to preside over the adoption of a constitution and executive secretariat. MEHSOG completed its registration in 2009 (P. Yaro, interviewed November 2011).

MEHSOG is made up of representatives from the district associations and some community groups. Its members participate in meetings with government officials to solicit their support for upholding the human rights and dignity of those with mental illness

and epilepsy. At the group level, they help register members with the National Health Insurance Scheme, advocate for assistance from development organizations to provide funds for medicines, and support group members (A. Yakubu, interviewed February 2012). MEHSOG has built connections with other civil society organizations, such as the Network for Women's Rights in Ghana and the Ghana Federation of the Physically Disabled, which helps provide critical mass as they promote their collective causes. Newspapers, television, and radio stations have been supportive and provide a mouthpiece for spreading the message of the movement. Ghana's movement has grown and has since expanded its reach to both regional and global mental health networks (Yaro & Menil 2005). As of December 2010, over 13 000 people with mental illness and epilepsy or their carers were involved in self-help groups across 35 districts from four regions of Ghana (Raja *et al.* 2010).

Achievements and challenges

The groups are a place for people with mental illness and epilepsy and their carers to share their experiences and challenges. Some groups have participated in financial credit programs, which provide economic support. Members are thus encouraged to tackle their poverty as well as their mental illness. Historically this was difficult for someone with a mental illness, but as these individuals make contributions in their communities, stigma reduces. The movement in Ghana is different from the movement in the UK in that it exists in the context of poverty, presenting a unique challenge for its members. Daily needs and survival can often take priority over advocacy or becoming involved in a movement. However, as group members receive help through treatment, peer support, and livelihood training, their confidence improves and they are in a better position to advocate for themselves. One member, who first joined a community group but has since been elected to a leadership role in his district association as part of MEHSOG, explained how his life has improved:

> Participating in MEHSOG has earned me recognition and respect in the community. It has given me a lot of exposure and increased my confidence to discuss issues that affect mentally ill people with authorities in the district . . . I got funds to undertake secure livelihood activities and this has improved my earnings. I used the funds to engage in farming in addition to my work as a teaching assistant and this has improved my income.
>
> (A. Yakubu, interviewed February 2012)

While the movement in Ghana has been significant, challenges at the grassroots level are ever-present. People with mental illness and epilepsy must first receive treatment and begin recovery before they can focus on advocacy or fueling a movement. Support on a very personal basis is key for many individuals, and healing is the first priority, but the shortage of qualified mental health workers and medicines, and the lack of funding present major barriers. Unfortunately, stigma does still persist, and many suffer from low self-esteem as a result (P. Yaro, interviewed November 2011). The movement still has a long way to go, but continues to take steps to improve human rights, beginning in the communities and expanding its reach nationally and even globally.

> MEHSOG is concerned about the frequent shortage of psychotropic and antiepileptic medicines . . . [We] will intensify [our] campaign for people with mental illness or epilepsy and their primary carers to be consulted on mental health issues, to be included in all levels of planning, and for a fair distribution of mental health professionals and infrastructure throughout Ghana.
>
> (A. Yakubu, interviewed February 2012)

PANUSP

We wish for a better world in which all people are treated equally, a world where human rights belong to everyone. We invite you to walk beside us. We know where we want to go.

(PANUSP 2011)

One of the regional mental health organizations in which MEHSOG participates is PANUSP, now known as the Pan African Network of People with Psychosocial Disabilities. It provides an example of how mental health movements can expand beyond country borders and local advocacy. In the 1970s, as affected individuals in North America and Europe were growing their own movements, a few scattered groups decided that there should be a worldwide network. In 1991, members from these groups met at the World Federation for Mental Health (WFMH) conference in Mexico, and the World Network of Users and Survivors of Psychiatry (WNUSP) was formed. WNUSP continued to spread, holding its second conference in Denmark in 2004. At this conference, members from mental health groups in Africa were present, and it was agreed that a regional organization specific to Africa was needed. A coordinator was appointed from Uganda to help establish PANUSP, and the next year, in 2005, a conference with representatives from various countries was held in Kampala, Uganda. It was here that PANUSP was officially established and a chairperson elected (Amegatcher 2007).

Growth of the movement

The main aim of PANUSP was to work with groups across Africa to establish more organized branches in different countries. For example, in Ghana, three delegates present at the WNUSP conference in Denmark were challenged to start a local group, which they did in 2005 in partnership with MindFreedom Ghana and BasicNeeds Ghana (Amegatcher 2007). For Kenya, there was not a formal mental health organization in existence before 2007. At a psychiatry conference in Nairobi, Kenya, Susan Keter was speaking about her family's personal experience with mental health, and some PANUSP delegates who were present were impressed by her story. They spoke to her about setting up a local program in Kenya, which was done under the name of Users and Survivors of Psychiatry – Kenya (USP-Kenya). There are now nine African countries participating in PANUSP: Uganda, Kenya, Tanzania, Rwanda, South Africa, Ghana, Guinea, Zambia, and Malawi. The network promotes the rights to dignity, participation, and self-determination. It provides support to the local projects such as USP-Kenya, in the form of technology, legal support, and expertise. Participating country programs also collaborate with each other to plan campaigns, hold events, and devise different initiatives (Susan Keter, interviewed by Jordan Pfau, February 2012).

At the country level, the PANUSP branches have been able to grow through advocacy and grassroots outreach. Through targeted campaigns using newspapers and magazines, they are encouraging members from local groups to speak out. One USP-Kenya newspaper advertisement that targeted working professionals with mental illness received over 200 responses. The movement aims to generate awareness that people with mental illness or epilepsy can substantially contribute to society, and that, should they wish for it, they should have access to treatment as a basic human right.

Achievements and challenges

> There can be no mental health without our expertise. We are the knowers and yet we remain the untapped resource in mental health care. We are the experts. We want to be listened to and to fully participate in our life decisions. We must be the masters of our life journeys.
> (PANUSP 2011)

In October 2011, an international congress was held under PANUSP's leadership in Cape Town, South Africa, to discuss mental health reform in Africa. Delegates from member organizations debated challenges and issues they were facing, and the event culminated with the Cape Town Declaration (PANUSP 2011). The declaration calls for full inclusion of people with psychosocial disabilities and an end to discrimination. It is an exceptionally beautiful piece of writing.

PANUSP is achieving much throughout Africa. USP-Kenya was invited to participate in the Kenya National Human Rights Commission, to assess human rights needs of the mentally ill and provide an avenue to report violations. In 2010, youth ambassadors, NGOs, and students partnered with USP-Kenya to spearhead the "One Mind, Lend Your Voice" campaign. It was aimed at gathering 1 million signatures on a petition to demand a government policy on mental health. In Ghana, a similar awareness campaign involving street marches, TV programming, and published articles has led to

discussions with the government about the needs of the mentally ill in the country (Amegatcher 2007). The movement continues to see successes, but is also facing challenges.

One of the major challenges that PANUSP faces is ensuring that its stance is not overshadowed by an agenda that is overly influenced by Western mental health movements, which are often very preoccupied with educating people about the problems with psychiatry. In the West, people have often been overtreated, overmedicated, and not given a voice in their treatment. However, for PANUSP member countries, it is the opposite. There is a shortage of care and the problems lie more in stigma and family abuse. Michael Njenga, Administrator at USP-Kenya, explains:

> There was one case where a person at a mental hospital became stable and well, so the hospital took him back to live with his family. The family members told the staff that if they left the person they would kill him. People are rejected by their families and communities and have nowhere else to go. This is the biggest human rights challenge that the movement is facing.
> (Michael Njenga, Administrator at USP-Kenya, interviewed by Jordan Pfau, February 2012)

In the end, the issue is not merely a medical one, but in fact it is a problem of development. While people may seek treatment, they also need a host of other practical matters addressed to enable them to thrive and prosper. In many cases, the medical system itself is generally not hostile towards those with mental illness. They are, however, often ignorant of the wider landscape into which the treatment they offer fits. Rather than fighting against the psychiatric system, the movement in Africa continues to focus on reducing stigma, so that people with mental illness and epilepsy can be included in society and accepted by their families (S. Keter, interviewed February 2012).

Reflections

From the varied perspectives highlighted in this chapter we can draw several key points for grassroots movements for mental health.

- Grassroots movements are most powerful when led by the vulnerable groups directly affected by the injustices these movements seek to change. At the heart of each movement lie marginalized individuals who, through simple actions, refused to fall in line with society's expectations of them.

Groups of people who have historically been isolated and disempowered have found strength. The process empowers the group, giving them a sense of purpose, solidarity, and collective strength, which grows the movement (Shakespeare 1993).

- Grassroots mental health movements are fundamentally about realizing basic human rights. While the orientation, focus, and agendas of mental health movements vary in different contexts across the world, each of these movements seeks to ensure that people with mental illness have the right to live with dignity and respect. As individuals recognize their entitlement to basic human rights, they are inspired to act – to challenge attitudes and reform society's failures towards them. Ultimately, gaining basic human rights and entitlements is the fundamental focus of each of these movements.

- Grassroots movements do not always share the same ideological perspective. While each movement discussed has been directed by affected individuals, contrasting viewpoints towards treatment sometimes put grassroots groups and individuals at odds with each other. The fundamental goal to establish basic human rights is there, but the ways to reach this goal are debatable. It is crucial that a variety of perspectives is expressed and heard.

- Membership in support groups, such as self-help groups, can catalyse the growth of a movement as individuals interact with one another. One key network of affected individuals – the self-help group – has been particularly useful in developing countries such as Ghana. Links to self-help groups provide members with a place for gaining practical support, sharing experiences and stories, as well as building confidence and capacities. Through these groups, people with mental illness and epilepsy are doing their own advocacy work and breaking down barriers.

- A charismatic leader representing the movement can motivate people on a grassroots level, and can also be very influential in spreading the word on a national level. While significant progress has been made in various grassroots mental health movements worldwide, the movement has had some difficulty organizing itself on national and international levels. The emergence of a dynamic leader could bring cohesion and increase the movements' influence on the global mental health movement.

- Individuals with mental illness are best prepared for self-advocacy when they have been allowed to heal through treatment and have had poverty issues addressed. Self-led movements, while powerful, can present challenges, particularly when the movement is centered around a highly marginalized group such as people with mental illness. People have difficulty focusing on self-advocacy when they do not have basic access to treatment or the ability to earn a living, as is true for many people with mental illness in developing countries. This is compounded by the challenges that accompany poverty, such as low education, low literacy rates, and poor health. In Ghana, fostering an environment where an interest in self-advocacy can develop has been critical to the success of the movement. Addressing the poverty of individuals with mental illness and their caregivers through livelihoods interventions helped individuals to feel ready to participate in self-advocacy.

- The individual and collective empowerment of a group of marginalized people can be achieved through different methods, but "empowerment" is essential to the sustainable growth of a mental health movement. One technique that was largely utilized in the disability movement, and has been used by BasicNeeds among people with mental illness, is animation. Animation acts under the assumption that if a group is sufficiently challenged, inspired, motivated, and encouraged, it will develop an analysis of its own problems and act upon this analysis (Underhill 1996).

- A mental health movement is most cohesive and influential when linked to a national or overarching organization. In Ghana, the mental health movement has grown by linking people with mental illness into strong partnerships with mental health professionals. These networks provide the movement with access to local and national policy makers. While the UK movement has suffered from a lack of a national forum, the Ghana movement has been developing in influence by strategically tying itself to the national government. While varying dynamics and challenges are ever-present, Ghana's large network of self-help groups for people with mental illness has helped create cohesion across communities and regions, allowing the groups to advocate for change on the national level. The Mental Health Society of Ghana has been able to engage with policy makers because of its size and cohesion.

- Fighting stigma is crucial to the sustainable growth of a movement. Stigma looms as an ever-present barrier for people with mental illness in these case studies, and efforts to educate people and combat community-level stigma have been shown to be crucial to the sustainable growth of a movement. Grassroots movements are uniquely placed to fight stigma, starting at the community level. As learned from the UK movement, the growth of a movement depends upon fighting stigma even from within the movement itself.

- Personal stories shared through various forms of media can be a very powerful form of self-advocacy. The media has been a powerful tool to combat stigma, and this has been strategically used in the UK movement. PANUSP also has relied heavily on the media to educate the public about mental illness. Relaying oral histories can be a powerful advocacy tool, both for the individual with mental illness telling the story and for the audience. Sharing personal stories, through books, television programs, radios and newspapers, has helped to changed attitudes towards people with mental illness and gain recognition of the movement at higher levels.

Conclusion

In summary, a number of key lessons can be learned from grassroots mental health movements:

- Grassroots mental health movements are most effective when fueled by those directly affected by it.
- Groups that initiate these movements form and expand through a shared sense of purpose.
- Differences of opinion often exist within movements, but common purpose should be centered on human rights and contextual relevance.
- Self-advocacy is best fostered through a supportive environment where treatment and poverty concerns are also being addressed.
- Without any central organizational structure or leadership, movements can become disjointed and make little progress.
- Dialog with decision makers at every level is a key aspect as a movement begins and expands.
- Personal experiences of affected individuals who are in the movement, when shared effectively, can be very powerful in influencing governments and civil society.

Grassroots movements in mental health are fueled by the tireless efforts of passionate individuals who often have overcome great personal injustices to advocate for change for themselves and others. Their successes and struggles remind us, through all of the back-and-forth policy discourse, that at the heart of this battle lie real people who desire to have the same rights and entitlements as others.

> I used to think I was useless ... But my life has now changed ... I am a member of a self-help group that cares for me. We have been able to start working together and improving our lives and this is the greatest gift.
>
> (Resty – affected individual, Uganda: Raja *et al.* 2010)

References

Amegatcher J (2007) The UN Convention on the Rights of Persons With Disabilities: a rights-based approach to development. *WNUSP News*, June 2007. http://www.wnusp.net (accessed July 2013).

Desai NG (2005) Antipsychiatry: meeting the challenge. *Indian Journal of Psychiatry* 47: 185–7.

Hervey N (1986) Advocacy or folly: the Alleged Lunatics' Friend Society,

1845–63. *Medical History* 30: 245–75.

International Disability Alliance (2012) About us. http://www.internationaldisabilityalliance.org/en/about-us (accessed July 2013).

International League Against Epilepsy (2010) 2010 Annual Report. http://www.ilae.org/Visitors/Documents/ILAEAnnual-Report2010Final_000.pdf (accessed July 2013).

Klein E (1984) *Gender Politics.* Cambridge, MA: Harvard University Press.

Kleinman A (2009) Global mental health: a failure of humanity. *Lancet* 374: 603–4.

Mind (2008) England's first mass participation event boosting wellbeing and breaking down the barriers of mental health stigma on 4–12 October 2008. http://www.mind.org.uk/news/257_get_moving_for_mental_health (accessed July 2013).

MindFreedom International (2012) About David W. Oaks, MindFreedom International

Executive Director. http://www.mindfreedom.org/about-us/david-w-oaks (accessed July 2013).

PANUSP (2011) Cape Town Declaration. http://www.panusp.org/wp-content/uploads/2013/01/Cape-Town-Declaration-2011.pdf (accessed July 2013).

Raja S, Sunder U, Mannarath S, *et al.* (2010) *Annual Impact Report.* Leamington Spa: BasicNeeds.

Shakespeare T (1993) Disabled people's self-organisation: a new social movement? *Disability, Handicap, and Society* 8: 249–64.

Shapiro J (2010) Advocate for people with mental illness dies. *National Public Radio*, January 19, 2010. http://www.npr.org/templates/ story/story.php?storyId=122706192 (accessed July 2013).

Underhill C (1996) Defining moments: a qualitative enquiry into perceptions of the process of community development practice with disabled people in Uganda. Masters thesis, University of Bristol School for Policy Studies.

Wallcraft J, Bryant M (2003) The mental health service user movement in England. Sainsbury Centre for Mental Health, Policy paper 2. http://www.centreformentalhealth.org.uk/pdfs/policy_paper2_service_user_movement.pdf (accessed July 2013).

World Health Organization (2007) UN Convention on the Rights of Persons with Disabilities: a major step forward in promoting and protecting rights. Geneva: WHO. http://www.who.int/mental_health/policy/legislation/4_UNConventionRightsofPersonswithDisabilities_Infosheet.pdf (accessed July 2013).

Yaro P, Menil V (2005) Lessons from the African user movement: the case of Ghana. In A Barbato, M Vallarino, eds., *Community Mental Health Care in Low-Income Countries: A Way Forward.* Milan: Press Milan.

Yaro P, Truelove A, Dokurugu A, Bernard A (2005) *Report on Baseline Study on Mental Health in Northern Ghana.* Leamington Spa: BasicNeeds.

Chapter

11

The rise of consumerism and local advocacy

Dinesh Bhugra, Norman Sartorius, and Diana Rose

Introduction

In the first quarter of the twenty-first century, the clinical practice of psychiatry is a continuation of how psychiatry developed in the last century. However, this is likely to change dramatically, with new developments on the horizon including the development and growth of epigenetics, psychopharmacogenomics, and therapies without therapists, such as web-based therapies that are becoming available on mobile devices. It is theoretically possible that in due course there may well be individualized and personalized medications available. In addition, changes at political, economic, and social levels across the globe are likely to influence the availability and accessibility of various treatments. With the additional impact of economic factors, not only will the resources providing healthcare change, but access to services itself will change. West and Western used in this chapter refer mainly to ideas and values of Western European countries and the Anglophone developed countries elsewhere (USA, Canada, Australia).

In this chapter, we highlight some of the changes occurring in services around the globe in the context of and as a result of political and economic changes. We describe some examples of how expectations of clinical services are changing and emerging. We do not aim to provide an exhaustive list of user/carer/patient campaigns and involvement from around the globe (see Chapter 10). We offer a background understanding of some of the changes that will affect the way patients and their carers are seen by clinical services. We describe some of the potential barriers and challenges that the stakeholders, especially service providers and policy makers, need to be aware of. The involvement of patients, their carers, and families is crucial in developing sensitive, effective, and accessible services. It must be emphasized that in different countries terms such as *patients*, *users*, and *survivors* are used, but we will simply use the term *patient*. Disease and illness models by themselves do not provide the whole answer, as each individual responds in a different way, and *patient* does not always explain social and psychological factors. However, for the purposes of this chapter we use the conventional term *patient*, nonetheless emphasizing that medicine and psychiatry are largely social enterprises as well.

Issues in global mental health

Global mental health describes an interlinking of mental and physical health around the globe, especially as the global village is shrinking rapidly. However, it is important that Western ideas and norms are not exported blithely and blindly in a missionary manner, indicating that the West knows best. This is particularly relevant in the delivery of psychotherapies, as most of the therapies are ego-based – but it can also be applied to medication, since there are differences in pharmacodynamics and pharmacokinetics across cultural groups. In the context of psychotherapies, there are further issues separating collectivist societies from individualistic societies and responsibilities which need careful thought. At the same time, it is evident that with globalization societies and cultures are changing at a frantic pace.

Sartorius (2009), while highlighting the recent trends in the development of medicine and its delivery, points out that these are affected by social as well as medical factors. Social factors include the processes of globalization, decivilization, commodification, decentralization of social services, changes in the middle class, technological revolution, and population movements

Essentials of Global Mental Health, ed. Samuel O. Okpaku. Published by Cambridge University Press. © Cambridge University Press 2014.

related to globalization and migration, especially urbanization-led rural-to-urban migration. These processes are occurring all over the world and have an impact on individuals and societies.

Medicine and its practitioners have a social contract with society. Within this implicit social contract, there is an expectation that society will offer medicine and its practitioners a degree of freedom embedded within self-regulation. Society expects physicians to provide impartial advice, services as a healer, altruism, morals, high levels of integrity and competence, accountability and transparency (Cruess & Cruess 2010). In return, medicine expects trust, autonomy, a value-driven and well-funded healthcare system, shared responsibility for health, and financial and status rewards (Cruess & Cruess 2010; see also Bhugra *et al.* 2011). Changes in society will inevitably lead to changes in the practice of medicine, and vice versa. The trends, which are immediate and strong, are described here. Of these, globalization is perhaps the most significant.

Globalization

An economic definition of globalization is the worldwide process of homogenizing prices, products, wages, profits and rates of interest (Shariff 2003). Within and outside this economic aspect, globalization is seen as the process by which traditional boundaries between cultures and societies on the one hand, and individuals on the other hand, are blurring (Okasha 2005). The impact of this transformation may be slow in some settings but fast paced in others, and leads to changes in relationships, expectations and functioning at individual, local, national, regional and supra-regional levels. There is an influence on cultural beliefs, values and behaviors, especially in the context of understanding and dealing with illness. The use of economic definitions may be at a broader level, but its impact on individuals and their roles cannot be underestimated. A classic example of this change is the role of call-center workers, who work according to time zones in another part of the world, and who also have parallel identities. These identities involve pretending to be living in another country, with different accents, names and functions. This outsourcing not only affects the country which is providing these services but also impacts upon the country from which labour has been lost. The growth of information technology and high technology sectors in this context will bring additional

factors into play. Thus de-industrialization in one nation state with an increase in soft service jobs in another state will bring tension across boundaries. Perceived to lead to the free circulation of people and goods across boundaries, globalization certainly has not delivered what it had promised. Mutual sharing and learning has not occurred and has not produced the anticipated results. Thus in the context of globalization, not only do the nation states consuming the goods produced by some nation states have to be understood, but significantly also the states which provide the raw materials and resources. This triangular relationship is often squeezed into a bi-polar contract between countries.

Globalization thus far has not reduced overall parity, but in newly emerging economies such as Brazil, South Africa, China, Russia, and India has created massive middle classes who have different expectations, as discussed further below. Traditional values are changing, but in some settings more extreme positions are being taken as a result of globalization. Globalization has influenced inequality both positively and negatively, added acculturative stress and the impact of shifting/parallel/alternative identities on the individual and on social mental health. It also tends to impose value systems of the highly developed and economically powerful countries on the developing countries creating a variety of processes.

The impact of globalization

Globalization might lead to a globalized culture in which cultural values become more homogenized and cultural relativism gives way to a uniform view. However, this fear remains unfounded; as a response to globalization many cultures as a whole, or cultures within cultures, are becoming rigid in attempting to preserve a distinct cultural identity. Cultural globalization occurs at different levels and simultaneously. The upper echelons of society may be exposed more, and will also be more likely to change. As a result, the idioms of distress and potential explanatory models may change. As Tseng (2001) has argued, the explanations of mental disorder may vary from supernatural to social or psychological, and this shift is reflected in the way the cultures evolve. Thus more traditional cultures explain mental illness in terms of supernatural or natural causative factors. Furthermore, it is also likely that as a result of closer contact with other cultures through globalization, these idioms may well change rapidly. The patient's presentation may change, and clinicians, if not aware, may misdiagnose, adding yet another dimension to the consumerist experience. There may also be a generation issue in the case of migrants, where older people retain traditional views of mental distress while younger people reject this in favor of the dominant view. The globalization process is not uniform, and certainly not an either/or phenomenon. Some aspects may change rapidly and others more slowly. Both internal and external factors may play a role in dealing with the impact of the process. Yet there will also be tensions on both sides, which will be reflected in the varying expectations of the therapeutic encounter.

On symptoms

In the past, it has been argued that those who somatize their symptoms are psychologically inferior (Leff 1988). However, there are arguments against this observation, indicating that the use of metaphors in expressing distress may well be psychologically more sophisticated. Another possibility is that psychology itself is a product of the West, and therefore psychologization of symptoms may be a reflection of acculturation. It is for these reasons that ego-centric psychotherapies should not and cannot be applied blindly elsewhere, which is one of the ironies of the concept of the global mental health perspective. It is also possible that culture-bound syndromes are becoming more diffuse and should be seen as culturally influenced syndromes (Sumathipala *et al.* 2004, Bhugra *et al.* 2007). The emergence of new conditions such as eating disorders in an adolescent population in Fiji as a result of exposure to television is a remarkable example of this development (Becker *et al.* 2002, Becker 2004). Other symptoms can also emerge as a consequence of exposure to other cultures.

On help-seeking and expectations

Cultures define normality and deviance and also dictate resources going into health services, thereby directing pathways into care. Help-seeking will be determined not only by explanatory models but also by resources needed. It is possible that social and cultural expectations will guide patients and their carers, especially in the early stages. Early encounters, irrespective of conditions, are likely to be in personal, social, or folk sectors, so there will be a different type

of consumerism at play. When patients reach allopathic healthcare systems, especially if they have to pay charges for consultation, investigations, and management, consumerism may influence therapeutic adherence and alliance. It is entirely possible that poor experiences by others in the personal, folk, or social sector will also play a role in sticking with or even initiating treatment. However, the use of the term *consumer* should be treated with caution where there are states with mental health legislation which can coerce service users into treatment, leaving them without choice.

On urbanization

There is no doubt that globalization has led to an increase in urbanization, which by itself brings a number of problems. Urbanization is the phenomenon by which there is a relative increase of urban population as a proportion of the whole population (Blue *et al.* 1995). The WHO (1991) has estimated that, by 2025, 61% of the world's population will be in urban areas, and the speed of such change is phenomenal. Kasarda and Crenshaw (1991) noted that it took 150 years for the population of New York to expand by 8 million residents, but it will take São Paolo and Mexico City less than 15 years. Urbanization is not simply a physical phenomenon but carries with it social, cultural, economic, and political changes. The differences in urbanization between high-income and low-income countries are many. In addition to stressors related to chronic difficulties, changes to the cash economy and violent life events – which may be linked to a single loss or series of losses – may affect an individual's adjustment.

Changes in social support

As a result of internal migration from rural to urban areas, overcrowding may result and social support networks will change. A reduction in support with low levels of joint families and a resulting increase in nuclear families will also affect social support (Harpham & Blue 1995). This in turn will affect help-seeking, and statutory services may be seen as critical. Environmental health hazards will influence rates of illness, but will affect help-seeking and will generate expectations that individuals want to go back to work quickly.

The development, practice, and training of medicine and its delivery are strongly influenced by the society in which these take place. Sartorius

(2009) highlights some of these factors. Of these, decivilization is perhaps the most invidious. He argues that the level of civilization of a society can be measured by the amount of care its vulnerable members receive. He notes as a symptom of decivilization that levels of child morbidity and mortality have increased disproportionately even in high-income countries. Part of the response therefore has been that these societies have become very risk-averse – a facet which is affecting clinical practice in countries such as the USA and the UK. For example, every patient in the UK now has to be assessed for purposes of child protection and every healthcare professional has to undergo a criminal review board check. Shortages of resources or increased awareness of risk may have further contributed to this. However, at a broader level, when professionals are treated as tradesmen they are likely to behave as such. The financial meltdown in the global economy has further added to difficulties experienced by vulnerable groups. In certain economies a closer focus on centralization, and in others localization, has produced similar effects, with vulnerable groups not only ignored but marginalized further. Burnout of healthcare professionals, penny pinching, and newer expensive treatments have added further dimensions. Some of these factors are acute and sudden, say with more people living longer requiring more support, but supply is not keeping pace with demand. Other factors are insidious and slow, but planners have not responded in time to these changes.

Commodification of health

Commodification of health is defined as the tendency to consider health care and related social care and services as commodities that can be bought or sold like other commodities such as sugar or cotton (Sartorius 2009). This phenomenon is not necessarily new, but with increased technological advances it has taken on another dimension. The trade in commodities is based on the intent to make profit, thus getting good-quality products at a low price or selling these for more than they are worth. With the establishment of guilds in Western Europe, where guilds controlled training, materials, and the input and output of training, health care had different dimensions. With the state emerging in the context of capitalist ideas, the role of healthcare providers started to shift. This led to further commodification, going as far back as the nineteenth century, but the rise of professionalism and professional ethics

ensured that ethical imperatives continued, certainly until the latter third of the last century. With increasing demands, shortage of providers, and technological advances, the demand for cheaper health care, especially by insurance companies, produced an increased emphasis on budgets. In this battle of budgets, the specialty that lost most was psychiatry. This is due to a number of reasons, including the labor-intensive nature of the subject and the perceived likelihood that this group of patients is not likely to be economically productive. As some of the psychiatric conditions are long-term, it is inevitable that those who can command resources will be able to access services.

Expectations from the therapeutic encounter

In psychiatry, more than in any other specialty, there remains a clear power differential between the treating clinician and the patient. Patients present with illnesses, but doctors are used to and are trained to diagnose and manage diseases. Furthermore, social, economic, and educational status influence help-seeking.

The middle classes are increasing as a result of globalization, and so is economic inequality. Deregulation of labor markets has played an increasing role in creating social inequalities (Katz 2000). The expectations of health care have also changed as a result. Modern socioeconomic processes are exacerbating wealth inequalities instead of diminishing them (Bhavsar & Bhugra 2008). The middle classes, in view of their increased awareness of their purchasing capability, may see the purchase of health and social care in the same way. This in itself may well create a further inequality in access to health care. This will obviously be influenced by the type of healthcare system and healthcare policy.

Poverty and its impact

The role poverty plays in healthcare delivery and the need for health care is well known. However, if the healthcare system provides basic care through the statutory sector and the rest comes from the private sector, it is entirely possible that the poor will receive a lower quality of health care; this will intensify the vicious cycle of poor health, leading to poor health care, producing poor outcomes. In newly emerging economies, the differential between the poor and the middle classes is increasing, creating disparity between social expectation and reality. As Sartorius (2009) points out, in many countries it is the middle class which defends the morals of the society, providing help to the vulnerable and those in need, but this is changing.

Consumerism

In many countries, for example in India, the practice of medicine and delivery of health care has been brought under consumer legislation, where patients are seen as consumers and have no rights of protection as consumers. Rather than medicine being a profession and physicians being professionals, this approach of consumerism takes medicine back to the seventeenth century, when in Western Europe medicine was a trade. It is inevitable that if the profession turns into a trade, professionalism is likely to give way to more financial aspects of the therapeutic encounter. Furthermore, with patients becoming more aware through the use of the internet of their illness, its management, and the side effects of drugs, "specialized" knowledge is also becoming more accessible, and the power differential between the physician and the patient is beginning to change.

There are, however, limits to consumerism and commodification. In states with mental health legislation, people with a diagnosis of mental illness can be detained and treated against their will. As such, they have no right to change providers, as "consumers" can. This is why some call themselves "service users" and some "survivors." There are European and worldwide movements to end forced detention and treatment (www.enusp.org, www.wnusp.org). These organizations are critical of the power differential between doctor and patient and would not necessarily agree that it is shifting in favor of the patient.

Political responses

Politicians appear to take ambivalent views towards health and health care. Some political systems allow politicians, as representatives of society, to take a rather laissez-faire approach, whereas in other systems politicians continue to interfere both at the macro level (in setting the policy) and at the micro level (in delivery itself). Political responses are often not based on scientific evidence but on political ideology and will. Often wants and needs get conflated, and special groups who are able to shout the loudest tend to receive better and bigger resources.

The social contract of medicine in general and psychiatry in particular has specific features that politicians, as representatives of the society, negotiate with the profession. For psychiatry, this contract is especially important, as psychiatrists have the power to enforce treatment and detain patients against their will, as argued above (see Bhugra *et al.* 2011 for a detailed discussion). As Bhugra (2011) argues, the role of autonomy in clinical practice is changing, and the disillusionment among health professionals – particularly in the UK – perhaps reflects society's interference as well as expectations, although these are represented by the politicians. There is no doubt that society expects value for money; this is where health professionals feel persecuted, as often these values are difficult to measure, and particularly so in psychiatry, where there is a further tension in the form of uncertainty as to whether the focus is on symptom reduction or on better functioning.

Patient responses

Patients distrust the healthcare system partly because of stigma but also because of its coercive powers. Some groups in some countries may see the role of psychiatric health care as part of the long arm of the government and control. In many situations in the past, psychiatrists have not covered themselves in glory either. Physicians may choose evidence-based therapies, but the more vocal patients may well demand their personal favorites. As Freddolino and Knapp (2011) have argued, the influence of the efficiency criterion can be seen in clinical decision making. It is inevitable that all healthcare systems are inequitable, but some are more so than others. Bhugra *et al.* (2011) noted that patients' and carers' expectations of the therapeutic encounter are related directly to the therapeutic process and to the characteristics of their psychiatrist rather than the system. These may include the physical environment or the therapeutic milieu. It is possible that expectations will also vary according to how the therapeutic encounter is initiated and where it takes place. The therapeutic encounter is part of the psychotherapy process, but will also affect pharmacotherapy.

Doctor responses

Doctors respond to patient attitudes in a number of ways, from confrontation to collusion. Consumerist values may produce different responses. The role of the doctor is shifting towards a more equitable relationship. The technological revolution, in terms of communication, has moved the interaction forward. Investigations may be available but are not always affordable, either by the system or by the individual. It is also likely that doctors have become more defensive in their clinical practice, leading to more, perhaps unnecessary investigations. The use of technology has occasionally led to the dehumanization of medicine. Social media and their use in daily life have created another dimension where both ethical and clinical dilemmas take place. Recent spates of suicides among the young through contact on social media make it clear to physicians and healthcare providers that there are difficulties which need to be addressed. Doctors' responses to migrants or to those whose cultures may not be familiar play a key role in therapeutic engagement. Such an approach raises fundamental questions about the therapeutic encounter and potential outcomes. Communication where the patient may convey a threat through a text message to commit suicide needs to be unpicked and understood.

Politicians often talk at length about choice. Choice is central to classical economic thought, and freedom of choice ensures that producers of goods and services deliver what consumers actually want at a price they are willing to pay. Health services may offer limited choice, especially if the patient is unable to pay or if payment is not required. And some patients are treated against their will under coercion. As Freddolino and Knapp (2011) point out, mental health services are more complex than grocers, and differ in many and profound ways. It is much more difficult for patients to determine what they need, what will be most appropriate, and who is the best person to provide it. Glasby *et al.* (2003) identified five reasons for involving patients and the general public in decision making: accountability, developing local understanding, strengthening public confidence, encouraging services to become more responsive, and challenging paternalistic models of provision. However, in many cultures patients like the paternalistic approach where they expect the doctor to make the decisions for them. These changes in patient expectations and the role of doctors, along with changes in the nature of medicine, produce another dimension. The use of complementary and alternative medicine is increasing, and as virtually all of these medications are available off the shelf without requiring any prescription, patients or their families can choose them and their consumption may further

cause drug interaction with prescribed drugs. Changes in professional values, tightening of regulatory control, and the rise of complementary medicine may well lead to a reduction in the prestige of allopathy. The changes in healthcare delivery systems in countries such as the USA and the UK, where doctors are increasingly seen as especially expensive, mean that it is possible that using psychologists and nurses to prescribe (as they may be more affordable) may become the norm. On the other hand, in low- and middle-income countries, a lack of doctors and other health professionals may lead to prescription by other health professions such as health visitors and midwives. The transformation from a profession to a trade will add to the expansion of consumerism.

As patients are living longer with disability, changes in society and social expectations lead to collaborative therapeutic encounters rather than paternalistic ones. Sartorius (2009) points out that in many cultures the physician's primary obligation was to work with the patient and their family and carers. The latter will dictate admission, and in various countries will be admitted along with the patient. But increased urbanization and an increase in nuclear families makes this more difficult, changing the relationship between the patient and the physician. Thus the patients become responsible for themselves and their own ability to function. With an increasing interest in mental health promotion and the prevention of mental illness, it is inevitable that there will be an introduction to further commodification of health. Outcomes need to be defined clearly, and symptom reduction may give way to a focus on functional improvement, which by itself is laudable. However, there is a danger that this switch may well give way to more consumerism.

Sartorius (2009) also argues that the introduction of community medicine presumes that communities exist and are supportive of each other. Changing demographic trends and movements of people have altered the shape of communities, and are changing the role of primary care physicians (who are expected to be specialists in many areas), the strategies of healthcare delivery and perhaps more importantly the expectations of the population and of healthcare providers. Illnesses of healthcare systems include increased pressures on staff, who may feel unable to deal with patients with kindness. The imposition of value systems across cultures will lead to further alienation of patients, turning them into consumers.

Conclusions

The changes in social expectations, and in society at large, have put medicine and healthcare systems in great difficulty. As medicine becomes more deprofessionalized, it is inevitable that patients will turn into consumers, at least where their freedom is not restricted. Consumerism can affect health care as a whole or psychotherapy or pharmacotherapy. The profession, if it is to survive, must work with stakeholders to ascertain what is needed and who will provide it, what the expectation of society is and how that it is met. Current health strategies need to be revised urgently, with a clear sense direction and clear milestones.

References

Becker A (2004) Television, disordered eating and young women in Fiji: negotiating body image and identity during rapid social change. *Culture, Medicine and Psychiatry* 28: 533–55.

Becker A, Bunwell R, Herzog D, Hamburg P, Gilman S E (2002) Eating behaviours and attitudes following prolonged exposure to television among Fijian adolescent girls. *British Journal of Psychiatry* 180: 509–14.

Bhavsar V, Bhugra D (2008) Globalization: mental health and social economic factors. *Global Social Policy* 8: 378–96.

Bhugra D (2011) Medical leadership in changing times. *Asian Journal of Psychiatry* 4: 162–4.

Bhugra D, Sumathipala S, Siribaddana S (2007) Culture-bound syndromes: a re-evaluation. In D Bhugra, K Bhui, eds., *Textbook of Cultural Psychiatry*. Cambridge: Cambridge University Press; pp. 141–56.

Bhugra D, Malik A, Ikkos G (2011) *Psychiatry's Contract with Society*. Oxford: Oxford University Press.

Blue I, Ducci M, Jaswal S, Ludermir A and Harpham T (1995) The mental health of low income countries. In T Harpham T, I Blue, eds., *Urbanisation and Mental Health*. Aldershot: Avebury.

Cruess SR, Creuss RL (2010) Medicine's social contract with society: its nature, evolution and present state. In D Bhugra, A Malik, G Ikkos, eds., *Psychiatry's Contract with Society*. Oxford: Oxford University Press; pp. 123–46.

Freddolino P, Knapp M (2011) Economics and society: efficiency, equity and choice. In D Bhugra, A Malik, G Ikkos, eds., *Psychiatry's Contract with Society*. Oxford: Oxford University Press; pp. 43–58.

Glasby J, Lester H, Clarke M *et al.* (2003) *Cases for Change in Mental Health Services*. Colchester: National Institute for Mental Health.

Harpham T, Blue I (1995) *Urbanisation and Mental Health*. Aldershot: Avebury.

Kasarda JD, Crenshaw E (1991) Third world urbanization: dimensions, theories, and determinants. *Annual Review of Sociology* 17: 467–501.

Katz HC (2000) *Converging Divergencies: Worldwide Changes in Employment Systems*. Ithaca, NY: Cornell University Press.

Leff J (1988) *Psychiatry Around the Globe*. London: Gaskell.

Okasha A (2005) Globalization and mental health: a WPA perspective. *World Psychiatry* 4: 1–2.

Sartorius N (2009) Medicine in the era of decivilization. *Works of Croatian Academy of Sciences and Arts* 504, vol. XXXIII, Medical Science. Zagreb: Hrvatska Akademija Znanosti I Umjetnosti; pp. 9–28.

Shariff I (2003) Global economic integration: prospects and problems. *International Journal of Development Economics and Development Review* 1: 163–78.

Sumathipala A, Siribaddana SH, Bhugra D (2004) Culture-bound syndromes: the story of dhat syndrome. *British Journal of Psychiatry* 184: 200–9.

Tseng W-S (2001) *Handbook of Cultural Psychiatry*. San Diego, CA: Academic Press.

WHO (1991) *World Health Statistics Quarterly* 44 (4). Geneva: WHO.

Chapter

12

Programs to reduce stigma in epilepsy and HIV/AIDS

Rita Thom

Introduction

In the final chapter in this section, stigma in epilepsy and HIV/AIDS is reviewed in terms of its origins and consequences, as well as stigma-reduction efforts in these conditions. Since the impact of these conditions is felt particularly in low- and middle-income countries, the discussion in this chapter largely focuses on literature from these regions.

Epilepsy-related stigma

It is estimated that some 50 million people suffer from epilepsy globally (World Health Organization 2005). Epilepsy is one of the leading brain disorders in the developing world, and it is estimated that 80% of sufferers live in low- and middle-income countries (Diop *et al.* 2003). There is a significant treatment gap, with less than half of the total population of people with epilepsy accessing treatment. The treatment gap in low- and middle-income countries is particularly wide (up to 80%). In these countries there are many preventable causes of epilepsy, in particular those related to perinatal events and infectious causes. In these countries too, there are insufficient trained healthcare providers to diagnose and treat epilepsy appropriately, and often erratic supplies of antiepileptic drugs. In many countries, people are ignorant of the medical causes of epilepsy. In one study, even some Zambian healthcare workers were found to hold some unfounded prejudicial views concerning people with epilepsy (Chomba *et al.* 2007).

Epilepsy has been associated with stigma since the earliest times. This is likely to be due to the fact that epileptic seizures are commonly highly visible, unpredictable, and may be frightening to onlookers. Epilepsy has been attributed to supernatural causes

such as demon possession or witchcraft. It has also been associated with fears of contagion, mainly through contact with saliva or other body fluids of a person having a seizure. People with epilepsy have been excluded from education, employment, marriage, and from being allowed to drive vehicles (de Boer 2010). The consequences of stigma for people with epilepsy include depression, anxiety, impaired physical health, somatic symptoms, reduced self-esteem, and poor quality of life (Jacoby & Austin 2007).

In a detailed exploration of epilepsy-associated stigma in sub-Saharan Africa, Baskind and Birbeck (2005) describe how stigma particularly affects people living in rural settings, because of communal living situations and traditional belief systems. People with uncontrolled epilepsy in a rural setting, where fire is a source of heat and cooking, often sustain burns during seizures. This may then be seen as a mark or "stigma" of epilepsy which is difficult to hide. Traditional treatments for seizures include bush teas. In children these may result in oral burns or aspiration if given during a convulsion. Courtesy stigma is described as the stigma that is experienced by the family associated with a person with epilepsy. Traditional healers exert considerable influence in rural settings, which may be positive or negative for the individual concerned. For example, it is commonly believed that breaking taboos can cause seizures, and that when ancestors are angered they may send seizures as a punishment. This may result in punitive attitudes towards people with epilepsy. In addition, seeking traditional treatment may delay accessing care for treatable conditions that cause seizures (cysticercosis, malaria, etc.). On the other hand, when traditional explanations of seizures incorporate the family

Essentials of Global Mental Health, ed. Samuel O. Okpaku. Published by Cambridge University Press. © Cambridge University Press 2014.

as victim, this may produce protective attitudes towards the person with epilepsy.

It has been found that there is a higher rate of disability from epilepsy in rural areas than in urban areas, due to delays in seeking treatment or difficulty in accessing treatment. People with uncontrolled epilepsy may not be able to fulfill daily manual tasks such as cutting and collecting firewood, fetching water, and growing food that are central to survival in a rural area. This may result in them being seen as less valuable. During times of food insecurity or famine, people with epilepsy may be at greater risk of malnutrition as priority is given to the fittest and "most useful" members of a social group.

Epilepsy also impacts on educational opportunities, where parents may choose to invest in the child with the greatest potential, and children with epilepsy may be excluded from education as a result. Teachers may also expel children from school because of a seizure disorder. It has been found that children with epilepsy receive less education, even when they are of normal intelligence.

Epilepsy also impacts on intimate relationships, marriage, and childcare. In some cultures, people with epilepsy cannot marry. In these same societies, unmarried women are vulnerable to sexual exploitation, increasing their risk for HIV, another stigmatized health condition.

HIV-related stigma

HIV is another illness that continues to attract significant stigma. The fact that it is predominantly sexually transmitted, and that certain high-risk groups, such as men who have sex with men, injection drug users, and sex workers, are socially unacceptable, probably has contributed to stigma. In addition, early in the epidemic, it was invariably fatal, and it therefore also carried the "taboo of death." It became a disease of shame, there was considerable fear of contagion, and it became the "new leprosy." People infected with HIV were also often made to feel guilty and responsible for infecting themselves and for spreading the virus.

As the epidemic expanded, it became a predominantly heterosexual disease, particularly in the developing world. Structural inequity, particularly in relation to the role of women in society, as well as the biologically determined increased risk of infection in women, has resulted in women being particularly vulnerable to HIV infection. Because of the unequal

power relations between men and women in many developing countries in particular, women have often been afraid to disclose their HIV status when they test positive. In some cases, rejection by their partners, abandonment, and intimate partner violence have been a result of such disclosure (Parker & Aggleton 2003). Conspiracy theorists and AIDS denialists fueled the fear of the illness in some countries, most notably South Africa, and this resulted in reluctance to access diagnostic and treatment services (Chigwedere & Essex 2010). People who were infected were afraid to speak out and their families hid their ill family members and denied that AIDS was a cause of death in their loved ones.

Maman *et al.* (2009) compared HIV-related stigma and discrimination in five international sites, four in sub-Saharan Africa and one in Southeast Asia, and found many similarities at all sites. Stigma was related to fear of transmission, fear of suffering and death, and the burden of caring for a family member infected with HIV. They found that a supportive family, access to antiretroviral treatment, and self-protective behaviors protected against stigma. Nthomang *et al.* (2009) found that HIV-related stigma is deeply embedded in societal structures and culture in Botswana. Monjok *et al.* (2009) found pervasive negative attitudes towards people living with HIV and AIDS in Nigeria amongst the general public as well as amongst health workers. Brickley *et al.* (2009) in their qualitative study among pregnant and postpartum women in Vietnam found an association between HIV-related stigma and sex work and drug use. The women who were interviewed described the need to manage disclosure, as those who disclosed their status experienced both stigma and support.

In their South African study Cluver and Orkin (2009) found that AIDS-orphaned children are more likely to experience mental disorders, as a result of food insecurity, bullying, and AIDS-related stigma. Interestingly, stigma reduction efforts were found to be less effective than interventions on child nutrition in reducing the psychological impact of AIDS-orphanhood. Interventions on bullying showed some promise, but with mixed results.

Early in the epidemic, treatment for HIV and AIDS was not affordable or available in many low- and middle-income countries. Whereas the availability of treatment in high-income countries changed the face of HIV from an invariably fatal disease to a

111

chronic condition, where people live with the virus for many years, people in poorer countries continued to die in large numbers, with long-term social, economic, and mental health consequences for their families and communities. As antiretroviral treatment has become more widely available in developing countries globally, evidence is beginning to emerge of improved survival in people infected with HIV (Abaasa *et al.* 2008, World Health Organization 2012). It has been suggested that access to treatment and improved survival will result in decreased stigma. However, currently the literature highlights more the impact of HIV-related stigma as a barrier to treatment access and retention in care (Assefa *et al.* 2010), rather than the impact of treatment on stigma.

Programs to reduce stigma in epilepsy and HIV/AIDS

Initiatives that have been used to address stigma and discrimination in these disorders (as well as in mental illness) tend to have many features in common. These can be summarized as follows:

(1) Initiatives to decrease ignorance and prejudice by **increasing knowledge** about the specific disorder being targeted. These may target the general public, consumers, or specific target groups such as family members, healthcare workers, employers, or landlords. It is hypothesized that increasing accurate knowledge about a stigmatized disorder will decrease prejudice and therefore also decrease discriminatory behavior. Education can take the form of public service announcements in mainstream media, campaigns, the production of pamphlets and posters, or the use of drama productions (live or recorded). In anti-stigma initiatives in any medical condition, it is important to balance the message that people with the condition are no different from anyone else in the general public, with the message that they have a disorder that needs treatment (Jacoby 2008). Despite this type of intervention being the most commonly employed anti-stigma initiative, the results of systematic evaluations have been disappointing (Brown *et al.* 2003).

(2) It has been hypothesized that **personal contact** with individuals with stigmatized health conditions is more effective than educational programs alone. However, personal contact that leads to stigma reduction needs to be in a situation of equality between the individuals with the stigmatized condition and the target audience. The aim is to provide stereotype-inconsistent information. It is preferable for contact to occur over a period of time and in a supportive environment (Bos *et al.* 2008).

(3) **Empowerment** of people suffering from stigmatized disorders is another strategy used to decrease felt and enacted stigma (Sunkel 2012). It is closely linked with the strategy of personal contact as part of educational efforts. It is critical to address internalized stigma by providing accurate information about the condition and its treatment, specifically addressing fears and concerns, and providing tools to deal with discrimination when it occurs. It has been suggested that skills building is an important component of these interventions, in order to build self-confidence, and in enabling income generation (Earnshaw & Chaudoir 2009). In addition, providing guidance on legitimate discrimination and practical support and solutions for illegitimate discrimination may empower consumers to become involved in advocacy, protest, and legislation review themselves (de Boer 2010).

(4) Part of the problem with epilepsy and HIV has been the scarcity of resources for effective treatment. Programs to **increase access and provide resources for treatment** have also been seen as a stigma-reduction strategy. Through the provision of treatment, people with these disorders improve in terms of their health and behavior, and therefore do not conform to the negative stereotypes of people with these particular disorders. Some strategies have included treatment access as part of stigma-reduction interventions: for example, the Global Campaign Against Epilepsy.

(5) Advocacy to **address systemic, structural, or institutionalized stigma**. Advocacy can take many different forms. It includes efforts to address specific instances of discrimination or abuse, as well as lobbying to change discriminatory policies or legislation. It can include legal action, protest, interpersonal contact, engaging with the media, writing letters to politicians, and many other forms of social action.

Again, consumers are often at the forefront of such programs (Treatment Action Campaign 2012). Many authors have highlighted the importance of social and political factors such as poverty, sexism, and racism in reinforcing stigma in various health conditions (Campbell *et al.* 2005, Bos *et al.* 2008). Understanding the specific mechanisms underlying stigma in different health conditions is also important (Alonzo *et al.* 1995, Link & Phelan 2001). If stigma is understood as a form of social control it cannot be addressed without addressing these other factors. It is suggested that critical thinking programs that address the more generic inequities are important if the problem of stigma is to be attacked at its root (Parker & Aggleton 2003, Campbell *et al.* 2005, Earnshaw & Chaudoir 2009).

Examples of stigma-reduction programs in epilepsy and HIV/AIDS

Epilepsy-associated stigma

The Global Campaign Against Epilepsy ("epilepsy out of the shadows") was launched in 1997 (Diop *et al.* 2003, de Boer 2010). This is a partnership between the International League Against Epilepsy, the International Bureau for Epilepsy, and the World Health Organization. The campaign aims to inform the public, various target groups (including employers and healthcare workers), and people with epilepsy about epilepsy and the management of the disorder. The provision of appropriate management for people with epilepsy is a central focus of the campaign, and therefore it also aims to increase the skills of healthcare workers in diagnosis and treatment, to ensure the availability of modern equipment for diagnosis, and to ensure the provision of a full range of antiepileptic drugs. The campaign aims primarily to provide practical assistance to countries with underdeveloped epilepsy services (Birbeck 2006).

Several regional meetings have been held, resulting in the development of regional declarations on epilepsy, and this has been followed by changes in discriminatory legislation in some countries. Certain countries in Africa were selected for interventions to improve the identification and management of epilepsy and to integrate care for people with epilepsy into primary care services. Because epilepsy is often associated with mental disorders, it has also been included in the mhGAP program (World Health Organization 2002). Interventions aimed at people with epilepsy include improving access to treatment, providing emotional support, and engaging in social policy-making/advocacy.

HIV-related stigma

The development and availability of treatment for HIV changed the lives of people infected with HIV. Activists and advocates for treatment did much to reduce stigma in many countries. It was people who were infected with the virus that led the fight to obtain access to antiretroviral treatment in South Africa (Heywood 2004). Nevertheless, stigma continues to pervade the world that people living with HIV inhabit. Public awareness campaigns, led by consumers, including high-profile individuals, helped to demystify the illness and its treatment. Psychosocial support for people living with HIV has been a mechanism for overcoming internalized or felt stigma. Once treatment became available, the Treatment Action Campaign and other non-governmental organizations (NGOs) continued to focus their efforts on addressing stigma and discrimination against people living with HIV (Treatment Action Campaign 2012).

Nyblade *et al.* (2009) reviewed interventions used to combat HIV stigma in healthcare settings and argued that interventions need to focus on the individual, environmental, and policy levels, and discussed a number of hospital-based studies. One study described was an intervention in four Vietnamese hospitals. The interventions included:

(1) a brief survey to document the prevailing attitudes, environment, and policies in the hospital, which informed the design of the intervention

(2) establishment of a steering committee to plan the intervention

(3) short-course training of all hospital staff (clinical, administrative, and support staff)

(4) participatory drafting of a hospital policy to foster staff safety and a stigma-free environment

(5) provision of materials and supplies to facilitate the practice of universal precautions

In the review of these interventions, there was a significant decrease in both fear-based and value-based stigma among hospital workers, there was a significant reduction in reported discriminatory behaviors and practices, and positive changes such as improvement in the use of universal precautions and an increase in voluntary HIV testing were noted.

Evidence of the effectiveness of various stigma-reduction programs

Most of the literature reviewing the effectiveness of stigma-reduction interventions highlights the lack of proper planning and evaluation of interventions (Jacoby 2008, Sengupta *et al.* 2011), as well as the lack of appropriate and valid stigma measures with which to monitor outcomes of interventions (van Brakel 2006, Bos *et al.* 2008). Earnshaw and Chaudoir (2009) suggest that although stigma measures may be psychometrically sound, they may still fail to discriminate between distinct stigma mechanisms if they are not based on a sound theoretical understanding of the various different ways in which stigma may develop and manifest. Jacoby (2008) noted that there was a lack of consistency regarding measures of stigma in epilepsy, and that there was a need to measure both internalized stigma and enacted stigma (overt discrimination).

Various measurements have been suggested to assess stigma change in various conditions, including mental illness, HIV, and epilepsy (Link *et al.* 2004, Corrigan & Shapiro 2010, Svensson *et al.* 2011). They include measures of penetration of public service announcements, measures of changes in knowledge, attitudes, and reported behaviors, measures of directly observable behavior, and more recently the use of physiological and information processing linked to cognitive measures of stigma, in order to counter the social desirability bias in many measures of stigma.

General principles in addressing stigma in epilepsy and HIV

(1) The importance of a **sound theoretical understanding** of stigma in general, as well as in specific conditions and contexts, is highlighted in the literature.

(2) A **framework for planning** stigma-reduction programs is essential. Evaluation of programs should be rigorous, with validated and specific stigma assessment tools and the use of randomized controlled trials of interventions to demonstrate effectiveness of interventions (Bandstra *et al.* 2008, Sengupta *et al.* 2011).

Bos *et al.* (2008) suggested a systematic approach in four major phases:

   (a) diagnosis (accurate and thorough situational analysis, based on theory as well as local context)

   (b) development (with attention to designing appropriate measures and clear interventions)

   (c) implementation (in a systematic and planned way)

   (d) evaluation (using pre- and post-intervention assessment tools)

(3) The **individual in context** is an important principle for stigma-reduction interventions. Heijnders and van der Meij (2006) suggest a patient-centered approach to stigma reduction in general. However, Scambler (2009) suggests that this is an inadequate "top-down" approach that needs to also include attention to the structural factors that maintain or entrench stigma and discrimination in societies. The UNAIDS publication (2007) offers a resource for addressing stigma and discrimination at a national level.

(4) "Nothing about us without us" is another important principle in planning, designing, implementing, and evaluating interventions. **Partnerships between consumers and professionals** are essential in living out (rather than just speaking about) an anti-stigma approach.

(5) **Link anti-stigma campaigns with treatment.** Addressing stigma should be an integral part of the management of stigmatized health conditions. While it is critical that medication is available and accessible to treat these disorders, it is essential to address the psychosocial needs of individuals with these disorders, in order to improve well-being, adherence, and treatment outcomes (Mahajan *et al.* 2008). It is critical to include psychosocial interventions, empowerment, and advocacy as part of the management of these conditions (Corrigan & Shapiro 2010).

(6) **Global campaigns.** As mentioned above, global campaigns for health-related stigma can produce significant change (de Boer 2010). The global campaigns in epilepsy and mental health are examples of this. It is often difficult to overcome stigma-related problems on an individual basis, but joining with other like-minded people can be a powerful force for change.

References

Abaasa AM, Todd J, Ekoru K, *et al.* (2008) Good adherence to HAART and improved survival in a community HIV/AIDS treatment and care programme: the experience of The AIDS Support Organization (TASO), Kampala, Uganda. *BMC Health Services Research* 8: 241.

Alonzo AA, Reynolds NR (1995) Stigma, HIV and AIDS: an exploration and elaboration of a stigma trajectory. *Social Science and Medicine (1982)* 41: 303–15.

Assefa Y, Van Damme W, Mariam DH, Kloos H (2010) Toward universal access to HIV counseling and testing and antiretroviral treatment in Ethiopia: looking beyond HIV testing and ART initiation. *AIDS Patient Care and STDs* 24: 521–5.

Bandstra NF, Camfield CS, Camfield PR (2008) Stigma of epilepsy. *Canadian Journal of Neurological Sciences* 35: 436–40.

Baskind R, Birbeck GL (2005) Epilepsy-associated stigma in sub-Saharan Africa: the social landscape of a disease. *Epilepsy and Behavior* 7 (1): 68–73.

Birbeck G (2006) Interventions to reduce epilepsy-associated stigma. *Psychology, Health and Medicine* 11: 364–6.

Bos AER, Schaalma HP, Pryor JB (2008) Reducing AIDS-related stigma in developing countries: the importance of theory- and evidence-based intervention. *Psychology, Health and Medicine* 13: 450–60.

Brickley DB, Hanh DLD, Nguyet LT, *et al.* (2009) Community, family, and partner-related stigma experienced by pregnant and postpartum women with HIV in Ho Chi Minh City, Vietnam. *AIDS and Behavior* 13: 1197–1204.

Brown L, MacIntyre K, Trujillo L (2003) Interventions to reduce HIV/AIDS stigma: what have we learned? *AIDS Education and Prevention* 15: 9–69.

Campbell C, Foulis CA, Maimane S, Sibiya Z (2005) "I have an evil child at my house": stigma and HIV/AIDS management in a South African community. *American Journal of Public Health* 95: 808–15.

Chigwedere P, Essex M (2010) AIDS denialism and public health practice. *AIDS and Behavior* 14: 237–47.

Chomba EN, Haworth A, Atadzhanov M, Mbewe E, Birbeck GL (2007) Zambian health care workers' knowledge, attitudes, beliefs, and practices regarding epilepsy. *Epilepsy and Behavior* 10 (1): 111–19.

Cluver L, Orkin M (2009) Cumulative risk and AIDS-orphanhood: interactions of stigma, bullying and poverty on child mental health in South Africa. *Social Science and Medicine* 69: 1186–93.

Corrigan PW, Shapiro J (2010) Measuring the impact of programs that challenge the public stigma of mental illness. *Clinical Psychology Reviews* 30: 907–22.

de Boer HM (2010) Epilepsy stigma: moving from a global problem to global solutions. *Seizure* 19: 630–6.

Diop AG, de Boer HM, Mandlhate C, Prilipko L, Meinardi H (2003) The global campaign against epilepsy in Africa. *Acta Tropica* 87 (1): 149–159.

Earnshaw VA, Chaudoir SR (2009) From conceptualizing to measuring HIV stigma: a review of HIV stigma mechanism measures. *AIDS and Behavior* 13: 1160–77.

Heijnders M, Van Der Meij S (2006) The fight against stigma: an overview of stigma-reduction strategies and interventions. *Psychology, Health and Medicine* 11: 353–63.

Heywood M (2004) The price of denial. *Development Update* 5 (3). http://www.tac.org.za/Documents/PriceOfDenial.doc (accessed July 2013).

Jacoby A (2008) Epilepsy and stigma: an update and critical review. *Current Neurology and Neuroscience Reports* 8: 339–44.

Jacoby A, Austin JK (2007) Social stigma for adults and children with epilepsy. *Epilepsia* 48 (Suppl 9): 6–9.

Link BG, Phelan JC (2001) Conceptualizing stigma. *Annual Review of Sociology* 27: 363–85.

Link BG, Yang LH, Phelan JC, Collins PY (2004) Measuring mental illness stigma. *Schizophrenia Bulletin* 30: 511–41.

Mahajan AP, Sayles JN, Patel VA, *et al.* (2008) Stigma in the HIV/AIDS epidemic: a review of the literature and recommendations for the way forward. *AIDS (London, England)* 22 (Suppl 2): S67–79.

Maman S, Abler L, Parker L, *et al.* (2009) A comparison of HIV stigma and discrimination in five international sites: the influence of care and treatment resources in high prevalence settings. *Social Science and Medicine* 68: 2271–8.

Monjok E, Smesny A, Essien EJ (2009) HIV/AIDS-related stigma and discrimination in Nigeria: review of research studies and future directions for prevention strategies. *African Journal of Reproductive Health* 13 (3): 21–35.

Nthomang K, Phaladze N, Oagile N, *et al.* (2009) People living with HIV and AIDS on the brink. Stigma: a complex sociocultural impediment in the fight against HIV and AIDS in Botswana. *Health Care for Women International* 30: 233–54.

Nyblade L, Stangl A, Weiss E, Ashburn K (2009) Comabating HIV stigma in health care settings: what works? *Journal of the International AIDS Society* 12 (15).

Parker R, Aggleton P (2003) HIV and AIDS-related stigma and discrimination: a conceptual framework and implications for action. *Social Science and Medicine* 57: 13–24.

Scambler G (2009) Health-related stigma. *Sociology of Health and Illness* **31**: 441–55.

Sengupta S, Banks B, Jonas D, Miles MS, Smith GC (2011) HIV interventions to reduce HIV/AIDS stigma: a systematic review. *AIDS and Behavior* **15**: 1075–87.

Sunkel C (2012) Empowerment and partnership in mental health. *Lancet* **379**: 201–2.

Svensson B, Markström U, Bejerholm U, *et al.* (2011) Test–retest reliability of two instruments for measuring public attitudes towards persons with mental illness. *BMC Psychiatry* **11**: 11.

Treatment Action Campaign (2012) About the Treatment Action Campain. http://www.tac.org.za/about_us (accessed July 2013).

UNAIDS (2007) *Reducing HIV Stigma and Discrimination: a Critical Part of National AIDS Programmes, Joint United Nations Programme*. Geneva: UNAIDS.

van Brakel W (2006) Measuring health-related stigma: a literature review. *Psychology, Health and Medicine* **11**: 307–34.

World Health Organization (2002) *Mental Health Global Action Programme (mhGAP)*. Geneva: WHO.

World Health Organization (2005) *Epilepsy Atlas*. Geneva: WHO.

World Health Organization (2012) *Global HIV/AIDS Response: Epidemic Update and Health Sector Progress Towards Universal Access: Progress Report 2011*. Geneva: WHO.

Chapter 13

The challenges of human resources in low- and middle-income countries

David M. Ndetei and Patrick Gatonga

Introduction

Human resources are the most valuable asset of mental health services (World Health Organization 2005). In recognition of this the WHO in 2001 listed development of human resources as one of its 10 recommendations for mental health (Box 13.1). In spite of this, lack of or inadequate planning and prioritization of human resources by governments or, until recently, unavailability of training facilities in several low- and middle-income countries (LMICs) is rampant. Many LMICs have few trained human resources, and often face distribution difficulties within the country or region. For instance, there may be too few staff in rural settings or too many staff in large institutional settings. Moreover, staff competencies may be outdated or may not meet the population's needs. In addition, available personnel may not be used appropriately, and many of the staff may be unproductive or demoralized, and experience burn-out. This situation demands that mental health human resources in LMICs be given

> **Box 13.1:** Ten recommendations for mental health
>
> (World Health Organization 2001)
> (1) Provide treatment in primary care
> (2) Make psychotropic drugs available
> (3) Give care in the community
> (4) Educate the public
> (5) Involve communities, families, and consumers
> (6) Establish national policies, programs, and legislation
> (7) Develop human resources
> (8) Link up with other sectors
> (9) Monitor community and mental health
> (10) Support more research

importance in global health and the public health agenda of different countries.

Despite the growing public health burden of neuropsychiatric disorders, there is still widespread neglect of human resources for mental health care in LMICs. The evidence that is available highlights an alarming scarcity and inequitable distribution of professionals available in such countries (Horton 2007, Jacob *et al.* 2007, Saraceno *et al.* 2007). This includes not only a scarcity of staff numbers, but also a shortage of appropriate training and supervision in mental health care (Ghebrehiwet & Barrett 2007, Saxena *et al.* 2007). Nearly 90% of African countries have less than one psychiatrist per 100 000 people, and the median density of professionals for low-income countries is 0.06 per 100 000, compared to 10.5 for high-income countries (Jacob *et al.* 2007). Such shortages have been attributed to the lack of financial incentives for professionals to receive mental health training (Ghebrehiwet & Barrett 2007); poor working conditions (Saraceno *et al.* 2007); widespread stigma of mental health professionals; frequent migration of professionals to high-income countries; and a grossly inadequate number of mental health training facilities and institutions (Saxena *et al.* 2007). Globally, inadequate human resources have been identified as one of the most tangible barriers to scaling up and improving mental health services (Saraceno *et al.* 2007).

Low-income countries are mainly concentrated in Africa and Asia. The former takes the bulk of these countries. Middle-income countries are concentrated in the Americas, Southeast Asia, the Western Pacific, and some parts of the Eastern Mediterranean and Eastern Europe (World Health Organization 2005). It is important to note that while dire shortages of

Essentials of Global Mental Health, ed. Samuel O. Okpaku. Published by Cambridge University Press. © Cambridge University Press 2014.

Box 13.2: The case of Kenya illustrates the human resource situation in low-income countries

In 2012, Kenya had a population of about 38 million people. In that year, the number of psychiatrists practicing in the country was about 150, about double that recorded in 2006 – giving a psychiatrist-to-population ratio of 1:253 333. This scenario is likely to persist over a long period of time despite the apparent growing popularity of psychiatry training among medical students in the country.

mental health human resources exist in each of these countries, the degree of this problem varies from country to country. Low-income countries are the most affected by this problem. A case of this problem is illustrated in Box 13.2.

Factors causing poor human resource availability

Several studies have contributed to the body of knowledge on the root causes of poor availability of the mental health workforce. These have been conducted in many LMICs across the world.

Poor implementation of mental health policies and guidelines

The training and distribution of human resources requires good will from political and administrative circles. These higher authorities are responsible for the creation of sustainable programs that churn out mental healthcare workers. Even where specialist training is not available, it is important to train lower cadres of healthcare workers on the basic principles of mental healthcare provision. This in turn would equip them with skills to tackle common mental illnesses such as anxiety and depression. This training requires resources that can only be made available by governments in respective countries.

Further, in most countries, even after training has been carried out, many mental healthcare workers disperse to areas where populations with high incomes are concentrated. It is understandable that given the economic difficulties facing most countries, many of these professionals opt to make a better living from the higher income earners. Indeed, it must be remembered that healthcare workers are individuals with various financial responsibilities

to take care of. Therefore it would be unrealistic to impart knowledge to them and expect them to provide services with little income.

This challenge can, however, be tackled by policies and government incentives. In order to improve retention of these workers in public service, incentives such as salary allowances, opportunities for further training, and better salaries would not only improve their availability to the larger public, but would equip them with better skills to grow and develop the profession further (World Health Organization 2005).

Brain drain

The emigration of mental health professionals from countries of low and middle income, along with rural-to-urban migration, constrains development of human resources for mental health. Professional isolation, social amenities, implements, insecurity, and better training and career opportunities are key reasons for emigration. The UK, the USA, New Zealand, and Australia employ 9000 psychiatrists from India, the Philippines, Pakistan, Bangladesh, Nigeria, Egypt, and Sri Lanka. Without this migration, many source countries would have more than doubled (in some cases 5–8 times) the number of psychiatrists per 100 000 population.

Lack of evidence in mental health

For a long time, there has been scarcity of research evidence on the burden of mental illness in many developing countries. This knowledge gap has been neglected, and therefore little has been known about the magnitude of the problem.

However, recently a lot of effort has been put into filling this gap. There is a continuing search for evidence on the impact of mental illness on affected individuals, families, and communities. One example is provided by the Africa Mental Health Foundation (AMHF), an organization based in Kenya. Its work has yielded overwhelming evidence of a high burden of mental health in Africa. Similarly, other individual and institutional researchers are reporting findings to support that mental illness does not spare developing countries.

The long period during which there was no supporting evidence led to neglect of this important aspect of health. Few policies were drafted, and even fewer of those few were implemented, and often only to a limited extent.

Education of mental health service providers

Ongoing development of a workforce with appropriate skills is essential to strengthen human resources for mental health. Training should be relevant to the mental health needs of the population and include in-service training and strengthening of institutional capacity to implement training programs effectively. However, training programs for psychiatrists are present in only 55% of low-income countries, 69% of middle-income countries, and 60% of upper-middle-income countries (Kakuma *et al.* 2011). Approaches to this training also vary among different countries. For example, in Nigeria a specialist training program has been in place for over 25 years, yet only half of the country's tertiary mental health facilities have enough psychiatrists to provide accredited training, implying that enrollment and accreditation processes are not optimally efficient.

Establishment of local training programs is especially important to reduce the likelihood of outmigration. International collaborations have been an important strategy in the scaling up of human resources for mental health. For example, by means of providing training in Ethiopia, the number of psychiatrists rose from 11 to 34 between 2003 and 2009. This has led to the expansion of the initiative. Indeed, this phenomenon should be replicated in several other affected parts.

Current interventions to improve mental health education among health workers include training primary healthcare workers, who are increasingly being delegated the role of mental health care. Increasingly, therefore, mental health is being integrated into general health care.

Stigma

While the main victims of stigmatization of mental health have been patients, healthcare professionals have not been spared either. Some people find it difficult to go into a profession where they will be dealing with societal outcasts. Even though it is known that mental health is largely manageable, a large population from LMICs is yet to understand this. They regard these illnesses and anyone involved with them as outcasts.

Perceived complexity of the mental health subject

Among the least understood subjects in health training institutions is neurological health. The perceived complexity of this subject ranges from the complex neuronal interactions to the fact that there is still much unknown about neuronal and mental functioning. Reasons for this include poor teaching in neurology and complex curricula. The result of this is that mental health is among the least favorite career options among students. Again, few attempts have been made to demystify this myth in most developing countries.

Poor mentorship programs

In order to nurture students into a future career, mentorship is important in helping the students appreciate the role of the profession, as well as in cultivating their interest (McCord *et al.* 2009). Yet, in many developing countries, mentorship has remained theoretical, with few attempts to put it into practice.

Current human resource improvement models

The need to shift models for mental health human resources

During the past 50 years, mental health has undergone major changes towards community-based care in most developed countries. Institutionalized mental health care systems, limited to a few large mental asylums in the main urban areas, disconnecting hospitalized people with mental disorders from their family and community, and run by a small number of overburdened health workers, are no longer acceptable.

Newer models of mental health care involve delegating tasks to existing or new cadres with either less training or narrowly focused training to increase access to lower-cost services. It can include delegating tasks to professionals with less training, or even non-professionals, or a combination of these. In a mental health setting, task shifting might include transferring tasks from a psychiatrist to a non-specialist medical doctor. This occurs in some countries where there are psychiatrist shortages.

This concept might also include the development of a new cadre. For instance, in the Lady Health Worker Programme in Pakistan, it was demonstrated that female community health workers who were trained in cognitive behavioral techniques had the ability to significantly lower depression prevalence among new mothers (Rahman *et al.* 2008).

The challenge with new models is that they require good management and supervision. For instance, higher-skilled mental health workers and/or professionals outside of mental health have to acquire these skills for the task-shifting approach to be successful.

Governments also need to do more to help develop informal resources, such as family and consumer associations, which play a key role in the care and rehabilitation of people with mental disorders.

The new models

In recognition of the enormous treatment gap for mental health, and in particular the poor availability of human resources, incorporation of mental health into primary health care has been adopted. Four main models are used:

(1) **Mental health in primary care** – Mental health is fully integrated with primary-level general health care with staffing by generalist health workers, e.g. doctors and nurses, as part of their routine function or as part of other healthcare programs operating at the primary care level. An example is the case of Uganda's mental health strategy. Here, primary health services are provided by general nurses, midwives, and clinical officers, supplemented by nursing assistants at parish level and medical doctors at county level. These primary healthcare services are supported by district general, regional, and national referral hospitals (Kakuma *et al.* 2011).

(2) **Mental health at primary health care** – Mental health care is located on site at, but not integrated with, primary-level general healthcare services, with staffing by specialist mental health practitioners (whether professional or auxiliary workers). The case of Brazil is an example of this model. This country has centers for psychosocial care, which are established in both urban and rural areas (Mateus *et al.* 2008). Another example is the case of India. This example is located in Thiruvananthapuram, a district of Kerala state. This district has an extensive network of decentralized primary health care centers, ranging from village-level centers serving about 20 villages. First-level referral services are offered at community health centers and taluk hospitals.

(3) **Mental health community outreach** – Mental health care is provided in community settings by staff such as community/village health workers

based in the community or operating on outreach from a health service.

(4) **Mental health care provided through other sectors** – Statutory and non-statutory services in areas other than health may provide mental health care. Staffing may be generalist staff, e.g. social workers, police officers, volunteer counselors, or on-site or on-call mental health professionals.

> **Box 13.3:** Cluster-randomized controlled trials (CRCTs)
>
> These are prospective studies in which groups of individuals or clusters are randomized to intervention groups. They are frequently used in evaluation of service delivery interventions, primarily to avoid contamination but also for logistic and economic reasons (Murray 1998).

Tested interventions

Assessing the efficacy of new models is a complex process. For instance, mental health interventions involve large prospective studies that require follow-up for a long time. An even more complex characteristic is the fact that it is difficult to blind participants in these studies. Hence the concept of cluster-randomized controlled trials, whose design has inherent difficulties (Box 13.3). Various interventions that have been tested through research are discussed below.

Integrated services

Integration of mental health with general health care is important in LMICs. Furthermore, mental disorders and physical health problems are closely associated and often influence each other. Therefore, by integrating mental health into general health care, overall health outcomes will be improved. This has multiple implications for human resources, mainly in the following:

(1) The need for training general healthcare staff in basic mental health competencies to enable them to detect mental disorders, provide basic care, and refer complex cases to specialist psychiatrists.

(2) The need to train mental health specialists to work collaboratively with general health workers, and to provide them with supervision and support.

Community focus and deinstitutionalization

In many developed nations, mental health human resources have been closely drawn from the community. This is in contrast to earlier times when mentally ill patients were confined to institutions. Then, the situation in these institutions was deplorable. Patients were forcefully admitted with little exercise of their due human rights. This situation is still seen in many developing countries. However, changes are beginning to be seen in some countries such as Brazil and Chile. As these changes continue spreading across the world, the community is assuming a major role in the human resource structure for mental health. Personnel drawn from the community are being integrated into mental health care. These local people such as community health workers and lay mental health workers have a much better community acceptance and are important in stigma alleviation efforts. Indeed, the concept of mental health technicians (mhTech) is gaining popularity in many countries. A model to assess the effectiveness of this approach has been tested in Kenya and Liberia, and it has shown positive though as yet unpublished results.

Government incentives

Increasing worker incentives can also improve productivity. The primary financial incentive is the payment system in the form of fees for services and capitation of salary (Scheffler 2008). Healthcare payment systems are increasingly being augmented with pay-for-performance programs, which use financial and non-financial incentives to better align provider and payer objectives, where the payer could be the government, a private insurer, or a patient. For example, Rwanda's pay-for-performance program includes a fee-for-service payment for specific maternal and child health services, and the payment is adjusted based on quality-of-care indicators (Basinga et al. 2010). Facilities with the program have higher probability of institutional deliveries and of children aged 0–23 months receiving a preventive care visit, and better prenatal care quality when compared with healthcare facilities without the program. Pay-for-performance programs are less common in mental health, but the United Kingdom's Quality and Outcomes Framework pay-for-performance program, for example, includes mental health quality-of-care measures, including whether a practice can produce a registry of people with schizophrenia, bipolar disorder, and other psychoses, and whether these patients have had a review in the preceding 15 months.

Other possible interventions in low- and middle-income countries

Recruitment and retention

Mental health human resource systems in LMICs must develop systems to attract staff and retain them over a sustained period of time. Equally, strategies to lead and inspire workers must go hand in hand with retention strategies. This will provide a supportive environment for mental health workers, ensuring that their drive for personal career development is aligned with the overall system's strategy framework.

Deployment

This has been one of the most long-standing problems of human resources management for mental health in LMICs. In some countries, there appears to have been neglect for how the workforce is distributed across a country's regions. There are few staff deployed to remote, rural, or otherwise unpopular areas of the country where there is commonly a much greater treatment gap for mental health.

Engaging private-sector providers

Policy makers need to enhance partnership building between the public and private sectors. Health care in general is a dynamic area, and sooner or later LMICs are likely to experience changes in healthcare financing and health service provision. This is likely to happen at a fast rate in the currently emerging economies of Southeast Asia and the Americas. As economic globalization quickly takes place, the gap between public and private mental health sectors is likely to blur. Hence the need for policies that create an enabling environment for partnership between public and private players in the mental health workforce.

Developing partnerships with non-governmental organizations

Non-governmental organizations (NGOs) have been instrumental in mental health research and program development. This gathered experience enables them to understand the burden of mental illness as well as mental health workforce needs. Some of them have established grassroot connections with communities, therefore gaining acceptability in their respective areas of work. The government, on the other hand, has the mandate to ensure that all its population's mental health needs are met. It develops policies and provides services to the public. It is readily recognized by a people of any nation, and has control of players in the mental health field. This control needs careful execution in order to achieve optimal results. Thus, combining the efforts of government and NGOs is crucial to the success of mental health workforce improvement. An existing example is in Kenya, where AMHF, an NGO, conducts research and develops intervention programs, which when tested are adopted by the Ministry of Health and other stakeholders in order to be fully and widely implemented to improve the mental health workforce, among other benefits.

Deprofessionalization

This refers to the use of non-mental health professionals to provide mental health services, a concept that has been in use since the 1960s. It was first used in the now developed nations and is becoming increasingly popular in many LMICs. Non-professional workers or lay workers provide effective care because they have better knowledge of the language and customs of the community. It has also been found that service users identify with them more readily and form therapeutic alliances with them. The challenge, however, is to ensure that these lay workers are competent and that professional workers are easily accessible when needed. Another challenge lies in ensuring that professional workers are consulted even after non-professional staff are trained and employed. This will avoid the perception that non-professional staff are undermining professional staff, lowering standards of care, and providing service managers with a less costly workforce.

Multidisciplinary approaches

The development of a competent mental health workforce requires coordination of multiple professional and non-professional disciplines. This ensures that staff are able to work in a variety of community, residential, and inpatient settings. They are also able to work across agencies linking service users to a range of statutory and other services. Teamwork enhances the ability to work across service levels.

Intersectoral collaboration

This complements multidisciplinary approaches. It is important to note that patients with mental illnesses typically have multiple other needs related to health, welfare, employment, criminal justice, and education. Thus the promotion of mental health straddles a broad range of sectors and stakeholders, and is not limited to the activities of a ministry of health. The mental health workforce should be developed inter-sectorally, bearing in mind the need to offer mental health training to teachers, welfare workers, police officers, and prison staff, among other stakeholders. Obviously, such a wide scope of training requires concurrence between the government and training institutions such as universities about what types and numbers of mental healthcare workers are needed. Otherwise, mental health human resources policies are doomed to fail. The WHO recommends that countries establish a clearly designated body to coordinate the many sectors involved in the development of a mental health workforce.

Changing staff roles

The change in staff roles stems from the dynamics of change from hospital-based to community-based care, together with the new emphasis on multidisciplinary and intersectoral approaches. While this change is really addition and delegation of responsibilities, it is often perceived as change of roles by affected staff. This is indeed a major issue in mental health reforms, as professionals may be concerned about losing their professional identity, status, income, familiar work environments, and a familiar work culture.

The cost challenge

Rapid scaling-up of human resources available to attend to the mental health treatment gap will incur enormous costs. In a report by Scheffler *et al.* (2011), the costs of such an exercise were provided as shown in Table 13.1, which illustrates how much it would cost to scale up the services of psychiatrists, mental health nurses, and psychosocial care providers for only the eight most common mental illnesses in these regions, namely depression, schizophrenia and other psychotic disorders, suicide, epilepsy, dementia, disorders due to the use of alcohol, disorders due to the use of illicit drugs, and mental disorders in children.

Table 13.1 Annual wage bill to remove shortage of mental health workers by WHO region, 2005 (US$ million, 2005)

WHO region	Psychiatrists	Nurses in mental health settings	Psychosocial care providers	Total
Africa	29	74	104	207
Americas	2	102	20	125
Eastern Mediterranean	21	107	99	227
Europe	0	9	2	11
South east Asia	16	69	51	136
Western Pacific	12	59	37	109

Box 13.4: Group interpersonal therapy (IPT)

This is a promising innovation developed in Uganda (Bolton *et al.* 2003). The focus of IPT is on depression in relation to interpersonal relationships, a focus that was considered congruent with Ugandan culture. This initiative was not part of formal primary mental health care, and group leaders were non-clinician, tertiary-level-educated employees of the sponsoring organization. This had remarkable success, mainly attributed to wide community acceptance following national commitment and the inclusion of mental health in the minimum healthcare package and in the health information system

The case of group interpersonal therapy in Uganda is a good example of how the cost challenge can be tackled (Box 13.4).

Developing mental health human resource strategies in low- and middle-income countries

One of the most critical processes in improvement and restructuring of a mental health workforce for LMICs is strategy development. This is a prerequisite, as it sets out a framework on which further processes are built. Not only is it an inherently critical task, but it also requires expert knowledge and experience for success to be achieved. The process is more than can be learned from books; thus practical experience from strategy developers is a key resource.

In many LMICs, mental health human resource strategists are rare professionals. Nevertheless, an outline of steps on how to restructure the mental health workforce will suffice for a brief overview.

Step 1: Evaluation

It is important to evaluate the existing workforce environment. This aims at establishing the interaction of key stakeholders and components, such as institutions, interest groups, and political processes, as well as the extent to which these elements interact. At the same time, it should be established whether services being delivered are efficient, effective, equitable, and accessible.

Step 2: Planning

The essence of this is to establish what human resources are needed for mental health, including the number of people required and their competencies. It is notable at this point that there is no gold standard as to the number of personnel required. Different countries must establish their own desired ratios, depending on their own unique needs and available resources. This step consists of a cycle of the following events (Figure 13.1):

(a) Situation analysis

This again has various tasks:

(1) Review of current human resource policy – The current policy informs the development of any new strategies.

(2) Assess current supply of staff – This is unique for every country, as every country has its own different level of supply. This also includes determining the competencies possessed by existing staff.

(3) Assess utilization of services – This involves reviewing the extent to which mental health services are currently being utilized. By doing so, human resource planners are able to establish

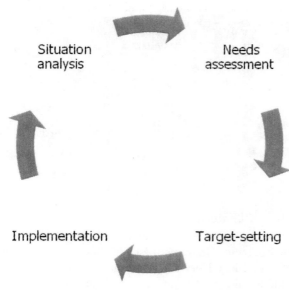

Figure 13.1 The planning cycle.

where staff are not able to meet population demands. For example, one may discover an undersupply of human resources.

(b) Needs assessment

This step acts as a supplement to situation analysis. While situation analysis provides a measure of current service utilization and staff supply, a needs assessment further enables planners to understand what staff are required to address the mental health needs of the community for services and care. In other words, community needs should dictate the required staff supply. The converse of this, which commonly occurs in many LMICs, should not apply. There are steps to follow when conducting a needs assessment:

(1) Determine the burden of psychiatric morbidity through community prevalence studies.

(2) Map the services required for identified population mental health needs.
(3) Identify the staff required for each established service level. This means identifying the functions and competencies of required staff.
(4) Identify the number of staff required at each level.

(c) Target setting

This entails comparing supply and need while utilizing gathered information on current supply of staff and information on existing needs.

(d) Implementation

Putting set targets into action and practice is perhaps the most difficult part of restructuring mental health human resources. It is a tedious, expensive, and challenging process that requires careful execution and patience. It also requires guided change management, as many staff may be reluctant to change from their old ways. Supporting staff members in this process is thus a critical role.

Conclusion

There is a urgent need to improve the mental health workforce in LMICs. While attempts have been made at this, a lot remains to be done. Intervention strategies must involve the government, NGOs, communities, families, affected individuals, and other stakeholders. Mental health human resource strategies should be streamlined, and emphasis should be put on stigma reduction as well as on the provision of accessible, acceptable, sustainable, and affordable care. The strategies should be formulated to address the different needs of specific population groups. They should be tailored in such a way as to address each of the needs of a country's population groups such as children, adolescents, adults, and vulnerable groups such as orphans, refugees, prisoners, and internally displaced persons.

References

Basinga P, Gertler PJ, Binagwaho A, *et al.* (2010) *Paying Primary Health Care Centers for Performance in Rwanda.* Washington, DC: World Bank (policy research working paper 5190).

Bolton P, Bass J, Neugebauer R, *et al.* (2003) Group interpersonal psychotherapy for depression in rural Uganda: a randomized controlled trial. *JAMA* **289**: 3117–24.

Ghebrehiwet T, Barrett T (2007) Nurses and mental health services in developing countries. *Lancet* **370**: 1016–17.

Horton R (2007) Launching a new movement for mental health. *Lancet* **370**: 806.

Jacob KS, Sharan P, Mirza I, *et al.* (2007) Mental health systems in countries: where are we now? *Lancet* **370**: 1061–77.

Kakuma R, Minas H, van Ginneken N, *et al.* (2011) Human resources for mental health care: current situation and strategies for action. *Lancet* **378**: 1654–63.

Mateus MD, Mari JJ, Delgado PG, *et al.* (2008) The mental health system in Brazil: policies and future challenges. *International Journal of Mental Health Systems* **2** (12). doi:10.1186/1752-4458-2-12.

McCord JH, McDonald R, Sippel RS, *et al.* (2009) Surgical career choices: the vital impact of mentoring. *Journal of Surgical Research* **155**: 136–41.

Murray DM (1998) *Design and Analysis of Group-Randomized Controlled Trials*. Oxford: Oxford University Press.

Rahman A, Malik A, Sikander S, Roberts C, Creed F (2008) Cognitive behaviour therapy-based intervention by community health workers for mothers with depression and their infants in rural Pakistan: A cluster-randomised controlled trial. *Lancet* **372**: 902–9.

Saraceno B, van Ommeren M, Batniji R, *et al.* (2007) Barriers to improvement of mental health services in low-income and middle-income countries. *Lancet* **370**: 1164–74.

Saxena S, Thornicroft G, Knapp M, Whiteford HA (2007) Resources for mental health: scarcity, inequity and inefficiency. *Lancet* **370**: 878–89.

Scheffler RM (2008) *Is There a Doctor in the House? Market Signals and Tomorrow's Supply of Doctors*. Palo Alto, CA: Stanford University Press.

Scheffler RM, Bruckner TA, Fulton BD, et al. (2011) *Human Resources for Mental Health: Workforce Shortages in Low- and Middle-Income Countries*. Geneva: WHO.

World Health Organization (2001) *The World Health Report 2001. Mental Health: New Understanding, New Hope*. Geneva: WHO.

World Health Organization (2005) *Human Resources and Training in Mental Health* (Mental Health Policy and Service Guidance Package). Geneva: WHO.

Chapter

14

Integration of mental health services into primary care settings

Shoba Raja, Sarah Kippen Wood, and Jordan Pfau

The management and treatment of mental disorders in primary care is a fundamental step which enables the largest number of people to get easier and faster access to services – it needs to be recognized that many are already seeking help at this level. This not only gives better care; it cuts wastage resulting from unnecessary investigations and inappropriate and non-specific treatments.
(World Health Organization 2001)

Literature review

Background

Primary health care systems are increasingly relied upon to deliver a myriad of health services, especially in situations of scarcity. In low- and middle- income countries, where poverty and sickness are high, and access to health care is low, health professionals and policy makers have emphasized approaches that integrate the diverse roles of health care and social systems. In the past decade, communicable disease programs have been integrated into primary health care in many countries (Shigayeva *et al.* 2010).

For HIV programs, integration has enabled shared use of space and staffing through training of health-care workers and standardizing procedures, increasing the number of people who have receive care (Topp *et al.* 2010). After integrating HIV into primary care, some countries noticed a large number of co-infected tuberculosis (TB) cases among the HIV patients. Therefore, TB has been integrated into primary care alongside HIV, and has been especially effective in places where the disease burdens are high, such as sub-Saharan Africa. This is done through training and development of staff, implementing

new forms of testing (such as HIV testing within TB departments), and establishing referral systems. This has been shown to greatly increase the number of TB patients among those accessing HIV care. However, some challenges have arisen, including convincing people to receive additional testing, and overcoming stigma barriers that often accompany receiving HIV treatment (Harris *et al.* 2008).

Horizontal integration into primary care has been an effective approach to treating communicable diseases, and in many cases has proven more effective than standalone programs focused specifically on eradicating one particular disease (Maeseneer *et al.* 2008). However, these integrations have faced challenges relating to buy-in from primary care physicians and patients, stigma about certain diseases, and most significantly inadequate primary care systems to support the integration of other services.

Similar methods of integration have been recommended for mental healthcare service delivery. It is estimated that mental disorders now account for 14% of the global burden of disease, while existing health systems are not always adequately meeting this need (Prince *et al.* 2007). Because each country's health system is unique and depends on social, economic, and political contexts, the way in which mental health services are executed through primary care may vary widely. Primary care and mental health systems also tend to operate very differently. Where structured diagnosis procedures and attention to many health issues is standard in the delivery of primary care, group therapy and case management are important aspects of mental health care. In order to integrate the two, there must be systematic changes that utilize the strengths in each (Thielke *et al.* 2007). While

---

Essentials of Global Mental Health, ed. Samuel O. Okpaku. Published by Cambridge University Press. © Cambridge University Press 2014.

the experiences of both developed and developing countries vary, key issues with integrating mental health care into primary care remain.

Integrating mental health care: evidence from the literature

Integration to primary care was one of the World Health Organization's 10 recommendations in the World Health Report 2001 on mental health. WHO argues that while mental health issues are prevalent in every country, access to care is limited, and a more comprehensive health policy is the only way to increase access. Integrating mental health care into primary care is recommended for several reasons. First, services at the primary care level are usually the most accessible and affordable. The recognition of mental illness within the community also increases. Second, many patients prefer to see primary care doctors rather than specialists or psychiatrists. Additionally, when a patient has an existing and ongoing relationship with a care provider, the quality of treatment will be better. Finally, receiving mental health care at the primary level reduces stigma and promotes human rights, especially as it replaces hospital-based systems (World Health Organization & Wonca 2008).

While this is a step in the right direction, there are many challenges involved in enacting the WHO's recommendation, and many countries are still relying on outdated hospital-based psychiatric care. The lack of sufficiently efficient primary care systems in low- and middle- income countries, as well as a lack of political support and overburdened health systems, presents major barriers. Without a strong foundation of primary care, it will not be possible to effectively include mental health care. Even where primary care systems do exist in the developing world, primary care health workers often have limited or no training in recognizing and treating mental illness (World Health Organization & Wonca 2008). It is important to note that simply integrating into primary care alone is not believed to be effective, but a mix of services is recommended to provide greater access. This includes community mental health services, general hospital-based care, and informal mental health services at the community level through traditional healers, village elders, and so on (Funk *et al.* 2004). Mental health interventions at the community level, through the training of community health workers, have been shown to be an effective

first line of care, especially where doctors and nurses may be scarce (World Health Organization 2008, BasicNeeds 2009).

Mental health integration is taking place in many countries, both developed and developing, and has gained further prominence because of WHO recommendations. In Jamaica, mental health service integration into primary care happened through training primary care staff, making psychotropic medications available in primary health centers, expanding community mental health programs, and providing more beds at the community level. As a result, the mental hospital population has reduced and community-level services have increased (Abel *et al.* 2011).

A partnership between the Kenyan Ministry of Health, Kenya Psychiatric Association, and the WHO Collaborating Centre through King's College London recently piloted a training and supervision program in order to support the efforts to integrate mental health care into the primary care system. In addition to training, the integration has involved including mental health in the annual operational plans for the district and provincial healthcare facilities, supplying psychotropic drugs to the district facilities in collaboration with the district pharmacist, and maintaining a register for people with a continuing mental disorder. The training program used local trainers and small-scale funding to train front-line health workers and set up systems for supervision. It has been an effective example of working within the framework of the local health and policy system to promote a sustainable training program. Over 1471 primary care staff have already been trained, and an evaluative study showed improvements in many aspects of providing care, including assessment, diagnosis, medicine supply, and record keeping (Jenkins *et al.* 2010).

In Kerala, India, the national government's District Mental Health Programme (DMHP) initiative has been implemented through mental health clinics, which are held in primary care centers, community health centers, and larger hospitals. Psychiatrists are kept on staff at the hospitals. The district mental health team, consisting of a psychiatrist, a clinical psychologist, a psychiatric social worker, and a staff nurse, make monthly visits to the mental health clinics held at the primary care and community facilities. Primary and community health center staff members have received intensive training in identification, diagnosis, and treatment of mental disorders in order to augment the integration. Because of the training, community-based medical officers can actually diagnose and prescribe medications. This has also given primary healthcare staff the resources needed to periodically follow up with participants, and the program has been very successful in improving access to mental health care through primary and community health centers. One issue that has arisen from this mental health initiative has been inadequate funding for ongoing primary health worker training. Because state health workers are reassigned to different districts on a periodic basis, there is a need for ongoing mental health training, requiring additional funding that can be difficult to secure (World Health Organization & Wonca 2008).

In 1996, Uganda began to integrate mental health services into primary care, and to reform regional mental hospitals. New standards were implemented, health workers were trained from the community to institutional level, and the capacity of the national psychiatric hospital was to be reduced by half. The Mental Health Act was also revised, and mental health is now part of the Health Ministry budget. Psychotropic medicines were added to the Essential Medicines List, although the supply of these medicines, especially at the primary care level, is still unreliable (Raja *et al.* 2012). The Uganda program found primary health worker training to be difficult, because of limited human resources and the increased workload; however, setting up village health teams of volunteers has been a critical step toward integrating mental health care in Uganda (World Health Organization 2001).

There is also a growing trend toward mental health integration into primary care in high-income countries. In the USA, a recent study found that primary care patients treated for cardiovascular disease benefited from depression screening through primary care. This depression screening was beneficial when diagnosis, treatment, and follow-up services were offered through a collaborative care model implemented at the primary care level. In the model, the primary care physician works with a care manager, who may be a nurse, social worker, or psychologist, to implement a treatment plan. The care manager supports and educates the patient about depression and the prescribed medicines, and monitors the patient's symptoms. If patients do not respond to treatments as expected, the care manager and primary care physician consult with the psychiatrist (Whooley & Unutzer 2010).

While integrating mental health into primary care seems to be the direction taken by many countries in recent years, there are several factors in play that effect the success of such integration. This is the case in both high-income and developing nations. In order to get a more complete understanding of these factors, the following three case studies will provide an in-depth analysis. One is taken from a developed country and two from low- and middle-income countries. By examining the methods used to integrate mental health and primary care, and the successes and challenges faced, we can extract key messages about mental health integration.

Case studies
United States of America

Mental health care is particularly important for veterans of war. In the United States, one study showed that nearly a third of veterans returning from Iraq and Afghanistan were diagnosed with mental health or psychosocial ills. After the trauma of war, post-traumatic stress disorder, anxiety disorder, and other diagnoses are common (Department of Veterans Affairs 2009). In response to these needs, the President of the United States established the New Freedom Commission on Mental Health in April 2002, which presented goals and recommendations for reforming the healthcare system to better respond to the needs of the mentally ill. The commission called for mental illness to be responded to with the same urgency as physical illness, and because the two are so interrelated, sought to create a more coordinated system. In response, the US Department of Veterans Affairs adapted a Mental Health Strategic Plan (MHSP) in 2004 (New Freedom Commission on Mental Health 2003). The department serves over 23 million veterans in various capacities, as well as the quarter of the US population that is eligible for VA benefits (either veterans, survivors of veterans, or family members) (Department of Veterans Affairs 2009). Specifically, the Veterans Healthcare Administration (VHA) spends over US$40 billion a year on health care, and comprises the country's largest integrated healthcare system. Since the implementation of the MHSP, over US$3 billion of the annual budget is allocated to mental health, and the administration has been a leader in integrating mental health care into the primary care system (Zeiss & Karlin 2008).

The integration has taken place in the three major locations where veterans receive care: community-based outpatient clinics (CBOCs), home-based primary care (HBPC), and primary care outpatient clinics in VA medical centers (PCOCs). The CBOCs are each staffed with at least one mental health staff member, whether it be a psychiatrist, nurse, social worker, or other type of personnel. The community clinics fall under the leadership of a parent facility, and staff can use the parent facility for expertise and other resources. At the home-based level, teams consisting of a psychologist, nurse, social worker, and other professionals such as physical and occupational therapists, visit veterans in their homes. The role of the psychologist is to screen and respond to mental health needs for those in the team's region. They also work with caregivers and help facilitate conversations that will aid in the healing process (Zeiss & Karlin 2008).

In the PCOCs, the integration is executed in three different models: (1) colocated collaborative care, (2) care management, and (3) blended models that incorporate features of the two. In colocated collaborative care, both primary care and mental health practitioners must be present, and both share the responsibility for evaluation and treatment. In the care management model, care managers are present in the primary care facility and are responsible for the mental health treatment of primary care patients. Care managers are typically nurses, but can also by psychologists or social workers. In the blended model, the mental health practitioner is responsible for psychosocial care when needed, and care managers provide ongoing complementary treatment, management, and referrals as necessary (Post & Van Stone 2008).

So far, the integrated system appears to be working well and better addressing the needs of the mentally ill. A study by the Department of Veterans Affairs and the Substance Abuse and Mental Health Services Administration, part of the US Department of Health and Human Services, found that depressed patients were 2.86 times more likely to have at least one contact with a mental health specialist in the integrated care system than in a referral to specialist system (Post & Van Stone 2008).

Challenges faced

The Veterans Health Administration (VHA) has faced challenges with this project largely because of the magnitude of the undertaking. There are 21 regional management entities within the VHA, with hundreds of healthcare facilities affected by the changes, so coordination between all of the entities has been a challenge. In order to keep communication open and keep the project organized, national implementation conferences have been held annually since 2007. Monthly conference calls are also held between stakeholders to address administrative issues, workload monitoring, best practices, and key objectives. The National Primary Care Mental Health Integration Office provides oversight and technical assistance (Post *et al.* 2010).

Laos

Laos (the Lao People's Democratic Republic) is a country in economic transition, and as a result is still working on developing an adequate healthcare system. The country has a total population of 5.62 million, with 72.8% living in rural and 27% in urban areas (Laos Steering Committee of Population Census 2006). The mental health needs in Laos are great, but the government has historically paid too little attention to those needs. Medical professionals are not well trained to recognize mental health problems, so many symptoms of mental illness are dismissed as inconsequential. As in other developing countries, the government's primary focus for health has been on communicable diseases. However, more recently, it has shifted some of its focus to non-communicable disease such as mental illness (Morakoth 2008). The Mahosot Mental Health Unit and the Military Hospital have the only psychiatric clinics in the country, both of which are located in the capital, Vientiane, and are insufficient to meet the needs of the entire population. There are only two psychiatrists in the country (Dr. C. Choulamany, interviewed by Jordan Pfau, December 2011).

In order to address the gaps in access to care, the government partnered with BasicNeeds, an international mental health organization, to establish a community-based mental health and development program. Dr. Chantharavady Choulamany, one of the two psychiatrists in the country, was put in charge of the program implementation. The Ministry of Health, Mahosot Hospital, and Vientiane Capital Health Department have been key players in establishing the program in nine districts of Vientiane. During its launch in 2007, a committee on mental health was established at the Ministry of Health level.

It consists of 11 members, including high-ranking members of government, the Mahosot Hospital director and a handful of mental health practitioners. The committee now approves every decision that is made about mental health for the country (C. Choulamany, interviewed December 2011).

Mental health care is provided at several levels. First, the mental health teams from the Mahosot and Military hospitals assisted in setting up outreach clinics (ORCs). These clinics are held in either village health centers or district hospitals and help to expand access in the communities. Those with mental illness or epilepsy may come to the ORC to receive consultation, diagnosis, and prescription, and to access medicines. The government provides the venue and the staff for the clinic, and BasicNeeds provides transportation, the fees for health workers, and medicines. A member of the mental health team from the Mahosot or Military hospitals (sometimes one of the psychiatrists if they are available) will attend the ORCs to provide the mental health services.

Training on mental health and capacity building has also been provided to general practitioners (GPs), medical officers, general nurses, and volunteers, and mental health teams were set up at the district level. These trained practitioners may help provide care at the ORCs, and also assist with outpatient clinics (OPCs). OPCs are held on a weekly basis at the district hospitals, and trained practitioners will provide consultation, diagnosis, and medicines (paid for out of pocket by the patient). The government fully funds these clinics, providing the venue and the staff (BasicNeeds 2012). Finally, the Mahosot and Military hospitals are available to receive referrals of more serious cases (C. Choulamany, interviewed December 2011). All of these services are performed in primary care settings, and the training of primary care practitioners is a key component in expanding services in a place where mental health specialists are unavailable.

While the program has only been in place for a few years, it has had some successes. Local authorities in Vientiane recently decided that the mentally ill should be included and have access to the same social security benefits as everyone else (C. Choulamany, interviewed December 2011). Government officials in other sectors (such as agriculture, education, and welfare) have received training in mental health and development to help create awareness and reduce stigma within the government (BasicNeeds 2012). The Ministry of Health has also started including

mental health in awareness-raising activities and campaigns. Finally, psychotropic medicines were added to the revolving drug funds at the district hospitals so that people are able to purchase the needed medicines (C. Choulamany, interviewed December 2011).

Challenges faced

The establishment of a mental health system in Laos is in its early stages, and it has been challenging to create something where hardly anything existed before. The shortage of personnel has been a major barrier. It is often difficult to convince the existing practitioners to set aside one day per month for the ORCs. To add to this, there have been some problems with losing practitioners who have been trained in mental health through the program. They are often promoted or moved to other positions where they are no longer able to provide mental health care. There are other areas of health that are lacking sufficient staff, so all practitioners are spread thinly. Nevertheless, health staff trained in mental health by BasicNeeds provide on-the-job training for their colleagues, who are now interested and more involved in mental health services. District hospitals in Vientiane now invest in some psychotropic drugs to ensure that the medicines are available. However, the availability of medicines is another big concern, as diazepam (Valium) is currently the only drug available at the district levels where there is no mental health services delivery. There is an overall shortage of resources to address the needs of the country (C. Choulamany, interviewed December 2011).

India

It is estimated that there are approximately 58 million people with mental illness in India, and only treatment given in a few government hospitals is free. Most psychiatrists are concentrated in the cities, but 75% of the country's population lives in rural areas. For those living below the poverty line, getting long-term treatment for mental illness is often impossible, since virtually all of their money is spent on basic needs for survival. Bihar and Jharkhand, neighbor states in the northeast, are examples where mental health service access is particularly limited, but needs are high. Bihar is the poorest state in India, with key development indicators (such as education and malnutrition) falling well below average (World Bank

2005). Almost 90% of the population resides in rural areas, and over 30% live below the poverty line (Raja *et al.* 2011). Jharkhand's mineral and forest assets show potential for wealth and development, but the state is lacking infrastructure and has the highest rate of child malnutrition in the country (World Bank 2007).

The government of India instituted the National Mental Health Programme in 1982 in order to improve mental health services at all levels – primary, secondary, and tertiary. Primary care is provided at the primary health center (PHC), secondary care at the community health center (CHC), and tertiary care at the medical colleges and district hospitals. The District Mental Health Programme (DMHP) was established to integrate mental health care into the primary care system in all districts. The DMHP applies a public health approach in which people are encouraged to use district mental health services, beginning with PHCs. Services at the PHC level should include medical treatment, educational support, counseling services, and linkages with nongovernmental organizations (NGOs). As of 2010, there were 123 out of 640 districts implementing DMHP in India, covering 28 states and seven territories. The Indian government's goal is to have DMHP implemented in every district by the end of 2017. For Bihar and Jharkhand specifically, local development organization Nav Bharat Jagruti Kendra (NBJK), in partnership with BasicNeeds, is actively working to enhance mental health services through the DMHP. The partnership program aims to implement mental health services through government health facilities in seven districts in Jharkhand and two in Bihar by 2014 (Raja *et al.* 2011).

In Jharkhand, DMHP only exists in three districts, and it remains more of an outreach effort than an integrated aspect of public health. However, progress is being made. District mental health teams of 5–6 people, including a psychiatrist and clinical nurses, are being established in district hospitals. The Ranchi Institute of Neuro-Psychiatry and Allied Sciences (RINPAS) is a government-funded mental health institution in Jharkhand and is key in implementing the DMHP in that state. Six doctors recently received training by RINPAS, including two practitioners from the PHC. They also help facilitate mental health camps, which are held in PHCs. At these camps, a trained psychiatrist or mental health team will come to the PHC to provide diagnosis, medical treatment,

and some counseling on certain days of the month. In addition to clinical services, vocational training is also available at RINPAS. Therefore, there are several levels now where people can receive mental health treatment in the three districts in Jharkhand: the mental health camp at the PHC, the district hospital, or the central hospital at RINPAS. Serious cases are referred from the PHCs and district hospitals to RINPAS.

DMHP has not yet been implemented in Bihar. Prior to the year 2000, Bihar and Jharkhand were one state, so the people of Bihar had access to the services available at RINPAS. After the region separated into two states, there was no such facility for the people of Bihar. The government of Bihar has formed the State Mental Health and Allied Sciences Institute located at the Koilwar Hospital, which now offers inpatient and outpatient treatment. Apart from this hospital, none of the district hospitals has a psychiatrist (Raja *et al.* 2011).

Challenges faced

As in Laos, one of the major challenges has been a lack of focus by the government on mental health problems, as other issues such as malaria and HIV have taken priority. The political will is generally low when it comes to mental health. The establishment of the DMHP requires coordination and support from the government, so it is crucial that it be on their priority list. Evaluative studies of the execution of DMHP in India as a whole have shown problems with poor governance, underpaid and poorly motivated primary health workers, unrealistic expectations, and techno-managerial underperformance (Goel 2011).

In Jharkhand, the DMHP as it functions now does not greatly facilitate integration into primary care. Mental health services are not currently available at the community level, so people must go to district hospitals once a month or to RINPAS. Only one-day training workshops have been offered to doctors and other medical personnel, and the lack of training has impeded the program's success. In Jharkhand, the DMHP has benefited hugely from the support and financing from RINPAS. However, the Koilwar Hospital in Bihar has only recently begun offering inpatient treatment services, and aside from this hospital, none of the district hospitals has a psychiatrist. Therefore, most people have not been able to access mental health services at all. The availability of psychiatrists poses a major challenge. There is meant to be one for each DMHP, but this is proving to be difficult, as there are shortages in trained psychiatrists and those who are trained may move around or leave. Efforts to generate awareness around mental health have been limited, and stigma and discrimination plague the region (Raja *et al.* 2011).

Reflective analysis

There are certain elements that cut across the case studies and allow us to identify common characteristics of integrating mental health into primary care. In each case, there are different levels or steps for receiving treatment, as well as different types of human resources that provide care at each level. First, community-based clinics are utilized in both the developed and developing country examples as the first level for receiving care. In developing countries, community-based workers often identify people with mental illness, provide outreach, visit patients in their homes for follow-up, or provide other services as needed. In developed countries, such as the USA, social workers or other health professionals assist with identification and may provide in-home follow-up visits. Beyond the community level, primary care facilities are utilized as a place to receive basic mental health treatment in addition to general care. General practitioners and nurses are key in providing this care, and training in mental health is provided in order to help general practitioners with identification and diagnosis. Ongoing and consistent supervision is an important aspect of this process, as this helps to ensure that health workers and volunteers are using their mental healthcare skills effectively. Supervision was shown to be especially critical in situations where staff turnover is high. Finally, mental hospitals or mental health units at larger hospitals are used to address referral cases. These are usually located in more central areas and will employ a psychiatrist. While in some countries there may only be one or two such facilities (such as in Laos), it is still necessary that specialized care is available in some form.

The case studies demonstrate how government infrastructure and support are needed for the establishment of an effective primary care system, as well as for the integration of mental health into that system. Government-funded hospitals are the key location for receiving specialized mental health treatment in each example. As governments develop plans for other sectors, it is important that mental health be integrated with these plans so that sustained resources can be secured (World Health Organization 2008).

There are many challenges in the cases examined that demonstrate some of the difficulties with integrating mental health into primary care. The most glaring challenge, especially in the developing countries, is with personnel. Not only is there a shortage of psychiatrists and mental health practitioners, but there are also shortages of general physicians, without whom neither primary nor mental health care can be provided. As is evident in the case studies, there can also be difficulties in retaining trained staff in their posts. Staff are often rotated through posts or assigned to new responsibilities, as was a key issue in India, making training an ongoing process for new staff. The high demands placed upon available primary care staff can sometimes make it difficult for them to make mental health training a high priority. Furthermore, while many training approaches exist for integrating mental health into primary care, little emphasis has been placed upon evaluating the effectiveness of these training programs as well as the overall effectiveness of the integration approach in various settings. Much could be learned from rigorous evaluations of this work.

Finally, funding was a common theme across the case studies. Whereas in the USA example the necessary funding was allocated and dispersed, other countries have not had such support from the government. Funding is needed to provide training, medicines, facilities for clinics, personnel, and other needs. In Kerala, India, funding for the DMHP was provided by the central government for the first five years. After that time, the state government was expected to continue funding the program, but was not able to earmark sufficient funds. Funds have since been secured, but this caused a major strain on operations at the time. If the government cannot be fully relied upon to provide the funding needed for integration and continuation of services, other organizations may need to get involved until sustainable funding is established.

Conclusions

Based upon the case studies presented in this chapter, some shared lessons have emerged. First, an emphasis on developing the primary healthcare system as a whole can be very helpful to the integration process. This includes continuously building a network of both general and specialized heath workers, as well as developing facilities to receive primary care from the local to more regional or national levels. Some flexibility within the primary care system allows historically vertical treatment programs such as mental health to more fully integrate into the system in a sustainable way.

Second, training for general practitioners and other non-specialized health workers is a common aspect of integration. In developing countries, where mental health care is scarce, non-specialized health workers are often utilized to bring care to the larger population. These non-specialized workers can be trained in recognizing and diagnosing mental illness, and it may be useful to include such skills in the general curricula in medical education wherever possible. This allows for the best use of the available knowledge to reach the largest number of people (World Health Organization 2001).

In each of the case-study sites, non-specialized health workers were involved in identifying mental illness, and worked in collaboration with more specialized personnel when needed, and training has been used to expand the capacity of these workers. It is also important that there is ongoing supervision and a place in the system for those who are trained. Whether through a blended collaborative care model, or utilizing non-specialized workers as the first line of contact and referring patients to specialized mental health facilities when needed, non-specialized workers are important when integrating with primary care and expanding access.

Awareness raising and reduction in stigma is another important aspect of integration, as it helps to ensure mental health services are included in conversations and on government agendas. Education and awareness-raising activities have been shown to be helpful throughout the process. A plan for identifying new people who may need mental health services can be especially important in areas where treatment has not previously been available or where there is an inequitable distribution of services. As people with mental illness and epilepsy feel more empowered, they can be instrumental in informing community members and policy makers of their needs.

Dependable funding at multiple levels is also needed to provide the resources required for mental health treatment. This includes human resources, medicines, facilities, funding for livelihood and other training, and all other aspects of mental health care. Government funding is an important part of this, but resources from NGOs or other partners may also play a part.

And finally, in order to determine if integration is successful, monitoring will be needed. Evaluating the integration process in various primary care settings can provide useful insights for mental health practitioners and policy makers, so that improvements can be made and the same mistakes are not repeated.

Many countries are moving mental health care from a hospital-based system to one that is integrated with primary care. As this happens, there is greater opportunity for access to treatment and human rights to improve. Integration with primary care requires cooperation and participation at many levels. While each country's healthcare system is unique, there are common features that can contribute to the sustainability of integration.

References

Abel WD, Richards-Henry M, Wright EG, Eldemire-Shearer D (2011) Integrating mental health into primary care an integrative collaborative primary care model- the Jamaican experience. *West Indian Medical Journal* **60**: 483–9.

BasicNeeds (2009) *Community Mental Health Practice: Seven Essential Features for Scaling Up in Low- and Middle-Income Countries.* Bangalore: BasicNeeds.

BasicNeeds (2012) *Annual Evidence Based Assessment of Mental Health and Development Programmes.* Lao PDR: BasicNeeds.

Department of Veterans Affairs (2009) Facts about the Department of Veterans Affairs. http://www.va.gov/opa/publications/factsheets/fs_department_of_veterans_affairs.pdf (accessed July 2013).

Funk M, Saraceno B, Drew N, *et al.* (2004) Mental health policy and plans: promoting an optimal mix of services in developing countries. *International Journal of Mental Health* **33** (2): 4–16.

Goel DS (2011) Why mental health services in low- and middle-income countries are under-resourced, underperforming: an Indian perspective. *National Medical Journal of India* **24** (2): 94–7.

Harris JB, Hatwiinda SM, Randels KM, *et al.* (2008) Early lessons from the integration of tuberculosis and HIV services in primary care centers in Lusaka, Zambia. *International Journal of Tuberculosis and Lung Disease* **12**: 773–9.

Jenkins R, Kiima D, Njenga F, *et al.* (2010) Integration of mental health into primary care in Kenya. *World Psychiatry* **9**: 118–20.

Laos Steering Committee of Population Census (2006) Results from the population and housing census, 2005. http://www.nsc.gov.la/PopulationCensus2005.htm (accessed July 2013).

Maeseneer JD, van Weel C, Egilman D, et al. (2008) Strengthening primary care: addressing the disparity between vertical and horizontal investment. *British Journal of General Practice* **58** (546): 3–4.

Morakoth M (2008) *Baseline Study Report on Community Mental Health and Development: in Xaythani and Sikhottabong Districts Vientiane Capital, Lao PDR*. Lao PDR: BasicNeeds.

New Freedom Commission on Mental Health (2003) *Achieving the Promise: Transforming Mental Health Care in America. Executive Summary*. Maryland: U.S. Government.

Post EP, Van Stone WW (2008) Veterans Health Administration Primary Care–Mental Health Integration Initiative. *North Carolina Medical Journal* **69**: 49–52.

Post EP, Metzger M, Dumas P, Lehmann L (2010) Integrating mental health into primary care within the Veterans Health Administration. *Families, Systems, and Health* **28** (2), 83–90.

Prince M, Patel V, Saxena S, *et al.* (2007) No health without mental health. *Lancet* **370**: 859–77.

Raja S, Wood SK, Singh M, et al. (2011) *Respecting the Rights and Needs of People with Mental Illness*. BasicNeeds India.

Raja S, Kippen S, Reich MR (2012) Access to psychiatric medicines in Africa. In E Akyeampong, A Hill, A Kleinman, eds., *Culture, Mental Illness and Psychiatric Practice in Africa*. Bloomington, IN: Indiana University Press.

Shigayeva A, Rifat A, McKee M, Coker R (2010) Health systems, communicable diseases and integration. *Health Policy and Planning* **25**: i4–20.

Thielke S, Vannoy S, Unutzer J (2007) Integrating mental health and primary care. *Primary Care: Clinics in Office Practice* **34**: 571–92.

Topp SM, Chipukuma JM, Giganti M, *et al.* (2010) Strengthening health systems at facility-level: feasibility of integrating antiretroviral therapy into primary health care services in Lusaka, Zambia. *PLoS One*, **5** (7): e11522.

Whooley M, Unutzer J (2010) Interdisciplinary stepped care for depression after acute coronary syndrome. *Archives of Internal Medicine* **170**: 585–6.

World Bank (2005) *Bihar: Towards a Development Strategy*. World Bank.

World Bank (2007) *Jharkhand: Addressing the Challenges of Inclusive Development*. World Bank. Report No. 36437-IN.

World Health Organization (2001) *The World Health Report 2001. Mental Health: New Understanding, New Hope*. Geneva: WHO.

World Health Organization (2008) *mhGAP: Mental Health Gap Action Programme. Scaling up Care for Mental, Neurological, and Substance Use Disorders*. Geneva: WHO.

World Health Organization, Wonca [World Organization of Family Doctors] (2008) *Integrating Mental Health into Primary Care: a Global Perspective*. Geneva: WHO.

Zeiss A, Karlin B (2008) *Integrating Mental Health and Primary Care Services in the Department of Veterans Affairs Health Care System*. Washington, DC: Department of Veterans Affairs.

Chapter 15

Collaboration between traditional and Western practitioners

Victoria N. Mutiso, Patrick Gatonga, David M. Ndetei, Teddy Gafna, Anne W. Mbwayo, and Lincoln I. Khasakhala

Many people do not seek help from their GP or via their local mental health services when they become unwell for a number of different reasons. Some people seek advice and support via traditional healers, preferring possibly to enter into a therapeutic dialogue with someone who is from the same culture or who understands their cultural perspective and can facilitate some form of cultural re-integration. *(Ethnic Health Initiative 2010)*

Many people, including mental health professionals, are dismissive of traditional healers and their practices, citing a lack of evidence base to prove the effectiveness of healing interventions or their concerns about the amount of money some healers charge. *(Ethnic Health Initiative 2010)*

Introduction

Management of the mental health patient is a concept that has gradually evolved in many countries and cultures. Every society has developed its own way of viewing the mental health patient, and sometimes different ways of viewing the family of a mental health patient. Thus, over time, different theories on causes of mental illnesses as well as varied ways of managing those illnesses have developed.

Given the multiple cultures and people's origins that exist, there is bound to be a great diversity in the way each group of people approaches health in general and mental health in particular. This phenomenon has been complicated further by different environments surrounding these groups of people. Industrial and economic developments have vastly divided the world into a developed part and a developing part. These advancements have straddled many sectors, including health care. Concurrently, mental health care advances have occurred at different rates across the world. It is clear that many countries are developing modern strategies to tackle current mental health burdens. Of significance, however, is that many societies continue to value their cultural perceptions of mental health. They also continue to carry out their respective traditional mental health practices. While times may have changed, and many societies have adopted a modern lifestyle, the effectiveness and holistic nature of traditional practices are still highly valued. They form an important component of the mental health care system, particularly in the developing world. The importance of these practitioners, along with the promotion and adoption of Western-style practice in many countries, has brought forth the issue of collaboration between the two groups of practitioners.

The place of traditional practitioners

Perhaps before we delve further into this issue, we need to know what is meant by traditional medicine. This term at a global level has eluded precise definition or description as it contains diverse and sometimes conflicting characteristics and viewpoints. Thus the World Health Organization (2002) has provided a working definition for the purposes of clarity and global understanding of the term:

> WHO defines traditional medicine as including diverse health practices, approaches, knowledge and beliefs incorporating plant, animal and/or mineral based medicines, spiritual therapies, manual techniques and exercises applied singularly or in combination to maintain well-being, as well as to treat, diagnose or prevent illness.
>
> (World Health Organization 2002)

Essentials of Global Mental Health, ed. Samuel O. Okpaku. Published by Cambridge University Press. © Cambridge University Press 2014.

Traditional healers are an important source of psychiatric support in many parts of the world, including Africa. They offer a parallel system of belief to conventional medicine regarding the origins, and hence the appropriate treatment, of mental health problems (Ndetei 2007). In one instance, it was reported that patients went to hospital only to look for the cure of their illness, whereas they went to see traditional doctors both for the cure and also to find out the cause of their illness. The application of diagnosis and treatment methods is largely influenced by the culture and beliefs dominant in a particular community, to the extent that they may be ineffective when applied in a different context (Ng'etich 2005).

Research statistics from parts of Africa suggest that 25–40% of all people seeking medical care at primary health level have problems purely related to mental health, and another 25–40% have a combination of mental health problems and physical problems (Ndetei & Muhanji 1979). At the same time the distribution of modern medicine personnel is uneven, with most being found in the urban centers as opposed to the rural areas, with few being found in informal settlements. This mental health treatment gap is seen in many parts of the world, particularly in low- and middle-income countries (Horton 2007, Jacob *et al.* 2007, Saraceno *et al.* 2007). Traditional healers are the first professionals contacted for mental illness in many parts of Africa (Abiodun 1995, Ngoma *et al.* 2003). This is because they are sufficient in numbers in the communities, are accepted, do home visits, do not stigmatize mental illness, are often consulted, and have been demonstrated to see many people with mental disorders (Ndetei *et al.* 2008). They are also willing to learn and willing to collaborate with hospital-based health professionals for a holistic approach in the management of patients. They are enshrined in the minds of the people, are respected in their community, are often its opinion leaders, and are first responders in case of an emergency.

Traditional mental health practices are mainly prevalent in low- and middle-income countries. In these countries, traditional healers provide a rather unique kind of mental health care, with cultural-specific rituals characterizing them. Most developed countries employ Western-style mental healthcare practices. However, general traditional medical practice is common even in developed countries. For instance, various government and non-government reports show that the percentage of the population that has used traditional medicine is 46% in Australia, 49% in France, and 70% in Canada (World Health Organization 2002).

Traditional therapies
Herbs
Many traditional healers use herbs, and a wide range of herbs is used for treatment purposes. An example of a plant with psychiatric medicinal properties that has been used for treating severe psychotic conditions going back to 1925 is *Rauwolfia*, which is rich in reserpine (Ndetei 1988). This plant is found as an ornamental plant in many parts of the world, such as around the Mount Kilimanjaro area in Kenya and Tanzania, where it also grows in the wild. It is known for the treatment of "madness," by which is meant psychosis, regardless of the cause or type.

Psychotherapy
The practice of psychotherapy and behavioral therapy is so much advanced in traditional practice in East Africa that these therapies as practiced in the West are not a match for what happens in traditional Africa. This is illustrated by a statement by Rappoport and Dent (1979), who noted that psychotherapy as practiced in Tanzania was as effective as, if not more effective than, psychotherapy as practiced in the West. The same observation was made by Ndetei (2007).

Surgical
A classic example of a traditional surgical intervention is craniotomy as practiced by the Kisii and Turkana peoples of Kenya for the treatment of psychosis, related to diseases thought to be located inside the skull (Ndetei 1988). This is, however, not practiced today.

Spiritual therapy
Spiritual therapy attempts to bring peace and harmony between the living and the spiritual world, especially spirits of the ancestors, which are believed to live on after death and continue to influence events in the living world.

Recognized benefits of traditional practice

Attendance to both physical and mental illnesses

Traditional mental health care is critical in providing support to societies and communities that would otherwise have no one to attend to the coexisting physical and mental illnesses. This is mainly seen in rural areas of the world with few if any formally trained mental health practitioners. A substantial proportion of people seen by traditional practitioners suffer from mental health problems as well as other diseases. Peltzer *et al.* (2006) found that mental health problems were fourteenth on a list of the most common conditions seen by traditional practitioners, affecting 9% of their clients. These practitioners attend to both physical and mental illnesses.

Acceptability among communities

The provision of mental health care by traditional practitioners may, in certain instances, have a positive impact on individual and community mental health, particularly for common mental disorders (Hewson 1998, Berg 2003, Meissner 2004). The traditional practitioner provides psychosocial support as well as highlighting areas of conflict in a person's life that need to be addressed. It is, however, important to note that while many people with more severe mental illness, such as psychotic disorders, seek care from traditional healers, their capacity to effectively deal with these conditions has been questioned (Ensink & Robertson 1999).

Reduction of the mental health treatment gap

There are far more traditional practitioners than Western-trained mental health practitioners (Meissner 2004), particularly in rural areas in developing countries. Involving traditional practitioners to assist with the care of common mental health problems could help narrow the current treatment gap for common mental disorders in the world. Studies have shown that in both the Western and African societies people living with psychosocial disability seek treatments from both Western-style biomedically oriented practitioners and other alternative-based treatments, including traditional healers. Hence the suggestion that in low- to middle-income countries, "non-professionals," who include traditional practitioners, offer a potentially important human resource for the provision of mental health care.

Cultural appropriateness

In a world where global health care has been tailored to be both responsive and appropriate to culture, traditional practitioners are increasingly considered to play a role in bridging the gap between the community and the Western practices. In the Western practice, various explanatory models have been developed to aid in the understanding of mental health problems by understanding how a person interprets his or her illness in relation to causation, precipitating events, initial symptoms, the expected course of the illness, and treatment options.

However, as much as the Western-based models have contributed to the understanding of mental health problem, they have been criticized as not being culturally appropriate and sensitive. In order to meet that need, a push has risen for the development of indigenous explanatory models of mental health problems which incorporate spiritual understandings of causation, including the understanding of beliefs, traditions, and culture. This has necessitated the need to increasingly cooperate with the traditional practitioners in mental health service delivery.

The shift towards collaboration

Over the past few years there have been moves to facilitate collaboration between traditional practitioners and Western practitioners. This has taken place in countries such as South Africa and India, where national health policies have been amended to try and recognize the role of traditional practitioners (Ndhlalambi 2009). This has entailed attempts towards the formalization, regulation, and professionalization of the sector. However, a number of questions have been raised concerning the move in some countries to recognize and professionalize the traditional practitioners. The concerns pertain to issues of whether it is possible, or desirable, to have state regulation over a system so steeped in cultural and spiritual knowledge and practice. Further, how traditional practitioners would interface with the Western-based state health care system is also unclear (Devenish 2005). Both practices have powerful, well-developed systems of treatment based on deeply entrenched beliefs within their respective communities.

Consequently, the challenge that has emerged in the attempt to encourage collaboration is to avoid a situation that allows and entrenches conflict between the two modes of practice. For in the context where mental health service users utilize both systems concurrently, it becomes vital for collaboration between the sectors to be championed through the development of systems to facilitate collaboration between Western and traditional-based healing systems.

The attempt to increase interaction between traditional and Western practitioners has brought to the fore three terms: incorporation, cooperation/collaboration, and integration. These terms can all be used in the context of the interaction between traditional practitioners and Western practitioners, and each term is fraught with its own challenges in its application. Over the past few years a lot more attention has been paid to collaboration than to the other two terms.

However, researched opinions of various stakeholders, including mental health specialists and traditional practitioners, have shown that there is a bias towards the cooperation/collaboration option which provides for the two systems to remain autonomous and self-regulating, with practitioners cooperating, for example, through mutual referral. This dual approach to collaboration, which encourages interdependence, has been greatly encouraged, for it is believed that it gives the person living with psychosocial disability freedom to choose and to enjoy the benefits from twofold psychiatric and traditional treatments. This practice of seeking treatment from both systems of health care is viewed as unproblematic. The dual approach, it has been emphasized, is even easier to implement in countries' constitutions, because it takes into account an individual's rights – which is in line with the mhGAP campaign (World Health Organization 2008).

Similarities between traditional and Western mental health care

There are two major similarities between traditional and Western mental health care.

Multifactorial causation of mental illness

Current Western theories on causation of mental illness support a multifactorial basis for the illnesses. These theories propose that mental illness is a product of complex interaction between biological/genetic predisposition to illness and environmental factors. This understanding is the basis for the biopsychosocial model of treating mental illnesses. This model supposes that in order to manage mental illness, the practitioner should target management decisions on three patient aspects: biological, psychological, and social dimensions.

Similarly, many traditional healers believe that mental illness has a multifactorial basis. What varies among different cultures and peoples are the attendant factors in this model. In South Africa, for example, studies report that healers understand mental illness as being caused by several factors. Among these factors are traditional causes such as jealousy and bewitchment, psychosocial causes such as stress and conflictual relationships, and causes expressed in Christian religious terms.

Treatment methods

Traditional healers use a range of treatment modalities, including herbs, massages, heat and/or whips. Treatment by these practitioners also involves psychotherapy, in which, using cultural means and convictions, a patients' behaviors are altered by invoking their perceptions. Similarly, Western-style practitioners employ a biopsychosocial approach to the management of mental illnesses. This approach addresses the various possible disease-causing or disease-aggravating dimensions surrounding a patient.

Current views on collaboration between traditional and Western-style practitioners

There is a great deal of debate over the legitimacy of traditional healers and differing views on collaboration. The different views put forward can be roughly divided into three groups. The "classical" view holds that there is disjuncture between scientific Western medicine and the magical thinking of traditional healing (Stein 2008). One group advocating this position is Doctors for Life (DFL), an international organization that represents a large number of medical doctors, dentists, veterinarians, and other professionals, which views traditional medicine as ineffective and unsafe.

A second "critical" view argues that science and biomedicine reflect just one particular way of looking at the world, which is not necessarily privileged (Stein 2008). Some who hold this view argue that both Western medications and traditional agents can have therapeutic efficacy. Others are more skeptical about the value of any particular intervention. A third perspective might be termed "integrative." In this view, both Western medicine and traditional healing are social activities and therefore reflect particular cultural values. Both types of intervention act on underlying biopsychosocial mechanisms, explaining why both medical and traditional interventions can influence health (Stein 2008).

Possible areas for collaboration

Recognizing differences in the needs and context of people of different ethnic groups is important for developing culturally responsive and appropriate health services. The complexity of mental health systems in some countries may be increased by the parallel operation of traditional healers and Western-style practitioners. Finau and Tukuitonga (1999) reported that there is need for Western healthcare approaches to operate alongside traditional approaches, as long as suitable, mutually respectful and understanding attitudes are adopted. However, there is also potential for the two systems to work at cross-purposes or incompatibly. This could lead to a higher risk and poorer outcomes for their clients. Collaboration is therefore necessary to ensure optimal benefit of the care accorded by both traditional and Western practitioners.

Referrals

Mental illnesses are differently understood by different cultures and peoples of the world. It so happens that some illnesses such as anxiety are greatly influenced by the patient's cognitive behavior rather than mere biological or neurological disturbance. This makes many mental illnesses manageable by careful psychotherapy. Who provides the psychotherapy is mostly a matter of the patient's choice, or in some cases the family's choice. Some families would be more inclined to seek the care of Western-style practitioners, while others seek the care of traditional practitioners. The choice depends on the environment of the patient and the patient's and the family's perceptions about mental illnesses.

On the other hand, practitioners are able to gauge the effectiveness of the treatment they provide. For instance, a traditional practitioner would be able to know when a patient is not responding to treatment as would be desired. Even though their parameters of measuring response may not be standardized or scientific, experienced practitioners would offer fairly good judgment as to the progress of the patient. Similarly, Western-style practitioners can easily determine how successful their management approach is. For instance, scientific methods or tools for assessment of a patient's progress exist. In other words, both groups of practitioners can easily know when there is need to refer a patient for further assessment and management.

At the same time, some patients respond better to traditional methods of treatment while others respond better to modern treatment methods. The response to either of these is determined largely by the nature of the illness, including risk factors surrounding the illness episode. For instance, an acute manic episode would be well managed by pharmacotherapy in order to calm the patient down. A patient with an anxiety disorder can be managed by a traditional healer, especially if they come from a culture that strongly believes in a cultural etiology of disease. Thus, for both traditional and Western-style practitioners, there is need to have judgment skills on when it is prudent to refer a patient to either cadre.

Such a referral system is not easy to develop. It is important, therefore, that policy makers in mental health develop a means of fostering cooperation between the two groups of practitioners. In a well-developed system, synergy would be greatly achieved. Examples of countries where this has taken place include Uganda, Kenya, and South Africa. Though this collaboration is still in maturation stages, studies show a good response and potential for major impact in the treatment of mental illnesses.

Identifying factors associated with traditional healer referral of their patients with a mental illness is also important for developing and designing interventions to ensure traditional healers refer more frequently and appropriately. Behavioral theories can assist with identifying the determinants of a behavior, which is imperative when developing interventions, since interventions that address these determinants are more likely to be effective (Bartholomew et al. 2000).

Appreciation of patients' cultural perceptions of mental illness

Another process by which collaboration with traditional healers occurs in the clinic is directly through the patient. The psychiatrists in these clinics conduct a cultural assessment of patients that includes review of tribal languages spoken, spiritual history, attitude towards traditional healing practices, and past treatment by traditional healers. For patients who endorse an interest in or history of working with traditional healers, the psychiatrist further discusses the treatment options related to traditional healing that can address the patient's current mental health issues.

Formal collaboration

In addition to the informal collaboration described above, several ways of formal collaboration can be instituted between the healers and the medical practitioner. This may entail discussion with the community's leadership structure and agreeing on recognition of certain traditional healers. Once this is done, a list of traditional practitioners is developed. The respective practitioners then formally work with existing mental health services in order to improve access to mental health care. This basically means that these traditional practitioners are formally recognized and no longer have informal dealings with established Western-style mental health practice. This more formal approach is effective between the traditional and Western-style mental health practitioners.

Obstacles to collaboration

> The greatest obstacle to such collaboration has been the mutual suspicion between the two sectors and the concerns of the biomedical sector and the religious establishment regarding the "unscientific" and unorthodox practices of traditional healers.
>
> (Vikram Patel 2011)

In some countries, there is a general impression by local formally trained mental health professionals that traditional healers cannot cure serious mental illness. In such circumstances, it is reported that indigenous healers do not give their clients any information about the prognosis of their condition or the effects of treatment, and do not concern themselves at all with the social circumstances of their clients. In fact, healers such as diviners appear to have potentially adverse effects on patients with serious mental disorders by increasing their already existing financial stresses, by increasing anxiety and stigmatization through the diagnosis of bewitchment, and by not making timely referrals to psychiatrists.

Human rights concerns of traditional/faith healing practices

One of the main obstacles hindering collaboration between Western-style practitioners and traditional practitioners concerns human rights abuses that can occur in prayer camps and traditional shrines. In a study conducted in Ghana, reports of maltreatment, neglect, and exploitation were cited by study participants as human rights abuses inflicted by traditional healers (Ae-Ngibise *et al.* 2010). Some participants complained that traditional healers used forced fasting and exorcisms, which included physical beatings that were sometimes fatal, chaining to contain agitated patients, and forced confinement.

Safety and efficacy concerns of traditional/faith healing practices

Formally trained mental health care workers doubt the safety and efficacy of traditional healing practices, particularly for more serious mental disorders. This is because very little clinical evidence exists concerning the quality of such methods.

Skepticism around effectiveness of Western-style practice

Traditional healers are also skeptical about the value of Western-style practice. Given perceptions of the underlying spiritual cause of mental disorders, some traditional healers feel that Western-style treatment is not always appropriate. This view of traditional healers is depicted in the statement quoted below (Ae-Ngibise *et al.* 2010):

> I do not think that doctors really know the difference between demons and real madness. Because if somebody goes into a trance, they start speaking in tongues; that is not madness but spirituality, and it is demon possession. If someone is being haunted by a ghost, it is not madness; and so in these cases doctors' medicine won't make an improvement.
>
> (a Ghanaian traditional healer)

Lessons learnt from existing collaborative models

The debate on the best way to involve both traditional and Western-style mental health practitioners rages on. While there remains a lot to be studied and discussed, the following lessons have been learnt:

- As both traditional and Western practitioners fear an undermining of the underpinning systems of mental health care, a collaborative approach which does not encroach on the domain of Western biomedical approaches or the domain of traditional healing but finds those points of intersection that are mutually reinforcing needs to be adopted.

- In order to build mutual respect, Western healthcare practitioners need to be oriented from a purely biomedical discourse of care towards a "meaning-centered" approach (Kleinman 1980) which is accommodating of diverse cultural explanations of illness. Kleinman (1980) provides a practical framework for the facilitation of culture-centered care, which involves a process of illness negotiation between Western healthcare practitioners and their patients. This process requires that the Western healthcare practitioners understand the user's illness problem from the user's perspective as well as the disease problem from a biomedical perspective, and that through a process of illness negotiation they can reach a consensus with the user as to the treatment plan. The plan could potentially incorporate certain traditional treatment options together with Western-based interventions. Further, traditional practitioners would need to be acquainted with Western treatment modalities.

- While Wreford's (2005b) collaborative model, which involves both Western and traditional health practitioners operating out of one center, is not feasible within the existing resource constraints for mental health, there is a need for the development of alternative arrangements for bringing these different mental health service providers together to negotiate collaborative arrangements.

Conclusion

To plan the way forward for cooperation/collaboration with respect to mental health care, it is vital to learn from previous attempts at establishing collaboration between traditional practitioners and the formal healthcare system for other illnesses. Such collaborative arrangements have been developed for the care of HIV/AIDS and tuberculosis in South Africa and other parts of Africa (King 2000, Colvin et al. 2003, Wreford 2005a, Peltzer et al. 2006). These attempts have,

however, generally been small-scale, localized, and short-term projects with limited funding and insufficient reporting and evaluation (Wreford 2005a). One major shortcoming in all of them has been a process whereby traditional practitioners are expected to learn from Western medicine, apply these concepts in their practice, and refer more serious cases to the formal health services – with virtually no appreciation of the practices of traditional medicine (King 2000, Wreford 2005b). It is thus questionable as to how truly collaborative these arrangements are, as they appear more a case of the traditional practitioners assisting the biomedical health sector. Wreford (2005b) suggests that any attempt at collaboration must involve mutual respect and learning from both sides.

Additionally, there is a need for the development of evidence-based models of collaboration which promote a reciprocal collaboration at district level and which are respectful of both healing systems. Wreford (2005b) describes an ideal model of collaboration for South Africa, based on the efforts of Women Fighting AIDS in Kenya (WOFAK) (Anderson & Kaleeba 2002). This model incorporates both biomedical and traditional diagnosis, treatment, and prescription through referral between two different service providers, working in different modalities, in one HIV/AIDS treatment and counseling center. It was found that this close mutual relationship encouraged more trust, mutual respect, and learning and better working relations between the two sectors (Anderson & Kaleeba 2002). Studies have shown that traditional practitioners allude to the need for a similar arrangement for the treatment of mental health problems, suggesting that locating both traditional practitioners and Western health practitioners in the same treatment setting would facilitate collaboration, possibly even leading to some level of cross-referral. Further, professionalization of traditional practitioners is also viewed as a possible mechanism for increasing the recognition afforded to traditional practitioners.

Overall, a model that incorporates both traditional and western-style practices needs to be worked out. It will be crucial in alleviating the growing burden of mental illness. While no consensus on an ideal model has been reached yet at the time of writing, one thing remains clear, that neither of these two groups shall solely address the mental health burden. There is need for collaboration, until such a time as both practices merge into one.

References

Abiodun O (1995) Pathways to mental health care in Nigeria. *Psychiatric Services* **46**: 823–6.

Ae-Ngibise K, Cooper S, Adiibokah E, et al. (2010) Whether you like it or not people with mental problems are going to go to them: a qualitative exploration into the widespread use of traditional and faith healers in the provision of mental health care in Ghana. *International Review of Psychiatry* **22**: 558–67.

Anderson S, Kaleeba N (2002) *Ancient Remedies, New Disease: Involving Traditional Healers in Increasing Access to AIDS Care and Prevention in East Africa*. Geneva: UNAIDS.

Bartholomew L, Shegog K, Parcel R, et al. (2000) Watch, discover, think and act: A model for patient education program development. *Patient Education and Counseling* **39**: 253–68.

Berg A (2003) Ancestor reverence and mental health in South Africa. *Transcultural Psychiatry* **40**: 194–207.

Colvin M, Gumede L, Grimwade K, Maher D, Wilkinson D (2003) Contribution of traditional healers to a rural tuberculosis control programme in Hlabisa, South Africa. *International Journal of Tuberculosis and Lung Disease* **7**: 586–91.

Devenish A (2005) Negotiating healing: understanding the dynamics amongst traditional healers in Kwazulu-Natal as they engage with professionalisation. *Social Dynamics* **31**: 243–84.

Ensink K, Robertson B (1999) Patient and family experiences of psychiatric services and African indigenous healers. *Transcultural Psychiatry* **36**: 23–43.

Ethnic Health Initiative (2010) Traditional healers and mental health services. London

conference held on November 10, 2010.

Finau S, Tukuitonga C (1999) Pacific peoples in New Zealand. In P Davis, K Dew, eds., *Health and Society in Aotearoa, New Zealand*. Melbourne: Oxford University Press; pp. 99–112.

Hewson MG (1998) Traditional healers in southern Africa. *Annals of Internal Medicine* **128**: 1029–34.

Horton R (2007) Launching a new movement for mental health. *Lancet* **370**: 806.

Jacob KS, Sharan P, Mirza I, et al. (2007) Mental health systems in countries: where are we now? *Lancet* **370**: 1061–77.

King R (2000). *Collaboration with Traditional Healers in HIV/AIDS Prevention and Care in sub-Saharan Africa: a Literature Review*. Geneva: UNAIDS.

Kleinman A (1980) *Patients and Healers in the Context of Culture*. Berkeley, CA: University of California Press.

Meissner O (2004) The traditional healer as part of the primary health care team? *South African Medical Journal* **94**: 901–2.

Ndetei DM (1988) Psychiatric phenomenology across countries: constitutional, cultural, or environmental? *Acta Psychiatrica Scandinavica Supplementum* **344**: 33–44.

Ndetei DM (2007) Traditional healers in East Africa. *International Psychiatry* **4** (4): 85–6.

Ndetei DM, Muhanji J (1979) The prevalence and clinical presentation of psychiatric illness in a rural setting in Kenya. *British Journal of Psychiatry* **135**: 269–72.

Ndetei DM, Khasakhala L, Oginga A (2008) *Traditional and Faith Healers' Practices in Kangemi Informal Settlement*, Nairobi: Africa Mental Health Foundation and BasicNeeds UK in Kenya.

Ndhlalambi M (2009) *Strengthening the capacity of traditional health practitioners to respond to HIV/AIDS and TB in Kwazulu Natal, South Africa*. AMREF Case Studies.

Ng'etich KA (2005) Indigenous knowledge, alternative medicine and intellectual property rights concerns in Kenya. Council for the Development of Social Science Research in Africa (CODESRIA) 11th General Assembly, Maputo, Mozambique, December 2005.

Ngoma M, Prince M, Mann A (2003) Common mental disorders among those attending primary health clinics and traditional healers in urban Tanzania. *British Journal of Psychiatry* **183**: 349–55.

Patel V (2011) Traditional healers for mental health care in Africa. *Global Health Action* **4**: 10.

Peltzer K, Mngqundaniso N, Petros G (2006) A controlled study of an HIV/AIDS/STI/TB intervention with traditional healers in KwaZulu-Natal, South Africa. *AIDS Care* **18**: 608–13.

Rappoport H, Dent PL (1979) An analysis of contemporary East Africa folk psychotherapy. *British Journal of Medical Psychology* **52**: 49–54.

Saraceno B, van Ommeren M, Batniji R, et al. (2007) Barriers to improvement of mental health services in low-income and middle-income countries. *Lancet* **370**: 1164–74.

Stein S (2008) Promoting indigenous mental health: cultural perspectives on healing from native counselors in Canada. *International Journal of Health Promotion and Education* **48**: 49–56.

World Health Organization (2002) *WHO Traditional Medicine Strategy 2002–2005*. Geneva: WHO.

World Health Organization (2008) *mhGAP: Mental Health Gap Action Programme. Scaling up Care for*

Mental, Neurological, and Substance Use Disorders. Geneva: WHO.

Wreford J (2005a) A literature review of current practice involving African traditional healers in biomedical HIV/AIDS interventions in South Africa. *Social Dynamics* **31**: 90–117.

Wreford J (2005b) Problems and potential for collaborative efforts between biomedicine and traditional medicine in South Africa. *Transcultural Psychiatry* **40**: 542–61.

Chapter

16

Setting up integrated mental health systems

Manuela Silva and José Miguel Caldas de Almeida

Introduction

Mental, neurological, and substance use disorders are among the most common and disabling health conditions worldwide. Mental disorders are responsible for 14% of the global burden of disease expressed in disability-adjusted life years (DALYs), and about 30% of the total burden of non-communicable diseases is due to these disorders (World Health Organization 2008). Individuals with mental disorders are disproportionately affected by co-occurring general medical conditions, but, if they seek general medical care, are also more likely to report problems with access to care and are more dissatisfied with their medical care (Kilbourne *et al.* 2008). Mental health problems, therefore, place a substantial burden on individuals and their families worldwide, both in terms of diminished quality of life and reduced life expectancy, and it is important to consider mental health needs within the context of global health care. The integration of mental health care into all the levels of the general health system is consensually recognized as necessary to improve the quality of care and prevent the stigma associated with mental disorders (World Health Organization 2001).

This chapter summarizes the principles of mental health services organization, describes the different types of mental health services, and discusses the main issues related to the development of integrated mental health systems.

Principles of mental health services organization

Mental health services are the means by which effective interventions for mental health are delivered (World Health Organization 2003), and are vital in reducing some of the burden of mental disorders. An important issue for the effectiveness of services is the way they are organized and the principles on which they are based. The WHO recommendations for action are, among others, to provide treatment in primary care, to give care in the community and to link with other sectors (such as education, labor, welfare, law, and non-governmental organizations) (World Health Organization 2001).

The key principles of community-oriented mental care delivery are:

- **Accessibility** – Mental health services should be available across the lifespan, across all levels of severity and need, and in the communities in which people live, work, and receive other services. However, the gap between the number of people affected by mental disorders and the number receiving care and treatment, even for severe conditions, remains enormous. A large cross-country survey supported by WHO (WHO World Mental Health Survey Consortium 2004) showed that 35–50% of serious cases in high-income countries and 76–85% in low-income countries had received no treatment in the previous 12 months. Mental health services tend to occupy a low priority on the public health agenda, and the mental health budgets of the majority of countries constitute less than 3% of their total health expenditures (World Health Organization 2001).

- **Comprehensiveness** – Mental health services should focus on public health needs and should include all facilities and programs that are required to meet the essential care needs of the populations. The exact mix of services required varies from place to place, depending on social, economic, and cultural factors, the characteristics

Essentials of Global Mental Health, ed. Samuel O. Okpaku. Published by Cambridge University Press. © Cambridge University Press 2014.

of disorders and the way in which health services are organized and funded. There are five key categories of services (Thornicroft *et al.* 2008), all of which are necessary to provide a comprehensive range of local services: (1) outpatient/ambulatory clinics; (2) community mental health teams; (3) acute inpatient care; (4) long-term residential care in the community; (5) rehabilitation, work, and occupation.

- **Coordination and continuity of care** – Especially for people with severe mental disorders, it is extremely important that services work in a coordinated manner and attempt to meet the range of social, psychological, and medical care needs. This requires input from services that are not directly related to health, e.g., social services, non-governmental organizations, and housing services. One way of addressing the need for continuity of care is to apply the sectoral or catchment area method of organizing services.

- **Effectiveness** – Service development should be guided by evidence of the effectiveness of particular interventions.

- **Equity** – People's access to services of good quality should be based on need. All too often the people most in need of services are the least likely or the least able to demand services and are thus likely to be ignored when priorities are being set.

- **Respect for human rights** – Services should protect the fundamental human rights of the patients and ensure the highest attainable standard of care. Services should also respect the autonomy of persons with mental disorders, empower and encourage such persons and their families to make decisions affecting their lives, and use the least restrictive types of treatment.

Description of mental health services

Historically, in the more economically developed countries, mental health service provision has been divided into three periods (Thornicroft *et al.* 2010):

- The rise of the asylum (from around 1880 to 1955), which was defined by the construction of large asylums that were far removed from the populations they served.

- The decline of the asylum or "deinstitutionalization" (after around 1955), characterized by a rise in community-based

mental health services that were closer to the populations they served.

- The reform of mental health services according to an evidence-based approach, balancing and integrating elements of both community and hospital services.

In the module *Organization of services for mental health*, the WHO broadly describes the way mental health services are organized around the world (World Health Organization 2003). The various components of mental health services are categorized as mental health services integrated into the general health system (in primary care and in general hospitals), community mental health services (formal and informal), and institutional mental health services (specialist institutional services and mental hospitals).

(1) Mental health services integrated into the general health system

Mental health services in primary care include treatment services and preventive and promotional activities delivered by primary care professionals (e.g., general practitioners, nurses, and other health-care staff based in primary care clinics providing diagnostic, treatment, and referral services for mental disorders or making home visits for the management of mental disorders; or non-medical primary care staff involved in health promotion and prevention activities).

It is argued that primary care services are less stigmatizing to people with mental disorders and that they are generally easily accessible and acceptable, and have reduced costs. For most common and acute mental disorders, basic primary services may have clinical outcomes that are as good as or better than those of more specialized mental health services, but clinical outcomes are highly dependent on the quality of the services provided, as affected by the knowledge of primary care staff, their skills in diagnosing and treating common mental disorders, the time available to conduct interventions, and access to psychotropic medication and psychosocial treatment.

Mental health services in general hospitals include certain services offered in district general hospitals and academic or central hospitals that form part of the general health system. Such services include psychiatric inpatient wards, psychiatric beds in general wards and emergency departments, consultation-liaison programs, and outpatient clinics. There may also be some specialist services, e.g., for children, adolescents, and the elderly.

Mental health services in general hospitals may raise some problems of accessibility and cost, but usually they are acceptable to people with mental disorders. Their clinical outcomes can vary, depending on the quality and quantity of the services provided. In many countries, these services can manage acute behavioral emergencies and episodic disorders that require only outpatient treatment, but they do not provide comprehensive and continuous care. Psychiatric departments in general hospitals require adequate numbers and training of specialist mental health professionals (psychiatrists, psychologists, psychiatric social workers, and psychiatric nurses), and they can act as centers for undergraduate and postgraduate training in psychiatry.

(2) Community mental health services

Formal community mental health services provide a wide range of services to meet diverse clinical needs, such as community-based treatment and rehabilitation programs, mobile crisis teams, therapeutic and residential supervised services, and home help and support services. Community mental health services need to maintain close working links with other mental health services and with informal care providers working in the community. These services require some staff with a high level of skills and training, although many of their functions can be delivered by general health workers with some training in mental health. They are accessible, and have reduced likelihood of violations of human rights.

Informal community mental health services may be provided by local community members other than general health professionals or dedicated mental health professionals and paraprofessionals. Informal providers may be a useful complement to formal mental health services.

(3) Institutional mental health services

A key feature of these services is the independent standalone service style, although they may have some links with the rest of the healthcare system.

Specialist institutional mental health services are provided by certain outpatient clinics and by certain public or private hospital-based facilities that offer various services in inpatient wards, such as acute and high-security units, units for children and elderly people, and forensic psychiatry units. These services meet very specific needs that require institutional settings and a large complement of properly trained specialist staff. They are usually tertiary referral centers for difficult-to-treat patients. If well funded and well resourced, they provide care of high quality.

Dedicated mental hospitals mainly provide long-stay custodial services. In many countries they consume most of the available human and financial resources for mental health. Mental hospitals are frequently associated with poor outcomes attributable to a combination of factors such as poor clinical care, violations of human rights, the nature of institutionalized care, and a lack of rehabilitative activities. Stigma associated with mental hospitals also reduces their acceptability and accessibility.

Organization of mental health services in countries with different level of resources

Service planners have to determine the optimal mix of different types of mental health services. According to the WHO's organization of services pyramid (World Health Organization 2003), the most significant part of formal care should be provided by primary care services, followed by community-based mental health services and psychiatric services based in general hospitals, while the institutional mental health services should be responsible for the response to the very specific needs of a small number of patients.

The recommendations for the organization of mental health services should take into account the evidence base for mental health interventions, the unique needs of those with mental disorders, the way communities and patients access services, and structural issues such as the need for collaboration, both within and outside the health sector (Thornicroft *et al.* 2010).

Thornicroft & Tansella (2002) described an evidence-based "balanced care model," a conceptual model that integrates elements of community and hospital services that can be useful to formulate service plans (Semrau *et al.* 2011). This model is mainly community-based with hospital back-up, and the following issues are central to the development of balanced mental health services (Thornicroft & Tansella 2004): (1) services need to reflect the priorities of service users and carers; (2) evidence supports the need for both hospital and community services; (3) services need to be provided close to home; (4) some services need to be mobile rather than static; (5) interventions need to address both symptoms and disabilities; (6) treatment has to be specific to individual needs.

The material resources available will severely constrain how this approach is applied in practice, and the authors suggest a stepped-care model to develop a balance of services in any level of resources (Semrau *et al.* 2011). In countries with a low level of resources, the large majority of cases of mental disorder should be recognized and treated within primary health, with specialist back-up to provide training, consultation for complex cases, and inpatient assessment and treatment of cases that cannot be managed in primary care (step A: *primary care mental health with specialist back-up*). Countries with medium resources may additionally provide general adult mental health care, e.g., outpatient clinics, community mental health teams, acute inpatient care, community residential care, and forms of employment and occupation. The recognition and treatment of the majority of people with mental illnesses remains a task that falls mostly to primary care, with referral to a specialist when necessary (step B: *mainstream mental health care*). In high-resource areas each of the components of the mainstream model can be complemented by additional and differentiated specialized mental health services (step C: *specialized and differentiated mental health services*), such as specialized outpatient clinics and community mental health teams, assertive community treatment teams, early intervention teams, alternatives to acute inpatient care, alternative types of community residential care, and alternative occupation and rehabilitation programs.

Another useful model to guide the description and reform of mental health services and to clarify service evaluation is the "matrix model" (Thornicroft & Tansella 2002). The model consists of two dimensions, one temporal and one geographical. The temporal dimension comprises three phases: input (the resources which are used, phase A), process (how the resources are utilized, phase B), and outcome (the results obtained, phase C). The geographical dimension has three levels: regional/national (level 1), local or catchment area (level 2), and individual, meaning a patient or a group of patients (level 3). Nine cells are created by the intersection of these two

dimensions. The matrix can be used not only to deal with problems in the description of mental health services, but also to accurately interpret treatment outcomes.

Integrated mental health systems

Integrated care for mental disorders encompasses forms of collaboration with general health delivery systems at all levels (primary, secondary, and tertiary) and with other sectors (such as social services, justice, and housing) (Zolnierek 2008), aiming to provide the best possible care and to utilize scarce resources most efficiently. Integration can be pursued at the clinical, managerial, administrative, and financial levels.

The integration of mental health services into general health services is the most viable strategy for extending mental health services to underserved populations. Furthermore, in integrated care mental health, specialty, and general medical care providers work together to address both the physical and mental health needs of their patients, since mental disorders and physical health problems are very closely associated and often influence each other. Other potential benefits include possibilities for providing care in the community, opportunities for community involvement in care, and reduction of the stigma associated with seeking help from standalone mental health services.

At a basic level, integration into general health care involves:

- the integration of mental health services into primary care settings
- the integration of mental health services into general hospitals
- the development of links between primary care and secondary services based in general hospitals
- the integration of mental health care into other established health and social programs

Integration of mental health services into primary care settings

Mental health care in primary care, a key recommendation of the World Health Organization, has been defined as "the provision of basic preventive and curative mental health care at the first point of contact of entry into the health care system" (Bower & Gilbody 2005). Usually this means that care is provided by a non-specialist who can refer complex cases to a more specialized mental health professional. Integrated models offer an approach that considers common barriers to care (stigmatization, marginalization, and access), providing a comprehensive scope, coordination across providers, and continuity over time (Thornicroft & Tansella 2004).

The structure of mental health care in primary care is generally understood in terms of the pathways that patients can follow to seek care, the "pathways to care" model. The Goldberg and Huxley scheme (O'Sullivan *et al.* 2005) describes five levels, separated by four filters, and represents the relationship between total psychiatric morbidity in the general population (level 1), the proportion who are seen in primary care (level 2), those who are recognized by primary care staff as having a mental disorder (level 3), those who are seen by specialist mental health staff (level 4), and finally those who are admitted to psychiatric beds (level 5). This model highlights the importance of the primary care clinician, whose ability to detect disorder in presenting patients (filter 2) and propensity to refer (filter 3) represent key barriers to care. The model also highlights the decreasing proportion of the total population who access higher levels.

Models of mental health care in primary care

The different models of mental health care in primary care can be ordered along a key dimension relating to the importance of the primary care clinicians in the management of mental health problems and the degree to which the model focuses on improving their skills and confidence (Bower & Gilbody 2005).

- **Training primary care staff** – This involves the provision of knowledge and skills concerning mental health care to primary care clinicians. It might involve improving prescribing or providing skills in psychological therapy. Training can involve widespread dissemination of information and guidelines or more intensive practice-based education seminars.
- **Consultation-liaison** – This is a variant of the training model but involves mental health specialists entering into an ongoing educational relationship with primary care clinicians, to support them in caring for individual patients. Referral to specialist care is needed in a small proportion of cases.
- **Collaborative care** – Collaborative care can involve aspects of both training and

consultation-liaison but also includes the addition of case managers who work with patients and liaise with primary care clinicians and specialists in order to improve quality of care. Often based on the principles of chronic disease management, this model may also involve screening, education of patients, changes in practice routines, and developments in information technology.

- **Replacement/referral** – In this model the primary responsibility for the management of the presenting problem is passed to the specialist for the duration of treatment.

Benefits of the integration of mental health care in primary care

The evidence suggests that a more integrated approach to care has a number of benefits compared to usual practice:

- By diagnosing and treating both physiological and psychological illnesses, integrated care considers comorbidity and its effects on the individual as a whole, and meets the mental health needs of people with physical disorders, as well as the physical health needs of people with mental disorders. Furthermore, most mental and physical disorders are chronic in course and require approaches to management that are very similar: complex packages of care involving combinations of pharmacological and psychosocial interventions delivered in a stepped-care manner (Patel 2009).
- Patients are much more likely to see a primary care physician each year than a mental health specialist. Therefore, primary care physicians may be in the best position to recognize and improve rates of appropriate treatment. Integrated care is the best way of improving the skills of primary care providers in dealing with the psychosocial aspects of care. Therefore, primary care can assume a pivotal role in delivering integrated mental health care, and can move beyond providing a gatekeeper function for secondary specialist services (Lester *et al.* 2004), minimizing referrals to specialty mental health clinics.
- Mental health services delivered in primary care minimize stigma and discrimination, and promote respect for human rights.
- Integrated models of care offer the potential to improve access to treatment, and help close the treatment gap. Integrating mental health into

primary care settings brings the care to where the patient is. Primary care for mental health also facilitates community outreach and mental health promotion, as well as long-term monitoring and management of affected individuals.

- Primary care for mental health is affordable and cost-effective (Chisholm *et al.* 2000). Primary care services for mental health are less expensive than psychiatric hospitals, for patients, communities, and governments.

Factors affecting success

According to the WHO and the World Organization of Family Doctors, the success of a more integrated approach to care will depend on a number of factors (World Health Organization & Wonca 2008):

- Policy and plans need to incorporate primary care for mental health. Commitment from the government to integrated mental health care, and a formal policy and legislation that concretizes this commitment, are fundamental to success.
- Advocacy is required to shift attitudes and behavior. Time and effort are required to sensitize national and local political leadership, health authorities, management, and primary care workers about the importance of mental health integration. Estimates of the prevalence of mental disorders, the burden they impose if left untreated, the human rights violations that often occur in psychiatric hospitals, and the existence of effective primary care-based treatments are often important arguments.
- Adequate training of primary care workers is required (Gilbody *et al.* 2003). Mental health services in primary care require significant investment in training primary care professionals to detect and treat mental disorders, preferably as ongoing training programs. Health workers must also practice skills and receive specialist supervision over time. Collaborative or shared care models, in which joint consultations and interventions are held between primary care workers and mental health specialists, are an especially promising way of providing ongoing training and support. The training should include all categories of health workers and other workers whose work touches on the mental health of the community, e.g., security officers and receptionists in health facilities.

- Primary care tasks must be limited and doable. Decisions about specific areas of responsibility must be taken after consultation with different stakeholders in the community, assessment of available human and financial resources, and careful consideration of the strengths and weaknesses of the current health system for addressing mental health. Functions of primary care workers may be expanded as practitioners gain skills and confidence. Primary care staff are overburdened in many countries, and in such situations it is necessary to increase the numbers of primary care staff so that they can take on additional mental health work.
- Specialist mental health professionals and facilities must be available to support primary care. Primary care staff have to be adequately supervised if integration is to succeed. This support can come from community mental health centers, secondary-level hospitals, or skilled practitioners working specifically within the primary care system. Mental health professionals should be regularly available to primary care staff to give advice on the management and treatment of people with mental disorders. Referral criteria should be clear, and information and communications systems should be available.
- Patients must have access to essential psychotropic medications in primary care.
- Collaboration with other government non-health sectors, non-governmental organizations, village and community health workers, and volunteers is required.
- Financial and human resources are needed. Although primary care for mental health is cost-effective, financial resources are required to establish and maintain a service.

Limitations of integration

There are some barriers to integrated care, and several strategies for reducing these barriers. Integrated approaches to mental health care and new ways of working require role changes for clinicians, and can create potential tensions. Any changes, particularly those that impact on professional roles and boundaries, can be perceived as threatening the power base of an individual or team. Any changes need to be accompanied by carefully negotiated adjustments to the way primary and secondary healthcare professionals conceptualize their tasks, obligations, and responsibilities, and must be underpinned by new ways of learning together.

Another impediment for the implementation of integration is misconceptions within both the psychological and physiological healthcare professions (Hine *et al.* 2008). Primary care workers may be uncomfortable about dealing with mental disorders or they may ignore and withdraw from working with people who have such disorders, and clinical outcomes would consequently be unsatisfactory (World Health Organization 2001). Integrated care demands that mental health professionals become comfortable in working in the biopsychosocial model of care (World Health Organization & Wonca 2008), including the role of medication and pharmacological treatment. For each member of a multidisciplinary team, being integrated demands a sufficient comprehension about disciplines and trainings of one's colleagues in order to design collaborative interventions that will most appropriately meet patients' needs.

Barriers can also be administrative (e.g., lack of common medical records for mental health and general medical conditions), financial (e.g., lack of reimbursement codes to bill for mental health and general medical care in the same setting), and clinical (e.g., lack of an integrated care protocol) (Kilbourne *et al.* 2008).

Strategies to overcome barriers to integrated care may require cooperation across different organizational levels, including administrators, providers, and healthcare payers, in order for integrated care to be established and sustained over time (Kilbourne *et al.* 2008).

Integration of mental health services into general hospitals

Mental health services based in general hospitals can provide secondary-level care to patients in the community and services to those who are admitted for physical disorders and require mental health interventions.

Integration into general hospitals requires facilities and human resources. The required facilities include beds for the management of acute mental disorders, outpatient facilities, equipment for specialized tests (e.g. psychological tests), equipment for specialized treatments, and medication. The required human resources include specialist mental health staff

such as psychiatrists, psychologists, psychiatric nurses, and social workers. These staff have to take responsibility for the training and supervision of primary care workers. Some of these specialist staff may not be sufficiently oriented towards primary mental health care and community-based service delivery and will themselves require training.

As specialist services are scarce and expensive, they should target their skilled impact upon: (1) undertaking the assessment and diagnosis of complex cases, and those requiring an expert second opinion; (2) treating people with the most severe symptoms; (3) providing care for those with the greatest degree of disability consequent on mental illness; (4) making treatment recommendations for those conditions which have proved non-responsive to initial treatment.

The need for good linkages between primary health care and secondary mental health facilities is crucial. A clear referral and linkage system should be put in place.

Establishment of links between primary, secondary, and tertiary care

Primary health care is both an entry point and a referral point for mental health care and prevention. In order to address the needs of persons with mental disorders for health care and social support, a clear referral and linkage system should be in place. Regular meetings of service providers should be held in order to review and improve the referral system and to evaluate how the needs of patients are being met.

Even where specialist mental health services are well developed, it is important to improve coordination between them and primary care. If this is not done, care is often duplicated or poorly coordinated.

Integration of mental health care into other established health and social programs

Mental health policies in many countries have been remodeled to focus on providing comprehensive and integrated health and social care services for those people with the most severe illnesses, those at greatest risk, and those with the most complex problems (Huxley *et al.* 2008). Mental disorders, particularly severe mental disorders, are frequently associated with high levels of disability, affecting the ability to work, activities related to home management, social life, and the ability to maintain personal relationships (Ormel *et al.* 2008). For this reason, mental health care for these patients must include an important psychosocial rehabilitation component, involving social skills training, vocational training, employment support, and residential support. This requires close coordination, and in some cases joint funding and management of health and social care services, as well as the collaboration of health services with services of the employment sector. Integrated approaches are also needed in child and adolescent mental health, in which prevention and treatment programs have to be developed in schools through the collaboration of health and education programs.

References

Bower P, Gilbody S (2005) Managing common mental health disorders in primary care: conceptual models and evidence base. *BMJ* **330**: 839–42.

Chisholm D, Sekar K, Kumas KK, *et al.* (2000) Integration of mental health care into primary care. Demonstration cost-outcome study in India and Pakistan. *British Journal of Psychiatry* **176**: 581–8.

Gilbody S, Whitty P, Grimshaw J, Thomas R (2003) Educational and organizational interventions to improve the management ofdepression in primary care: a systematic review. *JAMA* **289**: 3145–51.

Hine CE, Howell HB, Yonkers KA (2008) Integration of medical and psychological treatment within the primary health care setting. *Social Work in Health Care* **47**: 122–34.

Huxley P, Evans S, Munroe M, Cestari L (2008) Integrating health and social care in community mental health teams in the UK: a study of assessments and eligibility criteria in England. *Health and Social Care in the Community* **16**: 476–82.

Kilbourne AM, Irmiter C, Capobianco J, *et al.* (2008) Improving integrated general medical and mental health services in community-based practices. *Administration and Policy in Mental Health* **35**: 337–45.

Lester H, Glasby J, Tylee A (2004) Integrated primary mental health care: threat or opportunity in the new NHS? *British Journal of General Practice* **54**: 285–91.

Ormel J, Petukhova M, Chatterji S, *et al.* (2008) Disability and treatment of specific mental and physical disorders across the world: results from the WHO World Mental Health Surveys. *British Journal of Psychiatry* **192**: 368–75.

O'Sullivan T, Cotton A, Scott A (2005) Goldberg and Huxley's model revisited. *Psychiatric Bulletin* **29**: 116.

Patel V (2009) Integrating mental health care with chronic diseases in low-resource settings. *International Journal of Public Health* **54** (Suppl 1): 1–3.

Semrau M, Barley EA, Law A, Thornicroft G (2011) Lessons learned in developing community mental health care in Europe. *World Psychiatry* **10**: 217–25.

Thornicroft G, Tansella M (2002) Balancing community-basedand hospital-based mental health care. *World Psychiatry* **1**: 84–90.

Thornicroft G, Tansella M (2004) Components of a modern mental health service: a pragmatic balance of community and hospital care: overview of systematic evidence. *British Journal of Psychiatry* **185**: 283–90.

Thornicroft G, Tansella M, Law A (2008) Steps, challenges and lessons in developing community mental health care. *World Psychiatry* **7**: 87–92.

Thornicroft G, Alem A, Santos RA, *et al.* (2010) WPA guidance on steps, obstacles and mistakes to avoid in the implementation of community mental health care. *World Psychiatry* **9**: 67–77.

WHO World Mental Health Survey Consortium (2004) Prevalence, severity, and unmet need for treatment of mental disorders in the World Health Organization World Mental Health Surveys. *JAMA* **291**: 2581–90.

World Health Organization (2001) *The World Health Report 2001. Mental Health: New Understanding, New Hope.* Geneva: WHO.

World Health Organization (2003) *Organization of Services for Mental Health.* Geneva: WHO (Mental Health Policy and Service Guidance Package).

World Health Organization (2008) *mhGAP: Mental Health Gap Action Programme. Scaling up Care for Mental, Neurological, and Substance Use Disorders.* Geneva: WHO.

World Health Organization, Wonca [World Organization of Family Doctors] (2008) *Integrating Mental Health into Primary Care: a Global Perspective.* Geneva: WHO.

Zolnierek CD (2008) Mental health policy and integrated care: global perspectives. *Journal of Psychiatric and Mental Health Nursing* **15**: 562–8.

Chapter

17

Integrated mental health systems: the Cuban experience

Ester Shapiro and Isabel Louro Bernal

Introduction

This chapter presents the Cuban integrative health/ mental health system as a widely recognized model grounded in local community and primary care, within a national health system emphasizing free universal health care. Cuba's mental health system, offering community-based mental health care grounded in integrative primary care, incorporates the full spectrum of health promotion, problem prevention, curative treatments, rehabilitation, and social integration (*promocion, prevencion, curacion, rehabilitacion, integracion social*) (Borrego 2008). The chapter draws on recent overviews and evaluations of Cuba's mental health systems of care (León Gonzalez 2006, 2008, Aparicio Basauri 2008, Borrego 2008, GOSMA 2008, PAHO & WHO 2011), published research conducted by both Cuban and global sources, and Cuban practice accounts and experiences.

Wherever possible this chapter will use both the Cuban terms (*in italics*) and published translations for medical and mental health systems terminology; other translations into English are our own. The term *salud integral* has been translated as "integrative health," which speaks to the multiple levels of health integration in Cuba addressed in this chapter: integration of health and mental health care, of specialized biomedicine and complementary/alternative practices, and of community-based health promotion and health services.

Cuba's integrative systems of mental health care

At the end of 1958, Cuba's public health system was deplorable, characterized by poverty and corruption, lacking qualified personnel and institutions (Sintes Jiménez 2011). Beginning in January 1959, the Cuban revolution initiated great changes, moving toward a comprehensive state health system. By the end of the 1960s, highly unequal private medical services were replaced with a national health system that was government-run, completely free of charge, and accessible to the whole population, integrating curative and rehabilitative care with illness prevention and health promotion and improving quality of life (Delgado García 2008). The Cuban leadership prioritized free, universal, equitable access to high-quality health services as indivisible from health and linked to human dignity, equitable access to education and employment, social inclusion and participation, and other life-course biopsychosocial determinants of health, making these hallmarks of Cuba's socialist revolution. Cuba's health system collects detailed disease-specific and mortality data for local, national, and international monitoring (MINSAP 2012).

Though ranked as a low-income country, Cuba has achieved health indicators equal to those of more economically developed nations through investment of significant economic resources in health systems (7.5% of gross national product), a socialist/humanist approach, and a scientific planning process engaging the nation as a whole (Aparicio Basauri 2008, PAHO & WHO 2011). Cuba has protected health while facing significant economic hardships due to the US blockade, which has continued for over 50 years, the collapse of the Soviet Union and the withdrawal of aid and trade agreements, a decade of devastating hurricanes, and global economic crises. Cuba's successes are best understood using health/mental health promotion and human development frameworks, recognizing both individual and population health as resulting from challenges and resources in multiple systems, requiring attention to public health, life-course community education and mobilization, as well as healthcare system reforms (León Gonzalez 2006, 2008, Ochoa & Visbal 2007, Borrego 2008, Whiteford & Branch 2008, World Health Organization 2008, Mason *et al.* 2010, Shapiro 2011). Cuba's integrative health system systematically promotes connections between health planning, implementation, and evaluation at national, provincial, and municipal levels, giving providers, governmental, and community-led organizations, alongside individuals and their families, critical roles in improving linked processes of personal, familial, and community health.

Cuba's integration of mental/behavioral health care into every level of intervention is grounded in community-based, family-centered primary health care emphasizing functional outcomes and social inclusion with a continuum of promotion/prevention/ treatment/rehabilitation interventions offered across multiple settings. Direct mental health services are offered in primary health care and polyclinics, in community mental health centers, and in general and psychiatric hospitals. Cuba's experience of creating community-based mental health systems integrated into primary care offers exemplary innovations in foundational health promotion frameworks, community-based health services delivery balancing primary and specialty care, transformed practitioner education for societal roles, public engagement through health promotion education, societal involvement in intersectoral participatory research for needs assessments and services design, implementation and evaluation, and international collaborations and solidarity.

The Cuban health system: an overview

The Republic of Cuba is an archipelago with an area of 110 922 km in 15 provinces and a population of 11 239 128, three-quarters of whom live in urban areas. Cuba's National Health System is organized under the Ministry of Public Health (Ministerio de Salud Pública, MINSAP) with three levels, national, provincial, and municipal, linked to levels of governmental organization. Cuba has 1837 institutions offering health services, including 498 polyclinics offering over 25 specialty healthcare services and provider training in community settings such as internal medicine, pediatrics, obstetrics/gynecology and psychology, with linkages to over 14 000 medical offices

(*consultorios*) in neighborhoods and 222 hospitals (PAHO & WHO 2011). Cuba has over 31 000 family doctors, with 64.4 physicians, 87 nurses, 9.7 dentists, and 113 ancillary health professionals per 10 000 population, distributed proportionately throughout the country and providing 100% access to primary care (Luna Morales *et al.* 2009, PAHO & WHO 2011).

From the start, Cuba conceptualized socialism in line with national sovereignty, social justice, and cultural values of *Cubanidad* (what it means to be Cuban: De la Torre 2009, Guanche Zaldivar 2011). Cuba's health and mental health innovations draw from national applications of multiple scientific sources, creating a unique synthesis (Delgado García 2008, De la Torre 2009). Cuba's socialist government emphasizes the importance of government responsibility, while increasingly shifting programs to municipal levels through local assessments and participatory planning. Neighborhood political organizations and planning councils are connected to health programs through a web of educational, workplace, and civic as well as governmental organizations (Castell-Florit Serrate 2007, Castell-Florit Serrate *et al.* 2007, Pagliccia *et al.* 2010). A government-owned media offers a substantial menu of targeted health educational campaigns as well as broad science and health education. Applying these ethical, knowledge-based, multisystemic partnership approaches, Cuba has achieved global leadership in family-based primary care as well as specialties including HIV/AIDS prevention and treatment, maternal/child health, targeted infectious disease response, and disaster response.

Cuba's accomplishments in integrative health and mental health have evolved through scientific and administrative review characterized by four major decade shifts (Delgado García 2008, Brotherton 2011). Prior to 1959, Cuba had some of Latin America's best health facilities and outcomes, but these were extremely unequal and concentrated in Havana. Psychiatric hospitals dominated care for the mentally ill, with some private practice, almost exclusively in Havana, available primarily to the wealthy (López Serrano 1985, Aparicio Basauri 2008). When half the island's physicians and most of its medical-school professors left after 1959, Cuba faced a challenging yet meaningful opportunity to reorganize health care in line with revolutionary goals, re-designing health systems and re-visioning provider education towards transformative social roles based in both professional/scientific training and national/international solidarity (León Gonzalez 2002, 2006, 2008, Louro Bernal *et al.* 2009, Marimón Torres & Martínez Cruz 2011). The 1960s saw the creation of the National Health System based in neighborhood polyclinics and corresponding health areas (*areas de salud*). During the 1970s, the national system was consolidated by enhancing primary and secondary care services in local polyclinics and hospitals with links to tertiary specialized research and care facilities. During the 1980s, the Family Doctors and Nurses program introduced primary health providers responsible for a neighborhood population, residing there when possible, providing care anchored in a deep knowledge of the patients and their community conditions. They offer the gateway for referral (*puerta de entrada*) into specialty services, ensuring coherence and continuity of care within primary health care. Primary and secondary care is provided in local polyclinics and municipal hospitals. In the 1990s, work focused on protecting health and public health achievements while facing severe economic crisis.

Márquez Morales (2010) describes the innovative Family Doctors and Nurses (FDN) program as a unique primary care/social medicine program characterized by an **integrative/holistic approach** to prevention, treatment, and rehabilitation; **sectorized**, responsible for a specific target population; **regionalized**, maintaining close connections to secondary/tertiary care facilities; **continuous**, caring for patients in homes and neighborhood clinics as well as specialized settings; **dispensarized**, systematically attending to the healthy as well as the ill; in **interdisciplinary** teams, and with **community participation**. Family doctors became specialists in primary holistic health, receiving additional training preparing them to conduct research responsive to population needs. The FDN program adapted dispensarization of health interventions, a concept from Soviet public health (Cuesta Mejías 2011) using biopsychosocial assessment to deliver a continuum of health services. According to Batista Moliner *et al.* (2001), dispensarization is conducted by primary health teams as the dynamic, organized, and continuous evaluation of people's health status in a circumscribed community, using registration, diagnosis, intervention, and follow-up for implementing appropriate interventions. The family doctor is responsible for evaluating the family unit using MINSAP criteria to assign one of four levels of health status: (1) presumed healthy,

(2) exhibits risk factors, (3) in a state of illness, (4) in a state of sequelae following illness or accident. Together with life-course vulnerability (e.g., adolescence, pregnancy) and other risk factors (e.g., smoking or social isolation), assessments indicate specific interventions protecting/improving individual and family health in a community context. Through an integrative health systems approach, mental health assessments are incorporated into the family's dispensarization continuum, and mental health consultation integrated into primary and specialized health care through referral pathways described later in the chapter.

Cuba's approach to integrated health/mental health care centered on primary health/family medicine required reorganization of medical and provider education. Cuban doctors and other providers are trained as experts on whole patients in family/community contexts, conducting home visiting in interdisciplinary teams, working in homes and community settings as well as polyclinics, and conducting assessments linking patient care to social epidemiology and practice-based research. Consistent with 2004 revisions of medical education emphasizing primary care in university polyclinics (*polyclinicas universitarias*) and provider-directed community-centered, practice-based research, health and mental health care proceed through an inquiry evaluating links between biopsychosocial risk and protective factors linking patient, family, and community contexts (Luna Morales *et al.* 2009). Health psychology and family-based behavioral health are integrated into every level of health care, forming part of the family doctor/family nurse curriculum (Louro Bernal *et al.* 2009). Additionally, many doctors, psychologists, and increasingly nurses are completing both primary care training and a master's degree in behavioral/mental health care, with advanced study offered at Cuba's medical universities, the National School of Public Health (*Escuela Nacional de Salud Pública, ENSAP*), and the university system nationwide. Cuba has also invested significant resources in a national health resources informatics network (*Infomed*) and the Virtual Health University (*Universidad Virtual de Salud*), facilitating practitioners all over the country to continue advanced education.

Cuba has also made significant investments in health research, conducted in primary care settings and specialty hospitals as well as in specialized biotechnology centers playing critical roles in developing affordable medications and equipment. A critical tool for health and mental health planning in practice settings is "health situation analysis" (*el análisis de situación de salud*), based on the World Health Organization approach (León González 2006, Martínez Calvo & Gómez de Haz 2008, Louro Bernal 2011). Health situation analysis offers a scientific method based in social epidemiology and participatory research to identify, prioritize, and develop action plans addressing community health problems and advancing health promotion. Community sectors led by health administration such as local Health Councils identify problems/risks affecting health by collecting health indicators data along with community experiences, informing action plans for targeted improvements (Martínez Calvo & Gómez de Haz 2008). Health situation analysis is conducted at least annually at national, provincial, and municipal levels. León González (2006, 2008) suggests that engaging communities in planning through their family doctor's office (*consultorio*) offers unique opportunities to transform health concerns because of patient/family provider intimacy and immediacy. Family doctors and local polyclinics display social/epidemiological health profiles, for example tobacco/alcohol use or families at risk, facilitating community education. Used this way, health situation analysis enhances collaborations between the health sector, civil society, patients, and families (León González 2006, Martínez Calvo & Gómez de Haz 2008, Louro Bernal 2011).

Theoretical approach and organization of Cuba's mental health system

Historically, mental health was administered as a specialty within MINSAP by the National Psychiatric Group (*Grupo Nacional de Psiquiatria*). Child psychiatry as a specialty and child-oriented services were systematically introduced, starting in 1959, with child and adolescent psychiatry and psychology growing as specialties emphasizing outpatient, community-based care (Aparicio Basauri 2008). The Operating Group for Mental Health and Addictions (*Grupo Operativo de Salud Mental y Addicciones*: GOSMA) was founded in 2003 within MINSAP, with oversight and training responsibilities for all mental health and addictions care. Organizationally, GOSMA supervises provincial psychiatric hospitals, municipal hospitals with psychiatric units, and community mental health centers. Community mental health centers also interface

significantly with family doctor and nurse teams and mental health teams within polyclinics. Cuba's current mental health guidelines follow the *Caracas Declaration* of 1990, using health promotion principles endorsed in the Latin American region, and the 1995 *Havana Letter*, building on both revolutionary achievements and regional reforms to emphasize community-based mental health promotion, prevention, and care within Cuba's system of integrative primary care (GOSMA 2008). The current system of community mental health centers works closely with every facet of primary care. Revisions to the mental health plan based on "salutogenic" approaches emphasizing wellness rather than psychopathology (León Gonzalez 2002, 2006, 2008) have been transformational. The most recent mental health guidelines and strategic plan were revised in 2008 to emphasize development of resources for community-based care, greater involvement of patients and their families, advocacy and mental health promotion, continued protection of human rights, attention to an aging population's mental health needs, and equal access for diverse groups and regions (PAHO & WHO 2011).

Cuban mental health services draw from a number of theoretical perspectives and modalities. Consistent with the founding principles of Cuban health care, mental health care is offered within primary, secondary, and tertiary settings, is prevention minded, family centered, and life-course oriented (Louro Bernal 2008). Psychodynamic perspectives have had a long history in the training of Cuban psychiatrists and psychologists, though these were significantly reconceptualized using dialectical materialist philosophy, family systems theories, cognitive behavioral therapies, and Latin American social psychiatry/psychology (De la Torre 2009). This theoretical synthesis considers both social contexts and individual subjectivities as contributing to emotional wellness or to potential conflicts or barriers. Interventions are biopsychosocially informed and multisystemic, and emphasize health promotion while addressing health holistically, so that individuals, families, and community groups may all contribute to intervention plans, reducing symptoms while enhancing positive processes such as family and social support. These approaches are brought to the full continuum of primary, secondary, and tertiary care across settings. Because of the emphasis on family-based primary care, family systems practice has significantly influenced the training of mental health and primary health practitioners.

Because the guiding principles for wellness emphasize individual capabilities in contributing to society, Cuba's approach to psychosocial rehabilitation targets restoration of functional outcomes and social integration alongside symptom relief (GOSMA 2008, Martínez González *et al.* 2010). Culturally meaningful rehabilitation emphasizes group modalities including occupational therapies, athletics and team sports, dance ("psychoballet"), and theater ("psychodrama"). Work-force participation and other contributions to family and society are highly valued, and trained occupational and rehabilitation specialists work in multiple inpatient and outpatient health system, as well as in workplace settings (GOSMA 2008, Martínez González *et al.* 2010). Stress-reduction education is emphasized in both individual and group treatment, offered to both patients and family caretakers to improve well-being while reducing the need for medication. Stress-reduction modalities include cognitive behavioral approaches and complementary/alternative treatments including massage, acupuncture, and yoga. The emphasis on community-based partnerships for assessment and intervention planning helps identify and mobilize local resources addressing patient and family needs.

Mental health services within primary and secondary care

Cuba's polyclinics, encompassing a neighborhood network of family doctors and nurses as well as specialty clinics and providers, form the foundation for mental health care integrated into primary health care. All primary health providers receive mental health training, and health psychologists receive training in behavioral health within primary health-care settings and specialized mental health care. Polyclinics are also a primary setting for training interdisciplinary providers on mental health factors in health, including physical and occupational therapists, speech/hearing pathologists, and social rehabilitation specialists. Social workers in clinical and community settings assist patients with access to social and material resources, including medication payments, transportation assistance, and social security payments for patients unable to work.

Outpatient mental health services

Outpatient mental health services were historically offered in Cuba's polyclinics, all of which offered either mental health services departments or specialized mental health teams (*equipos de salud mental*) (León Gonzalez 2002, 2006, 2008). Cuba's 1995 reorientation of psychiatry towards primary care recognized the need for specialized community mental health settings to provide follow-up services in psychosocial rehabilitation, reducing long-term psychiatric hospitalizations by providing community-based care. Critics of deinstitutionalization movements worldwide found that without comprehensive community-based care, patients with severe/chronic mental health concerns were highly vulnerable to becoming homeless or incarcerated. Cuba's community mental health centers were designed to bridge that gap.

In 2008, 12 years after the *Havana Letter* reorienting psychiatry towards primary care, Cuba reported having 421 outpatient mental health services centers available throughout the country, covering 100% of the population (León González 2008). According to 2008 data (León González 2008, PAHO & WHO 2011) outpatient mental health services were accessed by 247 975 patients, representing 2206 users for each 100 000 of the general population, with an average of three visits per patient per year. Cuba developed 113 community mental health centers throughout the country, with 67 accredited at national and provincial levels, 20 at provincial levels, and 26 in the process of seeking accreditation (PAHO & WHO 2011). Many of these community mental health centers include partial or day hospital services focused on psychosocial rehabilitation, designed for both acute and chronic symptoms/diagnoses (Martínez González *et al.* 2010). Additionally, 199 mental health areas and mental health teams are housed within a polyclinic or other setting, and 96 mental health teams are available to polyclinic staff in a consulting role. All mental health teams can conduct home visits and community-based assessments, directly or through consultation with family doctors, nurses, and other specialists involved with patients and families.

Cuba's community mental health centers are as unique as the communities they serve. Yet all are hubs of specific types of activities covering the full spectrum of mental health promotion, disease prevention, and psychosocial rehabilitation-oriented mental health treatment. A wide variety of community-based mental health promotion/psychoeducational workshops may be offered, including workshops for handling stress, whose curriculum includes stress management using cognitive behavioral and integrative/holistic approaches. Family mental health promotion education includes growing attention to problems of family violence on the continuum from overly authoritarian discipline to instances of psychological or physical abuse. In prevention, alcohol and substance abuse have become important target areas, and community mental health centers often house services on the full continuum of prevention, treatment, and social integration using mutual help and treatment groups, family and individual therapies (León González 2008).

The work of the Community Health Center in Playa, Havana (Bertot Gonzalez 2009) illustrates how a particular community mental health center uses an intersectorial, social-medicine approach mapping risks and resources, identifying vulnerable populations, while offering individual and group services and community mental health education and promotion. The community mental health center is responsible for carrying out broad community mental health assessments and mental health promotion and education, programs targeting groups at risk due to life course (childhood and geriatric programs) and behavioral factors (addictions, depression, and suicide), as well as clinical and rehabilitation care for patients diagnosed with mental health concerns. In addition, the center conducts interdisciplinary provider training and research. The center is staffed by two generalist psychiatrists, a psychiatric pharmacologist and a child psychiatrist, two psychologists, a developmental disabilities specialist, a primary health physician with a mental health specialty, a mental health nurse, a social worker, and two psychometricians conducting psychological testing. These providers offer individual and group treatment as well as psychoeducation and rehabilitation services using a full range of clinical and holistic/complementary practices. The center takes a strong intersectoral approach, with rehabilitation emphasizing workplace integration, featuring collaborations with labor unions and workplace health groups as well as school-based special education programs and specialized youth and elder care centers. They conduct a regular program of community workshops in stress reduction and in caring for a relative with a mental illness, as well as groups for addiction maintenance

and recovery. In addition to their ongoing health situation analysis, the staff conduct life-course health/mental health research including resilience and stress, emotional intelligence in school-age children, and Alzheimer's disease and dementia incidence and course.

Psychiatric inpatient services

Cuba's inpatient services include psychiatric hospitals housing both acute-care patients for short-term stays and longer-term patients, and local and regional general hospitals housing emergency and short-term care. Cuba has 31 psychiatric services units within general, pediatric, and specialty clinical/surgical hospitals, with a total of 10.2 beds per 100 000 population (PAHO & WHO 2011, MINSAP 2012). Admissions to these services were 47% women and 34% children or adolescents, with all children requiring hospitalizations housed in these general hospital units. All patients hospitalized in these settings received at least one psychosocial intervention in the following year. All psychiatric units have available at least one psychotropic medication appropriate for these disorders, including antipsychotics, antidepressants, mood stabilizers, anti-anxiety medications, and medications for epilepsy (PAHO & WHO 2011).

The *Havana Letter* reorienting mental health care significantly impacted organization and services in both psychiatric hospitals and psychiatric units within general hospitals. León González (2006) describes these impacts at the General Teaching and Surgical Hospital "October 10." This provincial hospital, serving one of Cuba's most densely populated municipalities, houses psychiatric services from eight area polyclinics, representing approximately 40–50 family doctor/nurses' offices for each polyclinic. Psychiatric services include a six-bed psychiatric unit for crisis care, and separate day-hospital services for neurotic and psychotic patients, each with 30 slots for day treatment and 10 beds for acute care. Services also include a stress clinic, a clinic dispensing neuroleptics, and clinics for treating mood disorders and alcoholism. The alcohol clinic works closely with a network of patients in recovery offering mutual-help groups. Twenty years earlier, the "October 10" municipal hospital housed 76 psychiatric treatment beds, demonstrating the impact of the community mental health center model alongside polyclinic mental health teams in reducing psychiatric hospitalizations by emphasizing short-term acute care transitioning to community-based care.

Cuba has a larger proportion of hospital capacity in its 23 psychiatric hospitals, which average 56.7 beds per 100 000 population, housing adults only. Average stay in psychiatric hospitals is 62.4 days, although this represents a wide treatment range, as the data include patients in on-site day hospitals (PAHO & WHO 2011). In a survey of patients hospitalized on December 31, 2007, 21% had been hospitalized for less than a year, 20% for 1–4 years, 17% for 5–10 years, and 41% for over 10 years (PAHO & WHO 2011). Continuing dedicated efforts transferring resources from psychiatric hospitals to community-based mental health care resulted in a 20% reduction in psychiatric hospital beds during 2002–07. Cuba has a range of residential settings for patients diagnosed with profound mental retardation and physical disabilities. Group housing for discharged psychiatric patients is not a modality used in Cuba. The emphasis is on community-based services supporting care within the home (Aparicio Basauri 2008, PAHO & WHO 2011). One innovation introduced to facilitate community care is inscription of chronically mentally ill patients experiencing periods of remission so that they can be quickly re-admitted for brief hospital stays as needed, returning to their home and the care of the community mental health center when restabilized (GOSMA 2008). Cuba has two dedicated forensic hospitals housing patients charged with drug or other criminal offences, in Havana and Santiago de Cuba, and additionally houses forensic patients in psychiatric hospitals (Aparicio Basauri 2008). Increased tourism and greater numbers of foreign visitors have increased drug access and the need for drug abuse prevention education as well as outpatient alcohol/drug treatment.

Global mental health applications: disaster response

One critical area in which Cuba's integrative health approach offers internationally recognized expertise is in minimizing adverse health/mental health impacts of disasters. Cuba has been particularly hard hit by hurricanes in the last decade, but because of its high degree of organization, linking neighborhood and governmental groups, it has minimized the health and safety impacts. Lorenzo Ruiz (2006) directs the child mental health program at the Tarara Center in Havana, providing free health and mental health services to children and their mothers impacted by the Chernobyl disaster. He describes Cuba's disaster response programs as integrating social/material and subjective/psychological dimensions, as every disaster presents unique physical characteristics, material impacts, health sequelae, and psychological dimensions. The Cuban revolution saw health care as a critical resource not only for individual well-being and national development, but also as offering a uniquely Cuban contribution to international solidarity, global health, and economic development (Feinsilver 2010, Marimón Torres & Martínez Cruz 2011). Cuban doctors and other health personnel offer training and direct services all over the world. In January 2010, after Haiti's devastating earthquake, nearly 500 Cuban health personnel already serving patients throughout Haiti were immediately joined by 1300 providers from the Henry Reeve Emergency Medical Contingent formed in the aftermath of Hurricane Katrina (although the USA refused Cuban assistance). In Haiti, a trained disaster mental health team consisting of four psychiatrists, four pediatric specialty psychiatrists, and four health psychologists organized provider training and direct service workshops emphasizing culturally meaningful protective factors including expressive arts and multisectorial partnerships (Gorry 2010).

Conclusions: Cuban health and mental health

The Cuban health and mental health systems of care have evolved through deliberative planning while also responding to economic and political challenges eliciting both creative responses and enduring contradictions. Understanding the Cuban health and mental health system in sociopolitical contexts inspires appreciation for the creativity and resilience which Cuban families and social networks bring to their everyday struggles for economic survival and shared wellness. The Cuban government's successes in offering its people high levels of overall education, committing to a substantial social safety net, and promising a world-class healthcare system, have resulted in a medically knowledgeable population with high expectations of providers. The importance of acquiring health promotion knowledge is reinforced throughout society, with educational campaigns using government media and community outreach, provider relationships, and a range of cultural and community groups engaged in improving health through exciting initiatives using culturally meaningful creative arts for education and mobilization. Family and social networks continue to offer Cubans culturally meaningful material resources for protecting personal, familial, and social wellness. Cuba's health and mental health planning currently focuses on anticipating care for a growing aging population, while continuing its commitments to early childhood and maternal health programs central to its gender equality and human development accomplishments (PAHO & WHO 2011).

As can be seen from this description of the Cuban system's integration of multidisciplinary mental health practitioners into primary and secondary care, the Cuban healthcare system is uniquely well positioned to address some significant health challenges faced worldwide. The growing global burden of chronic illnesses, including comorbidities and co-occurring health and mental health conditions, requires systems of care facilitating continuity focused on whole persons while addressing multifaceted biopsychosocial interventions (Shapiro 2013). Close linkages between family doctors, local polyclinics, interdisciplinary mental health and social services practitioners, neighborhood institutions including schools and workplaces, and informed patients and families, facilitate referrals and consultations offering continuity of care and complementing health services with broader community resources.

This chapter has argued that the world has a great deal to learn from the Cuban experience in striving to achieve global goals for mental health treatment embedded in primary health care and linked to societal goals of achieving health access and equity through both health care and attention to social determinants of health. In Cuba, a national project that has progressively connected healthcare system transformation with an intersectoral approach to health, linking local, municipal, and national efforts, has brought together providers, administrators, governmental organizations from many sectors, civic organizations, and the public to improve mental health as a critical component of health, with families in communities at its center. Recognizing economic limitations, the Cuban government continues to invest in health policies in which every Cuban enjoys good health as personal and societal responsibilities and as human rights.

References

Aparicio Basauri V (2008) Cuba: mental health care and community participation. In JM Caldas de Almeida, A Cohen, eds., *Innovative Mental Health Programs in Latin America and the Caribbean*. Washington DC, Pan American Health Organization.

Batista Moliner R, Sansó Soberats F, Feal Cañizare, P, Corratgé Delgado H (2001) Dispensarization: a strategy for evaluation of the health/illness process. (La dispensarización: una vía para la evaluación del proceso salud-enfermedad). *Revista Cubana de Medicina General Integral* **17** (2).

Bertot Gonzalez M (2009) *Organization of Mental Health Services in the Community (Organización de los Servicios de Salud Mental en la Comunidad: Centro de Salud Mental Comunitaria "Gustavo Torroella",*

Playa, La Habana, Cuba). Havana: CYTED/RIPSOL.

Borrego C (2008) Strategies for mental health and addictions in the country (Estrategias para salud mental en el pais). In GOSMA, *Mental Health: Cuban Experiences (La Salud Mental: Experiencias Cubanas)*. Havana: MINSAP/GOSMA & PAHO; pp. 38–59.

Brotherton S (2011) Health and health care: revolutionary period. In A West-Duran, ed., *Cuba*. Detroit, MI: Gale.

Castell-Florit Serrate P (2007) Conceptual frameworks and intervening factors in the development of inter-sectoriality (Comprension conceptual y factores que intervienen en el desarrollo de la intersectorialidad). *Revista Cubana de Salud Pública* **33** (2).

Castell-Florit Serrate P, Carlota Lausanne R, Jean-Claude MM, Santana Espinosa C, Cabrera

Gonzalez T (2007) *Study on Intersector Practices in Health in Cuba: Report to the Pan American Health Organization*. Washington, DC: PAHO.

Cuesta Mejías, L (2011). Dispensarization in the Polyclinic University at Playa one year after reorganization (La dispensarización en el policlínico universitario docente de Playa un año después de la reorganización). *Revista Cubana de Medicina General Integral* **27** (1).

De la Torre, C (2009) History of psychology in Cuba: 50 years of psychology, 50 years of revolution (Historia de la Psicología en Cuba: cincuenta años de psicología, cincuenta años de revolución). *Revista Latinoamericana de Psicologia* **17**. http://www.psicolatina.org/17/cuba.html (accessed July 2013).

Delgado García G (2008) Changes in outpatient health care in Cuba from 1959–1964 (Cambio en la atención médica ambulatoria en Cuba de 1959 a 1964). *Cuadernos de Historial de la Salud Pública* **103**.

Feinsilver J (2010) Fifty years of Cuba's medical diplomacy: from idealism to pragmatism. *Cuban Studies* **41**: 85–104.

Gorry C (2010) Once the Earth stood still (part II): mental health services in post-quake Haiti. *MEDICC Review* **12** (3): 44–7.

Grupo Operativo de Salud Mental y Addicciones (GOSMA) (2008) *Mental Health: Cuban Experiences (La Salud Mental: Experiencias Cubanas)*. Havana: MINSAP/GOSMA & PAHO.

Guanche Zaldivar JC (2011) Cuban thought and cultural identity: socialist thought. In A West-Duran, ed., *Cuba*. Detroit, MI: Gale.

León González M (2002) Community care in mental health (La atención comunitaria en salud mental). *Revista Cubana de Medicina General Integral* **18** (5).

León González M (2006) *Mental Health, Community and Community Interventions (Salud Mental, Comunidad y Técnicas de Intervención Comunitarias)*. Havana: Centro Comunitario de Salud Mental de Lawton, Municipio 10 de Octubre.

León González M (2008) Psychiatry and mental health in Cuba after the triumph of the revolution (La psiquiatría y la salud mental en Cuba después del triunfo de la revolución). In GOSMA, *Mental Health: Cuban Experiences (La Salud Mental: Experiencias Cubanas)*. Havana: MINSAP/GOSMA & PAHO.

López Serrano E (1985) Cuban medical milestones (Efemérides médicas cubanas). *Cuadernos de Historia de la Salud Pública* (**69**): 1–261.

Lorenzo Ruiz A (2006) Reflections on the evolution of psychological

interventions in emergencies and disasters: analysis of Cuban experiences (Reflexiones sobre la evolución del quehacer psicológico en el tema de emergencias y desastres: análisis de la experiencia en Cuba). *Cuadernos de Crisis* **5** (2): 7–37.

Louro Bernal I (2008) Family focus in integrative primary care (Enfoque familiar en la atención sanitaria integral). In R Álvarez Sintes, ed., *Medicina General Integral. Salud y Medicina*. Havana: Editorial Ciencias Médicas; p. 4378.

Louro Bernal I (2011) Family focus in health situation analysis (Enfoque familiar en el análisis de la situación de salud). *Revista Cubana de Higiene y Epidemiología* **49**: 151–3.

Louro Bernal I, Casal Sosa A, Martín Alfonso L, Hernández Gómez L, Aguilar García IC (2009) Formation of human resources in health psychology in Cuba since 1959 (Formación de recursos humanos en Psicología de la Salud a partir de 1959 en Cuba). *Revista Cubana de Salud Pública* **35** (1).

Luna Morales CE, Sierra Pérez D, Gandul Salabarría L (2009) Transformation of the polyclinic in Cuba in the 21st century (La transformación del policlínico en Cuba de cara al siglo XXI). *Revista Cubana de Medicina General Integral* **25** (2).

Márquez Morales N (2010) The family doctor and nurse model in Cuba (Modelo el médico y la enfermera de la familia en Cuba). *Cuaderno de Historia de la Salud Publica* **108**.

Marimón Torres N, Martínez Cruz E (2011) Cuban experiences in South/South cooperation (Experiencia cubana en Cooperación Sur-Sur). *Revista Cubana de Salud Pública* **37** (4).

Martínez Calvo S, Gómez de Haz H (2008) Health situation analysis (Análisis de situación de salud).

In R Álvarez Sintes, ed., *Medicina General Integral. Salud y Medicina*. Havana: Editorial Ciencias Médicas; p. 543.

Martínez González H, Vidal C, Alfonso Carrillo E, Rodríguez Machado I (2010) Rehabilitation in psychiatry: theoretical considerations and an integrative proposal (Rehabilitación en psiquiatría: consideraciones teóricas y una propuesta integral). *Revista Hospital Psiquiátrico de la Habana* **7** (1).

Mason S, Strug D, Beder J (2010) *Community Health Care in Cuba*. Chicago, IL: Lyceum.

Ministerio de Salud Pública (MINSAP) (2012) *Health Statistics Annual, 2011 (Anuario Estadistico de Salud, 2011)*. Havana: MINSAP.

Ochoa FR, Visbal LA (2007) Civil society and health system in Cuba. Case study commissioned by the Health Systems Knowledge Network of the WHO Commission on the Social Determinants of Health.

Pagliccia N, Spiegel J, Alegret M, *et al.* (2010) Network analysis as a tool to assess the intersectoral management of health determinants at the local level: a report from an exploratory study of two Cuban municipalities. *Social Science and Medicine* **71**: 394–9.

Pan American Health Organization (PAHO), World Health Organization (WHO) (2011) *Evaluation of Mental Health Systems in Cuba (Informe sobre el Sistema de Salud Mental en la República de Cuba)*. Havana: PAHO & WHO. http://www.who.int/mental_health/who_aims_country_reports/who_aims_report_cuba_es.pdf (accessed July 2013).

Shapiro E (2011) Health and health care: introduction. In A West-Duran, ed., *Cuba*. Detroit, MI: Gale.

Shapiro E (2013) Nurturing family resilience in response to

chronic illness: an integrative approach to health and growth promotion. In D Becvar, ed., *Handbook of Family Resilience.* New York, NY: Springer; pp. 385–408.

Sintes Jiménez M (2011) Evolution of the Cuban health system (Evolución del Sistema de Salud cubano). *Revista Médica Electrónica* **33** (4).

Whiteford L, Branch L (2008) *Primary Health Care in Cuba: the Other Revolution.* Lanham, MD: Rowman & Littlefield.

World Health Organization (2008) *The World Health Report 2008. Primary Care Now More than Ever.* Geneva: WHO.

Chapter 18

Poverty and perinatal morbidity as risk factors for mental illness

Feijun Luo, Xiangming Fang, Lijing Ouyang, and Deborah M. Stone

Introduction

Mental illness is very prevalent in the USA and worldwide. According to a report by the Substance Abuse and Mental Health Services Administration (2010), 45.1 million adults (19.9%) in the USA in 2009 had any mental illness, and among them 11 million adults (4.8%) had serious mental illness that substantially interfered with one or more major life activities. One of the most common mental illnesses is depression. Depression is a mood disorder characterized by a range of symptoms including a persistent sad or anxious mood, feelings of hopelessness, loss of pleasure in usual activities, difficulty concentrating, insomnia or excessive sleeping, appetite loss or over-eating, and thoughts of suicide (American Psychiatric Association 1994). According to the World Health Organization, depression is the leading cause of disability as defined by the number of years lived with disability and is the fourth leading contributor to the global burden of disease (World Health Organization 2008). Kessler et al. (2005b) estimated that the lifetime prevalence of depression among adults was roughly 16%. Depression is often associated with other mental disorders such as anxiety and substance abuse disorders (Kessler & Walters 1998, Kessler et al. 2003) and poor physical health (Scott et al. 2007, Gabilondo et al. 2012). Among adolescents, depression and depressive symptoms are associated with suicide, suicidal behavior (Beautrais et al. 1998, Beautrais 2000, Gould et al. 2003), being bullied (Nansel et al. 2001, Arseneault et al. 2006, Lemstra et al. 2012), and exposure to intimate partner violence (Lehrer et al. 2006).

Depression is thought to be caused by a combination of genetic, biological, environmental, and psychological factors (National Institute of Mental Health 2011). After decades of research documenting disparities in mental illness among people with lower socioeconomic status (SES) (Srole & Langner 1962, Dohrenwend 1990, Murphy et al. 1991), researchers in the 1990s began using larger population-based studies, some with nationally representative samples and longitudinal designs, to focus greater attention on causal pathways between childhood risk factors and health and mental health later in life (Kessler et al. 1994, Davey Smith et al. 1997, Marmot 2001).

The longitudinal association between SES and mental health can be understood from a life-course perspective. Kuh and Ben-Shlomo (1997, p. 285) defined the life-course approach as "the study of long-term effects on chronic disease risk of physical and social exposures during gestation, childhood, adolescence, young adulthood and later in adult life." A range of models identify specific mechanisms by which this approach broadly works. These include critical-period models, which propose that exposures to deprivation early in life, for example during the prenatal period, impact cognitive and psychosocial development later in life (Graham 2002, Raikkonen et al. 2013); accumulation models, whereby cumulative damage over time, for example by multiple adverse exposures (e.g., environmental, socioeconomic, behavioral), negatively influences body systems, ultimately impacting health and mental health (Kuh et al. 2003); and pathway models, where adverse exposures in early life set the stage for subsequent negative exposures and in turn poor health and mental health outcomes over the life course (Ben-Shlomo & Kuh 2002).

SES is multidimensional, and the commonly used dimensions are education, occupation, and income. The current study uses poverty as a measure of SES

Essentials of Global Mental Health, ed. Samuel O. Okpaku. Published by Cambridge University Press. © Cambridge University Press 2014.

and seeks to add to the discussion about early social factors and their impact on mental health in young adulthood. In the literature there are several noteworthy studies of the longitudinal association between poverty and mental health. McLeod and Shanahan (1996) indicated that children's early experience of poverty affected their future mental health regardless of their future poverty status, and persistently poor children had different mental health trajectories than did transiently poor and non-poor children. Lynch and colleagues (1997) concluded that sustained economic hardship led to poorer physical, psychological, and cognitive functioning. McDonough and Berglund (2003) showed that poverty history had a long-lasting effect on self-rated health, and current economic circumstances did not remove the health effect of earlier poverty experience.

In addition to early poverty experience, the current study also examines the association of perinatal morbidity with mental health in young adulthood. Perinatal morbidity covers a wide range of conditions. A report by Australia's National Health and Medical Research Council (1995, p. 2) describes the full spectrum of perinatal morbidity, which includes frequent events such as maternal/infant separation due to admission to a special care facility, common conditions such as prematurity, low birth weight, and intrauterine growth restriction, and sentinel events such as major neurological or physical disability. The current study uses low birth weight as a measure of perinatal morbidity. The past two decades have seen a surge in research linking low birth weight to a variety of adult health outcomes such as cardiovascular disease, hypertension, diabetes (Barker *et al.* 1989, Barker 2006, Whincup *et al.* 2008), and mental health conditions. In 2000, a study of men and women exposed in utero to the Dutch Hunger Winter in 1944–45 in their second or third trimester of pregnancy were at increased risk of affective disorders, such as depression, later in life. Studies since this time have examined less severe exposures. Among 18 studies included in their meta-analysis, Wojcik *et al.* (2012) found a weak association (OR = 1.15, 95% CI 1.00–1.32) between low birth weight (< 2500 g) and adult depression or psychological distress. This association became non-significant upon controlling for what the authors said was "probable publication bias." Similar results were found when studies were constrained to case-level depression (versus those including psychological distress). The authors also state that there was

significant heterogeneity across studies, as many did not control for confounding (e.g., none controlled for maternal socioeconomic status), and had low statistical power, underscoring that more research is needed.

There are only a few studies that simultaneously link early poverty experience and low birth weight to mental health later in life, and their results are mixed. Fan and Eaton (2001) reported that low family income at ages 7–8 did not portend excess risk of adult depression, while low birth weight (< 2500 g) significantly predicted adult depression among women. Anselmi *et al.* (2008) found that poverty in childhood increased the risk of mental disorders for women, while low birth weight was not associated with the risk of mental disorders for either men or women. Rodriguez *et al.* (2011) found that neither low family income nor low birth weight was associated with mental health problems. Because of their study sample limitations, these studies lack generalizability and their results provide little inference to the USA population. Fan and Eaton (2001) used a sample originated in the early 1960s from a prescribed inner-city area in Baltimore, Maryland, Anselmi *et al.* (2008) studied individuals born in 1982 from a southern city of Brazil, and Rodriguez *et al.* (2011) focused on a cohort born in 1997/98 from a poor Brazilian city.

Building on the existing literature, this chapter will present new evidence on poverty and low birth weight as risk factors for later depression, using a longitudinal study of a nationally representative sample of US youth. Specifically, it examines whether poverty experience in adolescence and low birth weight are associated with depression in young adulthood after controlling for sociodemographic factors.

Methods

Data source and study sample

The present study used data from the National Longitudinal Study of Adolescent Health (Add Health), a four-wave longitudinal study that followed a nationally representative probability sample of adolescents in grades 7 through 12 in the 1994/95 school year (Harris 2009). The first three waves of Add Health data were collected from April to December 1995, from April to August 1996, and from August 2001 to April 2002. The fourth wave of data was collected in 2007 and 2008. The full sample for Wave IV included 15 701 or 80.3% of the eligible participants from Wave I. The mean ages of participants during the four waves of data collection were 15.7 years, 16.2 years, 22.0 years, and 28.3 years, respectively. Of the 15 701 participants who participated in both Wave I and Wave IV interviews, 14 800 had a sampling weight at the Wave IV interview which could be used to compute population estimates.

Measures

Mental conditions

We use two depression measures from Wave IV to characterize the mental conditions of the surveyed youth. These two measures are defined as follows:

- CES-D scale – Our study makes use of an abridged version of the Center for Epidemiological Studies Depression (CES-D) scale, a widely used scale designed to measure depressive symptomatology (Radloff 1977). The complete version of the CES-D scale measures 20 symptoms of depression, and respondents are asked how often during the last seven days (0 = never or rarely, 1 = some or a little of the time, 2 = occasionally or a moderate amount of the time, 3 = most of the time or all of the time) they have had each of the 20 symptoms. The CES-D scale has a score from 0 to 60 in the complete version, with a higher score indicating the presence of more depressive symptomatology. The abridged version of the CES-D scale from the Add Health Wave IV measures the following five symptoms of depression: "being bothered by things that usually don't bother you," "being unable to shake off the blues, even with help from your family and friends," "having trouble keeping your mind on what you were doing," "feeling depressed," and "feeling sad." Responses from these five items were summed to produce a score between 0 and 15, with a higher score suggesting a greater level of depression.
- Diagnosed depression (called "Depression" here on out) – This is a dichotomous variable indicating self-reported clinical depression. It is drawn from a Wave IV survey question, "Has a doctor, nurse or other health care provider ever told you that you have or had: depression?"

Poverty and perinatal morbidity

We use estimated poverty status or welfare receipt status as a poverty measure, and low birth weight as a perinatal morbidity measure. Poverty status was

estimated from family-size-adjusted income level relative to the federal poverty threshold in 1994. There were 24% missing values of parent-reported family income in the Wave I survey. We imputed missing family income as a continuous variable on the basis of an equation predicting income based on race/ethnicity, region, urban/rural status, family structure, receipt of public assistance, and whether the residence was well kept (Ouyang *et al.* 2008). Welfare receipt status was based on the Wave I survey question of whether the surveyed parent received public assistance, such as welfare. Low birth weight was constructed from the Wave I parent survey question that assessed youth's birth weight in pounds and ounces. We classified birth weight less than 5 pounds and 8 ounces (2500 g) as low birth weight. For both variables welfare receipt status and birth weight, we created a "missing" category to retain observations whose values on welfare receipt or birth weight were missing.

Sociodemographic variables

Several sociodemographic variables collected during Wave I of Add Health that are commonly known to be associated in the literature with health outcomes were included to control for potential confounders. These sociodemographic variables included gender, race/ethnicity (Hispanic, non-Hispanic white, non-Hispanic black, and non-Hispanic other), family structure (intact family [both biological parents present] and non-intact family [all other family structures]), and parent's (mother/main caregiver's) education level (less than high school and high school or above). The age variable was collected from Wave IV.

Statistical analysis

The two depression measures, the CES-D scale score and the dichotomous variable Depression, are our dependent variables. We first used linear regression analysis to examine the relationships between the CES-D scale and poverty (measured by poverty status or welfare receipt status) and low birth weight. Because the distribution of the CES-D scale was highly skewed, we transformed the scale into the log form to reduce skewness. Before we made the log transformation, we added 0.1 to the CES-D scale to deal with responses whose scores were 0. For the dichotomous variable Depression, we used logistic regression analysis. For regressions on the two depression measures, we considered both a model that included poverty and low birth weight only and a model that included poverty, low birth weight, and sociodemographic variables. All analyses were performed using Stata SE version 10 (StataCorp LP, College Station, Texas), which controlled for the survey design effects of individuals clustered within schools and stratification by geographic region. Post-stratification weights were applied to generate nationally representative estimates.

Results

Table 18.1 presents the descriptive statistics of the study sample. The study sample included 14 800 participants who were interviewed in Wave I and Wave IV and had a sampling weight in Wave IV. The mean of the CES-D scale is 2.62 (95% CI 2.54–2.71). In the distribution table of the CES-D scale (table not shown), the vast majority of participants had a score between 0 and 3: 20.1% of participants had a score of 0, 21.3% a score of 1, 17.3% a score of 2, and 13.1% a score of 3. In contrast, only 2.4% of participants had a score of 10 or above. In this study sample, 16.4% (95% CI 15.2–17.6%) of participants self-reported diagnosed depression. As for poverty experience, 15.1% (95% CI 12.5–17.6%) of participants were from families whose incomes were below the federal poverty line and 21.9% (95% CI 19.2–24.6%) of participants were from families receiving welfare assistance. Among participants 6.4% (95% CI 5.6–7.2%) had a low birth weight (< 2500 g). The percentages of female and male respondents in the study sample are 49.3 (95% CI 48.1–50.5) and 50.7 (95% CI 49.5–51.9), respectively. Hispanic, non-Hispanic white, non-Hispanic black, and non-Hispanic other account for 12.0% (95% CI 8.6–15.3%), 67.3% (95% CI 61.6–73.1%), 15.9% (95% CI 11.8–20.0%), and 4.8% (95% CI 3.3–6.3%) of the study sample, respectively. Also among participants 45.5% (95% CI 43.0–48.1%) came from non-intact families, and 13.9% (95% CI 11.5–16.3%) of parents (mothers or main caregivers) attained an education below high school level.

Tables 18.2 and 18.3 report results from linear regression analyses of the CES-D depression scale and logistic regressions of the dichotomous variable Depression, respectively. For each table, the first two columns (Models 1 and 2 or Models 1′ and 2′) correspond to regressions in which poverty status is used as a poverty measure, and the last two columns (Models

Table 18.1 Characteristics of the study sample

Variable	Value (95% CI)
CES-D scale, mean	2.62 (2.54, 2.71)
Participants with diagnosed depression, % (95% CI)	16.4 (15.2–17.6)
Poverty status, %	
Yes	15.1 (12.5, 17.6)
No	84.9 (82.4, 87.5)
Welfare receipt status, %	
Yes	21.9 (19.2–24.6)
No	66.6 (63.9–69.3)
Missing	11.5 (10.2–12.9)
Birth weight, %	
≥ 2500 g	78.2 (76.5–79.9)
< 2500 g	6.4 (5.6–7.2)
Missing	15.4 (13.8–17.0)
Age, mean	28.3 (28.1, 28.6)
Sex, %	
Female	49.3 (48.1–50.5)
Male	50.7 (49.5–51.9)
Race/ethnicity, %	
Hispanic	12.0 (8.6–15.3)
Non-Hispanic white	67.3 (61.6–73.1)
Non-Hispanic black	15.9 (11.8–20.0)
Non-Hispanic other	4.8 (3.3–6.3)
Family structure, %	
Intact	54.5 (51.9–57.0)
Non-intact	45.5 (43.0–48.1)
Parent's education, %	
Below high school	13.9 (11.5–16.3)
High school or above	86.1 (83.7–88.5)

The study sample included 14 800 participants who were interviewed in Wave I and Wave IV and had a sampling weight in Wave IV.

3 and 4 or Models 3′ and 4′) correspond to regressions in which welfare receipt status is chosen as a poverty measure. In each pair of columns (the first two or the last two columns), the model that includes poverty and low birth weight only is presented first.

Table 18.2 Parameter estimates from linear regressions using the CES-D depression scale (log transformed) as the outcome variable

	Model 1	Model 2	Model 3	Model 4
Poverty status (reference group: No)	0.246 (0.064)***	0.068 (0.061)		
Welfare receipt status (reference group: No)				
• Yes			0.243 (0.051)***	0.119 (0.046)*
• Missing			–0.043 (0.071)	–0.026 (0.073)
Birth weight (reference group: ≥ 2500 g)				
• < 2500 g	0.211 (0.068)**	0.140 (0.068)*	0.206 (0.068)**	0.137 (0.068)*
• Missing	0.142 (0.046)**	0.079 (0.047)	0.181 (0.062)**	0.104 (0.063)
• Male		–0.246 (0.033)***		–0.247 (0.033)***
Race/ethnicity (reference group: non-Hispanic white)				
• Hispanic		0.094 (0.062)		0.094 (0.060)
• Non-Hispanic black		0.259 (0.057)***		0.249 (0.056)***
• Non-Hispanic other		0.164 (0.064)*		0.163 (0.064)*
Age		–0.076 (0.288)		–0.083 (0.291)
Age squared		0.001 (0.005)		0.001 (0.005)
Non-intact family		0.157 (0.041)***		0.148 (0.041)***
Parent's education below high school		0.206 (0.060)***		0.192 (0.060)**

Model 1: the CES-D depression scale (log transformed) is regressed on poverty status and birth weight variables.
Model 2: the CES-D depression scale (log transformed) is regressed on Model 1 variables + sociodemographic variables (gender, race/ethnicity, age, age squared, family structure, and parent's education).
Model 3: the CES-D depression scale (log transformed) is regressed on welfare receipt status and birth weight variables.
Model 4: the CES-D depression scale (log transformed) is regressed on Model 3 variables + sociodemographic variables (gender, race/ethnicity, age, age squared, family structure, and parent's education).
Standard errors are in parentheses.
* $p \leq 0.05$,** $p \leq 0.01$,*** $p \leq 0.001$.

Table 18.2 indicates that both welfare receipt status (poverty measure) and low birth weight (< 2500 g) are positive, significant predicators of the CES-D scale (log transformed), regardless of whether sociodemographic variables are controlled (Models 3 and 4). This suggests a significant longitudinal association between an adolescent's poverty experience (participants' mean age = 15.7 years in Wave I) and perinatal morbidity (low birth weight) with his/her depressive symptoms in young adulthood (participants' mean age = 28.3 years at Wave IV). Poverty status is a positive, significant predictor of depressive symptomatology when the sociodemographic variables are *not* controlled (Model 1); however, it loses significance after the inclusion of the sociodemographic variables (Model 2). Low birth weight (< 2500 g) is positively and significantly associated with the CES-D scale in all Models 1 to 4, regardless of which poverty measure is used and whether sociodemographic variables are controlled for or not. Besides findings on our key variables of interest, the results of some sociodemographic variables such as family structure and parent education are worth mentioning. Results of Models 2 and 4 show that a non-intact family structure during adolescence and a parent's education level below high school are positively and significantly associated with depressive symptoms in young adulthood. These findings are consistent with the existing literature (Lopez 1986, Quesnel-Vallée & Taylor 2012).

Table 18.3 reports odds ratios from models using self-reported diagnosed depression as the outcome variable. The adjusted odds ratios of welfare receipt status (1.21, 95% CI 1.00–1.47) and low birth weight (1.29, 95% CI 1.00–1.66) in Model 4' are both marginally significant ($p = 5.1\%$). This implies that

Table 18.3 Odds ratios from logistic regressions using self-reported diagnosed depression as the outcome variable

	Model 1′	Model 2′	Model 3′	Model 4′
Poverty status (reference group: No)	0.96 (0.79–1.16)	1.07 (0.87–1.31)		
Welfare receipt status (reference group: No)				
Yes			1.11 (0.93–1.32)	1.21 (1.00–1.47)~
Missing			1.02 (0.77–1.36)	0.98 (0.73–1.31)
Birth weight (reference group: ≥ 2500 g)				
< 2500 g	1.28 (0.99–1.65)~	1.29 (1.00–1.67)*	1.26 (0.98–1.63)~	1.29 (1.00–1.66)~
Missing	1.02 (0.87–1.21)	1.09 (0.93–1.29)	1.02 (0.80–1.29)	1.13 (0.90–1.42)
Male		0.39 (0.35–0.44)***		0.39 (0.35–0.44)***
Race/ethnicity (reference group: Non-Hispanic white)				
Hispanic		0.58 (0.45–0.77)***		0.58 (0.44–0.76)***
Non-Hispanic black		0.42 (0.34–0.52)***		0.41 (0.33–0.51)***
Non-Hispanic other		0.61 (0.46–0.81)***		0.61 (0.46–0.81)***
Age		0.98 (0.33–2.92)		0.97 (0.32–2.91)
Age squared		1.00 (0.98–1.02)		1.00 (0.98–1.02)
Non-intact family		1.45 (1.26–1.66)***		1.42 (1.24–1.62)***
Parent's education below high school		1.00 (0.78–1.28)		0.97 (0.75–1.24)

Model 1′: the Depression dummy variable is regressed on poverty status and birth weight variables.
Model 2′: the Depression dummy variable is regressed on Model 1 variables + sociodemographic variables (gender, race/ethnicity, age, age squared, family structure, and parent's education).
Model 3′: the Depression dummy variable is regressed on welfare receipt status and birth weight variables.
Model 4′: the Depression dummy variable is regressed on Model 3 variables + sociodemographic variables (gender, race/ethnicity, age, age squared, family structure, and parent's education).
95% CIs are in parentheses.
~ $p \leq 0.10$,* $p \leq 0.05$,** $p \leq 0.01$,*** $p \leq 0.001$.

both welfare receipt status and low birth weight are marginally significantly associated with depression in young adulthood after adjustment for sociodemographic factors (Model 4′). The odds ratios for poverty status are not significant, whether unadjusted (0.96, 95% CI 0.79–1.16) or adjusted (1.07, 95% CI 0.87–1.31) for socidemographic variables as shown in Models 1′ and 2′, respectively. The odds ratios for low birth weight are either marginally significant (1.28, 95% CI 0.99–1.65, $p = 5.7\%$) when sociodemographic variables are not controlled (Model 1′) or significant (1.29, 95% CI 1.00–1.67) when sociodemographic variables are controlled for (Model 2′). Table 18.3 also indicates that adolescents from non-intact families are more likely to develop depression than those from intact families, controlling for other sociodemographic factors, and the odds ratios of the non-intact family structure are very close in Models 2′

and 4′ (1.45, 95% CI 1.26–1.66 vs. 1.42, 95% CI 1.24–1.62, respectively).

Discussion

This study sheds some light on poverty and perinatal morbidity as risk factors for mental illness, specifically the association of poverty experience in adolescence and low birth weight with depression in young adulthood. Two depression measures are examined: the CES-D scale of depressive symptoms and self-reported clinically diagnosed depression. Welfare receipt status, a measure of poverty experience, is significantly, positively associated with depressive symptoms regardless of whether sociodemographic variables are controlled (Models 3 and 4). It is only marginally significantly associated with diagnosed depression after the sociodemographic variables are controlled (Model 4'). Poverty status, another measure of poverty experience, is significantly and positively associated with the CES-D scale scores when sociodemographic variables are not controlled (Model 1); however, it loses significance after the inclusion of these variables (Model 2). Poverty status is found to have no association with diagnosed depression, regardless of whether sociodemographic variables are controlled for (Models 1' and 2').

The difference between results based on welfare receipt status and those based on poverty status may be partly attributed to the determination of poverty status. Poverty status was estimated from family-size-adjusted income level relative to the federal poverty threshold. However, several potential limitations of this threshold have been noted. For example, it is determined on the basis of food consumption rather than consumption of overall goods and services by households (Slesnick 1993) and it fails to account for the regional cost-of-living difference (Fass 2009). Another reason for the difference between results based on welfare receipt status and those based on poverty status may be that the threshold for welfare eligibility is often lower than the poverty threshold (Urban Institute Welfare Rules Database 2012), so that the welfare receipt status may measure the "poorest of the poor." We also tested whether our imputation of missing family income might help explain the difference. Instead of imputing missing family income, we created a missing income category in the same way we did for welfare receipt status and birth weight. The findings on poverty status are the same as before – poverty status is not significantly associated with the CES-D scale after the inclusion of sociodemographic variables, and it is not associated with diagnosed depression regardless of whether sociodemographic variables are included. Altogether, we conclude that adolescents' poverty experience in the form of welfare receipt status acts as a risk factor of mental illness in their young adulthood.

The association between low birth weight and depression exists for both the CES-D scale and diagnosed depression. Low birth weight is significantly and positively associated with the CES-D scale regardless of whether sociodemographic variables are controlled for (Models 1–4). It is significantly or marginally significantly associated with diagnosed depression regardless of whether sociodemographic variables are controlled for (Models 1'–4'). As with results reported for poverty and welfare receipt, the

results for low birth weight are consistently significant only for the CES-D measure and not for diagnosed clinical depression. While the original CES-D (Radloff 1977) and shorter variations have been found valid (Kohut et al. 1993, Irwin et al. 1999), a five-item scale may not accurately or reliably measure the same degree of depression as indicated by a clinical diagnosis. Alternatively, many people with clinical depression may not have yet been diagnosed (the average age of onset is 32: Kessler et al. 2005a), reflecting potential bias in the measure of clinical depression.

Mental health is an important facet of overall health in adulthood, yet relatively little research has taken a life-course approach to understanding how illnesses such as depression develop. Most data on the topic using this approach come from birth cohort studies (Fan & Eaton 2001, Anselmi et al. 2008, Rodriguez et al. 2011). In lieu of a birth cohort, this study adds to the dialog by taking advantage of unique US survey data; that is, a nationally representative sample of adolescents followed over time. It simultaneously examines measures of poverty and low birth weight and their associations with later mental health. Unlike in most studies, the poverty data used here come from early adolescence and so add a new element to the discussion, which typically focuses on earlier poverty as a risk factor. This study also provides evidence on the non-intact family structure as an independent risk factor for depression. Given the large array of risk-factor data available in Add Health, this study provides ample opportunity for future examination of the mechanisms linking early contributing factors to later mental health.

This chapter is subject to a number of limitations. First, we chose low birth weight as the only measure of perinatal morbidity because of data availability. Perinatal morbidity includes many conditions other than low birth weight, and some conditions, such as infants born small for gestational age, may have stronger associations with later depression than does low birth weight (Berle et al. 2006). From this point of view, the choice of low birth weight as the only measure of perinatal morbidity may underestimate the impact of perinatal morbidity on mental illness. Second, we used data from Waves I and IV of Add Health in this study – two mental health measures from Wave IV and poverty and perinatal morbidity measures and most sociodemographic variables from

Wave I. Although we can test the longitudinal associations of poverty and perinatal morbidity with mental illness using this approach, we cannot give a clear answer on how poverty and perinatal morbidity may contribute to mental illness. Whether a critical period exists, whether risks of living in poverty accumulate over time, or whether a pathway model exists is uncertain. For example, adolescents with experiences of poverty and/or perinatal morbidity may be more likely to live in poverty, have poor academic performance, engage in risky behaviors, suffer more physical and mental health problems, lack access to healthcare resources, etc. These adversities may in turn influence their mental health from adolescence to adulthood. A future study will integrate all four waves of Add Health and explore how adolescent poverty experience and low birth weight may have contributed to the development of the aforementioned problems that may influence young adults' mental health. Third, in this study neither the CES-D scale nor diagnosed depression is a perfect measure of survey participants' current mental health conditions. One measure may measure less severe depression (CES-D five-items)

than the other (diagnosed depression). Also, self-report bias may impact results, and finally having a previous depression diagnosis may not accurately reflect current mental health, especially given that the onset of depression diagnosis is unknown.

Results from the current study suggest that welfare receipt status in adolescence and low birth weight are associated with mental health in young adulthood. Continued research on these associations using a life-course perspective is recommended, however. Longitudinal studies with expanded measurement of these relationships over time, and with the ability to test multiple pathways such as environmental (e.g. family stability) and behavioral (e.g. alcohol and drug use) pathways, can help inform public health approaches to improved mental health.

Disclaimer

The findings and conclusions in this report are those of the authors, and do not necessarily represent the official position of the Centers for Disease Control and Prevention.

References

American Psychiatric Association (1994) *Diagnostic and Statistical Manual of Mental Disorders, Fourth Edition (DSM-IV)*. Washington, DC: APA.

Anselmi L, Barros FC, Minten GC, *et al.* (2008) Prevalence and early determinants of common mental disorders in the 1982 birth cohort, Pelotas, Southern Brazil. *Revista de Saúde Pública* 42 (Supl. 2): 26–33.

Arseneault L, Walsh E, Trzesniewski K, *et al.* (2006) Bullying victimization uniquely contributes to adjustment problems in young children: a nationally representative cohort study. *Pediatrics* 118: 130–8.

Barker DJ (2006) Birth weight and hypertension. *Hypertension* 48: 357–8.

Barker DJ, Osmond C, Golding J, Kuh D, Wadsworth ME (1989) Growth in utero, blood pressure in childhood and adult life, and mortality from cardiovascular disease. *BMJ* 298: 564–7.

Beautrais AL (2000) Risk factors for suicide and attempted suicide among young people. *Australian and New Zealand Journal of Psychiatry* 34: 420–36.

Beautrais AL, Joyce PR, Mulder RT (1998). Psychiatric illness in a New Zealand sample of young people making serious suicide attempts. *New Zealand Medical Journal* 111: 44–8.

Ben-Shlomo Y, Kuh D (2002) A life course approach to chronic disease epidemiology: conceptual models, empirical challenges and interdisciplinary perspectives. *International Journal of Epidemiology* 31: 285–93.

Berle JO, Mykletun A, Daltveit AK, *et al.* (2006) Outcomes in adulthood of children with foetal growth retardation. A linkage study from the Nord-Trondelag Health Study (HUNT) and the Medical Birth Registry of Norway. *Acta Psychiatrica Scandinavica* 113: 501–9.

Davey Smith G, Hart C, Ferrell C, *et al.* (1997) Birth weight of offspring and mortality in the Renfrew and Paisley study: prospective observational study. *BMJ* 315: 1189–93.

Dohrenwend BP (1990) Socioeconomic status (SES) and psychiatric disorders. *Social Psychiatry and Psychiatric Epidemiology* 25: 41–7.

Fan AP, Eaton WW (2001). Longitudinal study assessing the joint effects of socio-economic status and birth risks on adult emotional and nervous conditions. *British Journal of Psychiatry Supplement* 40: s78–83.

Fass S (2009). *Measuring Poverty in the United States*. New York, NY: National Center for Children in Poverty, Mailman School of Public Health, Columbia University. http://www.nccp.org/publications/pub_876.html (accessed July 2013).

Gabilondo A, Vilagut G, Pinto-Meza A, Haro JM, Alonso J (2012)

Comorbidity of major depressive episode and chronic physical conditions in Spain, a country with low prevalence of depression. *General Hospital Psychiatry* 34: 510–17.

Gould MS, Greenberg T, Velting DM, et al. (2003) Youth suicide risk and preventive interventions: a review of the past 10 years. *Journal of the American Academy of Child and Adolescent Psychiatry* 42: 386–405.

Graham H (2002) Building an inter-disciplinary science of health inequalities: the example of lifecourse research. *Social Science and Medicine* 55: 2005–16.

Harris KM (2009) *The National Longitudinal Study of Adolescent Health (Add Health), Waves I & II, 1994–1996; Wave III, 2001–2002; Wave IV, 2007–2009.* Chapel Hill, NC: Carolina Population Center, University of North Carolina at Chapel Hill.

Irwin M, Artin KH, Oxman MN (1999) Screening for depression in the older adult: criterion validity of the 10-item Center for Epidemiological Studies Depression Scale (CES-D). *Archives of Internal Medicine* 159: 1701–4.

Kessler RC, McGonagle KA, Zhao S, et al. (1994) Lifetime and 12-month prevalence of DSM-III-R psychiatric disorders in the united states: Results from the national comorbidity survey. *Archives of General Psychiatry* 51: 8–19.

Kessler RC, Berglund P, Demler O, et al. (2003) The epidemiology of major depressive disorder: results from the National Comorbidity Survey Replication (NCS-R). *JAMA* 289: 3095–105.

Kessler RC, Berglund PA, Demler O, Jin R, Walters EE (2005a) Lifetime prevalence and age-of-onset distributions of DSM-IV disorders in the National Comorbidity Survey Replication (NCS-R). *Archives of General Psychiatry* 62: 593–602.

Kessler RC, Chiu WT, Demler O, et al. (2005b) Prevalence, severity, and comorbidity of 12-month DSM-IV disorders in the National Comorbidity Survey Replication. *Archives of General Psychiatry* 62: 617–27.

Kessler RC, Walters EE (1998) Epidemiology of DSM-III-R major depression and minor depression among adolescents and young adults in the National Comorbidity Survey. *Depressin and Anxiety* 7: 3–14.

Kohut FJ, Berkman LF, Evans DA, Cornoni-Huntley J (1993) Two shorter forms of the CES-D (Center for Epidemiological Studies Depression) depressive symptoms index. *Journal of Aging and Health* 5: 179–93.

Kuh D, Ben-Shlomo Y (1997) *A Life Course Approach to Chronic Disease Epidemiology; Tracing the Origins of Ill-Health from Early to Adult Life.* Oxford: Oxford University Press.

Kuh D, Ben-Shlomo Y, Lynch J, et al. (2003) Life course epidemiology. *Journal of Epidemiology and Community Health* 57: 778–83.

Lehrer JA, Buka S, Gortmaker S, et al. (2006) Depressive symptomatology as a predictor of exposure to intimate partner violence among us female adolescents and young adults. *Archives of Pediatrics and Adolescent Medicine* 160: 270–6.

Lemstra ME, Nielsen G, Rogers MR, et al. (2012) Risk indicators and outcomes associated with bullying in youth aged 9–15 years. *Canadian Journal of Public Health* 103: 9–13.

Lopez FG (1986) Family structure and depression: implications for the counseling of depressed college students. *Journal of Counseling and Development* 64: 508–11.

Lynch JW, Kaplan GA, Shema SJ (1997) Cumulative impact of sustained economic hardship on

physical, cognitive, psychological, and social functioning. *New England Journal of Medicine* 337: 1889–95.

Marmot M (2001) Aetiology of coronary heart disease – Fetal and infant growth and socioeconomic factors in adult life may act together. *BMJ* 323: 1261–2.

McDonough P, Berglund P (2003) Histories of poverty and self-rated health trajectories. *Journal of Health and Social Behavior* 44: 198–214.

McLeod JD, Shanahan MJ (1996) Trajectories of poverty and children's mental health. *Journal of Health and Social Behavior* 37: 207–20.

Murphy JM, Olivier DC, Monson RR, et al. (1991) Depression and anxiety in relation to social status. A prospective epidemiologic study. *Archives of General Psychiatry* 48: 223–9.

National Health and Medical Research Council (1995) *Perinatal Morbidity: Report of the Health Care Committee Expert Panel on Perinatal Morbidity.* Canberra: NHMRC. http://www.nhmrc.gov.au/guidelines/publications/wh18 (accessed July 2013).

Nansel TR, Overpeck M, Pilla RS, et al. (2001) Bullying behaviors among US youth: prevalence and association with psychosocial adjustment. *JAMA* 285: 2094–100.

National Institute of Mental Health (2011) *Depression.* Bethesda, MD: NIMH. http://www.nimh.nih.gov/health/publications/depression/depression-booklet.pdf (accessed July 2012).

Ouyang L, Fang X, Mercy J, et al. (2008) Attention-deficit/hyperactivity disorder symptoms and child maltreatment: a population-based study. *Journal of Pediatrics* 153: 851–6.

Quesnel-Vallée A, Taylor M (2012) Socioeconomic pathways to depressive symptoms in adulthood: evidence from the National

Longitudinal Survey of Youth 1979. *Social Science and Medicine* **74**: 734–43.

Radloff LS (1977) The CES-D scale: a self-report depression scale for research in the general population. *Applied Psychological Measurement* **1**: 385–401.

Raikkonen K, Kajantie E, Pesonen AK, *et al.* (2013) Early life origins cognitive decline: findings in elderly men in the Helsinki Birth Cohort Study. *PLoS One* **8**(1): e54707.

Rodriguez JD, da Silva AA, Bettiol H, *et al.* (2011) The impact of perinatal and socioeconomic factors on mental health problems of children from a poor Brazilian city: a longitudinal study. *Social Psychiatry and Psychiatric Epidemiology* **46**: 381–91.

Scott KM, Bruffaerts R, Tsang A, *et al.* (2007) Depression–anxiety relationships with chronic physical conditions: results from the World Mental Health surveys. *Journal of Affective Disorders* **103**: 113–20.

Slesnick DT (1993) Gaining ground: poverty in the postwar United States. *Journal of Political Economy* **101**: 1–38.

Srole L, Langner TS (1962) *Socioeconomic status groups: their psychiatric patient*. In L Srole, TS Langner, ST Michael, MK Opler, TA Rennie, eds., *Mental Health in the Metropolis: the Midtown Manhattan Study*. New York, NY: McGraw-Hill; pp. 240–52.

Substance Abuse and Mental Health Services Administration (2010) Results from the 2009 National Survey on Drug Use and Health (NSDUH): Mental Health Findings. http://store.samhsa.gov/product/SMA10–4609 (accessed April 2012).

Urban Institute Welfare Rules Database (2012) Welfare Rules Databook Tables by Year. http://anfdata.urban.org/wrd/tables.cfm (accessed October 2012).

Whincup PH, Kaye SJ, Owen CG, *et al.* (2008) Birth weight and risk of type 2 diabetes: a systematic review. *JAMA* **300**: 2886–97.

Wojcik W, Lee W, Colman I, Hardy R, Hotopf M (2012) Foetal origins of depression? A systematic review and meta-analysis of low birth weight and later depression. *Psychological Medicine* **43**: 1–12.

World Health Organization (2008) *Global Burden of Disease: 2004 Update*. Geneva: WHO.

Chapter

19

Maternal mental health care: refining the components in a South African setting

Sally Field, Emily Baron, Ingrid Meintjes, Thandi van Heyningen, and Simone Honikman

Introduction

In low- and middle-income countries (LMICs), competing health priorities, civil conflict, and a lack of political will mean that expenditure on mental health is a fraction of that needed to meet the mental health care needs of the population (Chisholm *et al.* 2007). For mothers, this treatment gap is most notable in regions where health agendas focus on maternal mortality indicators (Saxena *et al.* 2007).

The South African Stress and Health study indicates that in the general population, 9.8% of South Africans experience mood disorders, with a lifetime prevalence of 15.8% for anxiety disorders (Stein *et al.* 2008). However, research shows that, despite South African policy and legislation advocating for a community-based provision of mental health, mental health services are still not adequate (Lund *et al.* 2010). Untreated perinatal mental disorders can have significant impact on the well-being of the mothers, their children, and their community. The transgenerational effects have been well established, and are felt particularly in societies facing adversity (Talge *et al.* 2007, Hay *et al.* 2008).

This chapter briefly reviews the literature on common perinatal mental disorders, describes the activities of the Perinatal Mental Health Project (PMHP) based at the University of Cape Town (UCT), South Africa, and reports on lessons learnt regarding the integration of maternal mental health care within primary care settings.

Background to common perinatal mental disorders

A global perspective

Common perinatal mental disorders (CPMDs) refer to non-psychotic disorders, most commonly depression or anxiety, which are experienced during pregnancy (antenatally) and/or within the first 12 months after delivery (postnatally) (Fisher *et al.* 2012).

Data from high-income countries show prevalence rates of 13% for antenatal depression (Hendrick *et al.* 1998) and 10% for postnatal depression (O'Hara & Swain 1996). A literature review from LMICs, however, reported that CPMDs are more common in LMICs, particularly amongst poorer women (Fisher *et al.* 2012), with a mean prevalence of 16% and 20% for antenatal and postnatal CPMDs respectively.

Interventions for pregnant women in sub-Saharan Africa have primarily focused on physical aspects of maternal and reproductive health, neglecting mental disorders (Skeen *et al.* 2010).

CPMDs in South Africa

In South Africa, research has shown high prevalence rates of depression amongst pregnant and postnatal women. In an informal settlement outside Cape Town, 39% of pregnant women screened positive for depression (Hartley *et al.* 2011) and 34.7% of post-natal women were diagnosed with depression (Cooper *et al.* 1999). In a rural area with high HIV prevalence, 47% of women were diagnosed with depression (Rochat *et al.* 2011).

Consequences of CPMDs

Adverse consequences of CPMDs reported in women during pregnancy include non-adherence to maternal care, self-medication with alcohol or drugs, disturbed sleep and appetite, and poor weight gain. Maternal depression in HIV-positive pregnant women can result in reluctance to access healthcare services, which affects adherence to antenatal interventions,

Essentials of Global Mental Health, ed. Samuel O. Okpaku. Published by Cambridge University Press. © Cambridge University Press 2014.

critical to the prevention of mother-to-child transmission of HIV (Rochat *et al.* 2006). CPMDs are also associated with higher rates of miscarriage, cesarean section delivery and preterm delivery, and low infant birth weight (Lusskin *et al.* 2007, Grote *et al.* 2010).

Untreated CPMDs can lead to multiple negative health outcomes for the fetus, infant, and child (Meintjes *et al.* 2010). CPMDs have been associated with poor fetal brain and neuro-development (Oates 2002), as well as alterations in the internal hormonal environment, all of which have implications for postnatal information processing (Bonari *et al.* 2004). CPMDs have also been associated with delay in the initiation of breastfeeding, which in turn is associated with infant mortality and increased diarrheal episodes, particularly in low-income settings (Rahman & Creed 2007).

Finally, CPMDs are associated with negative cognitive and emotional development outcomes in infants and children. These include increased crying and irritability, hyperactivity, unsocial behavior, attention-deficit/hyperactivity disorder, inconsolability, and lower language achievements (O'Connor *et al.* 2002, Murray *et al.* 2003, Patel *et al.* 2004).

Context of the Perinatal Mental Health Project (PMHP)

For women living in adversity, it is challenging to engage with mental health services when, in addition to facing competing priorities relating to poverty, violence, and childcare, they are confronted with the stigma of mental illness. However, in South Africa, despite limited resources, women tend to access health care during their pregnancies: over 99% of pregnant women have at least one antenatal care visit at a maternity facility, with a mean of 3.7 visits per client (Padarath & English 2011). Obstetric services in South Africa provide antenatal care at a primary level, and women with obstetric risk or complications are referred to secondary or tertiary-level care. The antenatal period thus presents a unique opportunity for intervention for women who are experiencing mental disorders.

The Perinatal Mental Health Project (PMHP) was founded in 2002 as a new mental health service for pregnant and postnatal women in Cape Town, South Africa. The PMHP provides integrated screening, counseling, and psychiatric services in four primary-level maternity facilities around Cape Town. For the purpose of this chapter, only the clinical services of one of the facilities is described. Cape Town has a population of approximately 3.5 million, where 85% are literate, a quarter of the population is unemployed, and 12% of the general population access poverty grants (Provincial Government Western Cape 2010). The South African birth rate is reported to be 19.48/1000 population, with Cape Town reporting 68 180 births annually (Index Mundi 2011).

Aims of the PMHP

The aim of the PMHP is to develop a model of mental health services for pregnant and postnatal women that is integrated into primary obstetric services in low-resource settings.

Clinical services

Integrated stepped-care model

The PMHP's mental health service is based on a stepped-care model (Honikman *et al.* 2012), which has been shown to provide a useful framework for the integration of psychological treatment in primary settings (Araya *et al.* 2003, Patel *et al.* 2007). At the facility, screening for mental health among pregnant women is conducted by maternity nurses, who refer those identified with mental distress for counseling. Counselors can then refer clients to a psychiatrist if further intervention is needed. Clients can continue to receive counseling for up to one year postpartum.

Screening

With the women's consent, nurses or midwives offer women a mental health screening form, which consists of the Edinburgh Postnatal Depression Scale (EPDS: Cox *et al.* 1996) and the Risk Factor Assessment (RFA), designed by the PMHP (Meintjes *et al.* 2010). The RFA screens for the presence of 11 common risk factors for perinatal disorders (Josefsson *et al.* 2002, Husain *et al.* 2006, Lusskin *et al.* 2007, Robertson *et al.* 2007); these include lack of partner or family support, unintended pregnancy, and domestic violence.

The mental health screening is self-administered in private. It is available in three local languages – English, Afrikaans, and Xhosa – and in French, because there is a significant Francophone refugee population attending the facility. The screening form is scored by midwives, and if scores meet the cut-off

Table 19.1 Descriptors of women screened at PMHP in 2011 (n = 1708)

Mean age	26.6 years
Mean gestation	22.5 weeks
Mean gravidity	1.96
Mean parity	0.7
Mean EPDS score	8.5
Mean RFA score	1.5

EPDS, Edinburgh Postnatal Depression Scale; RFA, Risk Factor Assessment.

Table 19.2 Presenting problems for counseling clients of PMHP in 2011 (n = 291)

Clients' screening scores	
Mean EPDS score	13.8
Mean RFA score	2.9
Presenting problems	**% of clients**
Primary support problems	89
Social environment difficulties	51
Health/medical problems	31
Problems adjusting to life-cycle transition	65
Previous/present psychiatric condition	24
Presenting more than one problem	76

EPDS, Edinburgh Postnatal Depression Scale; RFA, Risk Factor Assessment.

on either the EPDS or RFA (> 12 on EPDS and/or > 2 on RFA), women are offered referral for counseling. These cut-offs were chosen on the basis of international convention (Cox *et al.* 1996) and a pragmatic approach to service capacity.

Table 19.1 provides demographic and mental health screening data for women screened in 2011. In that year, the majority of women booked their first antenatal appointment in their second trimester. Most women were primiparous.

Counseling

Individual face-to-face counseling is provided by counselors. The counseling component has changed over time in terms of employment status, qualifications, and the number of hours available for counseling. Details indicating these differences over three time periods can be found in Table 19.4. Counselors were oriented to the PMHP and trained to use a client-centered approach to overcome the clients' distress and address problems presented at screening.

Brief structured psychosocial treatments, including cognitive behavior therapy, interpersonal therapy, and problem-solving approaches, have been recommended as evidence-based interventions for depression (Dua *et al.* 2011). The PMHP counseling techniques include elements of these, and others such as containment, psychoeducation, bereavement counseling, debriefing of traumatic incidents, and suicide and impulse risk management. A research protocol is being developed to standardize the counseling intervention provided by lay counselors, based on one of these evidence-based interventions. Table 19.2 indicates mean screening scores and categories of problems presented by clients counseled in 2011.

Lack of primary support, which typically involves lack of partner or family support, was the most reported problem. Adjusting to life-cycle transition was also a commonly reported problem, and typically referred to clients who had unintended, unwanted, or adolescent pregnancies.

Though the total number of counseling sessions can be limited, with a mean of 2.8 sessions per client in 2011, additional support to counseled clients is provided by the counselors through liaison with external agencies, social services, or support organizations, as well as through additional counseling provided on the telephone. In 2011, more than 10% of counseled clients were referred to additional services, and 20% received one or more telephone counseling sessions, in addition to their face-to-face counseling sessions.

Psychiatric referral

As part of the stepped-care model, counselors can refer clients who require additional assessment and treatment to an on-site psychiatrist. The psychiatrist attends the clinic twice a month. Table 19.3 provides a summary of descriptors for clients who have been referred to the psychiatrist from 2003 to 2011.

The most common diagnostic category presented was major depressive disorder, followed by diagnoses of comorbid features of anxiety and post-traumatic stress disorder. Approximately 75% of clients were prescribed medication.

Table 19.3 PMHP clients referred to a psychiatrist, 2003–2011 ($n = 100$)

Descriptors of clients	
Mean age	27.4 years
Mean EPDS score	18.2
Mean RFA score	4.0

Presenting diagnostic categories	% of clients
Major depressive disorder	82
Comorbid features of anxiety	14
Generalized anxiety disorder	2
Post-traumatic stress disorder	12
Panic disorder	3
Adjustment disorder	1
Sleep disorder	2
Personality disorder	3
No diagnosis	6
Comorbid disorders	31
Medication prescribed	75

EPDS, Edinburgh Postnatal Depression Scale; RFA, Risk Factor Assessment.

Monitoring and supervision

PMHP's experience is that adequate emotional support and routine supervision for counseling staff is fundamental to ensuring a sustainable, high-quality maternal mental health service. The PMHP protocol requires all counselors to receive weekly individual supervision. In addition, the PMHP counseling team attends a clinical meeting every two weeks to debrief as a group, support each other, and receive guidance from the clinical services coordinator (CSC).

In addition, the project coordinator conducts comprehensive monthly monitoring and evaluation of screening and counseling activities, and consults with counseling and clinic staff to adapt aspects of the service and implement changes to improve service delivery.

Service user's perspective

The perspective of one service user was chosen to foreground the common experiences of clients using the PMHP's services. Her name has been changed for confidentiality purposes.

Zukiswa's score of 24 on the EPDS suggested that she was very distressed: she had not been able to get hold of her boyfriend since she found out she was pregnant, and had just learnt that she was HIV-positive. After screening, Zukiswa was referred to a PMHP counselor, who initially focused on containing her emotions through active listening, reflection, and empathy.

> He won't take my calls. And his friends say he has gone to Jo'burg. I've been going through hell. I am so afraid my baby will get the virus. And what if I get sick? Who will support this child? I'm afraid to ask my mother because she never liked my boyfriend. (First session)

> I don't know what is wrong with me. I'm bad. My memory is very poor. On Monday I lost money in the taxi. Yesterday, I lost my jacket. I don't know what I must do these days. Maybe this virus works in my mind, and I'm suffering. I'm always thinking about my future and my children. (Subsequent mobile text message)

With the counselor, Zukiswa worked on solutions to her problems. She identified the resources she had around her, and thought of ways to use these in the best way. Subsequently, her mood improved, and she no longer felt as depressed and anxious. Eventually Zukiswa felt ready to disclose her HIV status to her mother. This helped her to get more support and understanding at home, which gave her the strength to cope with her HIV status, her pregnancy, and her plans for the future.

> I finished my job application today. I want to say thanks for everything you did for me. God bless you. You must continue to help other people, other people who are suffering, just like I was. (Mobile text message one month after final session)

Preliminary evaluation

Once the counseling intervention has been standardized, an evaluation study is planned to assess the impact of the intervention. A six- to ten-week postpartum telephone or face-to-face follow-up was introduced in 2010 as part of continuity of care, and has been used as an opportunity to evaluate mood status, bonding with the baby, and breastfeeding. A preliminary evaluation of the follow-up calls made in 2011 ($n = 276$) indicated the following:

- 90% of clients reported that their primary problems had improved, including 65% which had "much improved" or were "resolved completely."
- Social environment issues and primary support problems were the most difficult to resolve.

- More than 85% of clients with primary support issues indicated that these issues improved. A subset of 63% of these clients reported that those problems were "much improved" or "resolved completely."
- 95% of mothers reported successful bonding with their baby.
- 71% of mothers reported to be coping at follow-up.
- 67% of mothers reported to have a positive mood at follow-up.
- 93% of women saw counseling sessions in a positive way.

In 2011, counselors were able to follow up 68% of counseled women postnatally, 97% of whom were followed up telephonically. This mode of follow-up is feasible in South Africa, where there is high mobile phone ownership, text messaging services are relatively cheap, and "please call me" messages can be sent free of charge (UNDP 2012). The same pattern is also true in other African countries (UNDP 2012).

Lessons learnt

Table 19.4 provides a summary of the PMHP organizational structure and service outputs over time:

Table 19.4 PMHP's organizational changes over time

Organizational descriptors	2003	2008	2011
Management	Director	Director Coordinator University oversight	Director Coordinator University oversight
Service staff	3 sessional volunteer counselors (social workers, counseling psychologist)	Full-time employed counselor – clinical psychologist	Clinical services coordinator (clinical psychologist) Full-time counselors (trained lay counselor, registered counselor with undergraduate counseling degree)
Pathways to care	Screening for mental disorders and risk at second antenatal visit Counseling provided in antenatal clinic Counselors refer to psychiatrist at antenatal clinic as required	As for 2003	Screening for mental disorders and risk at first antenatal visit Counseling and psychiatry as for 2003

Service use indicators	2003	2008	2011
No. of women attending the antenatal clinic	1164	1728	2198
No. of women screened	588	1436	1708
Coverage (no. of women screened / no. of women attending antenatal clinic)	50.5%	83.0%	81.0%
% of women screened who qualify for counseling	31.6%	32.9%	30.0%
% of women who decline referral among those who qualify for counseling	33.8%	34.5%	33.8%
No. of new clients seen in counseling	112	252	291
Total no. of counseling appointments booked	242	843	1039
Total no. of counseling sessions held	149	563	822
Average no. of counseling sessions per client	1.3	2.2	2.8
% appointments defaulted	42.0%	25.5%	17.0%
% of referred women lost to follow-up	6.0%	16.5%	0.0%
No. of clients attending psychiatry	15	13	7

2003 represents the first full year of service delivery, 2008 is the year the PMHP shifted management and funding structures into UCT, and 2011 represents the most recent full year of data collection.

Over the years, the number of women attending the antenatal clinic nearly doubled, yet the PMHP managed to increase its screening coverage, from 50% in 2003 to 81% in 2011. The rate of women qualifying for referral remained constant, and so did the rate of women declining referral to counseling. Finally, while the number of new clients seen per year and the average number of sessions held per client increased steadily, the number of women defaulting or being lost to follow-up decreased.

Organization of services and staff

In the PMHP's experience, community-based obstetric units have high patient volumes and significant mental health needs. Because counselors routinely have to deal with suicide risk management, extreme poverty, domestic violence and abuse, problematic social environments, and primary support problems, the PMHP has had to be conscious of the possibility of counselor burnout.

The employment of a CSC in 2011 was found to be crucial in avoiding burnout and ensuring the sustainability and quality of maternal mental health care provided. The CSC provides regular supervision, debriefing, and ongoing support to the counselors, who in turn provide the main client interface work.

Instituting an appointment and follow-up system has assisted with the management of increasing client numbers, ensuring continuity of care and reducing rates of loss to follow-up. The latter is the result of a tracking system which involves counselors' attempting telephone contact three times to re-schedule missed appointments.

Screening

Maternity nursing staff have successfully managed to incorporate mental health screening into routine history-taking procedures and have reported high levels of acceptability of this integration. Furthermore, by labelling the screening as the "maternal support questionnaire," clients have found the mental health screening acceptable. This is evidenced by the low rate of clients declining to be screened (4%).

Counseling

Though the demands may vary across maternity facilities, a full-time counselor can be more flexible with appointments and ensure that these coincide with women's antenatal visits, further improving uptake of the services and decreasing the number of women declining the services or being lost to follow-up.

Short interventions, which focus on improving the women's social support environment and their resilience, can have beneficial effects on women's mood and functioning. This is the case even in circumstances where women can only attend two or three counseling sessions.

The women attending South African maternity facilities are likely to represent a variety of cultural backgrounds, and many may also be refugees. The PMHP's experience has shown that having a refugee as a counselor for refugee pregnant women is beneficial for this population. In addition to speaking the same language, a similarly located counselor can, for example, identify factors which may be masked to an "outsider," interpret cultural differences in expressions of distress, or understand how the local context may affect a displaced person.

Teaching and training

The aim of the training program is to prepare the service delivery environment to integrate maternal mental health care into routine practice. To reach this objective, the PMHP has three different strategies: increase awareness on CPMDs among health workers, attend to health workers' emotional well-being, and equip them with empathic engagement and basic counseling skills.

Rationale for training interventions

The PMHP has identified that nurses, as the initial – and often primary – interface between women and the primary health system, have the potential to exacerbate or alleviate mental distress among this vulnerable population.

However, nurses in South Africa's public health sector work in high-stress environments, because of insufficient staff, a lack of support from supervisors, long working hours, and task overload. The psychological phenomenon of "othering" as a form of "depersonalization" is routinely identified as a coping mechanism in this setting (Willets & Leff 2003,

Rothmann *et al.* 2006). This results in a significant number of cases of abuse and neglect of clients, particularly in maternity settings (Jewkes *et al.* 1998). For nurses and health workers to provide quality care and address women's mental distress in these settings, health workers' own emotional well-being and stresses must first be addressed (Rothmann *et al.* 2006, Pillay 2009).

Also, even among health workers, there is a poor understanding of the prevalence, etiology, and manifestations of mental illness, such as CPMDs. By raising awareness about CPMDs, the PMHP aims to shift attitudes and stigma around mental illness, so that health workers are more likely to accept and advocate for the need for maternal mental health services. This can facilitate the integration of screening, basic care, and management of mental health into maternal care, and the implementation of these services.

Emotional support for staff

PMHP's experience validates research findings reporting that nurses are overwhelmed, stressed, and traumatized, with little recourse to supportive services or debriefing opportunities. The CSC provides regular support and debriefing sessions with health workers to address their psychological needs. In addition, the training program has focused on designing training which allows health workers to develop insight into their own feelings and needs, whilst simultaneously gaining an awareness of and approach to the emotional state of the women in their care. One such method developed is called the "secret history."

The "secret history" training method

The PMHP's "secret history" training aims to shift attitudes and raise awareness among health workers about pregnant women's personal circumstances and how health workers' own personal problems can affect their interaction with other health staff and clients. The training, which lasts 2–3 hours, focuses on group role play, which immerses participants in the typical narratives of a pregnant mother and an overworked health worker, both experiencing social and emotional difficulties. Half of the group enacts the role of the health worker and the other half, the mother. Over time, new background information is revealed for each character and the facilitators enquire about what the participants are feeling and needing, as their assigned character. Participants are

encouraged to interact with one another in a naturalistic way. Halfway through the narrative, the participants swap roles. In the debriefing component of the training, interpersonal interactions and internal processes are examined in a participatory way.

Improving skills in empathic care and counseling

Training health workers in maternal mental health usually takes the form of workshops in counseling skills, didactic teaching on maternal mental health, and service development workshops. The PMHP teaches health practitioners who work in obstetric services, such as medical, nursing, midwifery, and postgraduate students. It provides in-service professional development for approximately 600 health workers per year and capacitates community-based practitioners working with vulnerable women.

> It [the training] opened our eyes. Sometimes we are doing things to patients, unaware of what we are doing. As nurses, we can talk and act in a way without thinking, but when you are in the shoes of the patient, you realize what you are doing. (Midwife)

Manuals on basic counseling skills and maternal mental health for general health workers have been developed to supplement the training.

Lessons learnt

The PMHP's experience is that a maternal mental health service requires foundational work to prepare the environment. Training health workers requires a synthesis of capacity building in empathic care and mental health knowledge, and requires regular debriefing to address their psychological needs.

By addressing health workers' emotional well-being, the PMHP found that mental health was destigmatized among staff, and, despite being located in busy, low-resource facilities, health workers were more willing and able to take on screening and referral responsibilities, as well as to provide high-quality, empathic care. The uptake of training was further enhanced when participative methodologies were used to draw on and emphasize health workers' existing knowledge, intuitive wisdom, and skills. They reported that this give them a sense of empowerment to address the psychological distress in their clients and in their own lives.

The PMHP has found it helpful to raise awareness among, and to collaborate with, complementary services at health facilities, such as HIV/AIDS peer counselors, social workers, or breastfeeding consultants. This provides more comprehensive care for mothers.

Research

The research program focuses on developing components of the PMHP's service model, as well as assessing its effectiveness and transferability to other low-resource settings. The PMHP is currently developing a short screening tool for CPMDs, and is engaged in developing and testing a standard counseling intervention. Future research plans are for an implementation study to assess PMHP's integration of services in other low-resource settings, and an amendment of the intervention accordingly, for scale-up.

Screening tool development study

The screening tool development study was initiated when health workers reported that the EPDS was too cumbersome to use and score for mental health screening in a busy clinical setting. The aim of the study was to develop and validate a brief screening tool for CPMDs, which would be more pragmatic and acceptable for use by health workers, thereby ensuring the sustainability and effectiveness of the screening services. The data for this study have been collected and are currently being analyzed.

Assessing the intervention's effectiveness

The PMHP has finalized a monitoring and evaluation framework which is implemented monthly across all clinical service sites. The framework facilitates the identification of clients' characteristics, risk profiles, and related care requirements, which can then be addressed effectively. It allows the PMHP to obtain thorough information to assess the PMHP service's impact and delivery.

However, developing a standard counseling intervention, which is consistent for all women receiving counseling, is necessary to assess whether PMHP's clinical services are effective or not. Feedback from clients and preliminary outcome analyses indicate that counseling is helpful in improving women's mood and functioning. However, prior to advocating

a model for scale-up, more rigorous effectiveness analyses must be undertaken.

Collaboration with national and international partners

Through collaboration with two global mental health research consortia, the PMHP has strengthened its capacity as a research partner and cross-country maternal mental health consultant. The focus of these research consortia is on strengthening mental health systems at primary care level, and developing capacity for scaling up mental health interventions in LMICs. PMHP's experience in service delivery has served to inform the design of these research protocols, which include a specific focus on CPMDs.

Lessons learnt

CPMDs remain under-recognized in low-resource settings, and the majority of those who need mental health care lack access to treatment (World Health Organization 2008). In South Africa, the limited availability of valid, feasible, and acceptable screening tools for maternal mental disorders, and increased demand from service providers, has generated demand for the development of a screening tool as a matter of priority. This is the first step towards the provision of universal maternal mental healthcare interventions at primary care level.

Regular monitoring and evaluation of screening, counseling, and follow-up procedures are important to be able to understand the patterns of service use, and identify existing barriers to accepting and attending mental health services. This is essential to be able to improve services and the effectiveness of counseling and referral mechanisms. The ongoing assessment of services is also valuable in accessing research grants and facilitating fundraising.

Advocacy

The PMHP's advocacy and communication program focuses on raising awareness among health officials, policy makers, and the public concerning the prevalence and impact of CPMDs, and on maternal mental health as a cross-cutting solution to several key health and development priorities. In addition, the advocacy program aims to increase demand for and utilization of services in communities, while simultaneously raising awareness and improving service delivery among health providers. The program promotes research uptake and policy implementation by disseminating PMHP's lessons and evidence through several channels and to the relevant stakeholders to present a "powerful case for sustainable social change" (Servaes & Malikhao 2010).

Advocacy activities

The PMHP has developed a website, which describes the role and objectives of the project and provides a resource portal for maternal mental health (www.pmhp.za.org). In 2011, the website generated over 23 000 hits. Also, public opinion is targeted through mainstream and community newsprint media, television, and radio. The PMHP's social media platforms, launched in 2012, are generating a substantial body of informed followers.

Psychoeducational pamphlets on maternal mental health aimed at service user groups (mothers, adolescents, refugees, and fathers) have been distributed at service sites and are regularly updated. Seven information briefs have been developed for dissemination to stakeholders engaged in maternal and mental health, early childhood development, women's rights, and public health policy. These briefs clarify the relationship between maternal mental illness and HIV/AIDS, violence and abuse, child outcomes, and adolescent pregnancy. In addition, the PMHP has outlined the costs of maternal mental illness to society, as well as produced a special issue on the mental health needs of pregnant refugee women.

Policy briefs are designed to expedite research uptake, and the PMHP has produced three policy briefs on the benefits of integrating maternal mental health services into the public healthcare system. These have been disseminated to a wide audience, including the Department of Health, health managers and planners, policy developers, partner organizations, and stakeholders at various local and international fora.

The project has also contributed to the development of the Draft National Mental Health Policy, and has developed input on maternal mental health and HIV for the HIV/AIDS and STI Strategic Plan for South Africa 2012–2016.

Targeted campaigns

A short film, *Caring for Mothers*, was produced in 2009, and outlined a service user's experience of maternal distress. In 2010, the PMHP embarked on a six-month "road show," screening the film to approximately 270 maternity staff and community-based carers across 12 sites in the Cape Town area.

Feedback from the film road show provided the opportunity for health workers to discuss with the PMHP team and reflect on their difficult circumstances. Health workers supported the PMHP's rationale for training, by explaining that they would be able to treat their patients better, and with better outcomes, if their own mental health issues were attended to.

> If other staff can see this, maybe they can understand why patients seem rude. Maybe they are just scared. If we understand this, we can treat them better. (Midwife)

Lessons learnt

Advocacy must engage at the policy level, producing original research and an evidence-based model for service integration, but this alone will not affect change. An increase in awareness among health workers *and* potential service users is also required. Through the use of advocacy materials and communication campaigns, demand for maternal mental health services becomes more widespread as health workers understand the benefits of an integrated and holistic health service, and women are empowered to know their rights and demand the services they need.

Institutional stigma is, however, a major challenge to providing mental health services in the public sector. Thus, at an institutional level, among decision makers at policy and facilities level, stigma against mental illness prevents effective interventions from being implemented. This is another arena in which PMHP advocacy has been active, and here research uptake strategies have been key in securing engagement at this level.

Cost and sustainability of the PMHP
The cost of integrated maternal mental health services

In 2011, it was calculated that it cost the PMHP R185 (US$22.50) to provide maternal mental health services to one woman for one year. This included as many counseling sessions as she needed, the counselor's liaison work with psychiatric services and social support agencies, and postnatal follow-up care. This can be compared to the average rate of private-sector psychotherapy, which is R700 (US$85.00) per hour for one individual counseling session alone (PsySSA 2012).

In low-resource settings, where women can face many barriers to accessing health care, providing integrated mental health care at the same time and same place as routine maternity and well-baby care can minimize travel costs or time away from employment or child-care responsibilities. Thus, these integrated interventions use existing services and resources and are likely to achieve better coverage, with minimal extra costs.

Longitudinal studies assessing the cost-effectiveness of the intervention, both at care and development levels of impact, are planned.

Sustainability

Though PMHP's mental health services were initiated with volunteers providing counseling, it became clear that, as uptake increased, a project coordinator and funding for basic costs, such as stationery and workshop materials, were necessary for the smooth running of the service. The PMHP's operations were formalized as it relocated into the University of Cape Town. This location provided PMHP with the infrastructure and means to access funding support from donor organizations.

Lessons learnt

The PMHP has identified three complementary pathways to support and sustain integrated maternal mental health care. This is vital in a health infrastructure with competing priorities and limited resources: (1) train for task shifting to equip the people who will be providing the service; (2) conduct ongoing research to develop and improve the healthcare package, and to inform the training and teaching programs; and (3) engage in advocacy, to convince health planners and policy makers that maternal mental health is not a competing priority, but a feasible solution that cuts across multiple sectors and serves key health priorities.

Key lessons learnt and replicability

Key lessons learnt

The overview of the four different programs at PMHP reflects how, over time and with regular feedback from counselors, service users, and health providers,

the programs have evolved and developed to improve the project's efficiency and reach. Table 19.5 summarizes the key lessons learnt over the 10 years.

Replicability to other settings: preparing the environment

PMHP's experience, developed through providing maternal mental health services in four different maternity facilities, is that preparing the environment is one of the key elements in developing such services. The public health environment is varied and diverse, with each health facility presenting challenges and opportunities specific to its context. The first step is then to undertake liaison work with facility staff, to get full support and buy-in at all levels within the hierarchy. Effective communication strategies and training programs aimed at service providers is required to ensure that they understand the need for the intervention. Rapport and respect is very important, especially in low-resource, busy clinical settings where health workers may already feel over-burdened.

Maternal mental health interventions require screening, which is ideally undertaken by maternity staff during routine antenatal care. Therefore, the second step in preparing the environment would be to equip health workers with the necessary skills to deliver the new intervention efficiently. The third step is to ensure that referral pathways are in place. Screening for mental illness alone is not sufficient and, for ethical reasons, adequate referral pathways and treatments must follow. Ideally, this would be a dedicated on-site mental health counselor. Where this is not possible, maternity staff may be supported in identifying and consolidating links with resources and organizations in their communities that offer support to pregnant women.

Adapting the clinical services to other environments

A situation analysis is essential to understand the economic and social demographics, as well as staffing profiles of a facility, as these may affect the organization and strategies of the screening, referral, and counseling services to be put in place.

For example, the types of questions raised in the situational analysis should establish where and how women access care during and after pregnancy (formal facility, traditional birth attendants, etc.).

Table 19.5 Key lessons from 10 years of PMHP

Clinical services: service organization	A clinical service coordinator, who provides supervision, debriefing, and ongoing support to counselors, ensures the sustainability of quality mental healthcare provision
	An appointment and follow-up system can improve service organization, continuity of care, and reduction in rates of women lost to follow-up
Clinical services: screening	A brief, valid screening tool is required for use in busy, low-resource settings
	Routine integrated screening destigmatizes mental health among health workers and pregnant women
	Discussing referrals with clients and their families optimizes service use and referral mechanisms
Clinical services: on-site counseling	On-site mental health services increase access for women who have scarce resources and competing health, family, and economic priorities
	The employment of full-time counselors (as opposed to sessional) is beneficial for meeting the mental health needs of mothers, and facilitates tracking and follow-up of clients
	Even a limited number of counseling sessions can help improve mood and functioning of distressed pregnant women
	A refugee counselor can gain a better understanding of pregnant refugees' situations and problems, and can improve the counselor–client relationship
	Telephone counseling is possible when women cannot attend face-to-face meetings for logistical or psychological reasons
Training	Training should focus on improving health workers' understanding of the need for the mental health intervention, so that they can become advocates for maternal mental health care
	Addressing the mental health needs of health workers helps them manage their workload, prevents burnout, and improves motivation and morale
	Training should equip health workers with skills to screen for mental distress and to provide basic counseling and empathic engagement to pregnant and postnatal women
	The support and buy-in from health workers, through training, ensures the sustainability of the task-sharing approach and of the integrated mental health model
	Improving maternal mental health knowledge and awareness among complementary services or other community-based organizations can facilitate referrals to other services and provide comprehensive care to women
Research	To integrate screening effectively and efficiently into low-resource primary care maternity settings, a new short screening tool for CPMDs must be developed
	Through regular monitoring and evaluation, patterns of service use and barriers to mental health service uptake can be identified
	Monitoring clinical services is important for understanding how to improve the effectiveness of counseling and referral mechanisms
	The effectiveness of integrated mental health services needs evaluation so that the model can be implemented in other low-resource settings
Advocacy	Awareness among decision makers at policy level alone will not affect change – awareness must also be improved among health providers and potential service users
	Stigma at the institutional level is a barrier to integrating maternal mental health services, and advocacy should focus on securing engagement at this level
	Advocacy materials and communication campaigns improve health workers' understanding of the benefits of maternal mental health services
	Advocacy materials and communication campaigns help empower women to know their rights and demand the service they need
Cost and sustainability	Teaching and training, research, advocacy, and communications programs are essential to support and sustain integrated maternal mental health care
	The integration of evaluation plans into service, teaching, and training programs is important for fundraising activities

The situation analysis should also establish information about obstetric and postnatal care facilities (how many in the area, how many women attend, how many visits are attended, staffing, etc.), and about existing support services available to mothers. Information on mental illness, prevalence, presentation, attitudes to mental illness, and care provision must also be collected.

The high antenatal attendance in South Africa has led the PMHP to identify women's first antenatal visit as a suitable and effective way to initiate contact with and screen pregnant women for mental distress. In contexts where women do not attend health facilities regularly in the perinatal period, a situation analysis would allow the identification of the optimal environment to reach, screen, and provide mental health care to women.

The birth rate in South Africa is considerably lower than in other African countries (e.g., 42.99/1000 in Ethiopia, 47.49/1000 in Uganda). Where higher birth rates exist, a greater number of women may require screening and, ultimately, mental health care. In this case, changes in the organization of the services, such as raised referral cut-offs or different referral strategies, may have to be put in place.

The literacy rate is also particularly high in South Africa compared to other African countries (e.g., 43% in Ethiopia, 70% in Uganda). Where the literacy rate is low, screening that is self-administered would not be feasible, and it may need to be administered by health workers instead. The screening tool development study may provide a tool that is effective and short enough for health workers to administer as part of their history taking.

Conclusion

The PMHP has been conducting training, research, and advocacy work in maternal mental health to improve the uptake and quality of integrated maternal mental health services in primary care settings. While awareness is growing among the community and health providers, advocacy and communication campaigns at policy level are still required if maternal mental health is to be accepted as a cross-cutting solution to several key health and development priorities. With 10 years of experience as a unique mental health service provider and an advocate for maternal mental health in South Africa, the PMHP envisions its future role as a facilitator for the Department of Health, strenghtening and supporting the public health sector to develop good practice and scaleable maternal mental health service models for low-resource settings.

References

Araya R, Rojas G, Fritsch R, et al. (2003) Treating depression in primary care in low-income women in Santiago, Chile: a randomised controlled trial. Lancet 361: 995–1000.

Bonari l, Bennett H, Elnarson A, et al. (2004) Risks of untreated depression during pregnancy. Canadian Family Physician 50: 37–9.

Chisholm D, Lund C, Saxena S (2007) Cost of scaling up mental healthcare in low- and middle-income countries. British Journal of Psychiatry 191: 528–35.

Cooper P, Tomlinson M, Swartz L, et al. (1999) Post-partum depression and the mother–infant relationship in a South African peri-urban settlement. British Journal of Psychiatry 175: 554–8.

Cox JL, Chapman G, Murray D, et al. (1996) Validation of the Edinburgh Postnatal Depression Scale (EPDS) in non-postnatal women. Journal of Affective Disorders 39: 185–9.

Dua T, Barbui C, Clark N, et al. (2011) Evidence-based guidelines for mental, neurological, and substance use disorders in low- and middle-income countries: summary of WHO recommendations. PLoS Medicine, 8 (11): e1001122.

Fisher J, Cabral de Mello M, Patel V, et al. (2012) Prevalence and determinants of common perinatal mental disorders in women in low- and lower-middle-income countries: a systematic review. Bulletin of the World Health Organization 80: 139–49.

Grote NK, Bridge JA, Gavin AR, et al. (2010) A meta-analysis of depression during pregnancy and the risk of preterm birth, low birth weight, and intrauterine growth restriction. Archives of General Psychiatry 67: 1012–24.

Hartley M, Tomlinson M, Greco E, et al. (2011) Depressed mood in pregnancy: Prevalence and correlates in two Cape Town peri-urban settlements. Reproductive Health 8: 9.

Hay DF, Pawlby S, Waters C, et al. (2008) Antepartum and postpartum exposure to maternal depression: different effects on different adolescent outcomes. Journal of Child Psychology and Psychiatry 10: 1079–88.

Hendrick V, Altshuler L, Cohen L, et al. (1998) Evaluation of mental health and depression during pregnancy. *Psychopharmacology Bulletin* **34**: 297–9.

Honikman S, van Heyningen T, Field S, Baron E, Tomlinson M (2012) Stepped care for maternal mental health: a case study of the perinatal mental health project in South Africa. *PLoS Medicine*, **9** (5): e1001222.

Husain N, Bevc I, Hudain M, *et al.* (2006) Prevalence and social correlates of postnatal depression in a low income country. *Archives of Women's Mental Health* **9**: 197–207.

Index Mundi (2011) Index Mundi: South Africa Birth rate demographics, http://www.indexmundi.com/south_africa/birth_rate.html (accessed February 2012).

Jewkes R, Abrahams N, Mvo Z (1998) Why do nurses abuse patients? Reflections from South African obstetric services. *Social Science and Medicine* **47**: 1781–95.

Josefsson A, Angelsioo L, Berg G, *et al.* (2002) Obstetric, somatic, and demographic risk factors for postpartum depressive symptoms. *Obstetrics and Gynecology* **99**: 223–8.

Lund C, Kleintjes S, Kakuma R, *et al.* (2010) Public sector mental health systems in South Africa: inter-provincial comparisons and policy implications. *Social Psychiatry and Psychiatric Epidemiology* **45**: 393–404.

Lusskin S, Pundiak T, Habib S (2007) Perinatal depression: hiding in plain sight. *Canadian Journal of Psychiatry* **52**: 479–88.

Meintjes I, Field S, Sanders L, *et al.* (2010) Improving child outcomes through maternal mental health interventions. *Journal of Child and Adolescent Mental Health* **22** (2): 73–82.

Murray L, Woolgar M, Murray J, *et al.* (2003) Self-exclusion from health care in women at high risk for postaprtum depression. *Journal of*

Public Health Medicine **25** (2): 131–7.

Oates, M (2002) Adverse effects of maternal antenatal anxiety on children: causal effect or developmental continuum? *The British Journal of Psychiatry*, **180**, 478–479.

O'Connor T, Heron J, Golding J, *et al.* (2002) Maternal antenatal anxiety and children's behavioural/emotional problems at 4 years: report from Avon Longitudinal Study of Parents and Children. *British Journal of Psychiatry* **180**: 502–8.

O'Hara MW, Swain AM (1996) Rates and risk of postpartum depression: a meta-analysis. *International Review of Psychiatry* **8**: 37–54.

Padarath A, English R, eds. (2011) *South African Health Review 2011.* Durban: Health Systems Trust.

Patel V, Rahman A, Jacobs KS, *et al.* (2004) Effect of maternal mental health on infant growth in low income countries: new evidence from South Asia. *BMJ* **328**: 820–3.

Patel V, Araya R, Chatterjee S, *et al.* (2007) Treatment and prevention of mental disorders in low-income and middle-income countries. *Lancet,* **370**, 991–1005.

Pillay R (2009) Retention strategies for professional nurses in South Africa. *Leadership in Health Services,* **22** (1): 39–57.

Provincial Government Western Cape (2010) Regional Development Profile: City of Cape Town. http://www.westerncape.gov.za/other/2011/1/city_of_cape_town.pdf (accessed July 2013).

PsySSA (Psychology Society of South Africa) (2012) Healthman Psychology Costing Guide 2012: comparative tariffs. www.psyssa.com/documents/Psychology%20Costing%20Guide%202012%20(HealthMan).pdf (accessed July 2013).

Rahman A, Creed F (2007) Outcome of prenatal depression and risk factors

associated with persistence in the first postnatal year: Prospective study from Rawalpindi, Pakistan. *Journal of Affective Disorders* **100**: 115–21.

Robertson E, Grace S, Wallington T, *et al.* (2007) Antenatal risk factors for postpartum depression: a synthesis of recent literature. *General Hospital Psychiatry* **26**: 289–95.

Rochat TJ, Richter LM, Doll HA, *et al.* (2006) Depression among pregnant rural South African women undergoing HIV testing. *JAMA* **295**: 1376–8.

Rochat TJ, Tomlinson M, Bärnighausen T, *et al.* (2011) The prevalence and clinical presentation of antenatal depression in rural South Africa. *Journal of Affective Disorders* **135**: 362–73.

Rothmann S, van der Colff JJ, Rothmann JC (2006) Occupational stress of nurses in South Africa. *Curationis* **29** (2): 22–33.

Saxena S, Thornicroft G, Knapp M, *et al.* (2007) Resources for mental health: scarcity, inequity, and inefficiency. *Lancet* **370**: 878–89.

Servaes J, Malikhao P (2010) Advocacy strategies for health communication. *Public Relations Review* **36** (1): 42–9. doi:10.1016/j.pubrev.2009.08.017.

Skeen S, Lund C, Kleintjes S, *et al.* (2010) Meeting the millennium development goals in Sub-saharan Africa: what about mental health? *International Review of Psychiatry* **22**: 624–31.

Stein DJ, Seedat S, Herman A, *et al.* (2008) Lifetime prevalence of psychiatric disorders. *British Journal of Psychiatry* **192**: 112–17.

Talge N, Neal C, Glover V (2007) Antenatal maternal stress and long-term effects on child neurodevelopment: how and why? *Journal of Child Psychology and Psychiatry* **48**: 245–61.

UNDP (2012) *Mobile Technologies and Empowerment: Enhancing Human*

Development Through Participation and Innovation. New York, NY: United Nations Development Programme Democratic Governance Group, Bureau for Development Policy.

Willetts L, Leff J (2003) Improving the knowledge and skills of psychiatric nurses: efficacy of a staff training programme. *Journal of Advanced Nursing* **42**: 237–43.

World Health Organization (2008) *mhGAP: Mental Health Gap Action Programme. Scaling up Care for Mental, Neurological, and Substance Use Disorders.* Geneva: WHO.

Chapter

20

Screening for developmental disabilities in epidemiologic studies in low- and middle-income countries

Maureen S. Durkin and Matthew J. Maenner

Introduction

Developmental disabilities include limitations in function and activities resulting from disorders of the developing nervous system in conjunction with unaccommodating environments or absence of assistive technologies. These limitations manifest during infancy or childhood as delays in reaching developmental milestones, and often persist throughout the lifespan affecting one or multiple domains, including cognition, behavior, motor performance, vision, hearing, and speech (Committee on Nervous System Disorders in Developing Countries 2001). Table 20.1 summarizes the major categories and provides examples of developmental disabilities that are classified and coded in the *International Statistical Classification of Diseases and Related Health Problems, 10th Revision* (ICD-10) (World Health Organization 2010). Although known causes and specific categories of developmental disability are relatively rare, when taken as a whole and including all levels of severity, developmental disabilities likely affect more than 10% of children worldwide, making them a major, if under-recognized, global public health priority (Durkin *et al.* 2006).

It is important to emphasize that the etiologies of functional limitations experienced by people with developmental disabilities include not only a diverse array of underlying causes of impairments or damage to the developing nervous system, but also social, economic, and physical barriers to participation experienced by people with neurodevelopmental impairments, and lack of access to necessary assistive devices and therapies (World Health Organization 2002, 2007). From a public health perspective, therefore, a comprehensive plan for prevention of

developmental disabilities must include not only strategies to prevent underlying causes (primary prevention) but also interventions and policies to enhance or preserve functioning (secondary prevention), as well as social and economic participation of individuals with developmental disabilities (tertiary prevention) (Durkin *et al.* 2006).

As with any public health concern, the first steps toward prevention of developmental disabilities include the collection and analysis of accurate information on their frequency and impacts, trends over time, and associated risk factors. Basic epidemiologic information serves to raise awareness; helps identify priorities, effective policies, and interventions; and provides a means to monitor progress over time.

Unfortunately, there is an enormous global imbalance in the capacity to conduct epidemiologic studies and in our understanding of the frequency and impacts of developmental disabilities. Most epidemiologic studies are conducted in high-income countries, where children are often routinely screened for disabilities, diagnostic tools are readily available, and systems exist to provide services for persons with disabilities and generate data. In low- and middle-income countries (i.e., countries with gross national income per capita in 2004 less than US$10 666: World Health Organization 2008), where some 90% of births occur each year globally (Population Reference Bureau 2012), basic information on the epidemiology of developmental disabilities is scant, and the limited information available suggests that the prevalence is higher than in wealthier countries and may be increasing rather than decreasing over time with improvements in child survival and longevity (Durkin

Table 20.1 Examples of ICD-10 classifications and codes for major categories of developmental disability

Developmental disability	ICD-10 code
Cognitive	
Intellectual disability (mental retardation)	F70–F73 (mild to profound levels)
Specific learning disabilities	F81–F81.2 (including dyslexia, dyscalculia)
Behavior	
Autism spectrum disorder (pervasive developmental disorder)	F84
Attention-deficit/hyperactivity disorder	F90.0
Motor	
Cerebral palsy	G80
Post-polio paralysis	B91
Muscular dystrophies	G71.0
Spina bifida	Q05
Spinal muscular atrophies	G12
Vision	
Refraction disorders	H52
Cataract, infantile and juvenile	H26.0
Chorioretinal infection	H32.0
Nightblindness (due to vitamin A deficiency)	E50.5
Hearing and speech	
Conductive and sensorineural hearing loss	H90
Specific speech articulation disorder	F80.0
Expressive language disorder	F80.1
Receptive language disorder	F80.2

2002, Gottlieb *et al.* 2008). This situation calls for global collaboration and increased capacity to conduct population-based studies of developmental disabilities, especially in low- and middle-income countries. Below we discuss some of the key principles and considerations in designing and implementing screening programs and epidemiologic studies of developmental disabilities.

Respect for people with disabilities

Persons with disabilities and their advocates have stressed the importance of the perspectives of persons with disabilities, and the need to incorporate these perspectives into research and policies related to disability. When this is done, the goals and objectives may shift away from a focus exclusively on primary prevention and away from policies that promote dependence. Instead, the goals and objectives shift toward research and policies to enhance the quality of life of persons with disabilities and to promote inclusion, self-determination, and economic opportunity (Carlton 1998). This perspective is in line with the capabilities approach, which emphasizes the need to enhance capabilities, level the playing field, and promote inclusive policies (Nussbaum 2002). It is also consistent with ideals expressed in the United Nations Convention on the Rights of Persons with Disabilities, which recognizes "the importance for persons with disabilities of their individual autonomy and independence, including the freedom to make their own choices," and states that "children with disabilities [should] have the right to express their views freely on all matters affecting them, their views being given due weight in accordance with their age and maturity, on an equal basis with other children" (United Nations 2006). With this perspective in mind, population-based studies of developmental disabilities can benefit by incorporating the perspectives of local experts, including individuals affected by developmental disabilities and their family members, from the initial planning and throughout the phases of the study.

Disability as a multidimensional concept

The World Health Organization's *International Classification of Functioning, Disability and Health* (known as the ICF) (2002), building on its predecessor the *International Classification of Impairment, Disability and Handicap* (World Health Organization 1980), provides a formal conceptual model with detailed classifications of disability along three dimensions: (1) impairments occurring at the level of bodily organ structure or functions (examples include neural tube defects, abnormal brain development due to chromosomal anomalies), (2) activity limitations or functional limitations at the level of the person (examples include limited walking ability,

Table 20.2 Examples of ICF or ICF-CY classifications and codes for impairments, activity limitations, and participation restrictions potentially associated with developmental disability (Durkin *et al.* 2006)

Examples of classifications and codes related to "impairment" (or bodily structures or functions)	Structure of brain (s110) Psychomotor control (b1470) Regulation of behavior (b127.4) Motor reflex functions (b750) Seeing functions (b210–b21029) Hearing functions (b230) Speech discrimination (b2304) Articulation functions (b320)
Examples of classifications and codes related to "activity limitation" and "participation restriction"	Learning to read (d140) Learning to calculate (d150) Focusing attention (d160) Thinking (d163) Sitting (d4103) Standing (d4104) Walking (d450) Using transportation (d470) Hand and arm use (d445) Toileting (d530) Listening (d115) Speaking (d330) Education (d810-d839) Play (d9200)
Examples of classifications and codes related to "environmental factors" affecting disability	Individual attitudes (e410–e455) Societal attitudes (e460) Social norms (e465) Mobility assistive technology (e120) Communication assistive technology (e1251) Health professionals (e355) Education systems and policies (e585)

limitations in cognitive skills such as reading), and (3) participation (examples include participation in school, recreational, social, and economic activities). According to the ICF, disability is not only a "medical" or "biological" dysfunction but also encompasses limitations in a person's functioning, activities, and roles that are affected by social, economic, and physical environmental factors.

The ICF includes extensive codes for aspects of disability within each of the three dimensions, and for environmental factors affecting disability. These codes could potentially be useful in epidemiologic studies of the frequency of disability and trends over time, much as ICD-10 codes are used to classify diseases or conditions that correspond to types of

developmental disability (Table 20.1). By expanding the definition of disability to include impairments, activity limitations, and participation restrictions, and pointing to opportunities for prevention and improvement at each level, the ICF is compatible with both the capabilities approach to human development (Mitra 2006, Trani 2009) and disability advocacy and human rights perspectives (Carlton 1998, United Nations 2006). Table 20.2 provides examples of ICF classifications and codes for impairments at the level of organ structures and functions (row 1), activity limitations and participation restrictions (row 2), and environmental factors (row 3) that are relevant to children with developmental disabilities.

Multifactorial nature of developmental disabilities and their causes

The epidemiology of developmental disability is complicated by the fact that developmental disability is not a single condition but includes a wide range of functional disabilities with onsets early in life. Known direct causes of developmental disability fall into at least eight categories, including specific nutritional deficiencies, genetic factors, infections, toxic exposures, trauma, perinatal complications, deprivation of cognitive stimulation, and multifactorial (Committee on Nervous System Disorders in Developing Countries 2001, Durkin 2002). Within each of these categories, there are numerous known specific causes and likely many causes yet to be discovered. In addition to direct causes, the complex web of known or hypothesized indirect causes of developmental disabilities includes factors such as poverty, maldistribution of resources, political instability and war, disasters, and parental mental health disorders (Brooks-Gunn & Duncan 1997, Murthy & Lakshminarayana 2006, Lung *et al.* 2009). Children born in low- and middle-income countries are likely to be at increased risk for disability due to some of these indirect causes. In addition to the diversity of causal mechanisms, the clinical and functional manifestations of developmental disabilities are extremely variable in type, severity, and comorbidity or presence of co-occurring conditions. Some of the variability in impairments and functional outcomes is due to variability in timing of exposures to causal agents vis-à-vis neurodevelopment. Other important determinants of outcomes include access to health care and early interventions or therapies (Peltola 2001, Adnams 2010, Bakare & Munir 2011).

Screening for the purposes of early intervention and prevalence estimation

Public health screening was first defined in 1957 as "the presumptive identification of unrecognized disease or defect by the application of tests, examinations or other procedures which can be applied rapidly" (Commission on Chronic Illness 1957). The authors of this definition further stated that "A screening test is not intended to be diagnostic. Persons with positive . . . findings must be referred . . . for diagnosis and necessary treatment." The concept of public health screening is integral to programs that provide early interventions for children with disabilities or those at high risk for developmental disabilities. A basic premise of early intervention programs for children at risk for disability is that neurodevelopment is especially malleable and responsive to environmental and therapeutic influences early in life. Developmental screening enables early detection and referral to treatments that can minimize or even prevent the occurrence and consequences of developmental disabilities (Clague & Thomas 2002, Nahar *et al.* 2009, Walker *et al.* 2010, 2011).

In addition to providing a basis for early identification and referral to services, screening can be a useful tool for estimating the prevalence of disability in the population. Whereas in developed countries studies of the prevalence of developmental disabilities are typically based on administrative records of children receiving therapeutic or educational services related to their disabilities (Kawamura *et al.* 2008, Barnevik-Olsson *et al.* 2010, Autism and Developmental Disabilities Monitoring Network 2012), in settings where children with disabilities do not necessarily receive formal services, the two-phase design incorporating rapid and low-cost screening for developmental disabilities (phase one) followed by diagnostic assessments of samples of children (phase two) has been shown to be a feasible and efficient strategy for estimating the prevalence of developmental disabilities and investigating their risk factors (Rutter 1989, Shrout & Newman 1989, Durkin *et al.* 2000, McNamee 2003). Specifically, the efficiency of the two-phase study design, relative to a single-phase design (diagnostic assessments for

everyone), is dependent on the validity of the screening test (the greater the sensitivity and specificity of the screen, the more likely the efficiency of a two-phase design will exceed that of a single-phase design); the rarity of the disease or disability (the rarer the disability, the greater the efficiency of a two-phase versus single-phase design), and the ratio of the cost of a diagnostic assessment to the cost of a screening test (the higher this ratio, the more efficient is the two-phase versus single-phase design) (Shrout & Newman 1989, McNamee 2003).

The use of screening to estimate the prevalence of developmental disabilities in settings where services are not available, however, raises an ethical dilemma. Public health screening should be done only if early detection can result in effective treatment options and improved outcomes. Yet until there is basic information about the prevalence of developmental disabilities in a population, it is unlikely that adequate services and treatment options will be available for those needing them. Researchers working in underserved populations in Bangladesh have overcome this ethical dilemma by implementing the two-phase design of broad-based screening for developmental disabilities followed by assessments of samples of children, and then using the information generated as a basis for developing necessary services. Children identified on the basis of screening to be at high risk for disability or to have a disability are then referred to those services (Committee on Nervous System Disorders in Developing Countries 2001, Danish Bilharziasis Laboratory 2004).

Paradoxical trends in disability prevalence

Within the field of public health, improvement is typically measured in terms of reductions over time in incidence or prevalence. Disability is paradoxical in that, at least in the short term, its prevalence appears to increase rather than decrease with improvements in health care and longevity. Examples of developmental disabilities that may increase over time in spite of, or perhaps because of, advances in health care and child survival include disabilities associated with very preterm birth (Hameed *et al.* 2004, Hack & Costello 2008, Schieve *et al.* 2011), those associated with improved child survival in low- and middle-income countries (Khan *et al.* 2010), and behavioral disorders such as autism spectrum disorders and attention-deficit disorders, for which apparent increases in prevalence are to some extent due to increases in awareness, diagnostic capabilities, and access to services (Barbaresi *et al.* 2005). Because of the paradoxical nature of disability prevalence and its association with improved survival and case detection, the contribution of screening programs and epidemiologic studies of disability is not simply the production of knowledge that leads to reductions in prevalence or the number of persons with disability in the population. Instead, it appears that in the field of disability, public health improvements can result in increased survival of children at risk for disability, and screening and epidemiologic studies may lead to greater awareness and recognition of the range of disabilities affecting children. With progress, therefore, we have seen increases in the prevalence of disability. For example, this has been documented in Bangladesh in recent decades, where, along with marked improvements in child survival and increased awareness of child development and disability, the prevalence of child disability has increased (Khan *et al.* 2010).

Ideally, epidemiologic studies of disability would monitor the multiple dimensions of disability (i.e., impairments, activity limitations, participation restrictions) as conceptualized in the ICF, generating information to plan and evaluate preventive interventions targeting each dimension. The hope is that, in the long term, this approach will enable both reductions in the prevalence of developmental impairments and improvements in functioning, quality of life, and participation of individuals with developmental disabilities.

Benefits of research for the populations under study

In the twentieth century, epidemiologic studies in low- and middle-income countries were frequently conducted by foreign researchers and sometimes characterized as "helicopter epidemiology," where the researchers "fly in ... collect descriptive data and biological specimens, fly out, process, and publish the information elsewhere" (Jamrozik 2006). In the field of developmental disabilities, Zena Stein (personal communication) has called this the "count and run" approach, and has stressed the need for epidemiologic research to benefit the communities providing the data. This can be done through community engagement, increasing research capacity in

host countries through provision of training in research methodology to local investigators and staff, using screening and epidemiologic surveys as a basis for developing and providing referrals to services for children with disabilities and their families (Danish Bilharziasis Laboratory 2004), and improving the accessibility of research tools and results globally.

Global availability of low-cost and accessible tools for screening, assessment, data analysis, and dissemination

An important barrier to conducting epidemiologic studies of developmental disabilities in low- and middle-income countries is the cost of proprietary screening and diagnostic assessment tools, as well as software for statistical analysis. Further, the results of many published studies are kept behind electronic "paywalls" and available only to institutions paying subscription fees that could be prohibitive for researchers in low- and middle-income countries. Some potential solutions to these barriers include the free availability in the public domain of a number of screening and assessment tools (Zaman *et al.* 1990, Thorburn *et al.* 1992, Durkin *et al.* 1994, Palisano *et al.* 1997, ICF CY Questionnaire 2003, Robertson *et al.* 2009, Gershon *et al.* 2010, Üstün *et al.* 2010), the emergence of open-source solutions for data management and statistical analysis (R Development Core Team 2011), and open-access publishing.

Cross-cultural appropriateness and comparability of disability screening, measures, and epidemiological data

One of the challenges of epidemiologic studies of disability is that case status is often based on information obtained from questionnaires or cognitive tests that are designed and validated for use in one language and culture, and may not be applicable for or capable of generating comparable data across cultures. The Ten Questions screen for child disability was designed to overcome this challenge (Durkin *et al.* 1995). It does so by querying in simple language about universal abilities or milestones that should be applicable to children in all cultures, and asking parents to rate their children's functional abilities or disabilities by comparing them to other children of similar age within the same cultural context. Psychometric analyses of the Ten Questions screen have found that it does have comparable measurement qualities across cultures and in settings where literacy is low (Durkin *et al.* 1995). Although this approach is effective for disability screening, still needed are low-cost and cross-culturally valid tools for assessing and diagnosing different types of developmental disabilities. One way to foster this is to follow the model of open-source technologies, and develop opportunities for international internet-based collaboration and sharing of assessment tools and other information.

It is also important to emphasize that even within many low- and middle-income countries, especially large countries such as India, there are vast regional and cultural differences that may affect the comparability of assessment practices, norms, and diagnostic results, even when common and standardized intelligence tests or other diagnostic tools are used (Girimaji & Srinath 2010, Madhavaram 2011). Moreover, it is likely that for the majority of the world's children with developmental disabilities, obtaining an accurate diagnosis, though an important step, comes with no

guarantee that coordinated services and appropriate services will be available.

Conclusion

Developmental disabilities and children's mental health are emerging yet still largely invisible public health priorities in low- and middle-income countries. Epidemiologic studies are needed to generate accurate information on the numbers of children with disabilities, trends over time, and risk factors for disability in these countries, where the vast majority of the world's children reside. For reasons discussed in this chapter, it would be overly simplistic to expect an expansion of epidemiologic studies of developmental disabilities in low- and middle-income countries to lead to reductions in the prevalence of these disabilities. However, increased capacity for conducting epidemiologic studies of the multiple dimensions of developmental disabilities globally is likely to raise awareness, empower communities, and provide a basis for planning appropriate service models and interventions to prevent disabilities and improve outcomes for future generations of children.

References

Adnams CM (2010) Perspectives of intellectual disability in South Africa: epidemiology, policy, services for children and adults. *Current Opinion in Psychiatry* 23: 436–40.

Autism and Developmental Disabilities Monitoring Network Surveillance Year 2008 Principal Investigators (2012) Prevalence of autism spectrum disorders: Autism and Developmental Disabilities Monitoring Network, United States, 14 Sites, 2008. *MMWR Surveillance Summaries* 61 (3): 1–29. http://www.cdc.gov/mmwr/pdf/ss/ss6103.pdf (accessed July 2013).

Bakare MO, Munir KM (2011) Excess of non-verbal cases of autism spectrum disorders presenting to orthodox clinical practice in Africa: a trend possibly resulting from late diagnosis and intervention. *South African Journal of Psychiatry* 17 (4): 118–120.

Barbaresi WJ, Katusic SK, Colligan RC, Weaver AL, Jacobsen SJ (2005) The incidence of autism in Olmsted County, Minnesota, 1976–1997: results from a population-based study. *Archives of Pediatrics and Adolescent Medicine* 159: 37–45.

Barnevik-Olsson M, Gillberg C, Fernell E (2010) Prevalence of autism in children of Somali origin living in Stockholm: brief report of an at-risk population. *Developmental Mediciine and Child Neurology* 52: 1167–8.

Brooks-Gunn J, Duncan GJ (1997) The effects of poverty on children. *The Future of Children* 7 (2): 55–71.

Carlton J (1998) *Nothing About Us Without Us.* Berkeley, CA: University of California Press.

Clague A, Thomas A (2002) Neonatal biochemical screening for disease. *Clinica Chimica Acta* 315: 99–110.

Commission on Chronic Illness (1957) *Chronic Illness in the United States, Volume I: Prevention of Chronic Illness.* Cambridge, MA: Harvard University Press, p. 45.

Committee on Nervous System Disorders in Developing Countries (2001) *Neurological, Psychiatric and Developmental Disorders: Meeting the Challenge in the Developing World.* Washington, DC: National Academies Press.

Danish Bilharziasis Laboratory (2004) *Disability in Bangladesh: a Situation Analysis. Final Report.* Dhaka: World Bank. http://siteresources.worldbank.org/DISABILITY/Resources/Regions/South%20Asia/DisabilityinBangladesh.pdf. (accessed July 2013).

Durkin MS (2002) The epidemiology of developmental disabilities in low-income countries. *Mental Retardation and Developmental Disabilities Research Reviews* 8: 206–11.

Durkin MS, Davidson LL, Desai P, *et al.* (1994) Validity of the ten questions screen for childhood disability: results from population-based studies in Bangladesh, Jamaica and Pakistan. *Epidemiology* 5: 283–9.

Durkin MS, Wang W, Shrout PE, *et al.* (1995) Evaluating a Ten Questions screen for childhood disability: reliability and internal structure in different cultures. *Journal of Clinical Epidemiology* 48: 657–66.

Durkin MS, Khan NZ, Davidson LL, *et al.* (2000) Prenatal and postnatal risk factors for mental retardation among children in Bangladesh. *American Journal of Epidemiology* 152: 1024–33.

Durkin MS, Schneider H, Pathania VS, *et al.* (2006) Learning and developmental disabilities. In World Health Organization, *Disease Control Priorities Related to Mental, Neurological, Developmental and Substance Abuse Disorders*. Geneva: WHO; pp. 39–56. http://whqlibdoc.who.int/publications/2006/924156332x_eng.pdf (accessed July 2013).

Gershon RC, Cella D, Fox NA, *et al.* (2010) Assessment of neurological and behavioural function: the NIH Toolbox. *Lancet Neurology* 9: 138–9.

Girimaji SC, Srinath S (2010) Perspectives of intellectual disability in India: epidemiology, policy, services for children and adults. *Current Opinion in Psychiatry* 23: 441–6.

Gottlieb CA, Maenner MJ, Cappa C, Durkin MS (2008) Child disability screening, nutrition, and early learning in 18 countries with low and middle incomes: data from the third round of Unicef's Multiple Indicator Cluster Survey (2005–06). *Lancet* 374: 1831–9.

Hack M, Costello DW (2008) Trends in the rates of cerebral palsy associated with neonatal intensive care of preterm children. *Clinical Obstetrics and Gynecology* 51: 763–74.

Hameed B, Shyamanur K, Kotecha S, *et al.* (2004) Trends in the incidence of severe retinopathy of prematurity in a geographically defined

population over a 10-year period. *Pediatrics* 113: 1653–7.

ICF CY Questionnaire (2003) ICF CY questionnaire, version 1.B, 3–6 years. http://www.ccoms-fci-cif.fr/ccoms/pagint/PDF/ICF_CY_Questionnaire_3_6_years.pdf (accessed July 2013).

Jamrozik K (2006) The epidemiology of colonialism: comment. *Lancet* 368: 4–6.

Kawamura Y, Takahashi O, Ishii T (2008) Reevaluating the incidence of pervasive developmental disorders: impact of elevated rates of detection through implementation of an integrated system of screening in Toyota, Japan. *Psychiatry and Clinical Neurosciences* 62: 152–9.

Khan NZ, Muslima H, Begum N, *et al.* (2010) Validation of rapid neurodevelopmental assessment instrument for under-two-year-old children in Bangladesh. *Pediatrics* 125: e755–62.

Lung FW, Chiang TL, Lin SJ, Shu BC (2009) Parental mental health and child development from six to thirty-six months in a birth cohort study in Taiwan. *Journal of Perinatal Medicine* 37: 397–402.

Madhavaram K (2011) Intelligence testing and its implication for disability evaluation in individuals with mental retardation. *Psychological Studies* 56: 289–94. DOI 10.1007/s12646-011-0093-y.

McNamee R (2003) Efficiency of two-phase designs for prevalence estimation. *International Journal of Epidemiology* 32: 1072–8.

Mitra S (2006)The capability approach and disability. *Journal of Disability Policy Studies* 16: 236–47.

Murthy RS, Lakshminarayana R (2006) Mental health consequences of war: a brief review of research findings. *World Psychiatry* 5: 25–30.

Nahar B, Hamadani JD, Ahmed T, *et al.* (2009) Effects of psychosocial stimulation on growth and development of severely

malnourished children in a nutrition unit in Bangladesh. *European Journal of Clinical Nutrition* 63: 725–31.

Nussbaum M (2002) Capabilities and disabilities: justice for mentally disabled citizens. *Philosophical Topics* 30: 133–65.

Palisano R, Rosenbaum P, Walter S, *et al.* (1997) Development and reliability of a system to classify gross motor function in children with cerebral palsy. *Developmental Medicine and Child Neurology* 39: 214–23.

Peltola H (2001) Burden of meningitis and other severe bacterial infections of children in Africa: implications for prevention. *Clinical Infectious Diseases* 32: 64–75.

Population Reference Bureau (2012) World population data sheet 2012. http://www.prb.org/Publications/Datasheets/2012/world-population-data-sheet.aspx (accessed July 2013).

R Development Core Team (2011) *The R Project for Statistical Computing*. http://www.r-project.org (accessed July 2013).

Robertson J, Hatton C, Emerson E (2009) The identification of children with or at significant risk of intellectual disabilities in low and middle income countries: a review. Lancaster: University of Lancaster Cenre for Disability Research. http://eprints.lancs.ac.uk/27956/1/CeDR_2009-3_Identifying_Children_with_ID_in_LAMI_Countries.pdf (accessed July 2013).

Rutter M (1989) Isle of Wight revisited: twenty-five years of child psychiatric epidemiology. *Journal of the American Academy of Child and Adolescent Psychiatry* 28: 633–53.

Schieve LA, Rice C, Devine O, *et al.* (2011) Have secular changes in perinatal risk factors contributed to the recent autism prevalence increase? Development and application of a mathematical assessment model. *Annals of Epidemiology* 21: 930–45.

Shrout PE, Newman SC (1989) Design of two-phase prevalence surveys of rare disorders. *Biometrics* **45**: 549–55.

Thorburn MJ, Desai P, Paul T, *et al.* (1992) Identification of childhood disability in Jamaica: evaluation of the ten question screen. *International Journal of Rehabilitation Research* **15**: 262–70.

Trani JF (2009) Screening children for disability. *Lancet* **374**: 1806–7.

United Nations (2006) *Convention on the Rights of Persons with Disabilities (A/RES/61/106)*. New York, NY: UN.

Ustün TB, Kostanjsek N, Chatterji S, Rehm J (2010) *Measuring Health and Disability: Manual for WHO Disability Assessment Schedule 2.0 WHODAS 2.0.* Geneva: WHO. http://whqlibdoc.who.int/publications/2010/9789241547598_eng.pdf (accessed July 2013).

Walker SP, Chang SM, Younger N, Grantham-McGregor SM (2010) The effect of psychosocial stimulation on cognition and behaviour at 6 years in a cohort of term, low-birthweight Jamaican children. *Developmental Medicine and Child Neurology* **52**: e148–54.

Walker SP, Wachs TD, Grantham-McGregor S, *et al.* (2011) Inequality in early childhood: risk and protective factors for early child development. *Lancet* **378**: 1325–37.

World Health Organization (1980) *International Classification of Impairment, Disability and Handicap*. Geneva: WHO.

World Health Organization (2002) *Towards a Common Language for Functioning, Disability, and Health. ICF: the International Classification of Functioning, Disability and Health*. Geneva: WHO (WHO/EIP/GPE/CAS/01.3). http://www.who.int/classifications/icf/en/ (accessed July 2013).

World Health Organization (2007) *International Classification of Functioning, Disability and Health: Children and Youth Version: ICF-CY*. Geneva: WHO.

World Health Organization (2008) *The Global Burden of Disease, 2004 Update*. Geneva: WHO.

World Health Organization (2010) *International Classification of Diseases and Related Health Problems, 10th Revision (ICD-10) Version for 2010*. Geneva: WHO. http://apps.who.int/classifications/icd10/browse/2010/en (accessed July 2013).

Zaman S, Khan N, Islam S, *et al.* (1990) Validity of the Ten Questions for screening serious childhood disability: results from urban Bangladesh. *International Journal of Epidemiology* **19**: 613–20.

Children's services

Margarita Alegría, Anne Valentine, Sheri Lapatin, Natasja Koitzsch Jensen,
Sofia Halperin-Goldstein, and Anna Lessios

Introduction

According to the United Nations Population Fund, there are an estimated 2 billion children and adolescents worldwide – the largest generation to date. Nine of 10 youth live in developing nations, countries which experience a majority of the world's conflicts and humanitarian crises (Women's Refugee Commission 2012), in addition to the daily risks of poverty, malnutrition, and poor health (Grantham-McGregor et al. 2007). War, internal displacement, and discrimination (Ladd & Cairns 1996) make them particularly vulnerable to exploitation, sex trafficking, and recruitment into armed conflict. Retrospective studies consistently identify higher rates of childhood adversity among individuals with a history of mental illness (Edwards et al. 2003), and prospective data confirm these associations. An estimated 22 million children and young people under the age of 24 years are either refugees or internally displaced, placing them at an elevated risk for mental health disorders and behavioral difficulties (Ladd & Cairns 1996). As mental disorders contribute to disability, poor interpersonal functioning, and reduced educational attainment, the public health implications are significant. This chapter describes challenges associated with the assessment of children's mental health and functioning, and identifies risk and protective factors, best practices for prevention, and promising interventions that can be utilized in resource-poor settings. Developmental disabilities and/or cognitive delays are not covered. Particular attention is paid to the importance of culture and context in discussing child mental health.

Assessment for children's mental health and functioning

The early identification of childhood mental health disorders is vitally important; research in Western nations suggests that one in five children is affected (Merikangas et al. 2010), and most do not receive the necessary help. Early identification may offer opportunities for effective treatment *prior* to the development of persistent and/or severe mental illness typically associated with suicide, substance abuse, academic failure, teenage pregnancy, and involvement with law enforcement (Luby et al. 2002). While an emerging body of research conducted in non-Western developing nations provides for a more nuanced understanding of mental health disorders, a dearth of reliable and valid assessment tools for child psychopathology has thwarted early identification efforts globally (Luby et al. 2002).

Cultural distinctions in development

Theories that have contributed to the West's understandings of child development do not necessarily translate across culture and context. Bowlby's attachment theory, for example: Bretherton (1997) suggests that infant attachment behaviors can be classified as secure, avoidant, ambivalent, or disorganized (Ziv et al. 2000), and that attachment insecurity increases the risk for mental disorders (Mikulincer & Shaver 2012). Yet the distribution of infants in these classification categories appears to vary from Europe and North America to Israel and Mali. Israeli samples tend to have a higher prevalence of ambivalent infants and practically no avoidant infants (Sagi et al. 1985,

Essentials of Global Mental Health, ed. Samuel O. Okpaku. Published by Cambridge University Press. © Cambridge University Press 2014.

Ziv *et al.* 2000), while among the Dogon of Mali there is a high frequency of securely attached infants and few infants classified as avoidant (True *et al.* 2001). This suggests that infant attachment varies by differences in child-rearing practices across countries, and that care practices may thwart the development of insecure attachment, which is common in Western countries.

Similarly, differences in child development have also been documented (Okamoto *et al.* 1996). Piaget theorized that cognition developed in four universal stages: sensorimotor (0–2 years), pre-operational (2–7 years), concrete (7–11 years), and formal logic (11+ years). However, evidence suggests differences in the formal logic stage sequence – particularly in cultures with a strong oral tradition (Okamoto *et al.* 1996). Some advanced intellectual activities that non-Western adults engage in are difficult to incorporate into Piaget's theory; children do not simply pass through a universal set of cognitive stages. Rather, sophisticated cognitions are based "on the mastery of systems that are cultural creations and not universal human attainments" (Okamoto *et al.* 1996). Further, recent work from Malawi suggests that measures of intelligence tend to be more closely associated with social and community integrity than with numeracy and literacy (Gladstone *et al.* 2010).

How culture affects child milestones and what is viewed as problematic behavior

The generation of global health knowledge about how culture affects developmental milestones and notions of problematic behavior is needed, because the social and cultural context in which behavior occurs can distinguish normal from disordered behavior (Canino & Alegría 2008). By implication, processes of development that differ from Western patterns may be considered abnormal or go unrecognized by outside observers (Zayas & Solari 1994). For example, Betancourt and colleagues (2010a) noted a roaming syndrome in their study of children that was considered unruly behavior in Sierra Leone, but could be considered normal in Western cultures. Efforts to understand the relationship between child development and culture require an informed and integrated perspective (Super & Harkness 2009); Western assessment tools used in developing countries may provide misleading information. Thus, some investigators have espoused the idea of developing and adapting cross-cultural assessment instruments to better understand not only mental health symptoms but their context (Betancourt *et al.* 2011).

Assessment of emotional problems in children

Accurate determination of whether diagnostic criteria for specific disorders have face validity among the population assessed is vital. For example, criteria for the measurement of time, simultaneity of symptoms, and comparative assessment (e.g., worries more than usual) may not have the same significance or relevance for different cultures. Asking diverse sets of parents whether behaviors occur more or less often than in a typical similar-aged child may be challenging; they might not share the same concept of typical behavior.

In order to effectively evaluate children, it is essential for clinicians to first comprehend the culture, local terminology, and commonly regarded psychopathology and distress symptoms (Weisner 1996). This includes words commonly used to label behavior, or signs that denote problems and how a community recognizes them. Clinicians must simplify the cognitive complexity of diagnostic assessment by incorporating questions that facilitate shared meaning across cultures. This means working to understand how behaviors impact a child's identity and social roles, as well as exploring the role of education, religion, sexual orientation, immigration history, and other factors of social position in the child's life (Canino & Alegría 2008).

Many researchers believe that the regulation of emotion in childhood through specific cognitions is tied to overall mental health. However, Garnefski and colleagues (2007) note a dearth of instruments worldwide to measure cognitive regulation and have focused on the development of a child version of the Cognitive Emotion Regulation Questionnaire (CERQ-k: Garnefski *et al.* 2007). Others suggest the importance of evaluating processes needed for youth to competently respond to social situations (Dodge & Price 1994), as some research suggests that children who have been socially rejected and aggressive tend to be less accurate in detecting peer intentions and more biased in generalizing hostile attributions. These findings are relevant particularly among youth exposed to chronic and extreme violence who might be at risk of post-traumatic stress disorder (PTSD) (Berman *et al.* 1996).

Identifying risk and protective factors

The development of mental health disorders in youth is multifactorial; risk and protective factors for mental health cross biological, psychological, and social domains (Patel *et al.* 2007). Early-life adversity is linked to individual differences in stress reactivity, cognitive deficits, and the development of psychopathology. There is also strong evidence for the role of genetic factors in the development of mental health disorders (Patel *et al.* 2007). However, attention must also be paid to individual, interpersonal, and neighborhood contextual risk/protective factors in concert with culture and context that shape self-identity and behavior.

Child rearing/family management (parenting)

The social developmental model has been used to explain the relationship between harsh discipline, poor parental monitoring, and risk for mental disorder. Bailey and colleagues (2009) report continuity between parenting practices and child externalizing behavior, whereby such behaviors during adolescence were associated with substance abuse in adulthood. Other research has shown that youth in families characterized by poor parenting practices are more likely to engage in violent behavior (Herrenkohl *et al.* 2006). In Palestinian children of the Intifada, discrepancies in mothering and fathering styles were also found to increase the risk for psychological maladjustment in children (Punamäki *et al.* 2001). Parenting behaviors are related to mental health disorders in youth, and therefore enhancing parental skills may reduce maladjustment in adolescence (Herrenkohl *et al.* 2006).

Parental mental health disorders

Poor parental mental health, aggressive or non-responsive behaviors, marital discord, and intimate partner violence are associated with the development of mental health disorders in youth. A meta-analysis examining maternal depression and child development in developing nations found that children of depressed mothers were at significantly increased risk for both stunting and being underweight (Surkan *et al.* 2011). Research suggests that not only parental mental health disorders, but how mental illness impacts child-rearing practices and the intergenerational transmission of certain behaviors, is relevant (Surkan *et al.* 2011).

Childhood maltreatment, violence and chronic stress

Exposure to maltreatment (e.g., physical, sexual, and emotional abuse), family violence, and parental instability have long-lasting detrimental effects on a child's mental health (Kessler *et al.* 1997, Green *et al.* 2010). Further, maltreatment during childhood has been associated with the onset of mental health disorders in adulthood. While estimates of both physical and sexual abuse vary, depending on the definitions used and the manner in which the data is collected, evidence from prevalence studies conducted in both Western and developing nations suggest that both are global problems. Chronic stress and exposure to violence and conflict can also increase vulnerability to child psychopathology. For example, Shen (2009) noted that 11.3% of Asian students in Taiwan who experienced interparental and child violence also scored high for internalizing disorders.

War and violence

More than 1 billion children have been exposed to armed conflict since 2008, and at least 20 million have been displaced (Unicef 2008). Elevated odds of psychiatric disorders and behavioral problems, such as depression and PTSD, have been reported among war survivors (Marfo *et al.* 2011). A study evaluating the effects of war on children in Bosnia and Herzegovina found that only 9% of the Bosnian children had experienced fewer than *seven* traumatic events (Dybdahl 2001). Among this sample of mothers and children, other stressors including poverty, resettlement, domestic violence, and alcohol abuse also contributed to children's mental health disorders.

Poverty

Poverty is associated with food insufficiency, malnutrition, inadequate clothing and shelter, and low educational attainment (Ravallion *et al.* 2008). Poor mental health may be both a cause and a consequence of the stresses associated with poverty. At the same time, dimensions of socioeconomic status, such as parental education and occupation, employment and social mobility, are also related to mental disorders in youth. In a recent study examining food insecurity and mental disorders among a large cohort of US adolescents, McLaughlin and colleagues (2012) found that both objective measures of household food insecurity and subjective social status measures were associated with past-year mood, anxiety, behavior, and substance disorders in youth. Thus, poverty and/or low socioeconomic status may influence youth mental health through both material deprivation and the individual's perception of social status (McLaughlin *et al*. 2012).

Neighborhood contextual factors and acculturation in the host country

Neighborhood contextual factors have been shown to exert influence on mental health outcomes among youth (Aneshensel & Sucoff 1996, Rutter 2009). Examining how experiences within the neighborhood result in feelings of alienation, rejection of conventional values, and the acceptance of maladaptive behaviors may elucidate which attributions augment risk. Exposure to violence, neighborhood residential instability, and attitudes which normalize deviancy have all been associated with mental health problems in youth (Green *et al*. 2005). Living in a US neighborhood deemed unsafe has been similarly associated with elevated risk of PTSD amongst Haitian immigrant students (Fawzi *et al*. 2009). Among a Canadian sample of immigrant youth, neighborhood quality assessed by items such as street garbage, burglaries, drug use and sale, public drinking, and bullying was predictive of emotional problems (Beiser *et al*. 2011).

Neighborhood contextual factors have also been linked with mental health disorders in developing nations. In the slums of Dhaka, Bangladesh, positive associations were found for mental well-being and contextual variables such as the natural environment, reduced risk of flooding, quality housing, and sanitation, whereas negative associations were found with higher population density (Gruebner *et al*. 2012).

Acculturation is associated with child and adolescent mental health outcomes, but the relationship is not straightforward. Among Asian-American youth, Yeh (2003) found that Chinese, Korean, and Japanese immigrant students who identified more strongly with American than Asian culture reported fewer mental health symptoms. Smokowski and colleagues (2009) found that for foreign-born parents, participation in US culture was associated with lower rates of anxiety and aggression in their adolescent children, while parent participation in native culture was not associated with *any* adolescent mental

health outcomes. Overall, adolescent involvement in culture of origin was positively associated with self-esteem but also with hopelessness, social problems, and aggression (Smokowski *et al*. 2009). Similar acculturation levels between parents and offspring have been found to influence child outcomes positively by reducing family conflicts (Lo 2010). Similar findings have been reported among Latino youth residing in the USA. These results underscore how the relationship between neighborhood contextual factors, experiences of acculturation, and the development of mental health disorders is contingent on multidimensional family and individual-level factors.

Protective factors

Most children do not suffer from psychopathology. Resilience research suggests that an early childhood characterized by strong emotional parental and familial ties, adequate nutrition, low levels of conflict, and community support facilitates the development of adaptive behaviors and good mental health (Jaffee *et al*. 2007). Protective factors include parental style and secure attachment, while community factors include a sense of connection to peers and other adults as well as school participation (Crews *et al*. 2007). Children facing maltreatment, poverty, and discrimination were found to have greater a chance of success when parental and familial relationships were strong (Jaffee *et al*. 2007, Bonanno & Mancini 2008). Neighborhood factors such as collective efficacy support and institutional resources can also serve as protective factors.

Prevention approaches and interventions

School readiness and educational initiatives

Efforts to improve literacy and numeracy skills may protect against mental illness (Jané-Llopis *et al*. 2004). Education may enhance opportunities, influence goals, and foster self-image (Patel 2001). Home-based interventions designed to facilitate school-readiness have been implemented throughout Western countries. While the effects of such initiatives implemented in developing countries have been described as modest, proponents maintain that they cannot be expected to compensate for the enduring effects of poverty and disadvantage that characterize the lives of many high-risk children (Liddell & McConville 1994). For example, an efficacy trial of a preventive low-cost school-readiness kit for youth and their families in urban South Africa reported small to medium effect sizes, although the differences between the intervention and control groups were not significant (Liddell & McConville 1994). Nevertheless, this approach may still be warranted; the researchers maintain that the kit was cost-effective and well accepted by families, and that the positive effects of the intervention may require a longer time period to determine its success. Other examples of preventive programs for early child development in Africa are discussed by Mwaura and Marfo (2011). Nonetheless, there is an incredible dearth of scientifically rigorous trials conducted in the developing world.

Child and adolescent mental health interventions

Substantive research and resources have been dedicated to understanding and ameliorating mental health service provision among children and adolescents in high-income countries, and thus effective evidence-based treatments for most mental health disorders exist (Saxena et al. 2006). In stark contrast, low-income and middle-income countries suffer from a lack of mental health resources and research (Saxena et al. 2006). Evidence for prevention and treatment is limited, as are skilled personnel (World Health Organization 2005). This is partly due to the failure to recognize the burden of child and adolescent mental health disorders by governments and policy makers. While youth mental health issues have received more attention in recent years (World Health Organization 2005), unmet need for treatment is very high in a majority of low- and middle-income countries (Omigbodun 2008, Patel et al. 2008).

Addressing child and adolescent mental health in these countries requires public health strategies that focus on both the promotion of mental health and the prevention of mental health disorders (Patel et al. 2008). This suggests the need for a public mental health framework targeting primary and secondary prevention (Jordans et al. 2009). Task-sharing approaches and non-specialty mental health workers may be critical for providing care to disenfranchised populations. Among preventive interventions with demonstrated efficacy, interventions in infancy and early childhood that enhance the mother–child relationship and school-based interventions hold particular promise since they tend to be cost-effective and target those who may be overlooked (Patel et al. 2008). Evidence from a long-term study of early psychosocial stimulation in Jamaica notes that children provided stimulation from infancy through age 2 exhibited less anxiety and depression, reported better self-esteem, and had fewer attention problems than their non-stimulated counterparts in adolescence (Walker et al. 2006). Universal interventions which promote capacity building in young children and adolescents through parent and/or teacher training have also proved efficacious (Mishrara & Ystgaard 2006, Patel et al. 2008). Results from a universal physical activity intervention for impoverished 15-year-olds in Chile suggest that important aspects of mental health status can be positively affected by attending to emerging risk factors common in many countries undergoing rapid economic and social transitions (Murray et al. 1997).

Among targeted interventions addressing internalizing disorders in children, significant improvements in symptoms of psychological distress were reported in a randomized trial of a school-based peer intervention for AIDS orphans, ages 10–15 years, in Uganda (Kumakech et al. 2009). Semi-structured exercises including theatrical play were designed to facilitate self-reflection, enable participants to connect their feelings, and promote self-determination. At follow-up, participants in the intervention group showed significant improvement in depression and anger (Bonhauser et al. 2005). In contrast, targeted interventions among children and adolescents with externalizing disorders in resource-poor countries are limited (Kieling et al. 2011), though many interventions, including pharmaceuticals, have been successfully used in developed nations. In high-resource settings, interventions with multiple targets (parents, teachers, and/or students) show promise, despite challenges associated with implementation and measurement (Domitrovich & Greenberg 2000, Hoagwood et al. 2007). Abbreviated training manuals have been utilized in some resource-poor settings; however, in environments characterized by a dearth of diagnosticians, correctly differentiating between problem behaviors remains challenging (Klasen & Crombag 2013).

Given that the context and intensity of trauma experienced by children and adolescents in high-resource countries is distinct from that of war-affected youth, evidence-based interventions from high-resource countries may not be particularly applicable (Klasen & Crombag 2013). Yet, comprehensive psychosocial and mental health care for youth affected by armed conflict and violence is of paramount importance, given evidence that a majority of interventions are not effective (Tol *et al.* 2008). A systematic review of intervention studies characterized most research as lacking scientific rigor and methodologically flawed, though some appear promising – mostly with respect to a diminishment of negative symptoms including depression, grief, emotional stress, and PTSD (Jordans *et al.* 2009). Dybdahl's targeted intervention provides evidence that a relatively inexpensive intervention for war-affected children *can* yield positive results. This psychosocial educational intervention sought to enhance maternal coping mechanisms and improve mother–child interactions, with positive outcomes including reduction in mental health problems among children in the intervention group (Dybdahl 2001). Tol and colleagues' randomized trial of a 15-week manualized classroom-based program for children in Indonesia suggests moderate improvement in PTSD symptoms and functional impairment, with boys evidencing increased optimism and girls maintaining hope (Tol *et al.* 2008), but also highlights the need for gender-based interventions (Kieling *et al.* 2011).

Although the number of rigorous studies addressing treatment outcomes among conflict-affected children is increasing (Tol *et al.* 2010), comparative inference about the relative strengths and weaknesses of discrete treatment approaches remains limited (Jordans *et al.* 2009). A synopsis of reviews examining children in complex and stressful life circumstances emphasizes: (1) the need for contextually valid assessment procedures; (2) the need to examine factors associated with *both* risk and resilience; (3) the dearth of specific treatment modalities; and (4) the scarcity of cost-effective, holistic, comprehensible interventions. Similarly, Betancourt and colleagues (2010b) propose a protective framework, call SAFE (Safety and security, Access to health care and physical needs, Family and others support, and Education for future support and hope) as a guideline for future interventions. While SAFE was developed specifically for Rwandan children affected by HIV/AIDS, the tenets of the interventions framework have useful application to all children facing adverse and difficult life situations.

Conclusion

Today's youth face unprecedented global challenges to their well-being and cognitive development. Many live in poverty without access to proper nutrition, health care, or education (Ravallion *et al.* 2008). A growing body of research documents adverse childhood experiences as major determinants of mental disorders that can persist throughout the life course. Yet research in developing countries has demonstrated extraordinary levels of resilience in children exposed to extreme poverty, natural disaster, and potentially traumatic events, with evidence of strong cultural and contextual variation in how youth respond to such events. A thorough understanding of protective and risk factors within these children, their families, and neighborhoods, and of the mechanisms by which these factors influence resilience or risk among children, is still lacking but necessary for the development of interventions that mitigate or eliminate known risk factors (Patel *et al.* 2007). Nonetheless, although advances have been made in our understanding of child development in diverse contexts, a great deal of current knowledge is based on the study of middle-class Western children (Ogbu 1988). Efforts to understand the relationship between child development and mental health problems require an informed and integrated perspective of the physical and social settings of daily life and customary childcare practices (Super & Harkness 2009) to be able to distinguish what is inappropriate development or harmful dysfunction. Also necessary is to explore the degree to which the child's emotional and behavioral problems fit along a continuum of adjustment and pathology within a specific culture. Risk and protective factors need to be established, as well as cultural and contextual factors that may help mitigate or exacerbate mental health problems. Preventive efforts and interventions to enhance coping mechanisms, improve mother–child interactions, and reduce symptoms of psychological distress including anxiety and depression all show promise.

References

Aneshensel CS, Sucoff CA (1996) The neighborhood context of adolescent mental health. *Journal of Health and Social Behavior* 37: 293–310.

Bailey JA, Hill KG, Oesterle S, *et al.* (2009) Parenting practices and problem behavior across three generations: Monitoring, harsh discipline, and drug use in the intergenerational transmission of externalizing behavior. *Developmental Psychology* 45: 1214–26.

Beiser M, Zilber N, Simich L, *et al.* (2011) Regional effects on the mental health of immigrant children: results from the new Canadian Children and Youth Study (NCCYS). *Health and Place* 17: 822–9.

Berman SL, Kurtines WM, Silverman WK, *et al.* (1996) The impact of exposure to crime and violence of urban youth. *American Journal of Orthopsychiatry* 66: 329–36.

Betancourt TS, Brennan RT, Rubin-Smith J, *et al.* (2010a) Sierra Leone's former child soldiers: a longitudinal study of risk, protective factors, and mental health. *Journal of the American Academy of Child and Adolescent Psychiatry* 49: 606–15.

Betancourt TS, Fawzi MKS, Bruderlein C, *et al.* (2010b) Children affected by HIV/AIDS: SAFE, a model for promoting their security, health, and development. *Psychology, Health and Medicine* 15: 243–65.

Betancourt TS, Rubin-Smith J, Beardslee WR, *et al.* (2011) Understanding locally, culturally, and contextually relevant mental health problems among Rwandan children and adolescents affected by HIV/AIDS. *AIDS Care* 23: 401–12.

Bonanno GA, Mancini AD (2008) The human capacity to thrive in the face of potential trauma. *Pediatrics* 121: 369–75.

Bonhauser M, Fernandez G, Klause P, *et al.* (2005) Improving physical fitness and emotional well-being in adolescents of low socioeconomic status in Chile: results of a school-based controlled trial. *Health Promotion International* 20: 113–22.

Bretherton I (1997) Bowlby's legacy to developmental psychology. *Child Psychiatry and Human Development* 28: 33–41.

Canino G, Alegría M (2008) Psychiatric diagnosis – Is it universal or relative to culture? *Journal of Child Psychology and Psychiatry* 49: 237–50.

Crews SD, Bender H, Cook CR, *et al.* (2007) Risk and protective factors for emotional and/or behavioral disorders in children and adolescents: a mega-analytic synthesis. *Behavioral Disorders* 32: 64–77.

Dodge KA, Price JM (1994) On the relation between social information: Processing and socially competent behavior in early school-aged children. *Child Development* 65: 1385–97.

Domitrovich CE, Greenberg, MT (2000) The study of implementation: current findings from effective programs that prevent mental disorders in school-aged children. *Journal of Educational and Psychological Consultation* 11: 193–211.

Dybdahl R (2001) Children and mothers in war: an outcome study of a psychosocial intervention program. *Child Development* 72: 1214–30.

Edwards VJ, Holden GW, Felitti VJ, Anda RF (2003) Relationship between multiple forms of childhood maltreatment and adult mental health in community respondents: Results from the adverse childhood experiences study. *American Journal of Psychiatry* 160: 1453–60.

Fawzi MCS, Betancourt TS, Marcelin L, *et al.* (2009) Depression and post-traumatic stress disorder among Haitian immigrant students: Implications for access to meantla health services and educational programming. *BMC Public Health* 9: 482.

Garnefski N, Rieffe C, Jellesma F, *et al.* (2007) Cognitive emotion regulation strategies and emotional problems in 9–11-year-old children. *European Child and Adolescent Psychiatry* 16: 1–9.

Gladstone M, Lancaster G, Umar E, *et al.* (2010) Perspectives of normal child development in rural Malawi: a qualitative analysis to create a more culturally appropriate developmental assessment tool. *Child: Care, Health and Development* 36: 346–53.

Grantham-McGregor S, Cheung YB, Cueto S *et al.* (2007) Developmental potential in the first 5 years for children in developing countries. *Lancet* 369: 60–70.

Green H, McGinnity A, Meltzer H, *et al.* (2005) *Mental Health of Children and Young People*. London: Palgrave Macmillan.

Green JG, McLaughlin KA, Berglund P, *et al.* (2010) Childhood adversities and adult psychopathology in the National Comorbidity Survey Replication (NCS-R) I: Associations with first onset of DSM-IV disorders. *Archives of General Psychiatry* 62: 113–23.

Gruebner O, Khan MMH, Lautenbach S, *et al.* (2012) Mental health in the slums of Dhaka: a geoepidemiological study. *BMC Public Health* 12: 177.

Herrenkohl TI, Hill KG, Hawkins JD, *et al.* (2006) Developmental trajectories of family management and risk for violent behavior in adolescence. *Journal of Adolescent Health* 39: 206–13.

Hoagwood KE, Olin SS, Kerker BD, *et al.* (2007) Empirically based school interventions targeted at academic and mental health functioning. *Journal of Emotional and Behavioral Disorders* 15: 66–92.

Jaffee SR, Caspi A, Moffitt TE, *et al.* (2007) Individual, family, and neighborhood factors distinguish resilient from non-resilient maltreated children: A cumulative stressors model. *Child Abuse and Neglect* 31: 231–3.

Jané-Llopis E, Muñoz R, Patel V (2004) Prevention of depression and depressive symptomatology. In C Hosman, E Jané-Llopis, S Saxena, eds., *Prevention of Mental Disorders: Effective Interventions and Policy Options*. Geneva: WHO.

Jordans MJD, Tol WA, Komproe IH, *et al.* (2009) Systematic review of evidence and treatment approaches: Psychosocial and mental health care for children in war. *Child and Adolescent Mental Health* 14: 2–14.

Kessler RC, Davis CG, Kendler KS (1997) Childhood adversity and adult psychiatric disorder in the US National Comorbidity Survey. *Psychological Medicine* 27: 1101–19.

Kieling C, Baker-Henningham H, Belfer M, *et al.* (2011) Child and adolescent mental health worldwide: Evidence for action. *Lancet* 378: 1515–25.

Klasen H, Crombag AC (2013) What works where? A systematic review of child and adolescent mental health interventions for low and middle income countries. *Social Psychiatry and Pscyhiatric Epidemiology* 48: 595–611.

Kumakech E, Cantor-Graae E, Maling S, *et al.* (2009) Peer-groups support intervention improves the psychosocial well-being of AIDS orphans: Cluster randomized trial. *Social Science and Medicine* 68: 1038–43.

Ladd GW, Cairns E (1996) Children: ethnic and political violence. *Child Development* 67: 14–18.

Liddell C, McConville C (1994) Starting at the bottom: towards the development of an indigenous school-readiness program for South African children being reared at home. *Early Child Development and Care* 97: 1–15.

Lo Y (2010) The impact of the acculturation process on Asian American youth's psychological well-being. *Journal of Child and Adolescent Psychiatric Nursing* 23: 84–91.

Luby JL, Heffelfinger A, Measelle JR, *et al.* (2002) Differential performance of the MacArthur HBQ and DISC-IV in identifying DSM-IV internalizing psychopathology in young children. *Journal of the American Academy of Child and Adolescent Psychiatry* 41: 458–66.

Marfo K, Pence A, LeVine RA, *et al.* (2011) Strengthening Africa's contributions to child development research: Introduction. *Child Development Perspectives* 5: 104–11.

McLaughlin KA, Green JG, Alegría M, *et al.* (2012) Food insecurity and mental disorders in a national sample of U.S. adolescents. *Journal of the American Academy of Child and Adolescent Psychiatry* 51: 1293–303.

Merikangas KR, He J, Burstein M, *et al.* (2010) Lifetime prevalence of mental disorders in U.S. adolescents: Results from the National Comorbidity Study-Adolescent supplement (NCS-A). *Journal of the American Academy of Child and Adolescent Psychiatry* 49: 980–9.

Mikulincer M, Shaver PR (2012) An attachment perspective on psychopathology. *World Psychiatry* 11: 11–15.

Mishara BL, Ystgaard M (2006) Effectiveness of a mental health promotion program to improve coping skills in young children: Zippy's Friends. *Early Childhood Research Quarterly* 21: 110–23.

Murray CJ, Lopez AD (1997) Global mortality, disability, and the contribution of risk factors. Global burden of disease study. *Lancet* 349: 1436–42.

Mwaura PAM, Marfo K (2011) Bridging culture, research, and practice in early childhood development: the Madrasa resource centers in East Africa. *Child Development Perspectives* 5: 134–9.

Ogbu JU (1988) Cultural diversity and human development. *New Directions for Child and Adolescent Development* 42: 11–28.

Okamoto Y, Case R, Bleiker C, *et al.* (1996) Cross-cultural investigations. *Monographs of the Society for Research in Child Development* 61: 131–55.

Omigbodun O (2008) Developing child mental health services in resource-poor countries. *International Review of Psychiatry* 20: 225–35.

Patel V (2001) Is depression a disease of poverty? *Regional Health Forum, WHO South-East Asia Region* 5(1): 14–23.

Patel V, Flisher AJ, Hetrick S, *et al.* (2007) Mental health of young people: a global public-health challenge. *Lancet* 369: 1302–13.

Patel V, Flisher AJ, Nikapota A, *et al.* (2008) Promoting child and adolescent mental health in low and middle income countries. *Journal of Child Psychology and Psychiatry* 49: 313–34.

Punamäki RL, Qouta S, El-Sarraj E (2001) Resiliency factors predicting psychological adjustment after political violence among Palestinian children. *International Journal of Behavioral Development* 25: 256–67.

Ravallion M, Chen S, Sangraula P (2008) *Dollar a Day Revisited*. World Bank Policy Research Working Paper WPS 4620.

Rutter M (2009) Understanding and testing risk mechanisms for mental disorders. *Journal of Child Psychology and Psychiatry* 50: 44–52.

Sagi A, Lamb ME, Lewkowicz KS, *et al.* (1985) Security of infant–mother–father, and metapelet attachments among kibbutz-reared Israeli children. Monographs of the society for research in child development.

Growing Points of Attachment Theory and Research **50**: 257–75.

Saxena S, Paraje G, Sharan P, Karam G, Sadana R (2006) The 10/90 divide in mental health research: trends over a 10 year period. *British Journal of Psychiatry* **188**: 81–2.

Shen ACT (2009) Long-term effects of interparental violence and child physical maltreatment experiences on PTSD and behavior problems: a national survey of Taiwanese college students. *Child Abuse and Neglect* **33**: 148–60.

Smokowski P, Buchman RL, Bacallao ML (2009) Acculturation of adjustment in Latino adolescents: How cultural risk factors and assets influence multiple domains of adolescent mental health. *Journal of Primary Prevention* **30**: 371–93.

Super CM, Harkness S (2009) *The Developmental Niche of the Newborn in Rural Kenya.* New York, NY: Wiley.

Surkan P, Kennedy C, Hurley K, *et al.* (2011) Maternal depression and early childhood growth in developing countries: Systemic review and meta-analysis. *Bulletin of the World Health Organization* **89**: 608–15.

Tol WA, Komproe IH, Susanty D, *et al.* (2008) School-based mental health intervention for children affected by political violence in Indonesia. *JAMA* **300**: 655–62.

Tol WA, Komproe IH, Jordans MJD, *et al.* (2010) Mediators and moderators of a psychosocial intervention for children affected by political violence. *Journal of Consulting and Clinical Psychology* **78**: 818–28.

True MM, Pisani L, Oumar F (2001) Infant–mother attachment among the Dogon of Mali. *Child Development* **72**: 1451–66.

Unicef (2008) *The State of the World's Children 2008.* New York, NY: Unicef.

Walker S, Chang SM, Powell CA, *et al.* (2006) Effects of psychosocial stimulation and dietary supplementation in early childhood on psychosocial functioning in late adolescence: follow-up of randomized controlled trial. *BMJ* **333**: 472.

Weisner TS (1996) *Why Ethnography Should be the Most Important Method in the Study of Human Development.* Chicago, IL: University of Chicago Press.

Women's Refugee Commission (2012) Children and youth: ensuring opportunities for displaced youth. http://www.womensrefugeecommission.org/programs/youth (accessed July 2013).

World Health Organization (2005) *Atlas: Child and Adolescent Mental Health Resources. Global Concerns, Implications for the Future.* Geneva: WHO.

Yeh CJ (2003) Age, acculturation, cultural adjustment and mental health symptoms of Chinese, Korean, and Japanese immigrant youths. *Cultural Diversity and Ethnic Minority Psychology* **9**: 34–48.

Zayas LH, Solari F (1994) Early childhood socialization in Hispanic families: Culture, context, and practice implications. *Professional Psychology: Research and Practice* **25**: 200–6.

Ziv Y, Aviezer O, Gini M, Sagi A, Koren-Karie N (2000) Emotional availability in the mother–infant dyad as related to the quality of infant–mother attachment relationship. *Attachment and Human Development* **2**: 149–69.

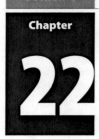

Chapter

22

Child abuse as a global mental health problem

Felipe Picon, Andrea Fiorillo, and Dinesh Bhugra

Introduction

Child abuse is an issue of major concern for the whole of society. It is a global mental health problem of epidemic proportion affecting children of all ages and races, and from all economic and cultural backgrounds. Even though it is not considered specifically a psychiatric disorder, it may be an important environmental risk factor for the genesis of many important and disabling psychiatric conditions. Depression and anxiety, for example, may make a person more likely to smoke, take alcohol or illicit drugs, or overeat. Not only do certain conditions, such as eating disorders, self-harm, and sexual dysfunction, occur more frequently in those who have been abused, but abuse also affects an individual's self-esteem, having long-term consequences for the individual.

Another complication in the twenty-first century arises from changing definitions of abuse, as well as the changing nature of the family. With sequential partners and secondary family relations, the likelihood of sexual abuse can increase. From a worldwide perspective, it is important to realize that of a total population now estimated to be above 7 billion, around 2.2 billion individuals are below the age of 18 years; a third of the world's population is either a child or an adolescent, with around 633 million being under 5 years old and consequently more vulnerable to abuse of all kinds (Unicef 2011).

Definitions

Abuse, whether it is sexual, emotional, or physical, can contribute to a variety of acts, as well as deprivation of care by those who look after children within settings such as schools, hospitals, and residential units (Rutter *et al.* 2008), and there are also recent reports suggesting links with ongoing abuse in church institutions. It is imperative that children grow up in a healthy environment, for a number of reasons. Firstly it is a matter of the growth of the individual, along with a reduction in circles of abuse, as those who are abused themselves are likely to abuse others. Furthermore, epidemiological data show that over half of psychiatric disorders in adulthood have an age of onset below the age of 18, and it is critical that clinicians also focus on resilience, which will ultimately lead to a better society. Much effort has been expended by mental health practitioners, educators, researchers, and policy makers in order to understand and treat the sequalae of child abuse – be it sexual, physical, or emotional. Various international organizations such as the World Health Organization (WHO), the United Nations Children's Fund (Unicef), and the International Society for the Prevention of Child Abuse and Neglect (ISPCAN) have focused on the betterment of dealing with sexual abuse of children. Annual reports from these agencies highlight various issues including estimated rates and associated factors, and they point to key differences across national policies in this area.

It is difficult to be certain about the definitions of abuse, as there will be cultural and social factors that will dictate the components of abuse. Actual physical abuse, sexual abuse, emotional abuse, and deliberate malnourishment can all be counted as abuse. The WHO attempts to define child abuse and neglect, or child maltreatment, as all forms of physical and/or emotional mistreatment, sexual abuse, neglect, or negligent treatment of children, as well as commercial or other exploitation resulting in actual or potential harm to the child's health, survival, development, or dignity in the context of a relationship of

Essentials of Global Mental Health, ed. Samuel O. Okpaku. Published by Cambridge University Press. © Cambridge University Press 2014.

responsibility, trust, or power. The perpetrators of child maltreatment may be parents and other family members; caregivers; friends; acquaintances; strangers; authority figures, such as teachers, soldiers, police officers, clergy; employers; healthcare workers; and also other children. There are four types of child maltreatment: physical abuse; sexual abuse; emotional and psychological abuse; and neglect, which can be both emotional and physical (World Health Organization 2006)

Child sexual abuse is probably the most deleterious form of child maltreatment, as it is a serious risk factor for the development of psychopathology in childhood, adolescence, and adulthood. Although it is an ancient phenomenon, it continues to remain a difficult challenge for society to deal with both in prevention and in management. Sexual abuse goes beyond incest, and frequently the abuser is a person known to the child. Despite several reports of very high rates of child sexual abuse, any disclosures are often regarded with suspicion.

As the primary unit of socialization, the family is where the cultural influences on child development are most significant, and also unfortunately where many types and instances of child abuse occur. Parents, family members, or other caregivers within the family are most likely to be responsible for subtle and/or severe forms of abuse. As mentioned above, with increasing rates of divorce and separation and subsequent attachments with other partners who may have children from other partners, the definition of core family needs to be recognized. In other cultures joint or extended families will have differing roles and expectations. The recent American television series *Modern Family* illustrates this remarkably well, where a gay couple have an adopted child, the father of the family is married to a woman who has brought a child into the relationship, and the daughter of the family has three children from her marriage.

Cultures determine child development patterns and the expectations of roles from both parents and children, which in turn raise specific issues about how abuse is defined and determined, and how it is dealt with. Evidence from 34 low- and middle-income countries revealed that physical punishment is common within families, even though it is not supported by the majority of parents in most countries surveyed (Cappa & Khan 2011). Thus the challenge is to see what is seen as normal and what is seen

as deviant. In the same survey, the percentage of mothers/primary caregivers who believed that physical punishment was necessary to raise a child ranged from 6% in Montenegro to nearly 92% in the Syrian Arab Republic. There are also rural/urban differences, which will be associated with educational attainments. Rural respondents were significantly more likely than urban respondents to believe that physical punishment is necessary to control a child. Thus it is not surprising that those with poor educational levels are more likely to believe in this behavior. Women with limited education (none or primary) were most likely to approve the use of physical punishment, compared with those who had a higher level of education. Surprisingly, and perhaps more interestingly, there was also an association with the economic status of the family, with an increased likelihood of physical punishment in the poorest families. In cultures where children are expected to start work at an early age to support the family, children and adolescents will often be seen as income generators, and if they do not deliver they may be seen as "deserving" of punishment. Not surprisingly, intimate partner violence was also a contributing factor. Those who physically abused their wives were also likely to abuse their children, and wives/mothers thought that the husband was justified in hitting or beating his wife in certain situations, such as if she went out without telling him, neglected the children, argued with him, refused to have sex with him, or burnt the food. Out of the 28 countries surveyed with these questions, an association between the two types of violence was reported in 20 countries. Women who justified wife-beating were significantly more likely to support the idea that children needed to be physically punished to be properly raised (Cappa & Khan 2011). This observation has significant impact on forming people's attitudes to violence and abuse in the family setting, and thus needs to be taken on board when planning any intervention and prevention strategies. In addition there are other factors such as low parental involvement with the child, early separation, low parental warmth, unwanted pregnancy, and maternal dissatisfaction with her child (Egeland & Bosquet 2002, Krueger *et al.* 1998). In certain cultures the gender of the child will also play a role.

Any form of physical and psychological violence between adults in the family, even if it is not directly focused on the child, may also be considered a form of child maltreatment. This exposure to domestic violence can be defined as a child witnessing physical or psychological violence, overhearing violence, or seeing its aftermath, such as resulting injuries or emotional harm. This was confirmed in a multisite study from Australia, Canada and the USA which showed that exposure to domestic violence is prevalent and common in child welfare cases, and that statistics on the phenomenon are likely to underestimate the problem because victims often under-report. This study noted that 7–23% of youths in the general population were exposed to domestic violence (Cross *et al.* 2012). Thus exposure itself can act as a contributing factor to further domestic violence.

Prevalence

It is important to note that the epidemiological data on the rates of child abuse vary dramatically, as there may be not only under-reporting but also varying definitions of abuse. The United States Department of Health and Human Services has reported, every year, for 21 years now, the rates of child maltreatment all over the country. A recent report shows that there was a total count of 688 251 child victims in 2010, accounting for 10% of the whole child population (Children's Bureau 2011). A study on physical abuse in high-income countries found prevalence rates varying from 4% to 16% (Gilbert *et al.* 2009). On the other hand, a study in 28 low- and middle-income countries using data from the Multiple Indicator Cluster Surveys (MICS) compared different forms of child abuse across countries and regions and showed that a median of 83.2% of children in the African region experienced psychological abuse, compared to 57.8% of children from transitional countries. This study showed that moderate physical abuse was also highest in African countries (64.3%) and lowest in transitional countries (45.5%) (Akmatov 2011). Such high rates raise serious questions about how to understand causation and management planning in social and school settings, as well as in clinical settings.

Sexual abuse

Child sexual abuse raises strong reactions, and its widespread prevalence is often ignored for a number of reasons which include social taboos surrounding adult sexual contact with children, the absence of a non-involved witness to this (secret) activity, and the potentially serious consequence for the alleged abuser (Rutter *et al.* 2008). Child sexual abuse includes variations such as trafficking of boys and girls for sexual activities by adults, whether or not the child is aware of what is happening. Thus any study of prevalence has to take into account these huge variations.

In a study from southern Brazil, responses by 1936 children and adolescents to a confidential questionnaire showed a prevalence of child sexual abuse of 5.6% among girls and 1.6% among boys, with 60% of this sample experiencing abuse under the age of 12 (Bassani *et al.* 2009). In the United States, in 2008, the state and local child protective services received 3.3 million reports of children being abused or neglected. Of those, 71% were victims of neglect, 16% of physical abuse, 9% of sexual abuse, and 7% of emotional abuse. There is an estimate that around 150 000 cases of child sexual abuse happen in the United States each year, reaching a rate of 1.1 cases per 1000 children. Approximately one in four girls and one in six boys are sexually abused before the age of 18 (Troiano 2011). A representative study on the frequency of maltreatment among children and adolescents in Germany studied 2504 respondents and reported a rate of 12.6% for sexual abuse (Häuser *et al.* 2011).

These studies are part of a growing body of well-designed studies from all over the world, and should be seen as an indication of trends. A review of the nature and occurrence of sexual abuse showed a geographically diverse selection of recent studies, with rates for penetrative child sexual abuse higher for girls than for boys. For female children/adolescents, rates for penetrative abuse ranged from 0.3% in China to 1.3% in France, 1.6–3% in South Africa, 2% in the UK, 4% in Israel, 4.9% in Swaziland, 5.6% in Ireland, 11% in Tanzania, and 18% in Ethiopia. The rates for penetrative sexual abuse are lower than the rates for other types of sexual abuse, such as fondling, kissing, fellatio, indecent exposure, or even asking or pressuring the child to engage in sexual activities regardless of the actual physical outcome (Lalor & McElvaney 2010).

A recent meta-analysis on childhood sexual abuse, comprising 217 publications from 1982 to 2008, studied a total of 9 911 748 participants from North America, South America, Europe, Africa, Asia and Australia/New Zealand and included boys and girls (Stoltenborgh *et al.* 2011). The combined prevalence for child abuse for the whole set of studies was 11.8%, with the combined prevalence for informant studies 0.4% and for self-report studies 12%. Significant differences were found between the continents of origin of the sample for both girls and boys. The highest combined prevalence was found in Australia for girls and in Africa for boys, whereas the lowest combined prevalence was found in Asia for both genders. Significant gender differences were found in Asia, Australia, Europe, and United States/Canada, with girls showing a higher combined prevalence than boys. It is possible that these are real differences, but it could also mean that the boys may be more reluctant to report abuse, as it may be seen as loss of masculinity. However, boys might not perceive sexual experiences with older women as sexual abuse, because of gender and masculinity stereotypes, thus complicating factors and explanations further. A male victim of male perpetrators might fear being regarded as homosexual and therefore not reveal the experience. In more collectivist societies in Asia, lower prevalence rates are reported than in the more individualistic countries; this may reflect a collective responsibility in keeping matters quiet. There may also be different notions of shame in disclosures. In addition, cultural values related to taboos on sexuality, found, for example, in Hispanic cultures, are likely to inhibit disclosure. Initiation rites of passage to adulthood in Africa, for example, may encourage sexual behavior between adults and early and mid-teenagers (Stoltenborgh et al. 2011).

An additional factor that often gets ignored in our exploration of these issues is the resultant HIV infections, which are more focused in countries with higher rates of prevalent infections such as those in Africa. A cross-sectional school-based community representative study in 10 countries in Africa (Botswana, Lesotho, Malawi, Mozambique, Namibia, South Africa, Swaziland, Tanzania, Zambia, and Zimbabwe) reported that 19.6% of female students and 21.1% of male students aged 11–16 years had experienced forced or coerced sex (Andersson et al. 2012). A qualitative study of girls from South Africa who were raped or forced to get married revealed the complex situation which intertwines severe poverty, the sale of the daughter by the family in exchange for money, and subsequent exposure to HIV infection (Banwari 2011). Thus clinicians and policy makers must take into account not only the abuse but also the associated physical sequalae.

Physical abuse

Children and adolescents are also the most vulnerable possible victims of physical violence, due to the development of body and brain and resulting psychological development. Physical abuse involves hitting, shaking, throwing, poisoning, burning, scalding, drowning, suffocating, or otherwise causing physical harm to a child. Fabricated or induced illness by a parent or caregiver is also a type of physical harm. Physical neglect comprises failing to provide adequate food, clothing, or shelter, or exclusion or abandonment. Physical abuse occurs in every country of the world, although its exact extent and severity may vary, as will forms of clinical presentation. The consequences also vary, and in extreme cases death may occur. In Canada, data from 2008 showed that 2.9 per 1000 children suffered from physical abuse (Afifi 2011). In India, a recent study carried out by the Ministry of Women and Child Development enrolled 12 447 children and reported that 69% were physically abused and 53% were subjected to one or more forms of sexual abuse (Srivastava 2012), which goes against the earlier-noted reports of lower rates in Asian countries. This may also reflect social and economic changes which are ongoing in the country. High rates for severe physical abuse are also reported from various African countries: Gambia (52.6%), Sierra Leone (51.8%), Ghana (43.3%), Guinea-Bissau (42.9%), Burkina Faso (37.1%), Côte d'Ivoire (36.9%), Togo (36.5%); also in other developing countries: Yemen (61%), Jamaica (41.6%), Guyana (40.7%), Iraq (32.6%), Belize (31.3%), Vietnam (29.3%), Syria (28.9%), Trinidad and Tobago (23.3%). Transitional countries show slight lower rates of physical abuse: Georgia (21.2%), Tajikistan (19.2%), Macedonia (16.8%), Belarus (10.6%), Serbia (10.1%), Albania (8.9%), Montenegro (7.6%), Ukraine (6.8%), Bosnia and Herzegovina (6.1%), Kyrgyzstan (4.9%), and Kazakhstan (2.2%). Clearly this phenomenon is a global health issue (Akmatov 2011).

Risk factors and protective factors
Child trafficking

Child trafficking is a major risk factor for child abuse and child prostitution. Child trafficking is a global problem and a heinous crime against children. It is defined as the recruitment, transportation, transfer, harboring, or receipt of a child for the purposes of sexual or labor exploitation, forced labor, or slavery. It is often damaging to the health, development, and well-being of the child, and in some cases even life-threatening. The most severe example is of those children trafficked into prostitution facing exposure to HIV and other sexually transmitted diseases. The exploitative and hidden nature of child trafficking makes it very hard to be properly studied, and consequently to be dealt with.

Child trafficking has been reported from all over the world, but more substantially in some regions, including west Africa, south Asia (India and Nepal), southeast Asia, central Asia, eastern Europe, Russia and the Commonwealth of Independent states, and Latin America (Colombia and Mexico). Most children are trafficked for cheap and controlled labour, but also for adoption, sexual exploitation, arranged marriages, and harvesting of organs. Many children, especially in sub-Saharan Africa, are also drawn to being trafficked as a result of becoming orphans of parents deceased from AIDS (Beyrer 2004). In Thailand it is estimated that between 60 000 and 200 000 girls are trafficked into prostitution annually. This is associated with factors such as poverty; the cultural acceptance of a girl raising money to support her family, even if it is through prostitution; low educational possibilities; growing demand for prostitutes for sex tourism; and also misconceived beliefs that sex with a virgin or a young child is rejuvenating, brings luck, strength, virility, and cures venereal diseases; and the idea that children are less likely to be infected with HIV (Lau 2008). Adding to the worldwide statistics on the matter, and asserting the global status of this problem, a report on human trafficking in the United States in 2009 suggests that between 14 500 and 17 500 individuals are trafficked annually into the country, many of them to work in the sex industry (Macy & Graham 2012).

Children and armed conflicts

Another important specific form of child abuse relates to an increasing use of children in armed conflicts as soldiers recruited by a number of official and other agencies. They may be abducted from school or from the local community, or they may enlist "voluntarily," usually because there is a lack of other employment opportunities. Although international law prohibits the participation in armed conflict of children and adolescents under 18, many boys and girls do so voluntarily or involuntarily and

are consequently killed or injured. This use of children in military activities takes one or more of three distinct forms: as fighters taking direct part in hostilities, being an actual soldier; or in several support roles such as cooks, spies, messengers, porters, servants, or to lay or clear land mines; or they can be also used for political advantage, either as human shields or in propaganda. Girls, in particular, are at severe risk of rape, serving as sexual slaves, but are also victims of other forms of sexual abuse. These children have their childhood stolen from them and are inevitably exposed to severe forms of psychological trauma and physical suffering (Amnesty International 2011). The use of children in warfare has happened many times in history and in many cultures, and although international organizations such as Child Soldiers International nowadays work every day to limit the participation of children in armed conflicts, it remains a widespread phenomenon.

In their 2008 triennial report, the Child Soldiers International organization revealed that children were recruited or used in hostilities, from April 2004 to October 2007, in a large number of countries. Details of these countries can be found in the report (Coalition to Stop the Use of Child Soldiers 2008). Following an earlier report in 2004, there is a decrease in the number of armed conflicts listed from 27 in 2004 to 17 by the end of 2007. Although it is a downward trend, the authors state that this fall is more due to conflicts ending rather than the impact of initiatives to end child soldier recruitment and use. Yet this list of countries is not complete, as recruitment still continues in at least 86 countries and territories worldwide. Some have their official armed forces using children, others use children in paramilitaries, militias, civilian defense forces or armed groups, and yet others use children as spies, informants, or messengers. There are also countries where there were child soldiers in non-state armed groups (Coalition to Stop the Use of Child Soldiers 2008).

Apart from the involvement of children in "official" armed conflicts, there is also the recruitment by gangs, organized crime, and criminal armed groups. In Brazil, for example, until recent government efforts cleared many areas from the influence of drug gangs, young boys were used to guard the "favelas" from the police and also to carry drugs and spread information through the alleys of the slums (Guardian 2010). A similar situation has been reported from Mexico, with its drug cartels, where some 30 000 children are said to be involved in some sort of organized crime, according to the Child Rights Network in Mexico – who also point out that many of these children are taking part because of death threats (to themselves or their families) or because of economic and social necessity (CNN 2010). In many countries in Europe, Gypsy gangs use children to steal and beg for money. In Madrid, children are taught to commit crime and escape punishment by law, as the age of criminal responsibility in Spain is 14. Although some of the small crimes carried out by children are driven by poverty, a worrying amount is the result of child exploitation, organized by professional criminals and gang bosses who traffic people, including children, from one European country to another to beg and steal and return them the profits (BBC News 2009). Often these children are much younger than the age limit for a criminal charge, and their role is to protect an adult from the risk of being caught, arrested, and prosecuted.

These exploitative acts by armed militias or gang bosses threaten and harm the very essence of childhood, and of society as a whole. Physical and psychological harm are not limited to the combat zones. The collapse of civil society around these children, during war times, exposes them to becoming orphans, unprotected and malnourished, and to suffer from many other health conditions such as cholera. Sexual abuse is also a frequent event, especially among girls (Humphreys 2009).

Child soldiers face several medical and psychological risks, from malnutrition, HIV, and exposure to other sexually transmitted diseases, to mutilation and premature death. Apart from the combat-zone wounds such as stabbing or gunshot injuries, they are also at greater risk of contracting malaria, cholera, and yellow fever, diseases that are common in crisis situations where the infrastructure of society has crumbled. And for those who survive all these threats, there is the extremely difficult task of dealing with the memories of the horror and coping with readjustment into their communities, compounded by all sorts of issues including shame and guilt. The physical and emotional healing of the young soldiers is a very difficult challenge for themselves, for those who support these survivors directly, and for the community at large.

Protective factors

Although most of the child maltreatment research has focused on negative outcomes associated with maltreatment, a growing literature has investigated protective factors related to resilience. These factors can be divided into those at the individual, familial, and community level. It is vital to understand resilience, so that appropriate measures can be put in place. Individual factors are personal characteristics, personality traits, intellect, self-efficacy, coping, appraisal of maltreatment, and life satisfaction. Family-level protective factors include resources and supportive relationships, such as family coherence, stable caregiving, parental relationships, and spousal support. Protective factors at the community level include peer relationships, non-family-member relationships, non-family-member social support, and religion (Afifi & MacMillan 2011). Children with hobbies, interests, good peer relationships, an easy temperament, a positive disposition, an active coping style, positive self-esteem, good social skills, an internal locus of control, and a balance between seeking help and autonomy are less prone to suffer abuse. Families with a supportive environment, a household with clear rules and monitoring of the child, family expectations of pro-social behavior, and high parental education are also protective factors. Other social protective factors are access to health care and social services, consistent parental employment, adequate housing, and access to good schools.

Consequences of abuse

The consequences of child abuse are multifaceted, varying from ongoing trauma to personality changes and even death. In 2010 there was a total of 1537 child fatalities registered in the United States, reaching a national fatality rate of 2.07 per 100 000 children in the population (Children's Bureau 2011). A dreadful total of 79.2% of child fatalities were caused by one or more parents, and of those 29.2% were perpetrated by the child's mother alone and 21.9% were caused by both parents. Perpetrators without a parental relationship to the child accounted for 12.5% of fatalities, and in the remaining 8.3% the perpetrator was unknown. The death of a child represents the extreme antithesis of what is expected to be a child's upbringing, and is the ultimate insult to the developing child's need for care and nurturing.

Emotional abuse or psychological abuse/maltreatment is another important form of abuse that produces severe consequences. This may occur in isolation or in conjunction with other types of abuse. Emotionally abusive or neglectful child-rearing methods include excessive and continuing criticism, denigration, terrorizing, repeated blaming, insults, and threats against children by their carers. For example, parents/caregivers may use extreme or bizarre forms of punishment, such as lengthy confinement of a child in a dark closet. Emotionally neglectful behaviors include gross indifference and inattentiveness to a child's developmental or special needs.

In a longitudinal study, 236 children exposed to maternal domestic violence, frequent bullying, victimization, and physical maltreatment by an adult had DNA samples taken at the age of 5 and followed up at the age of 10 (Shalev et al. 2012). This study showed significantly more telomere erosion between the ages of 5 and 10 in these children than in age-matched controls. The deleterious effects of stress on these children's DNA is clear evidence that abuse at an early age is linked with a DNA alterations and potentially with harmful impacts on lifelong health (Shalev et al. 2012). Any form of emotional abuse is intrinsically connected with the eliciting of stress responses, and beyond the emotional impact there is also damage at the molecular level, which may well lead to several psychiatric disorders or psychiatric vulnerabilities.

Physical health outcomes are affected in abused and neglected children, increasing the risk for diabetes, lung disease, malnutrition, and vision problems in a 30-year follow up study (Widom et al. 2012). The diagnosis of physical abuse also remains challenging, because of a lack of history, delayed presentation, and often vague and subtle external findings of abuse. Unexplained bruising remains one of the most common external signs of occult injury. Skin burns, occult fractures, occult abdominal trauma, and head trauma are other serious medical signs that may point to child physical abuse (Denton et al. 2011). Pediatricians are often the first professionals to be involved, and they have the responsibility of searching for further information and evaluation whenever the history and explanation for the bruises or complaints are not adequate for the clinical presentation. Physical abuse is associated with increased risk for disruptive and emotional psychopathology. Those who have been victims are likely to become perpetrators, and bullying may be the first step towards this. Other possible outcomes of child physical abuse are not only direct physical injuries or physical disability but also disruption of the hypothalamic–pituitary–adrenal axis,

growth reduction, under- immunization, and ultimately death. The consequences of physical abuse on the adolescent include an increased likelihood of risk-taking behaviors, early first sexual experience, multiple sexual partners, pregnancy before the age of 19, and drug and alcohol abuse (Children's Bureau 2011).

Possible interventions for prevention and treatment

Child abuse is linked to long-term deleterious effects on health and well-being, but separating the effects of child maltreatment from other often concomitant childhood adversities, such as poverty, has been challenging. Methodologically rigorous studies are able to show significant associations between child abuse and subsequent mental disorder diagnoses, such as mood disorder, post-traumatic stress disorder (PTSD), and anxiety disorder, after adjusting for demographic and socioeconomic factors (Denton et al. 2011).

Both prevention and treatment focus on the individual, but other actions must be at community and global levels, in order to abolish the burden of abuse and prevent the vicious cycle of abuse continuing. This circle of transgenerational passage of violence should be one of the key targets of governmental policies in the fight against child abuse.

Child abuse is multifaceted in nature, and therefore several professional systems have a stake in its detection, prevention, and response, including health, education, and justice systems. Child mental health practitioners, in spite of operating in different systemic levels, can plan and integrate services of child protection and child mental health, ensuring a developmental perspective and a culturally sensitive approach, responsive to impairment and disability. They can also bring a scientific perspective to planning services and research initiatives, and they have a role in teaching and training other professionals in the investigation, assessment, and treatment of child abuse. Pediatricians and physicians from other medical specialties are also often in charge of patients who have suffered from many forms of maltreatment, and they are therefore also responsible for the response to and care of this problem. Working toward reducing rates of abuse in childhood, it is crucial to work with other stakeholders such as teachers, police officers, activists, judges, attorneys, politicians, and policy makers. In dealing with child trafficking, mass education campaigns in source areas are only one way to deal with this menace, but the implementation of the policy is more important. The fight against transnational organized crime and drug cartels also deals indirectly with this problem, because usually these organizations also perform human trafficking alongside their original enterprise.

Another global approach is related to the military use of children. Child Soldiers International (www.child-soldiers.org), formerly known as the Coalition to Stop the Use of Child Soldiers, is an international coalition of human rights and humanitarian organizations, created in 1998, dedicated to preventing the recruitment and use of children as soldiers, to securing their demobilization, and to ensuring their rehabilitation and reintegration. They not only provide data but also research, advocacy of international campaigns, and lobbying of governments and armed political groups (Coalition to Stop the Use of Child Soldiers 2008).

Globally active organizations such as Unicef and ISPCAN promote effective action against child abuse, by promoting preventive strategies, supporting governments to establish formal legal child abuse policies and response systems, and promoting the emerging global agreements regarding child abuse and neglect, beyond possible culturally different views of what defines maltreatment. The work toward that goal has to be made within each country's national situation, which includes economic and social status. Much of the world's response to child abuse and neglect is inextricably linked to funding. Although the proportion of developing countries that are organizing effective response systems is growing, wide discrepancies remain in terms of service availability. Children living in countries facing extreme economic hardship and social disruption are at particular risk, although the professionals involved in the care of abuse victims in these countries are improving their ability to document the incidence of maltreatment and to provide effective avenues for children and families to be properly assisted (ISPCAN 2008).

Conclusions

Regrettably, because of the vulnerability of children, their abuse continues for several reasons. The development of an individual person is a complex process that takes many years to complete, and a suitable caring, nurturing, and loving environment is essential for every child in the world to avoid later development of psychopathology. As clinicians, it is critical that we play our part in therapeutic endeavors. We must also act as leaders in the prevention of such acts by working with parents, teachers, politicians, physicians, other mental health professionals, other stakeholders such as educational psychologists, and indeed the adults of society as a whole in order to provide the best settings possible for the safe and healthy development of the world's children. When faced with problems of such global dimensions, it is essential to have globally scaled forces ready to counter them. Many of these events are international, affecting children across national boundaries, and to tackle them will therefore require a major global initiative.

References

Afifi TO (2011) Child maltreatment in Canada: an understudied public health problem. *Canadian Journal of Public Health* **102**: 459–61.

Afifi TO, MacMillan HL (2011) Resilience following child maltreatment: a review of protective factors. *Canadian Journal of Psychiatry* **56**: 266–72.

Akmatov MK (2011) Child abuse in 28 developing and transitional countries: results from the Multiple Indicator Cluster Surveys. *International Journal of Epidemiology* **40**: 219–27.

Amnesty International (2011) *Amnesty International Report 2011: The State of the World's Human Rights.* http://www.amnesty.org/en/annual-report/2011 (accessed July 2013).

Andersson N, Paredes-Solís S, Milne D, et al. (2012) Prevalence and risk factors for forced or coerced sex among school-going youth: national cross-sectional studies in 10 southern African countries in 2003 and 2007. *BMJ Open*, **2** (2): e000754.

Banwari M (2011) Poverty, child sexual abuse and HIV in the Transkei region, South Africa. *African Health Sciences* **11**: 117–21.

Bassani DG, Palazzo LS, Béria JU, et al. 2009. Child sexual abuse in southern Brazil and associated factors: a population-based study. *BMC Public Health* **9** (1): 133.

BBC News (2009) How Gypsy gangs use child thieves. http://news.bbc.co.uk/2/hi/8226580.stm (accessed July 2013).

Beyrer C (2004) Global child trafficking. *Lancet* **364**: 16–17.

Cappa C, Khan SM (2011) Understanding caregivers' attitudes towards physical punishment of children: evidence from 34 low- and middle-income countries. *Child Abuse and Neglect* 35: 1009–21.

Children's Bureau (2011) *Child Maltreatment 2010*. Washington, DC: US Department of Health and Human Services. http://archive.acf.hhs.gov/programs/cb/pubs/cm10 (accessed July 2013).

CNN (2012) Children in Mexico: criminals or victims? http://edition.cnn.com/2012/01/17/world/americas/mexico-children-crime (accessed July 2013).

Coalition to Stop the Use of Child Soldiers (2008) *Child Soldiers Global Report 2008*. London: The Coalition.

Cross TP, Mathews B, Tonmyr L, Scott D, Ouimet C (2012) Child welfare policy and practice on children's exposure to domestic violence. *Child Abuse and Neglect* 36: 210–16.

Denton J, Newton AW, Vandeven AM (2011) Update on child maltreatment: toward refining the evidence base. *Current Opinion in Pediatrics* 23: 240–8.

Egeland B, Bosquet M (2002) Continuities and discontinuities in the intergenerational transmission of child maltreatment: Implication for breaking the cycle of abuse. In KD Browne, H Hanks, P Stratton, C Hamilton, eds., *Early Prediction and Prevention of Child Abuse: a Handbook*. New York, NY: Wiley.

Gilbert R, Widom CS, Browne K, *et al.* (2009) Burden and consequences of child maltreatment in high-income countries. *Lancet* 373: 68–81.

Guardian (2010) Rio de Janeiro police occupy slums as city fights back against drug gangs. http://www.guardian.co.uk/world/2010/apr/12/rio-de-janeiro-police-occupy-slums (accessed July 2013).

Häuser W, Schmutzer G, Brähler E, Glaesmer H (2011) Maltreatment in childhood and adolescence: results from a survey of a representative sample of the German population. *Deutsches Ärzteblatt International* 108 (17): 287–94.

Humphreys G (2009) Healing child soldiers. *Bulletin of the World Health Organization* 87 (5): 330–1.

ISPCAN (2008) *World Perspectives on Child Abuse*. Chicago, IL: ISPCAN.

Krueger RF, Moffitt TE, Caspi A, Bleske A, Silva PA (1998) Assortative mating for antisocial behavior: developmental and methodological implications. *Behavior Genetics* 28: 173–86.

Lalor K, McElvaney R (2010) Child sexual abuse, links to later sexual exploitation/high-risk sexual behavior, and prevention/treatment programs. *Trauma, Violence, and Abuse* 11 (4): 159–77.

Lau C (2008) Child prostitution in Thailand. *Journal of Child Health Care* 12: 144–55.

Macy RJ, Graham LM (2012) Identifying domestic and international sex trafficking victims during human service provision. *Trauma, Violence, and Abuse* 13 (2): 59–76.

Rutter SM, Bishop D, Pine D, *et al.* (2008) *Rutter's Child and Adolescent Psychiatry*, 5th edn. Oxford: Blackwell.

Shalev I, Moffitt TE, Sugden K, *et al.* (2012) Exposure to violence during childhood is associated with telomere erosion from 5 to 10 years of age: a longitudinal study. *Molecular Psychiatry* 18: 576–81.

Srivastava R (2012) Child abuse and neglect: Asia Pacific Conference and the Delhi Declaration. *Indian Pediatrics* 49: 11–12.

Stoltenborgh M, van Ijzendoorn MH, Euser EM, Bakermans-Kranenburg MJ (2011) A global perspective on child sexual abuse: meta-analysis of prevalence around the world. *Child Maltreatment* 16: 79–101.

Troiano M (2011) Child abuse. *Nursing Clinics of North America* 46: 413–22.

Unicef (2011) *The State of the World's Children 2011. Adolescence: an Age of Opportunity*. New York, NY: Unicef.

World Health Organization (2006) *Preventing Child Maltreatment: a Guide to Taking Action and Generating Evidence*. Geneva: WHO.

Widom CS, Czaja SJ, Bentley T, Johnson MS (2012) A prospective investigation of physical health outcomes in abused and neglected children: new findings from a 30-year follow-up. *American Journal of Public Health* 102: 1135–44.

Chapter 23

Child soldiers

Ruwan M. Jayatunge and Daya Somasundaram

Introduction

Using children in armed conflicts has been reported in many countries around the world. Various rebel groups, and occasionally states, in Africa, Asia, and Latin America exploit children in their armed conflicts. It is estimated that some 300 000 children – boys and girls under the age of 18 – are today involved in more than 30 conflicts worldwide (Coalition to Stop the Use of Child Soldiers 2008). Often these children are kidnapped from their parents and indoctrinated, given brief training, and, along with the adult rebel cadres, sent to fight against fully trained, fully equipped government forces. Many child soldiers are killed in the war. Those who survive suffer deep physical and psychological traumas. These traumas affect their social and cognitive development. When the war ends, or when they are released or escape, the children often try to reunite with their families. Some go through a process of demobilization and rehabilitation. Despite re-education, rehabilitation, and social integration processes, a large number of child soldiers continue to suffer from the adverse effects of war.

Despite the adoption of the Convention on the Rights of the Child (CRC) by the General Assembly of the United Nations in 1989, war is an adult male preoccupation that exploits children. According to the Report of Graça Machel to the United Nations on the *Impact of Armed Conflict on Children* (1996):

> In recent decades, the proportion of war victims who are civilians has leaped dramatically from 5 per cent to over 90 per cent ... With all standards abandoned, human rights violations against children and women occur in unprecedented numbers. Increasingly, children have become the targets and even the perpetrators of violence and atrocities ... War violates every right of a child: the

right to life, the right to be with family and community, the right to health, the right to the development of the personality and the right to be nurtured and protected ... Disrupting the social networks and primary relationships that support children's physical, emotional, moral, cognitive and social development in this way, and for this duration, can have profound physical and psychological implications.

At the same time, wars may be about these rights, growing out of discrimination, socioeconomic inequities, and repression of a section of the population, including children.

The phenomena of child soldiers can be found manifesting in situations of horizontal inequalities between groups with clearly defined cultural or ethnic identities (Stewart 2001). Social instability that can lead to violent conflict grows out of severe inequalities in political, economic, and social dimensions between groups. These could include unequal access by different ethnic groups to valuable resources, such as the distribution and exercise of political power, employment, education, land, health care, food, public goods, mineral profits, and infrastructure. Ethnic and cultural deprivations can then become powerful mobilizing agents. The weaker and less resourced rebel forces, but at times even states, can resort to using children as soldiers. Often in situations of manpower shortage, where adult fighters have been killed, or are unwilling or unavailable, leaders in the weaker party may turn to women and children in asymmetrical warfare (Hassan 2008). The proliferation of modern weaponry which allows even children to handle them with ease (the AK47 or T56 assault rifles or small landmines are so light and easy to handle that children can be easily trained in their use), and of the arms traders in ensuring their supply, is also

---

Essentials of Global Mental Health, ed. Samuel O. Okpaku. Published by Cambridge University Press. © Cambridge University Press 2014.

crucial in this complex equation. There are huge profits to be made from the arms trade, and the manufacture and route of supply often involve the international community. Further, the level of the conflict has reached considerable sophistication. Training and arms come from various developed countries. Children on the frontlines become the pawns in adult male games and economic profit.

The conscription of children is a form of physical, emotional, and moral abuse, more so in the case of "suicide by proxy" (de Silva *et al.* 2001). However, it may not be enough merely to condemn or prohibit the recruitment of children. We must ask the deeper question, "Why do children join?" It is important to understand the context, particularly the systemic factors under which children become soldiers, and to work to counter those factors, if we are to effectively prevent it. At the same time, better understanding of the causal factors and the condition of the child soldiers would lead to designing a more comprehensive and effective demobilization, rehabilitation, and

reintegration program for them. The underlying sociopolitical, economic, and psychological factors that compel children to fight can be quite complex. One way to try and understand the complex contexts under which children become soldiers is to use *push–pull* categorization (Figure 23.1), as used by the International Labour Organization's International Programme on the Elimination of Child Labour in relation to child labor, and more specifically child soldiers.

Push factors
Traumatization

In war and violent conflict, children are traumatized by such common experiences as frequent shelling, bombing, helicopter strafing, round-ups, cordon-off and search operations, deaths, injury, destruction, mass arrests, detention, shootings, grenade explosions, and landmines. Studies focusing on children in war situations, for example in Mozambique (Richman

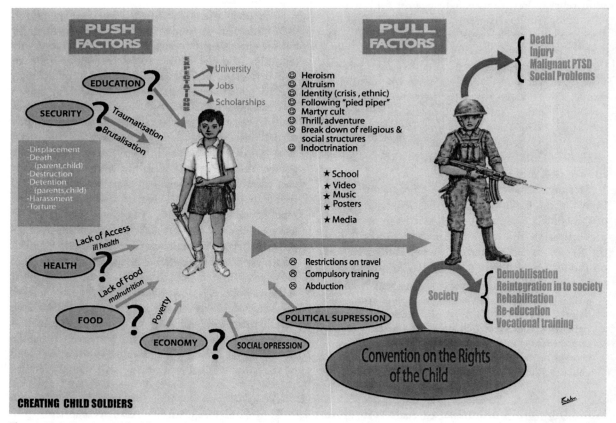

Figure 23.1 Creating child soldiers: understanding the context. Courtesy of Naguleswaran Srivigneswaran.

et al. 1988) and the Philippines (Children's Rehabilitation Center 1986), report considerable psychological sequelae. A detailed Canadian study of children in the Eastern Province of Sri Lanka found considerably more exposure to war trauma and psychological sequelae in the ethnic minority Tamil children (Health Reach 1996), similar to the same group's results from studies in Yugoslavia, Palestine, and Iraq. The impact of war on their growing minds, and the resulting traumatization and brutalization, is decisive in making them more likely to become child soldiers. In addition to the direct effects on children, war also results in collective trauma at the family and community levels (Somasundaram 2007). There is a breakdown of family and community processes, support structures and networks, ethical and moral values, cohesion and purpose. In this uncertain, insecure, and hopeless environment, children are more likely to look for alternative opportunities, follow alluring possibilities, and be compelled to make unwholesome choices. Brutalization resulting from growing up with violence and injustice, along with their vulnerability, their fear for their safety, and real threats would motivate them to protect themselves (and in their imagination, their families and community) with arms and training.

Deprivation

Many families that are displaced, without incomes, jobs, and food, may encourage one of their children to join so that at least they have something to eat. There is a higher incidence of malnutrition and ill health in the war-torn areas. Allocation and distribution of healthcare facilities (staff, drugs, equipment) to some areas may be markedly disproportional. Education and schools become disorganized. There are often real or perceived inequalities in opportunities for and access to further education, sports, foreign scholarships, and jobs for some groups compared to other more privileged groups. For the more conscious and concerned children, seeing or experiencing these deprivations for their family and community could push them into joining an armed resistance group.

Institutionalized violence

Discrimination and violence against certain groups become institutionalized, entrenched within the system, so much so that the terror and oppression are widely prevalent. Laws such as Prevention of Terrorism Acts and emergency regulations allow detention for long periods without judicial processing, torture, and "disappearance." The greatest impact of this kind of structural violence and oppression is on the younger generation. These conditions create a sense of fear, frustration, hopelessness, and general discontent. Joining becomes a means of putting things right.

Sociocultural factors

Another potent push factor is oppressive social practices, where the lower classes and castes are suppressed by the higher, who hold power and authority. For many from the lower classes, joining then becomes a way out of this oppressive system. Similarly, for younger females who experience the patriarchal oppression against their sex, it is a means of escape and "liberation."

Pull factors

Because of their age, immaturity, curiosity, and love of adventure, children are susceptible to "Pied Piper" enticement through a variety of psychological methods. Public displays of war paraphernalia, funerals and posters of fallen heroes; speeches and videos, particularly in schools; heroic, melodious songs and stories, drawing out feelings of patriotism and creating a martyr cult – all these create a compelling milieu. Severe restrictions on leaving areas create a feeling of entrapment, ensuring that there is a continuing source of recruits. Military-type training instills a military thinking.

In war and violent circumstances, sociocultural and religious leaders and institutions do not protect children or protest against child recruitment. The actions of the state in using indiscriminate violence such as heavy firepower, shooting, bombing, shelling, detention, and torture against a community is a powerful motivating factor.

Psychological consequences

Apart from death and injury, the recruitment of children becomes even more abhorrent when one sees the psychological consequences. In those that came for treatment, we found a whole spectrum of conditions from neurotic conditions such as somatization, depression, and post-traumatic stress disorder (PTSD) to more severe reactive psychosis and complex PTSD, which leaves the child a complete psychological and social wreck (Somasundaram 1998).

Numerous studies have shown that child soldiers are at high risk of developing PTSD and other disorders. Okello *et al.* (2007) found that 27–34.9% of Ugandan child soldiers suffered PTSD. Kohrt *et al.* (2008) found that 75 of 141 Nepali child soldiers (53.2%) met the symptom cut-off score for depression, 65 (46.1%) met the score for anxiety, 78 (55.3%) met the criteria for PTSD, 55 (39%) met the criteria for general psychological difficulties, and 88 (62.4%) were functionally impaired. A study conducted in Sri Lanka found higher rates of PTSD in children than adults who are conscripted (de Silva *et al.* 2001). The emotional consequences for the majority of the children interviewed included sad moods, preoccupations, suicidal thoughts and fears. Most of them experienced loss in relation to the death of members of their family and social status as a result of their actions. This study also found that while all children in Sri Lanka grew up as a generation knowing nothing but war, and being subjected to indoctrination so they would feel hatred against their enemy, the children who were conscripted were from families living in poverty. Children from privileged families either migrated out of the area or would have been released if they were conscripted.

Garvarino & Kostelny (1993) suggest that experiences related to political violence and war might constitute a serious risk for the well-functioning family. Most of the child soldiers were separated from their parents for a long period and many had lost the sense of family belongingness. Their family ties are wrecked. These children are separated from their cultural, social, and moral identity, and it makes them vulnerable to psychological and social ill effects. Those with PTSD have intrusive memories of the war, flashbacks, emotional arousal, emotional numbing, and various other anxiety-related symptoms. Many avoid places and conversations related to their past experiences. Some children are reluctant to go back to their native villages, maybe because of shame or guilt.

Avoidance, as described by the former child soldiers, included actively identifying social situations, physical locations, or activities that had triggered an emergence of post-traumatic stress symptoms in the past, and making efforts to avoid them in the future. One of the strongest traumatic re-experience triggers was physical location: some former child soldiers are now avoiding places where they witnessed or participated in violent and inhumane atrocities (Boothby *et al.* 2006).

War affects children in all the ways it affects adults, but also in different ways (Santa Barbara 2006). Combat trauma could affect children in all aspects of their lives, causing long-term effects that are now termed complex PTSD (Herman 1992). Common symptoms would include affect dysregulation characterized by persistent dysphoria, chronic suicidal preoccupation, self-injury, and explosive anger; dissociative episodes (which in African countries can be in the form of trance or possession states); somatization, memory disturbances, sense of helplessness and hopelessness; isolation and withdrawal, poor relationships, distrust, and loss of faith.

Our observation has been that children are particularly vulnerable during their impressionable formative period, leading to permanent scarring of their developing personality. Military leaders have expressed their preference for younger recruits as "they are less likely to question orders from adults and are more likely to be fearless, as they do not appreciate the dangers they face. Their size and agility makes them ideal for hazardous and clandestine assignments" (Amnesty International 2008).

Some of the child soldiers have managed to escape from their country but are still living with past memories of war. A study conducted by Kanagaratnam *et al.* (2005) focuses on ideological commitment and post-traumatic stress in a sample of former child soldiers from Sri Lanka living in exile in Norway. Using a sample of 20 former child soldiers, the researchers tried to find a correlation between ideological commitment and developing mental health problems.

Usually female child soldiers face hardships in the war front. Female child soldiers in Uganda, Sierra Leone, and Congo were frequently used as sex slaves, and they were repetitively raped by the adult fighters. The LTTE ("Tamil Tigers") used female child soldiers to commit murders when they attacked endangered villagers. There were groups of female LTTE cadres consisting mainly of underage girls called "clearance parties." The clearance party would advance after the assault group; their main task was to kill the wounded civilians or soldiers by using machetes. Gender appears to be a risk factor for PTSD; several studies suggest that girls are more likely than boys to develop PTSD (Hamblen 2007).

Attachment problems

When children were forcibly removed from their parents, many experienced separation anxiety. Some developed into full-blown symptoms of separation anxiety disorder (DSM-IV: American Psychiatric Association 1994). These children repeatedly cry, attempt to run away from the captors, have fear of being alone, and are sometimes troubled by nightmares. The senior cadres use physical violence and intimidation to train the newly recruited child soldiers. Bowlby (1969) believed that attachment behaviors are instinctive and will be activated by any conditions that seem to threaten the achievement of proximity, such as separation, insecurity, and fear.

Many child ex-combatants have apathy and poor attachment with their parents. The parents often feel that the child has changed dramatically and is unable to express love and warmth in return. Some express that there is an invisible wall between parents and child. The child seems to have lost the sense of trust in adults and feels that he has lost his identity as a valuable member of the society. The child becomes oppositional, defiant, and impulsive, and parents feel that the child acts as if adults do not exist in his world and does not look to adults for positive interactions. Some children created bonds with their abductors during their stay with them, and feel that they had a better time with the militants than with their parents.

Moral development

Children's moral development can be disrupted by their participation in armed conflicts. Normally children learn to conform to a number of social rules and expectations as they become participants in the culture (Nucci 1987). Children and adolescents who had been displaced by civil war in Colombia reported expecting that they and others would steal and hurt people despite acknowledging that it would be morally wrong to do so, and many of them, especially adolescents, judged that taking revenge against some groups was justifiable (Posada & Wainryb 2008).

Social learning theorists such as Albert Bandura (1990) claim that children initially learn how to behave morally through modeling. Many child soldiers had learned their social behavior through adult militants, and for a number of years these senior figures were their role models. They had learned that aggression and violence were acceptable behaviors and killing the enemy was correct. They were constantly taught that kindness, compassion, and forgiveness were signs of weakness. The senior members of the rebel forces killed and tortured in front of the

children, for them to observe and learn. According to Bandura's postulation, individuals acquire aggressive responses using the same mechanism that they do for other complex forms of social behavior: direct experience or the observation-modeling of others (Hart & Kritsonis 2006). For a number of years violence had become a way of life for these children. For years they believed that violence was a legitimate means of achieving one's aims, and it was an accepted form of behavior. They find it difficult to disengage from violent thoughts and transition to a non-violent lifestyle.

Participation in war and indoctrination into the ideologies of hatred and violence leaves children's moral sensibilities distorted. Children may hand over their guns, but they cannot so easily abandon the violent ways of thinking in which they have been trained. Part of demobilization is enabling the child to move away from violence and into a more inclusive and constructive way of life. The inclusion of peace education in curricula facilitates this process (Menon & Arganese 2007).

Cognitive development

Recruiting children for military purposes and exposing them to combat leads to problems in their cognitive development. When children are indoctrinated and forced to perform acts such as killings, destructions, and torture their cognitive schemas take a pathological shift. Their problem-solving skills are diminished, and logical thinking is suppressed by the ideology. They are taught to react instead of to think. They just obey orders from the senior militants and act like perfect killing machines. The time they spend in training and hiding in jungles, doing bunker duty and participating in various attacks, seriously limits them from having fruitful learning opportunities.

Lev Vygotsky's sociocultural theory emphasizes the role in development of cooperative dialogs between children and more knowledgeable members of the society (Woolfolk *et al.* 2011). The recruitment and military usage of children limits their associating with knowledgeable members of society such as teachers, clergy, and other community leaders. There were no educational or intellectual stimulations for the child soldiers. Vygotsky (1978) expressed the view that children learn the culture of their community through these interactions. For child soldiers, these interactions become restricted and their universe is limited to combat and violence. These children are deprived of cultural tools, with limited time to read or write. Their vocabulary mostly consists of war- and violence-based terms. Demobilized children have limited vocabulary and language skills. Children who start school with limited capacity in vocabulary develop more slowly than their peers who start with better vocabulary skills (Baker *et al.* 1997). It has been reported that many young child soldiers were unable to perform cognitive tasks such as reading comprehension, or to solve mathematical or word problems, during their stay with the rebels. Although many child soldiers wore wrist watches pompously, they were unable to read the time.

Learning difficulties

When rehabilitated, child soldiers go back to school once again. They have been away from the school environment for many years. Their cognitive and learning skills have been adversely affected by the war at a significant level. Despite all these odds, the children struggle to study and learn new social skills. The memories of war have not left them completely. Children prove most susceptible to anxiety and emotional problems. Teachers have observed a wide range of learning problems in former child soldiers. They have missed a vast amount of teachable moments with appropriate mentors, and instead have spent crucial time with rebels. Instead of reading, writing, and doing math they have been taught how to shoot and kill.

Some children have attention problems. Memory difficulties may be due to psychological distress that they experience. They continue to struggle with learning in the classrooms. In some schools peer rejection is recorded following their past history of war experience. The communities have not fully accepted back the former child combatants. When facing social rejection, former child soldiers experience embarrassment, confusion, and humiliation, and this could go hand in hand with falling behind their peers in school. Some are poorly motivated and show anger and frustration at school. The affected children become withdrawn, shy, anxious, and helpless, with a devalued sense of personal worth and lower personal expectations.

Experts believe that education is a form of powerful social integration and rehabilitative apparatus. Therefore education is the way out for most of these war victims. However, further research has found that although the majority of children greatly benefit from access to education, some former child soldiers are not interested in continuing their education (Boothby *et al.* 2006).

Appropriate help, including coaching in learning strategies, should be offered to the child ex-combatants with learning difficulties. Educational bridging programs work well in these settings, as they enable returning children to achieve some basic literacy and primary-level competencies in a relatively short time. Bridge programs effectively create a base from which the child can move to other learning options. In most cases, children proceed to vocational education. Vocational training exists to help children gain skills in agriculture, animal husbandry, baking, carpentry, crafting, masonry, mechanics, tailoring, and a variety of other trades (Menon & Arganese 2007).

Behavioral problems

Former child soldiers exposed to brutal episodes of war-related violence face a range of behavioral problems. In addition, post-conflict factors may contribute to varying degrees of vulnerability to adverse behavioral outcomes. According to Vygotsky (1978), the child's culture and the community that he or she lives in largely affects the child's development.

For a number of years child soldiers have spent time with adult militants under strict rules and regulations. The children were constantly exposed to hostile situations that had a negative impact on their psychosocial well-being. Their thinking patterns and cognitive schemas were changed into a more aggressive and violent direction. They were indoctrinated to perform atrocities without asking questions. They witnessed the gloomy realities of war, which made drastic changes in their behavior. The children who had committed atrocities in the past have a high risk of developing conduct disorders or anti-social personality disorder and addiction problems if their mental health issues are not appropriately addressed.

In Nepal, Kohrt *et al.* (2008) concluded that post-conflict factors such as stigma might contribute to adverse mental health outcomes. Former child soldiers in his sample showed significantly higher behavioral symptoms of depression and PTSD compared to matched controls, even after adjusting for exposure to traumatic events. Betancourt *et al.* (2010) did a prospective study to investigate psychosocial adjustment in male and female former child soldiers in Sierra Leone, using 156 male and female child soldiers. Over the two-year period of follow-up, children who had wounded or killed others during the war demonstrated increases in hostility. It has been reported that former child soldiers in Uganda had various behavioral problems, and some of them were charged with antisocial activity after their demobilization. Over 70% of prisoners in the juvenile crime unit in the Gulu District, Uganda, were former child soldiers, incarcerated on charges of rape, assault, and theft (Akello *et al.* 2006).

Social relationships play a key role in a child's behavior. Nested interacting spheres of social relationships that determine individual behavior and well-being are the fundamental components of analysis in social ecology (Bronfenbrenner 1979). When these children were abducted and kept in camps, they had no way of having healthy social relationships.

Problems of reintegration into society

Reintegration of the former child soldiers can be challenging. Some children have no families; either they have fled the country or they have been killed in the war. Child soldiers often face psychological and social problems. It has been reported that sometimes their community members ostracize these children, fearing their wartime activities. Some of these children had killed or tortured their relatives. These factors hinder the child soldiers' reintegrating back into society and living meaningful and productive lives.

A number of studies done in Asian, African, and Latin American countries show that the reintegration of child ex-soldiers faces similar challenges. In some countries the conflicts still prevail, and liberated child soldiers still have impending threats such as recapture by the rebels, persecution by the authorities, and attempts to harm them by the members of their community for past atrocities. The coordinators of Save the Children, Gulu, Uganda, found that three months after the rescue of 300 former child soldiers in 2004–05, none were found residing in the community in which they were supposed to have been reintegrated (Akello *et al.* 2006). It should be stressed that it is those responsible for the recruitment, training,

and deployment of child soldiers who should be charged as war criminals, not the child soldiers themselves who surrender or are captured. They should not be treated as criminals or juvenile delinquents, but offered appropriate psychological, socioeconomic, and educational opportunities for rehabilitation (Jareg & McCallin 1993).

Successful reintegration of child soldiers into society has been reported in many countries around the world. Angola's demobilization exercise, which lasted from 1995 to 1997, was one of the most extensive in the history of the United Nations. It was perhaps the first time that children were specifically included in a peace process. While not explicit in the 1994 Lusaka Protocol, their demobilization and reintegration was declared a priority in the first resolution adopted by the commission set up to implement the peace agreement. Partnerships among local civil society networks made it possible for many children to return to their homes (Verhey 2001). One longitudinal study documented that post-conflict experiences such as family support and economic opportunity played a role in the mental health of 39 Mozambican males re-interviewed 16 years after reintegration (Boothby *et al.* 2006). Post-conflict rehabilitation is crucial to the child ex-combatants. The society should be empathetic and create a healthy environment for these traumatized children, so that they can recuperate and reintegrate into society as productive members. Betancourt *et al.* (2010) are of the view that former child soldiers' acute war experiences have long-term consequences, but the nature and extent of these consequences are influenced by post-conflict risk and protective factors.

Verhey (2001) highlights that reintegration of child soldiers should emphasize three components: family reunification, psychosocial support and education, and economic opportunity.

Prevention

The only way to reduce the phenomenon of child soldiers is to work on the push and pull factors described above. Towards this end, civil society, the state, and the international community have an important role to play. The state must act to ameliorate the socioeconomic and political conditions that push children into becoming soldiers. The state will have to systematically dismantle the structures of inequity, discrimination, and violence. Particularly, it should create opportunity structures in education, employment, and development, opening the doors to children and youth for advancement. The international community can curtail the funding and support for war to all sides from international sources, both direct and indirect, as well as apply pressure to conduct war within some norms, such as the Geneva Conventions, its additional protocols, and the Convention on the Rights of the Child. The role of modern weaponry such as the AK47 or a hand grenade, which even children can handle with ease, and of the arms traders in ensuring their supply, is also crucial in this complex equation. The economic profit from the arms trade, including manufacture and route of supply, can be controlled. In her report to the UN on the impact of armed conflict on children, Graça Machel (1996) concludes that "the most effective way to protect children is to prevent the outbreak of armed conflicts."

Acknowledgments

Dr. Naguleswaran (Babu) prepared Figure 23.1. Some of the material in this chapter has been published perviously (Somasundaram 2002, Jayatunge 2012). The authors gratefully acknowledge interviews with many involved in the rehabilitation of child soldiers, and with child soldiers themselves.

References

Akello G, Richters A, Reis R (2006) Reintegration of former child soldiers in northern Uganda: coming to terms with children's agency and accountability. *Intervention* 4: 229–43. http://www.ourmediaourselves.com/archives/43pdf/akello.pdf (accessed July 2013).

American Psychiatric Association (1994) *Diagnostic and Statistical Manual of Mental Disorders, Fourth Edition (DSM-IV)*. Washington, DC: APA.

Amnesty International (1998) *Children in South Asia*. London: AI.

Baker SK, Simmons DC, Kameenui EJ (1997) Vocabulary acquisition: research bases. In DC Simmons, EJ Kameenui, eds., *What Reading Research Tells Us About Children with Diverse Learning Needs: Bases and Basics*. Mahwah, NJ: Erlbaum; pp. 183–218.

Bandura A (1990) Mechanisms of moral disengagement. In W Reich, ed., *Origins of Terrorism: Psychologies, Ideologies, Theologies, States of Mind*. Cambridge: Cambridge University Press; pp. 161–91.

Betancourt TS, Borisova II, Williams TP, *et al.* (2010) Sierra Leone's former child soldiers: a follow-up study of psychosocial adjustment and community reintegration. *Child Development* 81: 1077–95.

Boothby N, Crawford J, Halperin J (2006) Mozambique child soldier life outcome study: lessons learned in rehabilitation and reintegration efforts. Global Public Health 1: 87–107.

Bowlby J (1969) *Attachment and Loss*. New York, NY: Basic Books.

Bronfenbrenner U (1979) *The Ecology of Human Development: Experiments by Nature and Design*. Cambridge, MA: Harvard University Press.

Coalition to Stop the Use of Child Soldiers (2008) *Child Soldiers Global Report 2008*. London: The Coalition.

Children's Rehabilitation Center (1986) Psychological help to child victims of political armed conflict. Philippines: CRC.

de Silva H, Hobbs C, Hanks H (2001) Conscription of children in armed conflict: a form of child abuse. A study of 19 former child soldiers. *Child Abuse Review*, 10: 125–34.

Garvarino J, Kostelny K (1993). Children's response to war: what do we know? In L Leavitt, N Fox, eds., *The Psychological Effects of War and Violence on Children*. Hillsdale, NJ: Erlbaum.

Hamblen J (2007) PTSD in children and ddolescents. National Centre for PTSD fact sheet. Washington, DC: United States Department of Veteran Affairs. http://www.isu.edu/irh/projects/better_todays/B2T2VirtualPacket/Trauma/PTSD%20in%20Children%20and%20Adolescents%20-%20(National%20Center%20for%20PTSD.pdf (accessed July 2013).

Hart KE, Kritsonis WA (2006) Critical analysis of an original writing on social learning theory: *Imitation of Film-Mediated Aggressive Models* by Albert Bandura, Dorothea Ross and Sheila A. Ross (1963). *National Forum of Applied Educational Research Journal* 19 (3).

Hassan R (2008) *Suicide Bombings: an Analysis of Global Trends 1981–2006*. Adelaide: Flinders University.

Health Reach (1996) *The Health of Children in Conflict Zones of Sri Lanka*. Hamilton, Ontario: Centre for International Health and the Centre for Peace Studies, McMaster University.

Herman J (1992) *Trauma and Recovery*. London: Pandora.

Jareg E, McCallin M (1993) *The Rehabilitation of Former Child Soldiers*. Geneva: International Catholic Child Bureau.

Jayatunge RM (2012) Psychosocial problems of the Sri Lankan child soldiers. *Lankaweb*. http://www.

lankaweb.com/news/items/2012/03/28/psychosocial-problems-of-the-sri-lankan-child-soldiers (accessed July 2013).

Kanagaratnam P, Raundalen M, Asbjornsen AE (2005) Ideological commitment and posttraumatic stress in former Tamil child soldiers. *Scandinavian Journal of Psychology* **46**: 511–20.

Kohrt BA, Jordans MJD, Tol WA, *et al.* (2008) Comparison of mental health between former child soldiers and children never conscripted by armed groups in Nepal. *JAMA* **300**: 691–702.

Machel G (1996) *Impact of Armed Conflict on Children.* New York, NY: United Nations, Unicef.

Menon G, Arganese A (2007) Role of education and demobilization of child soldiers: aspects of an appropriate education program for child soldiers. USAID, American Institutes for Research (EQUIP1 LWA). Issue Paper 2. http://pdf.usaid.gov/pdf_docs/PNADI663.pdf (accessed July 2013).

Nucci L (1987) Synthesis of research on moral development. *Educational Leadership* February 1987: 86–92.

Okello J, Onen TS, Musisi S (2007) Psychiatric disorders among war-abducted and non-abducted adolescents in Gulu district, Uganda: a comparative study. *African Journal of Psychiatry* **10**: 225–31.

Posada R, Wainryb C (2008) Moral development in a violent society: Colombian children's judgments in the context of survival and revenge. *Child Development* **79**: 882–98.

Richman H, Kanji N, Zinkin P (1988) *Report on Psychological Effects of War on Children in Mozambique.* London: Save the Children Fund.

Santa Barbara J (2006) Impact of war on children and imperative to end war. *Croatian Medical Journal* **47**: 891–4.

Somasundaram D (1998) *Scarred Minds: the Psychological Impact of the War on Sri Lankan Tamils.* New Delhi: Sage.

Somasundaram D (2002) Child soldiers: understanding the context. *BMJ* **324**: 1268–71.

Somasundaram D (2007) Collective trauma in northern Sri Lanka: a qualitative psychosocial-ecological study. *Sri Lanka International Journal of Mental Health Systems* **1**: 5.

Stewart F (2001) Horizontal inequalities: a neglected dimension of development. Oxford: Centre for Research on Inequality, Human Security and Ethnicity (CRISE Working Paper, 1).

Verhey B (2001) Child soldiers: preventing, demobilizing and reintegrating. World Bank (Africa Region Working Paper Series, 23). http://www.worldbank.org/afr/wps/wp23.pdf (accessed July 2013).

Vygotsky LS (1978) *Mind in Society: Development of Higher Psychological Processes,* ed. VJ Steiner, M Cole, S Scribner, E Souberman. Cambridge, MA: Harvard University Press.

Woolfolk A, Winne P, Perry N (2011) *Educational Psychology,* 4th Canadian edn. Toronto: Pearson.

Chapter

24

Mental health and intellectual disability: implications for global mental health

Marco Bertelli and M. Thomas Kishore

Introduction

Intellectual disability (ID) is one of the severe neurodevelopmental disorders, affecting both intellect and adaptive behaviors, and it is included in the category of mental disorders in the international classification systems. ID is a permanent condition, associated with a high comorbidity of physical and mental disorders worldwide. It is associated with high levels of caregiving burden, and implies high service provision, producing high health and societal costs (Bertelli *et al.* 2009, Salvador-Carulla *et al.* 2011). Despite this, ID is a neglected area both in the field of general health and in mental health everywhere, but the problems are more evident in low- and middle-income countries (LMICs). In this context, this chapter highlights various issues related to mental health in ID, and the kind of solutions that may be provided to meet the challenges in global mental health.

Essential problems for intellectual disability, and implications for global health

ID is not a disease but a syndrome grouping, similar to the construct of dementia. It includes a heterogeneous group of typical clinical frames with different etiologies, ranging from genetic to environmental factors. A significant proportion of persons with ID may have multiple disabilities and other medical conditions (Bertelli *et al.* 2009). Furthermore, ID imposes a considerable burden on families and caregivers throughout the lifespan (Salvador-Carulla & Bertelli 2008). Therefore, ID requires full attention with regard to both general health needs and mental health needs.

The prevalence rate of ID in northern European countries is reportedly around 1.5%, but it may rise to 4–6% in deprived regions of the world (Durkin 2002). In LMICs, the excess rate of ID is related to fully preventable etiologies such as teratogens, diet deficiencies, pregnancy, and birth-related conditions (Persha *et al.* 2007, Bertelli *et al.* 2009). In at least 30–50% of cases, the etiology is not identified even after thorough diagnostic evaluation (Armatas 2009). The percentage of undetected etiology could be somewhat higher than this in LMICs, as indicated by the available data (Bhatt *et al.* 2008, Ahmad & Phalke 2009). Barring a few genetic and congenital problems, the causes of ID are usually not given full attention by the international agencies (Salvador-Carulla *et al.* 2000). Bertelli *et al.* (2009) identified four major factors that may be responsible for this situation: (1) lack of a reliable construct of intelligence and a common international procedure for IQ measurement; (2) lack of comprehensive epidemiological data, which would be crucial in raising public awareness and providing a roadmap to service delivery; (3) lack of adequate attention from the health sector, as ID is usually included not within the remit of the division of health but within the social or educational sector in many countries; and (4) low allocation of funds, as ID is not a key topic in many national health research programs.

The challenges start right at the level of terminology used to refer ID, as it is not uniform across the countries. The terms "mental retardation" (MR), "learning disabilities," and "intellectual disabilities" have coexisted during the past 15 years. Although still used in many diagnostic systems, MR and learning disabilities are considered outdated terms, whereas ID is increasingly accepted, as is evident in the titles of scientific journals (e.g., the *Journal of Intellectual*

Essentials of Global Mental Health, ed. Samuel O. Okpaku. Published by Cambridge University Press. © Cambridge University Press 2014.

Disability Research) and the names of international organizations (e.g., the International Association for the Scientific Study of Intellectual Disabilities, and the American Association on Intellectual and Developmental Disabilities). There are also lesser-known terms such as "developmental cognitive disability" used in some parts of the USA. At the same time the term MR continues to be officially used in many countries, with wide variations in the assessment and diagnostic processes. Although the terms ID and IaDD (intellectual and developmental disabilities) reflect the nature of the condition better than the other terms, none of them convey any additional information from the healthcare perspective.

Recently the World Health Organization International Classification of Diseases Working Group on the Classification of ID proposed to replace the term MR with the concept of "intellectual developmental disorders (IDD)." According to the working group, IDD and ID describe two different but related aspects of the same construct and have different scientific, social, and policy applications. IDD refers to a health condition – a syndromic grouping or meta-syndrome analogous to the construct of dementia – and has to be coded by the *International Classification of Diseases* (ICD), while "intellectual disability" refers to its functioning/disability counterpart and should be coded by the *International Classification of Functioning, Disability and Health* (ICF) (Salvador-Carulla et al. 2011). However, past trends strongly suggest that the debate on the terminology will continue in the years to come, and so we are left with the dilemma of whether ID is a health problem or a social problem. Meanwhile, it is desirable that the healthcare goals are guided more by the nature and needs of ID than by the labels.

Why the psychiatry of intellectual disability deserves a central place in general psychiatry

It is a general view that ID imposes considerable burden on families, caregivers, societies, not to mention the individual. Family burden is very high when there is a comorbidity of psychiatric disorders (Irazabal et al. 2012). Psychiatric and behavioral disorders are one of the main reasons for segregation and stigma associated with ID (McIntyre et al. 2002). Nearly 50% of people with ID need psychiatric care, far surpassing the mental health needs of the general

population (Cooper et al. 2007, Salvador-Carulla & Bertelli 2008). Globally there is a serious deficiency of mental health services and resources for persons with ID, especially in most LMICs. But at the same time it cannot be said that ID uniformly figures at the bottom of health care across LMICs. For example, in countries such as India, one finds state-of-art facilities for ID, primarily at national and regional level government agencies and in the private sector, though they are relatively few and are usually located at urban settings, while mental health or rehabilitation facilities are sparse in the rural settings where the majority of the disabled population lives.

A review conducted by Salvador-Carulla and Bertelli (2008) highlighted several dimensions of why ID should be given more attention in psychiatry. First, ID provides genetic models for scores of psychiatric disorders, as it is one among the few syndromes found at an increased frequency in other major psychiatric disorders such as schizophrenia, bipolar disorder, major depressive disorder, and autism spectrum disorders (Grayton et al. 2012, Van Den Bossche et al. 2012), which are now considered a unique group of disorders affecting neurodevelopment (Owen 2012). ID also provides models for the assessment, support, and diagnostic frameworks (e.g., provision for incorporating a developmental/ideographic approach) in severe mental and cognitive disorders. Further, models of care (e.g., residential care, respite care, multidisciplinary approach to care) and social issues of health (e.g., stigma and labeling, self-advocacy) were developed first in the ID field, and are now widely used in general psychiatry. The need for close interaction between various agencies within the social, educational, legal, and health sectors, to integrate services for holistic management of the individual, had its origins in the ID field. Therefore, the mainstream mental health field could benefit from the field of ID regarding successful models of identification, assessment, care, and support systems. At another level, more than any other mental health condition, ID provides ample opportunities to explore the clinical expression of the relaltionship between body and mind (Bertelli & Brown 2006).

Essential problems in the psychiatry of intellectual disability

A third of people with ID have comorbid psychiatric disorders, and another 10–20% have behavioral problems not related to psychiatric illness. Nearly one-half (0.75–2% of the total population) need psychiatric care, surpassing any known major psychiatric disorder (Salvador-Carulla *et al.* 2000). In spite of its global burden, ID is regarded as a second-level condition within psychiatry. The nature of ID, along with the expertise and attitudes of the mental health professionals and a lack of rigorous clinical trials, may partly explain the situation. The cognitive limitations of persons with ID pose greater challenges for assessment, diagnosis, and treatment. It is always a task to differentiate between the symptoms of mental health disorders and developmental problems in ID (Szymanski & King 1999, Ailey 2003). These issues highlight the importance of high-quality training for mental health professionals. In many countries, hands-on training in ID is not included in the psychiatric curriculum and there are limited clinical and practice guidelines to rely on. Several studies indicate that there is a need to enhance clinical training opportunities for psychiatrists to improve their knowledge, competence, and attitudes (Kwok & Chui 2008, Jeevanandam 2009, Werner & Stawski 2012). Furthermore, there is a need for information on rigorous research trials related to interventions to help health professionals to take appropriate decisions. But an extensive database search spanning over 16 years by Balogh *et al.* (2008) indicated that there were only six randomized controlled trials and virtually none on organizational interventions.

Evidence suggests that the settings in which evaluations are carried out may influence the diagnostic decisions (Nezu 1994). For example, in a psychiatric setting there will be a bias towards a psychiatric diagnosis while in educational settings the bias is to see every problem as an inappropriately reinforced maladaptive behavior. Even after accurate diagnosis, people with both ID and mental health problems may slip through the service delivery system in many countries, as the services are dichotomized into hospital-based services, usually meant for the general population, and rehabilitation and/or special education services, meant for people with disabilities including those with ID. This division is increased further when there is no coordination between the agencies managing these two systems. Evidently, we could find unmet mental health needs across the lifespan, and more so with increased severity levels of ID (Allerton *et al.* 2011).

Epidemiology and phenomenology of psychiatric disorders in intellectual disability

There are very few population-based prevalence studies, and hardly any studies on the incidence of mental health problems in persons with ID. Nonetheless, conventional estimates indicate that individuals with ID have at least the same prevalence of mental health disorders as the general population, and may have increased susceptibility to some types of mental health disorders (Ailey 2003). The existing data are limited by various methodological problems, making comparisons difficult. The methodological issues are mainly related to the operational definition of ID, representativeness of samples, and adaptation of standard diagnostic criteria (Smiley 2005). There is ample evidence to suggest that psychiatric comorbidity varies considerably depending on the diagnostic tools used (Kishore *et al.* 2004, Cooper *et al.* 2007). Even the results of standard diagnostic systems, namely the *Diagnostic Criteria for Psychiatric Disorders for use with Adults with Learning Disabilities/Mental Retardation*, the *Diagnostic and Statistical Manual of Mental Disorders Fourth Edition*, and the *ICD-10 Classification of Mental and Behavioral Disorders*, may not corroborate (Cooper *et al.* 2007).

The reliability of the information source, including the individual with ID, is often in question. Sovner (1986) identified several problems at the individual level. First, there could be "intellectual distortion," which refers to limitations in abstract thinking and verbal expressions interfering with the communicative content as well as intent. Further, the information given by the individual can be compounded by the social skill deficits and life experiences, leading to atypical presentation (a phenomenon referred to as "psychosocial masking"), stress-induced disruption of information processing ("cognitive disintegration"), and rise in pre-existing maladaptive behaviors ("baseline exaggeration"). Another frequent problem is diagnostic overshadowing, which refers to the difficulty clinicians have in distinguishing between psychiatric symptoms and behavioral alterations or expressive methods associated with ID in general and with certain phenotypes in particular (Reiss & Szyszko 1983). Other sources of information are usually limited, heterogeneous, and contradictory in this type of setting. Family members often have trouble answering questions aimed at understanding the presence of other disabilities in the subject's mental functioning. Furthermore, clinical files and other archived documentation are often incomplete and inexact. Understandably, the symptomatology can be intermittent, fluctuating, atypical, masked, mixed, poorly defined, or extremely rigid. For all of these reasons the application of rating scales developed for the general population to people with ID will have its limitations. This in turn stresses the need for specific tools to simplify the psychodiagnostic procedure and to aid epidemiological data in ID. In this context, it is apt to review some of the existing tools.

The first tool, PIMRA (Psychopathology Instrument for Mentally Retarded Adults: Matson *et al.* 1984), is still considered a benchmark. It is related to DSM diagnostic criteria. PIMRA is found to be very useful in research settings, in therapeutic planning, and in the evaluation of treatment outcomes (Swiezy *et al.* 1995).

The second tool, DASH (Diagnostic Assessment for the Severely Handicapped: Matson *et al.* 1991) and its revision (DASH-II: Matson 1995) are based mainly on the detection of key symptoms related to different syndromes, which could be defined by frequency, duration, and severity.

The PAS-ADD (Psychiatric Assessment Schedule for Adults with Developmental Disabilities Checklist: Moss *et al.* 1993) was designed for the diagnosis of psychiatric disorders in adults with ID according to ICD-10. There are mini versions of this tool intended for identification and screening (Prosser *et al.* 1998, Moss *et al.* 1998).

All these tools have certain limitations. PIMRA is more suitable for those who can communicate verbally (La Malfa *et al.* 1997), and has demonstrated problems of inter-rater reliability (Havercamp & Reiss 1996). There are some concerns on the criterion validity of DASH, and on the sensitivity and inter-rater reliability of PASS-ADD. Among the others, RSMB (Reiss Screen for Maladpative Behaviors: Reiss 1988) and SPAID (Psychiatric Instrument for the Intellectually Disabled Adults: Bertelli *et al.* 2012a) are used for screening and diagnosis, respectively. But RSMB is mainly meant for screening while SPAID is relatively new and has been standardized only on the Italian population.

A recent study indicates that the sensitivity of the tools for individual psychiatric disorders is quite varied (Myrbakk & von Tetzchner 2008), indicating that there is scope for refining the existing tools or developing new scales. It is desirable that there are screening tools for non-medical setting (e.g., schools, vocational centers, community centers) where the ID cohorts attend on a regular basis, so that caregivers or instructors can utilize them, and seek timely intervention. As far as the psychiatrists are concerned, many recent studies have indicated that the clinician's own experience, behavioral descriptions, and clinical observations are more helpful than the screening or diagnostic tools. Hence more emphasis is required on training.

Burden on caregivers and family quality of life

The predominant view is that ID is associated with considerable burden because it presents special challenges not only to the individual but also to the family (Neely-Barnes & Dia 2008, Kishore 2011). The challenges for the caregivers/families could be in the form of meeting special needs that the condition creates (e.g., meeting the healthcare needs if there is an associated condition such as epilepsy or hypothyroidism), or understanding and fulfilling age-appropriate needs (e.g. recreational, social, and educational needs) against the backdrop of a certain degree of intellectual impairment. In addition, families will face the continual demands of meeting their own needs. These issues may overwhelm the families, both on a daily basis and long term, and may affect the quality of life (QoL) of individuals with ID, caregivers, and family members. But it is not the case that every family will buckle under the pressure of caregiving. A few studies have reported that some parents and families will even experience a sense of purpose, psychological growth, tolerance, sensitivity, and heightened family functioning (Neely-Barnes & Dia 2008, Kishore 2011).

Studies focusing on the impact of ID on families point to the fact that the individual's characteristics (e.g., age, gender, and associated conditions) and family characteristics (e.g., educational and socioeconomic status) mediate the impact of the disability. But mental health problems in individuals with ID and caregivers' perceptions of disability have been consistently associated with high stress, negative impact, and low QoL (Miodrag & Hodapp 2010). A recent study confirms that behavioral problems and mental health disorders alone account for more than 61% of the variance in family burden (Irazabal *et al.* 2012). An equally important finding is that ID alone, irrespective of the associated conditions, can leave a negative impact on caregivers and families (Kishore 2011). Collectively these findings imply that intervention strategies should focus on reducing the disability associated with ID, altering the caregivers' perceptions of disability, and treating comorbid mental health disorders to strengthen both the individuals and the families. In this context, cross-cultural studies could be planned to explore the concept of disability in order to develop culturally relevant intervention models to facilitate positive coping in caregivers. It should be of special interest to study to what extent positive coping strategies and positive reappraisal are helpful in reducing the disability impact and family burden. Information generated in this way could be generalized to other developmental disorders and chronic psychiatric disorders where caregiving and family burden is a serious issue.

The rise of new person-centered outcome measures: quality of life

The concept of QoL, which originated in the broader fields of psychology and psychiatry, has successfully been applied in the field of ID. It is increasingly advocated that QoL should be a measure of treatment and intervention outcome in ID. Since QoL is widely understood and used as a multidimensional concept, contexts are essential to clarify the same (Bertelli *et al.* 2011a). Though the concept of QoL is considered too abstract and subjective to have sufficient precision to provide practical supports to people with ID, there is a considerable amount of substantive work both within and outside the system of health care (Renwick & Brown 1996, Wong *et al.* 2011). For practical purposes, the QoL approach is understood to be more about choosing a course that helps people to be satisfied with their own lives in ways that are customary to them and valued by them. Within this broad framework, QoL provides an alternative to the traditional medical approach in that it emphasizes understanding, respecting, and providing what is important to and valued by each individual, and what aspects of life or the environment contribute positively to life quality (O'Dell *et al.* 2012). One of the fundamental principles of QoL is that it is important for all people, and that all people are thus entitled to a life of quality (Brown & Brown 2003). This principle applies

equally to people with ID and to people who do not have ID.

Given that QoL depends on a host of individual and environmental factors that persons with ID either lack or are deprived of, the question of how we can ensure entitlement to a life of quality for people with ID who have mental health problems is an interesting and challenging one. First it is necessary that mental health professionals value the needs and choices of people with ID, and believe that it is possible to improve their life conditions. This in turn helps them recognize the use of positive interventions that view the health – and indeed the whole life – of people with ID in more holistic and integrated ways. When mental health professionals work with people who have ID, it is helpful to consider three aspects of QoL, in the form of (1) personal QoL, (2) shared QoL, and (3) family QoL.

All three are relevant in the context of care and service provision, but personal QoL ranks above the others, as ultimately it is the individual's perceptions, attitudes, values, and other attributes that determine how his or her life is experienced. At the same time, each individual is expected to be a social being, and hence shared QoL is also important. The shared QoL could be understood in terms of the social support made available by the family, work place, and community. Thus the QoL concept needs to be explored at both a personal and a shared level (Brown & Brown 2003). Similarly, family QoL is relevant for ID, as families can influence and be influenced by the nature of the disability (Turnbull *et al.* 2006). The number of people with ID living with their families and communities is on the rise worldwide, often without any entitlement to services. But families may need professional services and social support to achieve lives of quality. Therefore, family outcome needs to be determined with reference to the impact of a disability on the family. Speaking of the family outcome, "stress and caregiving burden," "impact on family functioning," and "eco-cultural adaptation" are important dimensions of the disability impact (Summers *et al.* 2005). However, there is a need for robust models to understand family QoL.

Of late, QoL measurement is gaining more importance, as there is growing support for evidence-based practice and QoL is being widely recognized as a key indicator of intervention outcomes (Brown & Brown 2003). It implies that there should be clear evidence that our mental health practices contribute positively to a person's QoL. Though there are conceptual differences between the generic and health-related QoL, the growing need for new, patient-oriented outcome measures has brought QoL to the center of mental health care in ID (Bertelli *et al.* 2009).

As far as measurement is concerned, the source and the tools applied need specific consideration. Several reviews on ID indicate that QoL should include both quantitative and qualitative aspects and interpretations should be according to both objective and subjective principles (Bertelli & Brown 2006). While the individual's views are important, they need to be corroborated with the caregivers' account, even though they may not necessarily match (Bertelli *et al.* 2011b). As Brown *et al.* (1997) found, significant others frequently make decisions on behalf of a person with ID, or are influential in helping the person with ID to make decisions, and thus the perspectives of the others are equally important. Additionally, proxy data can add clarity and depth to historical information, which might otherwise be missing due to individual skill deficits.

Another pertinent issue is how to quantify or measure QoL. Despite several advances in the conceptualization and measurement of QoL, there is a need for generic instruments that can be applied to individuals, irrespective of health condition, disability, culture, or socioeconomic status (Townsend-White *et al.* 2012). Currently there is no formula for assessing QoL, nor should there be. Rather, the QoL approach is above all a way to explore the rich intricacies of personal quality of life (see, e.g., the Life Satisfaction Matrix: Lyons, 2005). QoL assessment should guide personal and service choices, rather than representing a classification of individuals, services, or systems (Verdugo *et al.* 2005). It should help provide, within a given system of services and organizations, a value system that is consistent with those values held by people with ID. At a broader level, QoL can represent an integral and multidimensional view of health of the persons with ID that allows the multidisciplinary team to identify needs and wishes of the individual and plan interventions in the most useful way. Thus it is anticipated that the QoL approach mobilizes and reappraises resources that can help the individuals, and the systems they represent, to continue developing personal skills across their lifespan. For the field of mental health, understanding that the QoL concept can be applied to everyday practice in a way that is systematic, reliable, and helpful is the challenge for the near future. To address this challenge, we will need methodologically rigorous research and, more importantly, cross-cultural studies that evaluate the effectiveness of QoL in healthcare practice over a longer period.

Relationship between individual and family quality of life

There is abundant literature on both individual and family QoL in ID, but there is no empirical evidence to suggest that the relationship between them is robust (Summers *et al.* 2005). Rather, the relationship is influenced by the level of disability and behavioral problems in the individual (Baker *et al.* 2002, Wang *et al.* 2004). Bertelli and collaborators recently made an attempt to study the possible relationship between individual QoL and family QoL in a more structured way, with the help of standardized tools (Bertelli *et al.* 2011b, 2012b). They found significant negative correlation between all the main domains of individual QoL and the domains of family QoL (i.e., health, relationships, support, career, and family values). These findings may suggest that personal QoL and family QoL are different. Hence, it is desirable that all dimensions of QoL are assessed, with due recognition for variability across families and individuals, in order to make an effective intervention plan.

Future directions

A key public health function is to address health disparities and the social determinants of health, specifically as they relate to disability (Cameron *et al.* 2005). Using ID as a model, the following steps may be adapted for use in developing global mental health strategies more widely:

- To plan population-based, large-scale studies on the prevalence and incidence of mental health problems in ID. While doing so, it is important to make a distinction between psychosocially deprived and advantaged groups. Such data could be compared with data from the non-ID population to address health inequalities and ensure access to health care.
- To work out a universally acceptable framework for assessment and diagnosis of ID and associated mental health needs. Such efforts will hopefully broaden our insights into the mental health needs

of diverse population with developmental problems, communication difficulties, and cognitive deficits.

- To develop or validate screening tools for psychiatric problems and QoL through international collaborations, particularly for the use of frontline workers such as social workers, educators, and caregivers.
- To identify the preventable environmental determinants of health inequalities for people with ID, and to compare them with other developmental or chronic psychiatric disorders, in order to develop inclusive models of health care.

- To integrate general health services and mental health services within the available resources and policies, particularly in LMICs. Any research outcome in this regard could be extrapolated to meet the mental health needs of special groups.
- To identify the scope, methods, and challenges of involving individuals with ID, other severe developmental disorders, and cognitive disorders in healthcare decisions.
- To periodically review the quality of manpower training in the field of mental health and ID, recognizing that there is a need for further evidence and adapting evidence-based guidelines.

References

Ahmad N, Phalke DB (2009) Study of health status and etiological factors of mentally challenged children in schools for mentally challenged children. *Pravara Medical Reviews* **4** (1): 17–20.

Ailey SH (2003) Beyond the disability: recognizing mental health issues among persons with intellectual and developmental disabilities. *Nursing Clinics of North America* **38**: 313–29.

Allerton LA, Welch V, Emerson E (2011) Health inequalities experienced by children and young people with intellectual disabilities: a review of literature from the United Kingdom. *Journal of Intellectual Disabilities* **15**: 269–78.

Armatas V (2009) Mental retardation: definitions, etiology, epidemiology and diagnosis. *Journal of Sport and Health Research* **1**: 112–22.

Baker BL, Blacher J, Crnic KA, Edelbrock C (2002) Behavior problems and parenting stress in families of three-year-old children with and without developmental delays. *American Journal of Mental Retardation* **107**: 433–44.

Balogh R, Ouellette-Kuntz H, Bourne L, Lunsky Y, Colantonio A (2008) Organising health care services for persons with an intellectual disability. *Cochrane Database of Systematic Reviews* **4**: CD007492.

Bertelli M, Brown I (2006) Quality of life for people with Intellectual disability. *Current Opinion in Psychiatry* **19**: 508–13.

Bertelli M, Hassiotis A, Deb S, Salvador-Carulla L (2009) New contributions of psychiatric research in the field of intellectual disability. In GN Christodoulou, M Jorge, JE Mezzich, eds., *Advances in Psychiatry*. Athens: Beta Medical Publishers; pp. 37–43.

Bertelli M, Piva Merli M, Bianco A, et al. (2011a) A Battery of Instruments to assess Quality of Life (BASIQ): validation of the Italian adaptation of the Quality of Life Instrument Package (QoL-IP). *Italian Journal of Psychopathology* **17**: 205–12.

Bertelli M, Bianco A, Rossi M, Scuticchio D, Brown I (2011b) Relationship between individual quality of life and family quality of life for people with intellectual disability living in Italy. *Journal of Intellectual Disability Research* **55**: 1136–50.

Bertelli M, Scuticchio D, Ferrandi A, et al. (2012a) Reliability and vailidity of the SPAID-G checklist for detecting psychiatric disorders in adults with intellectual disability. *Research in Developmental Disabilities* **33**: 382–90.

Bertelli M, Bianco A, Scuticchio D, Brown I (2012b) Individual and family quality of life in intellectual

disability: a challenging relationship. In F Maggino, G Nuvolati, eds., *Quality of Life in Italy: Research and Reflections*. Amsterdam: Springer; pp. 305–19.

Bhatt C, Mishra Z, Goyel N (2008) Detection of inherited metabolic diseases in children with mental handicap. *Indian Journal of Clinical Biochemistry* **23** (1): 10–16.

Brown I, Brown RI (2003) *Quality of Life and Disability: an Approach for Community Practitioners*. London: Jessica Kingsley.

Brown I, Raphael D, Renwick R (1997) *Quality of Life-Dream or Reality? Life for People with Developmental Disabilities in Ontario*. Toronto: University of Toronto Centre for Health Promotion.

Cameron DL, Nixon S, Parnes P, Pidsadny M (2005) Children with disabilities in low-income countries. *Paediatric Child Health* **10** (5): 269–272.

Cooper SA, Smiley E, Finlayson J, et al. (2007) The prevalence, incidence, and factors predictive of mental ill-health in adults with profound intellectual disabilities. *Journal of Applied Research in Intellectual Disabilities* **20**: 493–501.

Durkin M (2002) The epidemiology of developmental disabilities in low-income countries. *Mental Retardation and Developmental Disability Research Reviews* **8**: 206–11.

Grayton HM, Fernandes C, Rujescu D, Collier DA (2012) Copy number variations in neurodevelopmental disorders. *Progress in Neurobiology* **99**: 81–91.

Havercamp SM, Reiss S (1996) Composite versus multiple-rating scale in the assessment of psychopathology in people with mental retardation. *Journal of Intellectual Disability Research* **40**: 176–9.

Irazabal M, Marsa F, García M, *et al.* (2012) Family burden related to clinical and functional variables of people with intellectual disability with and without a mental disorder. *Research in Developmental Disabilities* **33**: 796–803.

Jeevanandam L (2009). Perspectives of intellectual disability in Asia: epidemiology, policy, and services for children and adults. *Current Opinion in Psychiatry* **22**: 462–8.

Kishore MT (2011) Disability impact and coping in mothers of children with intellectual disabilities and multiple disabilities. *Journal of Intellectual Disabilities* **15**: 241–51.

Kishore MT, Nizamie A, Nizamie SH, Jahan M (2004) Psychiatric diagnosis in persons with intellectual disability in India. *Journal of Intellectual Disability Research* **48**: 19–24.

Kwok HW, Chui EM (2008) A survey on mental health care for adults with intellectual disabilities in Asia. *Journal of Intellectual Disability Research* **52**: 996–1002.

La Malfa GP, Notarelli A, Hardoy MC, Bertelli M, Cabras P (1997) Psychopathology and mental retardation: an Italian epidemiological study using the PIMRA. *Research in Developmental Disabilities* **3**: 179–84.

Lyons G (2005) The Life Satisfaction Matrix: an instrument and procedure for assessing the subjective wellbeing quality of life of individuals with profound multiple disabilities. *Journal of Intellectual Disability Research* **49**: 766–9.

Matson JL (1995) *The Diagnostic Assessment for the Severely Handicapped II*. Baton Rouge, LA: Disability Consultants.

Matson JL, Kazdin AE, Senatore V (1984) Psychometric properties of the Psychopathology Instrument for Mentally Retarded Adults. *Applied Research in Mental Retardation* **5**: 81–9.

Matson JL, Gardner WI, Coe DA, Sovner R (1991) A scale for evaluating emotional disorders in severely and profoundly mentally retarded persons: development of the Diagnostic Assessment for the Severely Handicapped (DASH) scale. *British Journal of Psychiatry* **159**: 404–9.

McIntyre LL, Blacher J, Baker BL (2002) Behaviour/mental health problems in young adults with intellectual disability: the impact on families. *Journal of Intellectual Disability Research* **46**: 239–49.

Miodrag N, Hodapp RM (2010) Chronic stress and health among parents of children with intellectual and developmental disabilities. *Current Opinion in Psychiatry* **23**: 407–11.

Moss S, Patel P, Prosser H, *et al.* (1993) Psychiatric morbidity in older people with moderate and severe learning disability. I: Development and reliability of the patient interview (PAS–ADD). *British Journal of Psychiatry* **163**: 471–80.

Moss S, Prosser H, Costello H, *et al.* (1998) Reliability and validity of the PAS–ADD checklist for detecting disorders in adults with intellectual disability. *Journal of Intellectual Disability Research* **42**: 173–83.

Myrbakk E, von Tetzchner S (2008) Screening individuals with intellectual disability for psychiatric disorders: Comparison of four measures. *American Journal of Mental Retardation* **113**: 54–70.

Neely-Barnes SL, Dia DA (2008) Families of children with disabilities: a review of literature and recommendations. *Journal of*

Early and Intensive Behavioural Intervention **5** (3): 93–107.

Nezu AM (1994) Introduction to special section: mental retardation and mental illness. *Journal of Consulting and Clinical Psychology* **62**: 4–5.

O'Dell R, Leafman J, Nehrenz GM, Bustillos D (2012) Health care decision making and adults with intellectual disability: a descriptive survey. *AJOB Primary Research* **3**: 8–13.

Owen MJ (2012) Intellectual disability and major psychiatric disorders: a continuum of neurodevelopmental causality. *British Journal of Psychiatry* **200**: 268–9.

Persha A, Ayra S, Nagar RK, *et al.* (2007) Biological and psychosocial predictors of developmental delay in persons with intellectual disability: retrospective case-file study. *Asia Pacific Disability Rehabilitation Journal* **18** (1): 85–93.

Prosser H, Moss S, Costello H, *et al.* (1998) Reliability and validity of the mini PAS–ADD for assessing psychiatric disorders in adults with intellectual disability. *Journal of Intellectual Disability Research* **42**: 264–72.

Reiss S (1988) *The Reiss Screen Test Manual*. Orlando Park, IL: IDS.

Reiss S, Szyszko J (1983) Diagnostic overshadowing and professional experience with mentally retarded people. *American Journal of Mental Deficiency* **8**: 396–402.

Renwick R, Brown I (1996) *Quality of Life in Health Promotion and Rehabilitation: Conceptual Approaches, Issues, and Applications*. Thousand Oaks, CA: Sage.

Salvador-Carulla L, Bertelli M (2008) "Mental retardation" or "intellectual disability": time for a conceptual change. *Psychopathology* **41**: 10–16.

Salvador-Carulla L, Rodríguez-Blázquez C, Rodríguez de Molina M, Pérez-Marín J, Velázquez R (2000) Hidden psychiatric morbidity in a vocational programme for people with intellectual disability. *Journal of Intellectual Disability Research* **44**: 147–54.

Salvador-Carulla L, Reed GM, Vaez-Azizi LM, *et al.* (2011) Intellectual developmental disorders: towards a new name, definition and framework for "mental retardation/ intellectual disability" in ICD 11. *World Psychiatry* **10**: 175–80.

Smiley E (2005) Epidemiology of mental health problems in adults with learning disability: an update. *Advances in Psychiatric Treatment* **11**: 214–22.

Sovner R (1986) Limitating factors in the use of DSM-III criteria with mentally ill/mentally retarded people. *Psychopharmacology Bulletin* **22**: 1055–9.

Summers JA, Poston DJ, Turnbull AP, *et al.* (2005). Conceptualizing and measuring family quality of life. *Journal of Intellectual Disability Research* **49**: 777–83.

Swiezy NB, Matson JL, Kirkpatrick-Sanchez S, Williams DE (1995) A criterion validity study of the schizophrenia subscale of the Psychopathology Instrument for Mentally Retarded Adults (PIMRA). *Research in Developmental Disabilities* **16** (1): 75–80.

Szymanski L, King BH (1999) Summary of the practice parameters for the assessment and treatment of children, adolescents, and adults with mental retardation and comorbid mental disorders. *Journal of the American Academy of Child and Adolescent Psychiatry* **38**: 1606–10.

Townsend-White C, Pham ANT, Vassos MV (2012) Review: a systematic review of quality of life measures for people with intellectual disabilities and challenging behaviours. *Journal of Intellectual Disability Research* **56**: 270–84.

Turnbull A, Turnbull R, Erwin E, Soodak L (2006) *Families, Professionals, and Exceptionality: Positive Outcomes Through Partnerships and Trust*, 5th edn. Upper Saddle River, NJ: Merrill/ Prentice Hall.

Van Den Bossche MJ, Johnstone M, Strazisar M, *et al.* (2012) Rare copy number variants in neuropsychiatric disorders: Specific phenotype or not? *American Journal of Medical Genetics Part B: Neuropsychiatric Genetics* **159B**: 812–22.

Verdugo MA, Schalock RL, Keith KD, Stancliffe RJ (2005) Quality of life and its measurement: Important principles and guidelines. *Journal of Intellectual Disability Research* **49**: 707–17.

Wang M, Turnbull AP, Summers JA, *et al.* (2004). Severity of disability and income as predictors of parents' satisfaction with their family quality of life during early childhood years. *Research and Practice for Persons with Severe Disabilities* **29**: 82–94.

Werner S, Stawski M (2012) Mental health: knowledge, attitudes and training of professionals on dual diagnosis of intellectual disability and psychiatric disorder. *Journal of Intellectual Disability Research* **56**: 291–304.

Wong PK, Wong DF, Schalock RL, Chou YC (2011) Initial validation of the Chinese Quality of Life Questionnaire-Intellectual Disabilities (CQOL-ID): a cultural perspective. *Journal of Intellectual Disability Research* **55**: 572–80.

Chapter

25

Adolescent alcohol and substance abuse

Julia W. Felton, Zachary W. Adams, Laura MacPherson, and Carla Kmett Danielson

Introduction

Adolescence is a time marked by significant biological, psychological, and social growth and upheaval. Alongside more positive aspects of maturation come notable increases in rates of teen substance use and substance use disorders (SUDs) (Johnston *et al.* 2007, SAMHSA 2006, 2008). Early onset and increased frequency of substance use during adolescence are problematic, given their relation to addiction and other psychological disorders in later life (Brook *et al.* 1999, Riggs *et al.* 2007, Behrendt *et al.* 2008) as well as a host of other potentially lethal correlates, including impaired driving (Shope *et al.* 2001), self-harm (Nock *et al.* 2006), and risky sexual behaviors (Guo *et al.* 2002). Although prevalence estimates for alcohol and drug use are most often drawn from samples of youth from the United States, similar trends over this developmental period have been observed consistently across several cultural groups and geographic regions (e.g., Hassan *et al.* 2009). Yet despite the heavy toll of adolescent substance use, relatively limited empirical attention has been paid to the prevalence and treatment of these disorders outside the developed world. This chapter outlines the literature on the prevalence of adolescent substance use worldwide and describes empirically supported treatments for adolescent substance abuse. These findings are discussed with regard to promoting a better understanding of adolescent substance use internationally and addressing the current barriers and opportunities for disseminating effective interventions on a global scale.

International prevalence data

The largest literature on the prevalence of adolescent substance use is drawn from nationally representative data collected in the United States, Europe, and Australia. Recently, there have been efforts to create multinational surveys that allow for direct comparisons across countries and, ultimately, the capacity to track adolescent substance use trends across geographic regions and over generations. Data from these and other studies are described below.

Adolescent substance use and abuse in developed countries

United States

The Monitoring the Future (MTF) study, a collaboration between the National Institute on Drug Abuse (NIDA) and the University of Michigan, is one of the largest surveys of adolescent substance use in the United States. The survey uses a nationally representative sample of approximately 50 000 US students in the 8th, 10th, and 12th grades (aged approximately 13–18 years) and provides prevalence data on a wide range of substance use behaviors, as well as attitudes and beliefs regarding alcohol, tobacco, and illegal drugs. Conducted annually since 1975, the MTF study allows researchers to examine the development of substance use across age groups and track changes in use over time. Prevalence estimates reported below are from the most recent available data, collected in 2010 (Johnston *et al.* 2011).

Alcohol remains the most frequently consumed substance among teenagers since the MTF study began. The report suggests that between 8th and 12th grades, estimates of lifetime alcohol use double from 35.8% to 71%. Among all students in the study, 27% reported using alcohol in the last month and 14.6% reported having gotten drunk during that time period. Encouragingly, these numbers show a steady decline in prevalence of alcohol use since the early

Essentials of Global Mental Health, ed. Samuel O. Okpaku. Published by Cambridge University Press. © Cambridge University Press 2014.

1990s, suggesting that the recent emphasis on alcohol prevention and intervention programs is evincing some success.

Evidence from the MTF report illustrates similar declines in tobacco use in the United States over recent years. The most recent findings suggest that 30.9% of youths have tried smoking during their lifetimes. In the last 30 days, 12.8% of students reported having a cigarette and 6.5% reported consuming smokeless tobacco products.

In contrast, the MTF report suggests that illicit drug use has been increasing in recent generations, largely due to a rise in adolescent marijuana use. Prevalence of daily marijuana use across all three grade levels increased by 1.4% from 2009 to 2010 and by 7.7% since the beginning of the MFT study. Prevalence of lifetime marijuana or hashish use was 17.3% among 8th graders and 43.8% among 12th graders; 14.8% of respondents indicated they had used marijuana within the past month.

Illicit drugs other than marijuana constitute a considerably smaller portion of total substance use among American high-schoolers. Still, rates of lifetime reported use of illicit substances (not including marijuana) more than double from 10.6% in 8th grade to 24.7% in 12th grade. Inhalant use is the second most common illicit drug surveyed and is the only drug to be more commonly used by 8th graders than 12th graders (lifetime rates are 14.5% and 9%, respectively). Amphetamines are the third most common drug reported, followed by hallucinogens, ecstasy, tranquilizers, and sedatives, all endorsed by less than 10% of the sample.

Europe

The European School Survey Project on Alcohol and Other Drugs (ESPAD) is the largest multinational study of adolescent substance use in the world. Modeled after the MTF, the ESPAD was initiated in the early 1990s and involves collection of self-reported alcohol, tobacco, and drug use from adolescents between the ages of 15 and 16 every four years. Prevalence estimates reviewed below are based on the most recent ESPAD survey, conducted in 2007 (Hibell *et al.* 2009).

Estimates of teen drinking in European countries are, on average, significantly higher than in the USA. This may be related to the younger legal drinking ages in European countries, which range from 16 to 20 years old (median age 18, compared to the US legal

drinking age of 21). The mean lifetime prevalence of teen alcohol use reported in the study was 90%, with all participating countries indicating rates over 66%. Estimates of previous-month alcohol use were also high. Across all ESPAD regions, 62% of students indicated having used alcohol within the past month. Reports of alcohol use have remained relatively consistent since the inception of the study.

European teens also endorse significantly higher levels of tobacco use than American adolescents. Unlike laws governing the minimum legal age to purchase or consume alcohol, age restrictions for tobacco use are similar between the USA and most European countries, with most countries requiring people to be 18 years or older to purchase tobacco products. Few European countries have a legal *smoking* age, however, which means that children under 18 may smoke, but not purchase, tobacco in those countries. The highest estimates of lifetime tobacco use in adolescents come from Eastern European countries, including Latvia (80%), the Czech Republic (78%), and Estonia (75%). With regard to developmental trends, ESPAD found that cigarette use starts earlier in Europe than in the USA, with 7% of all European students reporting that they began daily smoking at or before the age of 13. Compared to previous waves of data collection, rates of cigarette use appear relatively stable over time across European countries.

Similar to their American counterparts, marijuana is the most commonly used illicit drug among European adolescents. Across ESPAD countries, 22% of boys and 16% of girls report having used marijuana in their lifetime. Only 7% of European teens endorse having used marijuana within the past month. Although estimates of marijuana use vary widely among countries in Europe, there appears to be a general trend of increasing use over the course of the survey. After marijuana, ecstasy was the second most commonly used drug, with an average of 3% of students reporting having tried the drug during their lifetime. Prevalence of cocaine and amphetamines also were approximately 3% across all participating countries. Because of the relatively low prevalence estimates of illicit drug use other than marijuana, changes in use of these other drugs over time are difficult to determine.

Australia

As in the USA and Europe, the Australian government collects large-scale survey data at regular intervals to

Table 25.1 Comparison of substance use by 15-year-olds: USA, Australia, and Europe (percentage prevalence)

Country or region	Alcohol use, past 30 days	Cigarette use, past 30 days	Drug use, lifetime
United States[a]	28.9	13.6	37.0
Australia[b]	52.2	15	(marijuana only) 20.3
Europe[c]	61.9	28.7	20.3
Armenia	35	7	4
Austria	80	45	22
Belgium	70	23	25
Bulgaria	66	40	24
Croatia	64	38	19
Cyprus	62	23	7
Czech Republic	76	41	46
Denmark	80	32	28
Estonia	60	29	28
Faroe Islands	—	33	6
Finland	48	30	8
France	64	30	33
Germany	75	33	23
Greece	71	22	9
Hungary	59	33	15
Iceland	31	16	10
Ireland	56	23	22
Isle of Man	76	24	35
Italy	63	37	25
Latvia	65	41	22
Lithuania	65	34	20
Malta	73	26	15
Monaco	62	25	29
Netherlands	69	30	29
Norway	42	19	6
Poland	57	21	18
Portugal	60	19	14
Romania	52	25	5
Russia	52	35	20
Slovak Republic	63	37	33
Slovenia	65	29	24
Sweden	44	21	8
Switzerland	67	29	34
Ukraine	61	31	15
United Kingdom	70	22	29

Data from Monitoring the Future (Johnston et al. 2011), European School Survey Project on Alcohol and Other Drugs (Hibell et al. 2009), and the Australian National Survey (White & Smith 2009).
[a] Estimates from 10th graders only.
[b] Unweighted average.
[c] Estimates computed from unweighted averages of 15- and 16-year-olds.

gauge current adolescent substance use and generational trends. The most recent data come from 2008 and include reports from over 24 000 students aged 12–17 (White & Smith 2009). Results from the study suggest that 37.1% of all students drank alcohol in the past month. Consistent with other national surveys, prevalence of alcohol use rises significantly from early to late adolescence. Total estimates of past-month alcohol consumption increased from 20.3% at age 13 to 63.4% by age 17. Estimates for tobacco use among Australians are fairly consistent with same-aged American peers. Prevalence of past-month smoking averaged 10.1% across the sample, with estimates rising steeply over adolescence, from 4.2% at age 13 to 18.3% by age 17.

In line with findings from other developed countries, marijuana use constitutes the most commonly used illicit drug among Australian teens. Lifetime marijuana use rises over the course of adolescence from 4.1% to 26.2% between ages 13 and 17. Rates of drug use excluding marijuana are considerably lower. For 12- to 15-year-olds, lifetime use of non-marijuana illicit drugs is 5.4%. This estimate represents a significant drop from the two previous waves of data collection in 2002 and 2005.

Comparing developed countries

Table 25.1 summarizes data from the MTF, ESPAD, and Australian national surveys. Despite methodological differences between these studies (e.g., slight differences in age groups, recruitment methods, item content), there are several notable points of comparison. First, rates of adolescent alcohol and tobacco use in Australia and Europe are considerably higher than in the USA. This disparity may reflect different national policies and attitudes toward these substances. Drinking alcohol specifically may be more socially acceptable in developed nations outside the USA, as evidenced by the younger drinking age across most of these countries. Disparities in tobacco use are especially evident between the USA and European countries. These differences may be due to declines in American teen cigarette use as a result of significant tobacco control efforts aimed at reducing youth tobacco consumption. Conversely, estimates of lifetime illicit drug use are considerably higher in the USA than in Europe or Australia, and these trends are driven by marked increases in marijuana use among American teens. This growth in marijuana abuse represents a troubling trend, and suggests that targeting marijuana use among teenagers should be a national priority in the USA.

Adolescent substance use and abuse in developing countries

Efforts to establish estimates of adolescent substance use levels in developing countries have increased in recent years through partnerships between multinational organizations, such as the World Health Organization (WHO), and community-level agencies. One of the broadest initiatives is the Global School-based Student Health Survey (GSHS), a collaborative surveillance project including the WHO, the United Nations, and the US Centers for Disease Control and Prevention (CDC), aimed at tracking adolescent health and health behaviors across the globe (World Health Organization 2009). The study currently comprises 73 countries and reports data from students aged 13–15. GSHS surveys include both universal core components that measure alcohol, drug, and tobacco use, and country-specific questions that assess distinctive regional health behaviors. Although much work remains to be done, these partnerships are leading the way in improving our understanding of rates of teen substance use across the globe.

Western Pacific Region

Of the 37 countries classified by the WHO as the Western Pacific Region, the GSHS reports data from only nine countries (as well as four locations within

China). Such limited participation rates highlight that, despite the vast population of Western Pacific countries, relatively little is known about adolescent substance use in this area. From the available data, there is some suggestion that prevalence of drug and alcohol use are on the rise, particularly in China where expanding international ties have also opened the door to drug trafficking and the spread of substance use among adults and teens (Hassan *et al.* 2009). Estimates of drug and alcohol use vary widely among Western Pacific countries, perhaps owing to the disparate cultures and religions that make up the region. For example, prevalence estimates of teen alcohol, cigarette, and drug use are particularly low in Mongolia (approximately 6%, 5%, and 2% respectively). These low rates may be attributed to the country's sparse population, harsh climates, and limited infrastructure, which has left the country relatively isolated from the spread of substance use from larger neighboring countries such as China and Russia (Mathers *et al.* 2009). In contrast, data from the small island nation of Kiribati indicates that the country leads the region in prevalence of adolescent alcohol and tobacco use. Over 30% of children aged 13–15 from this region endorsed past-month alcohol use, and more than a quarter stated they had smoked at least one cigarette in the past month. Risk factors associated with adolescent substance misuse, such as poverty, lack of education, and being raised in single-parent homes, are common in Kiribati and may explain, in part, the elevated prevalence of teen drinking and smoking in that country (Unicef 2010).

Data from the most recent GSHS suggest that types of illicit drugs used also vary nationally. Some of these differences in prevalence estimates may reflect regionally specific preferences and access to specific classes of drugs. For instance, due to its expansive poppy seed resources, opioids (specifically heroin) are very common in China and its neighboring countries (Hao *et al.* 2002). These factors should be considered and assessed when measuring and interpreting substance use trends across countries.

African Region

The WHO Africa Region includes 46 countries, encompassing a wide range of cultures, religions, and laws. Of these, 16 countries are represented in the GSHS. The majority of data on adolescent substance use come from the sub-Saharan region.

Cross-national studies of this area suggest lower prevalence estimates of alcohol and drug use than are observed in the USA and Europe (Jernigan 2001, Peltzer 2009). Alarmingly, however, the prevalence of substance misuse in this area appears to have steadily increased over the past decade. Factors contributing to this rise include swelling unemployment and greater social tolerance towards drug use (e.g. Adelekan et al. 2001, Peltzer et al. 2010). Prevalence of adolescent substance use in other parts of the region varies widely, owing to differences in the way substances are regulated and perceived socially across the continent. For instance, the percentage of teens who report using alcohol in the last month is over 60% in the Seychelles, where the relative ease of purchasing alcohol and more liberal social attitudes towards alcohol are unique in the region (Alwan et al. 2011). Poverty also appears to be a strong predictor of substance use in Africa, with poorer countries exhibiting higher rates of adolescent substance misuse (Peltzer 2009).

The types of drugs used by teens in Africa vary widely. For example, khat, a flowering plant that produces stimulant-like effects when chewed, and kola nut, a caffeinated nut specific to tropical environments, are native to this region and are commonly ingested in different parts of Africa. These regionally specific substances are often viewed as a "safer" alternative to other drugs (Hassan et al. 2009). Marijuana has also, historically, been widely used in the region, particularly in South Africa, where it plays an integral role in traditional cultural activities (Peltzer et al. 2010). More recently, marijuana has spread to Africa's tropical climates, where the plant can be easily cultivated and exported to other areas (Hassan et al. 2009).

Region of the Americas

The WHO Region of the Americas includes 35 countries, 22 of which participated in the GSHS (not including the USA). While there are significant intra-regional differences in the prevalence of adolescent substance use, this region reports the highest average levels of teen alcohol use. Data from the GSHS suggest that rates of past-month alcohol use range from 16% in Guatemala to nearly 60% in Uruguay. Illicit drug use also appears to be on the rise as countries transition from substance producers to consumers (Medina-Mora & Rojas Guiot 2003).

With the exception of Mexico, Costa Rica, and Chile, researchers have been slow to describe and understand these trends because of the lack of national surveys (Aguilar-Gaxiola et al. 2006). Throughout the region, marijuana remains the most popular drug of choice among teens (Hassan et al. 2009). Of particular concern, however, is the uptick in inhalant use among South American teens. One recent study found that 12–13% of school-aged youth had been offered an inhalant, and 5% had used this drug on one or more occasions (Dormitzer & Gonzalez 2004).

Southeast Asia Region

The WHO Southeast Asia Region includes 11 member states, of which five participated in the GSHS. Limited information is available regarding alcohol and drug use, particularly in India, due to cultural and religious taboos regarding substance use (Hassan et al. 2009). Regional estimates of substance misuse are based on small samples from only a handful of countries. The limited data available from the GSHS indicate that, among participating countries, alcohol, tobacco, and drug use are relatively low compared to developed nations. Alarmingly, recent research suggests that rates of alcohol use among Indian teens are on the rise and that the average age of alcohol use initiation has dropped from 19 to 13 over the past two decades (Prasad 2009). Other research on drug abuse in the region indicates that while marijuana remains the most abused drug, opioid and heroin use have been steadily increasing since the 1970s (Suwanwela & Poshyachinda 1986).

Eastern Mediterranean Region

The Eastern Mediterranean Region includes 22 countries, 12 of which participated in the GSHS. The majority of countries did not respond to questions about alcohol and illicit drug use, however, because most religious groups common to the region and local governments ban substance use of any kind (Hassan et al. 2009). Surveys utilizing smaller samples, however, suggest that adolescents in this region do indeed use alcohol, tobacco, and illicit drugs, although rates are considerably lower than in developed countries. Recent research from Iran indicates that, among male high-school students, 12.7% indicated they had used alcohol and 2% reported illegal drug use during their lifetime (Poorasl et al.

2007). Tobacco use is more common. A survey of Saudi Arabian secondary-school students found that over 20% of adolescents were current smokers (Amin *et al.* 2011). In other regions, including Lebanon, Syria, and the West Bank, over 30% of students indicated using shisha, a type of water pipe used for smoking tobacco (Khader *et al.* 2009). Larger multinational studies are necessary, however, to compare rates between this and other regions.

Comparing developing countries

Table 25.2 reports data from the GSHS as well as rates from comparably aged students from the MTF and Australian national surveys. The ESPAD survey was not included because it used a sample of 15- to 16-year-olds exclusively, while the GSHS used slightly younger students (aged 13–15), making rates difficult to compare. In comparing GSHS data to US and Australian estimates, several differences stand out. First, past-month alcohol use is significantly higher in the Americas than in all other geographic areas. This may reflect a greater cultural acceptance of alcohol use among young people, similar to attitudes in many European countries. Early alcohol use, however, is often predictive of later alcohol dependence (Dawson *et al.* 2008) and these estimates may also indicate a need for greater intervention and prevention efforts in the region. A second notable finding is that average tobacco use in Western Pacific countries is greater than in any other region included in the study. This estimate, however, may not accurately reflect the complex pattern of rates of tobacco use in the area. While the prevalence of cigarette use in specific countries is concerning, there is significant variability among countries in the region. Further, the GSHS study did not consider tobacco products other than cigarettes (e.g., shisha or hookah), which may be more common in other regions. A final important finding is that reported rates of illicit drug use are considerably higher in developed nations than in developing regions. Indeed, of the countries included in the GSHS study, only adolescents from Jamaica and St. Lucia had higher prevalence of lifetime drug use than America and Australia. Alarmingly, rates of illicit substance use appear to be rising among developing nations, underscoring the need for international intervention efforts targeting the prevention and treatment of adolescent drug use.

Treatment for adolescent substance use disorders

Since the mid-1990s, a growing body of literature has established support for a variety of treatment approaches targeting adolescent SUDs. Interventions for adolescent SUDs are organized around the target of intervention, including individual-level, family-level, and community-level approaches. Most of this work has taken place within the USA, although recent research suggests that many of these interventions are adaptable to other regions.

Individual-level approaches

Contingency management (CM) refers to treatment approaches couched in basic reinforcement theory. Specifically, substance use is viewed as a behavior that is maintained by the direct reinforcing effects of a drug (e.g., euphoria) as well as by other secondary sources of reinforcement (e.g., non-pharmacological effects), and thus principles of learning theory can be applied to reinforce behaviors consistent with abstinence from drugs (Higgins & Petry 1999, Petry 2000). CM interventions seek to influence a target behavior (e.g., smoking) by monitoring the behavior over time and applying a consequence (reinforce or punishment) for changes in that behavior. While CM has received considerable support in reducing substance use among adults (e.g., Petry 2000), only recently have researchers begun to use CM with adolescents (Roll & Watson 2006), with several studies supporting CM approaches as both efficacious and cost-effective with adolescents (e.g., Dennis *et al.* 2004, Stanger & Budney 2010).

Individual **cognitive behavioral therapy** (CBT) has demonstrated success among adolescents with SUDs (Waldron & Turner 2008). CBT approaches tend to be multicomponent and integrate strategies based in classical, operant, and social learning frameworks. CBT often includes both cognitive strategies, such as identifying distorted thought patterns (e.g., "I am not a worthwhile person"), and behavioral strategies, such as problem solving, communication skills, planning for and responding to high-risk situations, and managing cravings (Waldron & Turner 2008, Slesnick *et al.* 2008). A recent meta-analysis (Waldron & Turner 2008) of psychosocial treatments for adolescent SUDs indicated that individual CBT, as compared to minimal treatment control, could be

Table 25.2 Comparison of substance use by 13- to 15-year-olds: USA, Australia, and developing countries (percentage prevalence)

Country	Alcohol use, past 30 days	Cigarette use, past 30 days	Drug use, lifetime
United States[a]	13.8	7.1	21.4
Australia[b]	22.3	9.1	(marijuana only) 20.7
Western Pacific[c]	19.0	16.4	6.3
China[c]	14.9	6.3	1.8
Philippines	18.7	11	—
Cook Island	29.1	19.7	(marijuana only) 9.2
Fiji	16.4	11.7	—
Kiribati	30.3	26.1	(marijuana only) 4
Mongolia	5.6	5.4	(marijuana only) 1.8
Nauru	21.9	22.1	—
Solomon Islands	18	24	(marijuana only) 14.3
Tonga	16.4	21.6	(marijuana only) 6.5
African Region[c]	22.6	9.8	12.6
Algeria	—	9.2	2
Benin	16.4	2.8	1.5
Botswana	20.6	7	7.5
Ghana	28.1		25
Kenya	14.6	13.9	13.2
Malawi	3.9	4.9	—
Mauritania	—	17.3	8
Mauritius[c]	25.7	14.5	5.9
Namibia	32.8	16.1	28.8
Senegal	3.2	6.5	1.4
Seychelles	61.6	17.2	13
Swaziland	16	—	7
Uganda	—	4.3	8.5
Tanzania	5.8	3.8	5.8
Zambia	42.3	—	38.1
Zimbabwe[c]	17.5	8.1	11.1
Region of the Americas[c]	41.1	12.0	12.5
Anguilla	45.8	6.1	—
Antigua & Barbados	45.1	7.4	—
Argentina	51.8	21.0	9.0
British Virgin Islands	33.4	5.7	—
Cayman Islands	39.4	10.9	15.6
Chile[c]	29.1	25.4	8.6
Columbia[c]	54.8	16.2	12.0
Costa Rica	23.6	9.5	—
Dominica	54.5	—	—
Ecuador[c]	34.2	14.8	5.4
Grenada	45.6	4.7	13.9
Guatemala[c]	16.2	—	—
Guyana	39.2	12.0	
Jamaica	52.5	—	23.9
Montserrat	33.4	—	17.2
Peru	27.1	17.3	3.8
Saint Lucia	55.4	7.8	22.0
Saint Vincent and the Grenadines	53.2	8.5	19.9
Suriname	32.6	10.4	—
Trinidad and Tobago	41.0	9.3	12.8
Uruguay	59.6	17.7	8.4
Venezuela[c]	36.7	—	—
Southeast Asia[c]	6.0	6.4	2.3
Maldives	4.9	8.9	—
Myanmar	0.8	2	0.4
India	—	1.2	—
Indonesia	2.6	11.1	0.5
Thailand	15.6	8.8	6.1
Eastern Mediterranean[c]	18.0	8.3	3.9
Djibouti	—	3.3	6.6
Egypt	—	—	—

Table 25.2 (cont.)

Country	Alcohol use, past 30 days	Cigarette use, past 30 days	Drug use, lifetime
Jordan	—	12.3	—
Kuwait	—	15.9	2.8
Lebanon	28.5	—	3.5
Libya	—	4.2	—
Morocco	—	5.2	3
Pakistan	—	6.3	—
Syrian Arab Republic	7.4	10.6	—
Tunisia	—	7.5	3.8
United Arab Emirates	—	9.8	—
Yemen	—	—	—

Data from the Global School-based Student Health Survey (World Health Organization 2009).
[a] Estimates from 8th graders only.
[b] Estimates computed from unweighted averages of 13- to 15-year-olds.
[c] Unweighted average.

classified as well-established according to criteria outlined by Chambless et al. (1996). Additionally, group-based CBT approaches may also be effective and carry the additional benefit of greater cost-effectiveness (Waldron & Turner 2008).

To our knowledge, the field has yet to examine the feasibility, transportability, or efficacy of these individual-level approaches with adolescent substance users in other countries. These interventions represent a potentially fruitful avenue for further research, yet several concerns with regard to disseminating individual-level approaches outside the USA should be noted. For instance, careful attention must be paid to cultural values regarding use of "external reinforcers" for abstinence and concerns surrounding the effects these factors may have on internal motivation for change. With regard to reward-based approaches, cultures that value autonomy/personal responsibility, or that are not accustomed to routine provision of rewards, may be uncomfortable integrating an intervention approach that relies on contingencies. Despite these potential pitfalls, individual-level approaches also offer considerable promise. Indeed,

both approaches are cost-effective and may be particularly well suited for developing countries with limited numbers of trained providers and restricted economic resources.

Family-level approaches

Some of the most thoroughly researched treatment models for adolescents with SUDs target the family as the focus of intervention. Several family-based approaches have yielded promising results, including **brief strategic family therapy** (Robbins & Szapocznik 2000, Szapocznik & Williams 2000) and **multidimensional family therapy** (MDFT: Liddle et al. 1992). Here, we will focus on MDFT because of the rigorously designed studies that have tested its efficacy, as well as ongoing transnational trials that can speak to the feasibility of translating family-level approaches at an international scale (Rigter et al. 2010).

MDFT is a multicomponent approach that incorporates traditional family systems framework to change interactional patterns within family and social systems (Liddle et al. 1992). MDFT is manualized with specific assessment and treatment modules that target four areas: (1) the adolescent's interpersonal functioning with parents and peers; (2) the parents' parenting practices and personal level of functioning separate from their parenting role; (3) parent–child interactions in treatment sessions; and (4) communication between family members and pertinent social systems, including school and child welfare, etc. (Liddle et al. 2004). Among adolescents with SUDs, MDFT may be more effective than adolescent group therapy, family education, enhanced services as usual (Liddle et al. 2001, 2009), and individual CBT (Liddle et al. 2008), and equivalent in its effectiveness to group CBT (Liddle et al. 2004, 2009) and the adolescent community reinforcement approach (Dennis et al. 2004).

Based on support for MDFT in the USA, a major international initiative has been undertaken in five European countries (Belgium, France, Germany, the Netherlands, and Switzerland) known as the International Cannabis Need of Treatment Project (INCANT) (Rigter et al. 2010). Significant hurdles existed at first with this initiative, particularly concerns raised by policy makers and by the therapeutic community that adolescents with marijuana use disorders and their families would not be interested in taking part in a randomized trial as a "(real-world)

RCT was still exotic and controversial in Western European youth care at the time." (Rigter *et al.* 2010). Other potential hurdles included incompatibility of time-limited, manualized treatments in countries with long histories of psychoanalytic approaches or countries where longer-term treatment (e.g., > 1 year) for adolescent SUDs was standard care (Rigter *et al.* 2010). However, following initial piloting and extensive transnational consultation, INCANT is under way and provides a unique example of the intersection of national policy and healthcare systems, clinical trials, and cultural/therapeutic values regarding adolescent SUD treatment.

Community-level approaches

Multisystemic therapy (MST) is a well-validated, ecologically based intervention that targets multiple systems in which the adolescent lives, including family, school, neighborhood, and peer group (Henggeler *et al.* 1998). Originally developed for adolescents with SUDs who were serious juvenile offenders, the primary goals of MST are to: (1) reduce criminal and antisocial behaviors including substance use, and (2) decrease incarceration and other forms of "out-of-home" placement (Schoenwald *et al.* 2008). MST incorporates structural and strategic family therapy with CBT in an intensive home-based delivery model in which therapists are available 24 hours a day, seven days a week, with an average treatment length of 60 hours across multiple months (Schoenwald *et al.* 2008). Although a meta-analysis by Waldron and Turner (2008) indicated it remained probably efficacious, more recent investigations have highlighted the substantial impact of MST with some of the most severely delinquent youth (e.g., Sawyer & Borduin 2011).

Consistent with the potential impact of such findings at a societal level, other nations have exhibited considerable interest in implementing MST. To date, MST has been transported to Australia, Canada, Denmark, Ireland, the Netherlands, New Zealand, Norway, and Sweden (Schoenwald *et al.* 2008), and results of an RCT with a large, diverse sample of youth offenders has been published from the United Kingdom (Butler *et al.* 2011).

Discussion and conclusions

Adolescent substance abuse is an international public health burden, associated with a host of costly and potentially harmful behaviors. Several intervention approaches have proven efficacious in Western societies; however, few have been tested in developing countries, where rates of illicit drug use appear to be on the rise. Although the current picture appears bleak, this review highlights several opportunities for both improving our understanding of drug and alcohol use worldwide and developing strategies to reduce rates of teen substance use globally.

First, significant strides have been made recently in documenting the patterns of adolescent substance use on a global scale. Collaborations between multinational institutions, such as the CDC and the WHO, and local organizations have yielded the first cross-national epidemiological data on adolescent alcohol, tobacco, and drug use. Despite these initial successes, more data still need to be collected. Given that rates of illicit drug use are rising in several developing countries, it will be especially important to sustain efforts to track changes in patterns of substance use over time. Future research also should focus on elucidating the pathways to initiation and escalation of substance misuse among developing countries, as understanding the mechanisms of early substance use is imperative for creating effective interventions. For example, understanding how early trauma and post-traumatic stress disorder (PTSD) may lead to adolescent substance misuse has significant implications for intervention and prevention in areas where war, famine, and natural disasters are common.

Second, despite recent achievements in the treatment of adolescent drug and alcohol use inside the United States, most empirically supported interventions have not yet been adapted for use on an international scale. A recent review of 670 RCTs examining mental health interventions for youth found that only 58 came from middle-income countries and only one came from a low-income country (Kieling *et al.* 2011). This may be due in part to regional barriers associated with implementing treatments "as-is." For instance, CM techniques may not be as successful, or as easily adapted, in collectivistic cultures. Alternatively, MST may necessitate the use of entirely different types of "systems" in rural and resource-poor regions, and CBT approaches may need to consider regional differences in attitudes and behaviors associated with substance use. Although it is difficult to fully anticipate all of the barriers to implementing evidence-based treatments, the field should encourage research on issues related to disseminating empirically supported interventions on a global scale.

Even less research has been dedicated to examining the utility of existing traditional or indigenous approaches to treating adolescent substance use. Developing such treatments to be "scaled up" has intuitive appeal and may overcome barriers associated with more "top-down" approaches (such as disseminating treatments developed in the USA internationally). Undertaking any of these avenues of future research requires the creation and fostering of partnerships between organizations on the international and local levels. Developing these collaborations will be essential to both broadening our understanding of worldwide adolescent substance use and successfully intervening to reduce rates on a global scale. Future researchers should focus on creating the "research infrastructure" necessary to achieve these goals and promote healthy adolescent development throughout the world.

References

Adelekan ML, Makanjuola AB, Nolam RJ, *et al.* (2001) 5 yearly monitoring of trends of substance use among secondary school students in Ilorin, Nigeria, 1988–1998. *West African Journal of Medicine* 20 (1): 28–36.

Aguilar-Gaxiola S, Medina-Mora ME, Magana CG, *et al.* (2006) Illicit drug use research in Latin America: Epidemiology, service use, and HIV. *Drug and Alcohol Dependence* 84: S85–93.

Alwan H, Viswanathan B, Rousson V, Paccaud F, Bovet P (2011) Association between substance use and psychosocial characteristics among adolescents of the Seychelles. *BMC Pediatrics*, 11 (85). doi: 10.1186/1471-2431-11-85.

Amin TT, Amr MA, Zaza BO (2011) Psychosocial predictors of smoking among secondary school students in Al-Hassa, Saudi Arabia. *Journal of Behavioral Medicine* 34: 339–50.

Behrendt S, Wittchen HU, Höfler M, Lieb R, Beesdo, K (2009) Transitions from first substance use to substance use disorders in adolescence: is early onset associated with a rapid escalation? *Drug and Alcohol Dependence* 99: 68–78.

Brook JS, Balka E, Whiteman M (1999) The risks for late adolescence of early adolescent marijuana use. *American Journal of Public Health* 89: 1549–54.

Butler S, Baruch G, Hickey N, Fonagy P (2011) A randomized controlled trial of multisystemic therapy and a statutory therapeutic intervention for young offenders. *Journal of the American Academy of Child and Adolescent Psychiatry* 50: 1220–35.

Chambless DL, Sanderson WC, Shoham V, *et al.* (1996) An update on empirically validated therapies. *Clinical Psychologist* 49: 5–18.

Dawson DA, Goldstein RB, Chou SP, Ruan WJ, Grant BF (2008) Age at first drink and the first incidence of adult-onset DSM-IV alcohol use disorders. *Alcoholism: Clinical and Experimental Research* 32: 2149–60.

Dennis M, Godley SH, Diamond G, *et al.* (2004) The Cannabis Youth Treatment (CYT) study: main findings from two randomized trials. *Journal of Substance Abuse Treatment* 27: 197–213.

Dormitzer CM, Gonzalez GB, Penna M, *et al.* (2004) The PACARDO research project: youthful drug involvement in Central America and the Dominican Republic. *Revista Panamericana de Salud Publica* 15: 400–16.

Guo J, Chung IJ, Hill KG, *et al.* (2002) Developmental relationships between adolescent substance use and risky sexual behavior in young adulthood. *Journal of Adolescent Health* 31: 354–62.

Hao W, Xiao S, Liu T, *et al.* (2002) The second National Epidemiological Survey on illicit drug use at six high-prevalence areas in China: prevalence rates and use patterns. *Addiction* 97: 1305–15.

Hassan A, Csemy L, Rappo MA, Knight JR (2009) Adolescent substance abuse around the world: an international perspective. *Adolescent Medicine: State of the Art Reviews* 20: 915–29.

Henggeler SW, Schoenwald SK, Borduin CM, Rowland M, Cunningham PB (1998) *Multisystemic Treatment of Antisocial Behavior in Children and Adolescents. Treatment Manuals for Practitioners.* New York, NY: Guilford Press.

Hibell B, Guttormsson U, Ahlström S, *et al.* (2009) The 2007 ESPAD report: Substance use among students in 35 European countries. Stockholm, Sweden: the Swedish Council for Information on Alcohol and Other Drugs. http://www.espad.org/documents/Espad/ESPAD_reports/2007/The_2007_ESPAD_Report-FULL_090617.pdf (accessed July 2013).

Higgins ST, Petry NM (1999) Contingency management incentives for sobriety. *Alcohol Research and Health* 23: 122–7.

Jernigan DH (2001) *Global Status Report: Alcohol and Young People.* Geneva: World Health Organization.

Johnston LD, O'Malley PM, Bachman JG, Schulenberg JE (2007) *Monitoring the Future National Results on Adolescent Drug Use: Overview of Key Findings, 2007.* Bethesda, MD: National Institute on Drug Abuse.

Johnston LD, O'Malley PM, Bachman JG, Schulenberg JE (2011)

Monitoring the Future National Results on Adolescent Drug Use: Overview of Key Findings, 2010. Ann Arbor, MI: Institute for Social Research, University of Michigan.

Khader A, Shaheen Y, Turki Y, *et al.* (2009) Tobacco use among Palestine refugee students (UNRWA) aged 13–15. *Preventive Medicine* 49: 224–8.

Kieling C, Baker-Henningham H, Belfer M, *et al.* (2011) Child and adolescent mental health worldwide: evidence for action. *Lancet* 378: 1515–25.

Liddle HA, Dakof G, Diamond G, *et al.* (1992) The adolescent module in multidimensional family therapy. In GW Lawson, AW Lawson, eds., *Adolescent Substance Abuse: Etiology, Treatment, and Prevention.* Gaithersburg, MD: Aspen Publishers; pp. 165–86.

Liddle HA, Dakof GA, Parker K, *et al.* (2001) Multidimensional family therapy for adolescent substance abuse: results of a randomized clinical trial. *American Journal of Drug and Alcohol Abuse* 27: 651–88.

Liddle HA, Rowe CL, Ungaro RA, Dakof GA, Henderson C (2004) Early intervention for adolescent substance abuse: pretreatment to posttreatment outcomes of a randomized controlled trial comparing multidimensional family therapy and peer group treatment. *Journal of Psychoactive Drugs* 36: 36–7.

Liddle HA, Dakof GA, Turner RM, Henderson CE, Greenbaum PE (2008) Treating adolescent drug abuse: a randomized trial comparing multidimensional family therapy and cognitive behavior therapy. *Addiction* 103: 1660–70.

Liddle HA, Rowe CL, Dakof GA, Henderson CE, Greenbaum PE (2009) Multidimensional family therapy for young adolescent substance abuse: twelve-month outcomes of a randomized controlled trial. *Journal of*

Consulting and Clinical Psychology 77: 12–25.

Mathers B, Wodak A, Shakeshaft A, Khoei EM, Dolan K (2009) *A Rapid Assessment and Response to HIV and Drug Use in Mongolia.* Sydney: National Drug and Alcohol Research Centre, University of New South Wales.

Medina-Mora ME, Rojas Guiot E (2003) Demand of drugs: Mexico in the international perspective. *Salud Mental* 26 (2): 1–11.

Nock MK, Joiner TE, Gordon KH, Lloyd-Richardson E, Prinstein MJ (2006) Non-suicidal self-injury among adolescents: Diagnostic correlates and relation to suicide attempts. *Psychiatry Research* 144: 65–72.

Peltzer K (2009) Prevalence and correlates of substance use among school children in six African countries. *International Journal of Psychology* 44: 378–86.

Peltzer K, Mzolo T, Mbelle N, *et al.* (2010) Dual protection, contraceptive use, HIV status and risk among a national sample of South African women. *Gender and Behaviour* 8 (1): 2833–45.

Petry NM (2000) A comprehensive guide to the application of contingency management procedures in clinical settings. *Drug and Alcohol Dependence* 58: 9–25.

Poorasl M, Vahidi R, Fakhari A, Rostami F, Dastghiri S (2007) Substance abuse in Iranian high school students. *Addictive Behaviors* 32: 622–7.

Prasad R (2009) Alcohol use on the rise in India. *Lancet* 373: 17–18.

Riggs NR, Chou CP, Li C, Pentz MA (2007) Adolescent to emerging adulthood smoking trajectories: when do smoking trajectories diverge, and do they predict early adulthood nicotine dependence? *Nicotine and Tobacco Research* 9: 1147–54.

Rigter H, Pelc I, Tossmann P, *et al.* (2010) INCANT: a transnational

randomized trial of multidimensional family therapy versus treatment as usual for adolescents with cannabis use disorder. *BMC Psychiatry*, 10: 28. doi: 10.1186/1471-244X-10-28.

Robbins MS, Szapocznik J (2000) Brief strategic family therapy. *Juvenile Justice Bulletin.* Washington, DC: US Department of Justice, Office of Justice Programs, Office of Juvenile Justice and Delinquency Prevention.

Roll JM, Watson D (2006) Behavioral management approaches for adolescent substance abuse. In HA Liddle, CL Rowe, eds., *Adolescent Substance Abuse: Research and Clinical Advances.* New York, NY: Cambridge University Press; pp. 375–95.

SAMHSA (2006) *Results from the 2005 National Survey on Drug Use and Health: National Findings.* Rockville, MD: Substance Abuse and Mental Health Services Administration.

SAMHSA (2008) *Results from the 2007 National Survey on Drug Use and Health: National Findings.* Rockville, MD: Substance Abuse and Mental Health Services Administration.

Sawyer AM, Borduin CM (2011) Effects of multisystemic therapy through midlife: a 21.9-year follow-up to a randomized clinical trial with serious and violent juvenile offenders. *Journal of Consulting and Clinical Psychology* 79: 643–52.

Schoenwald SK, Heiblum N, Saldana L, Henggeler SW (2008) The international implementation of multisystemic therapy. *Evaluation and the Health Professions* 31: 211–25.

Shope JT, Waller PF, Raghunathan TE, Patil SM (2001) Adolescent antecedents of high-risk driving behavior into young adulthood: substance use and parental influences. *Accident Analysis and Prevention* 33: 649–58.

Slesnick N, Kaminer Y, Kelly, J (2008) Most common psychosocial interventions for adolescent substance use disorders. In Y Kaminer, OG Bukstein, eds., *Adolescent Substance Abuse: Psychiatric Comorbidity and High-Risk Behaviors*. New York, NY: Taylor & Francis.

Stanger C, Budney AJ (2010) Contingency management approaches for adolescent substance use disorders. *Child and Adolescent Psychiatric Clinics of North America* **19**: 547–62.

Suwanwela C, Poshyachinda V (1986) Drug abuse in Asia. *Bulletin on Narcotics* **38** (1–2): 41–53.

Szapocznik J, Williams RA (2000) Brief strategic family therapy: twenty-five years of interplay among theory, research and practice in adolescent behavior problems and drug abuse. *Clinical Child and Family Psychology Review* **3**: 117–34.

Unicef (2010) *I Feel I Can Never Get Infected: Understanding HIV and AIDS Risk and Vulnerability Among Kiribati Youth*. Kiribati: Unicef & Government of Kiribati. http://www.unicef.org/pacificislands/Kiribati_part_1.pdf (accessed July 2013).

Waldron H, Turner CW (2008) Evidence-based psychosocial treatments for adolescent substance abuse. *Journal of Clinical Child and Adolescent Psychology* **37**: 238–61.

White V, Smith G (2009) *Australian Secondary School Students' Use of Tobacco, Alcohol, and Over-the-Counter and Illicit Substances in 2008*. Victoria: Drug Strategy Branch, Australian Government Department of Health and Aging.

World Health Organization (2009) Global school-based student health survey (GSHS) 2009. [April 17 through August 12, 2009]. http://www.who.int/chp/gshs/en (accessed July 2013).

Chapter 26

Women's mental health

Samuel O. Okpaku, Thara Rangaswamy, and Hema Tharoor

In the nineteenth century, the central moral challenge was slavery. In the twentieth century, it was the battle against totalitarianism. We believe that in this century the paramount moral challenge will be the struggle for gender equality around the world.
(Kristof & WuDunn 2009)

Introduction and background

Women's mental health as an intersectoral matter has drawn the attention of major international organizations such as the United Nations (UN) and its agencies, the International Monetary Fund (IMF), the World Bank, non-governmental organizations (NGOs), and major foundations. This trend is likely to expand as the definition of health extends into the realms of human rights, dignity, autonomy, and equal access and opportunities for education, employment, and health care, especially for women. This concern for the status of women worldwide has gradually evolved over time.

In 1995, at the Fourth World Conference on Women, sponsored by the UN in Beijing, an action statement was made that "women have the right to the enjoyment of the highest attainable standard of physical and mental health. The enjoyment of this right is vital to their life and well-being" (United Nations 1996). In 1999, women's mental health leaders in Europe, Asia, Africa, USA, and Australia began to explore the social determinants of women's mental health and illness. In 2001, during the First World Congress on Women's Mental Health in Berlin, there was an interdisciplinary discussion that rank-ordered the above social determinants of women's mental health. In 2004, the Second World Congress on Women's Mental Health was held in

Washington DC. This led to the publication of an international consensus report of women's mental health. Similarly, a consensus statement on interpersonal violence against women had been written by the World Psychiatric Association (WPA).

These statements of consensus have been approved by influential organizations such as the American Psychiatric Association (APA), the American Psychological Association, and the WPA (Stewart 2006). Perhaps more important, however, was the passage of the Millennium Development Goals in 2000. The passage of this declaration was a crowning point for Kofi Annan who was then the Secretary-General of the UN. The declaration was signed by 189 members of the UN. It entailed considerable background diplomacy in obtaining agreement on such sensitive issues as women's rights even among traditional political enemies and strange bedfellows. The activities of four female ministers of state and their contributions to the development of the Millennium Development Fund (MDF) have been chronicled. These women were Clare Short (UK), Evelvn Herfkens (the Netherlands) Hilde Johnson (Norway), and Heidemarie Wieczorek-Zeul (Germany) (Hulme 2009).

The history of the development of the Millennium Development Goals (MDG) provides an excellent background to global diplomacy. An examination of the eight goals of MDG will show their relevance to women and mental health. However, four of the goals (1, 3, 4, and 5) have great significance for women and mental health (United Nations undated):

Goal 1: Eradicate extreme poverty and hunger
Goal 3: Promote gender equality and empower women

Essentials of Global Mental Health, ed. Samuel O. Okpaku. Published by Cambridge University Press. © Cambridge University Press 2014.

Goal 4: Reduce child mortality

Goal 5: Improve maternal health

Education, availability of family planning, economic opportunities, and access to care all impinge on a woman's health and mental health. There are unique sex and gender risks for women in terms of poverty, literacy, HIV/AIDS infection, and partner violence. Women are more likely to be subjected to such cultural practices as female genital mutilation. Women are also at greater risk for poverty. While there is an emphasis on access to education and economic opportunities, we must not lose sight of the fact that women may have unique needs because of biological, cultural, and demographic factors that require special attention. It cannot be easy to balance the demands of work, income production, and child bearing and rearing.

In this chapter we attempt to describe various psychosocial issues, specific risks, and diagnostic and service biases that relate to women. We will make some reference to the role of education, family planning availability, and economic opportunities, as illustrated by experience from microfinancial strategies.

Women's mental health and risk factors

A variety of factors have been identified as likely to impinge on the mental health of women and girls. These factors include financial and economic stressors, poverty, socioeconomic status, violence, education, and family of origin, as well as refugee, immigration, and minority status.

The above factors generally act in unison, but for heuristic reasons we will attempt to separate them. The association of poverty and mental health status has been amply documented (Patel *et al.* 1999). Women are at greater risk of poverty than men. We can add the risks of the consequences of divorce and single heads of families.

Low academic achievement has been identified as a risk factor for physical abuse by men (Moffitt *et al.* 2001). Higher levels of education by both spouses appear to protect against poor mental health, but intimate partner violence has been found to be worldwide, and intimate partner violence and its concomitants contribute to mental illness (Counts *et al.* 1992).

Higher socioeconomic status coupled with good social support appears to be protective of spousal physical violence (Jeyaseelan *et al.* 2007). An inverse relationship has been identified between social position and health outcomes. Negative health outcomes occur at a rate of two to two-and-a-half times higher in the most disadvantaged compared with the most privileged. Such observations have been made in Scandinavia and other countries. Similarly, the association between poor mental health and low income in urban-dwelling women has been observed in Bombay, India, and Santiago, Chile (World Health Organization 2000).

Another contributing factor to women's mental health is the woman's family of origin. The family is the crucible for raising a child. The family's expectation of the girl and the family stereotypes have been shown to influence subsequent social behavior and adjustments (Cheng 2009). Lastly, minority status conferred by being a refugee, an immigrant or a member of a racialized or gendered minority may lead to discrimination in terms of opportunities and access to services.

Sex/gender, psychopathology, and diagnosis

Although sometimes used interchangeably, the terms sex and gender have different connotations. Social scientists and other workers have commented on these two terms since the disreputable publication of Sigmund Freud's observation that "anatomy is destiny." Margaret Mead, in *Sex and Temperament in Three Primitive Societies* (1935), observed that sex roles in one society may differ from sex roles in another society. In one group the men could carry out certain roles, while in another the identical roles could be carried out by women.

Generally, sex refers to a construct that emphasizes the biological and psychological characteristic of an individual. Until recently, an individual's sex assignment was fixed. However, with the somewhat more common practice of sex-change surgery, there is now the possibility that some individuals may have a sex change. Gender, on the other hand, is a social construct that emphasizes roles and role assignments and the various expectations and interpersonal interactions that may occur in that society.

Meanwhile, at least partially as a result of feminist influences, the whole idea of what constitutes gender is shifting. Also there appear to be more liberal attitudes and greater recognition of the rights of individuals who are lesbian, gay, bisexual, and transgender. Recently I heard a radio commentary in the United States that some university students preferred not to categorize themselves by their gender. However, for this chapter we will adopt the traditional definitions of sex and gender and their relevance in research activities.

Sex/gender and epidemiological data

Epidemiological data frequently allude to:

(1) Females being at a disadvantage in terms of health status, while males have earlier mortality (Kruger & Nesse 2004).

(2) The apparently consistent observation that with some psychiatric disorders females have a greater prevalence, while in other psychiatric disorders males have a higher prevalence, but that overall both sexes have the same prevalence of psychiatric disorders (Astbury 1999).

This observation has become refined with the use of longitudinal strategies and the application of structured and more comprehensive interview instruments in place of the previous simplistic counting techniques. The relationship between sex/gender and diagnosis now appears to be more complex than previously thought (McDonough & Walters 2001). For example, schizophrenia in women tends to occur later than in men (Astbury 1999).

There are other aspects of gender relationships to psychiatric diagnosis. Earlier versions of the *Diagnostic and Statistical Manual of Mental Disorders* (DSM) did not pay very close attention to gender-based factors in their psychiatric nosology. In a document on *Age and Gender Considerations in Psychiatric Diagnosis: a Research Agenda for the DSM-V*, the editors, while recognizing that some strides have been made in taking into consideration the effects of sex and gender in the revisions, suggested that more research is needed (Narrow *et al.* 2007).

In addition, attention has been drawn to a discriminating bias in the criteria requirements in depression, for example, which condition occurs in a ratio of 2:1, women to men (Astbury 1999). Common symptoms of mood reactivity, weight gain, elevated appetite, hyperinsomnia, and long-standing interpersonal rejection sensitivity are the diagnostic criteria for "atypical depression." This suggests that men's symptom profiles are being used for

diagnostic criteria for a condition that occurs more in women (American Psychiatric Association 1994).

From a historic perspective, hysteria, nymphomania, and neurasthenia have reflected women's conformity or lack of social norms. Also male homosexuality has been blamed on mothers' close, binding, and intimate tendencies. Premenstrual dysphonic disorder (PMDD) suggests that womens' emotions are governed by their reproductive functions (Johnson & Stewart 2010).

In an attempt to explore the variation in lifetime mental disorders across cultures in 15 countries, the WHO conducted a worldwide mental health survey, the World Mental Health Survey. This was a face-to-face household survey of 72 933 community-dwelling adults. A variable used was the "female gender role traditionality as measured by the aggregate patterns of female education, employment, marital timing, and use of birth control." A major finding was that gender differences in most lifetime mental disorders were fairly stable, but significant inter-cohort narrowing of differences in major depressive disorder is related to changes in the traditionality of several gender roles (Seedat *et al.* 2009).

Furthermore, while not ignoring the biases in research on gender, as it focuses mainly on the reproductive function of women versus that of men, as this chapter is on the female gender it behoves us to re-examine the traditional beliefs about sex/gender in psychopathology and diagnosis. It is highly suspect that considering the variations worldwide in psychosocial factors, economics, traditions, the presence of conflicts, and different sex roles that overall the prevalence of mental illness in different countries and different segments of society appears more or less consistent. This same question is now being addressed by some researchers. For example, McDonough and Walters (2001) found evidence for a variable pattern of gender disparity in health outcomes and therefore recommended the use of several measures for recording health status. In a review on "Gender and mental health," Jill Astbury (1999) pointed out that "with serious mental illness, where there is little evidence of gender differences in prevalence rates, gender differences do exist along other dimensions within these mental disorders." She concluded that general differences in psychiatric disorders go beyond the mere rates of these conditions, their time of onset, and their course. She suggested that a variety of factors may influence the risk or susceptibility, diagnosis, treatment, and adjustment to mental disorders. These factors may intervene at the individual, group, or the environmental level.

To summarize, the link between gender and mental health is complex and the different pathways require further exploration.

Gender risk factors: a developmental approach

Childhood

Poverty, maternal depression, exposure to violence, and family of origin are some of the major risk factors of this stage of development. The pervasive effect of poverty has previously been alluded to. The depressed mother cannot optimally provide emotionally for her offspring. There are long-term effects of physical abuse and sexual abuse of children. Exposure to violence also has negative consequences (Mullen *et al.* 1996).

Adolescence

This is an important transition for girls as they begin to negotiate becoming adults. There are significant concomitant psychological changes with consequences for interpersonal relationships, school adjustments, and acquisition of skills. Some specific risk factors in this period include adolescent pregnancy, school bullying, exposure to violence, female genital mutilation, and premature marriage. For some women, their depression begins to emerge during this period. Suicide is the third leading cause of death in adolescents and young adults (Kallon 2003). The United Nations Population Fund (UNFPA) is active in this area.

Reproductive stage

This period within the life cycle is crucial in terms of societal and relationship expectations. The stressors and demands can be great. Hence, limited resources as in poverty, low socioeconomic status, unemployment, lack of domestic help, and violence can be major sources of psychic distress to the female. Depression in women occurs at a rate of 2–3 times that in men. Its causation appears to be multifactorial. Suicide attempts and completion are significant events in this life phase. Women attempt suicide more frequently than men, but complete suicide less often than men (Washington University 1998).

Trauma, wars, and women

The plight of women in conflict areas and war zones is generally indescribable. For a variety of reasons, civilian casualties may rise to as high as 90% of all casualties (Ahlstrom 1991). Both civilian men and women are severely traumatized physically and psychologically. However, there are specific gender traumas that women suffer. They are sexually traumatized, raped, and humiliated. Sometimes the trauma is incessant and occurs multiple times. This harassment may even continue in refugee camps. All this may be coupled with multiple losses and bereavements.

Intimate partner violence

This is a major problem in developed and non-developed countries. We have previously referred to some of the risk factors for intimate partner violence. The UN's UNiTE campaign is active in this area. Intimate partner violence has gained prominence in the last few decades. This is most probably a long-standing phenomenon which is now in the open as a result of advocacy, education, and health promotion. Intimate partner violence can be emotional, psychological, physical, and sexual. It is most often domestic, and the perpetrators are usually men known to their female victims. Intimate partner relationships can also occur between individuals in homosexual relationships, and with older children. This phenomenon occurs across cultures in both developed and developing countries (Harway undated).

Sometimes the violent behavior of the perpetrators is as widespread as it is blatant. In a recent UN study of rape in six countries in the Asia–Pacific region, one in four men admitted to raping a woman. The study further reported that 23% of these men in Papua New Guinea and 16% in Cambodia were teenagers when they committed these violent crimes (Fulu *et al.* 2013). The recent incidents of egregious and public rape in India are inexplicable.

A variety of pathologies have been linked to intimate partner violence. These include chronic pain syndrome, post-traumatic stress disorder, depression, suicidal behavior, and, in extreme cases, suicide, sati, and murder. Intimate partner violence can also expose the victim to sexually transmitted diseases and HIV/AIDS. Several studies have linked current domestic violence to past violence. Chronic abuse correlates with increased psychosocial distress, chemical dependency, and negative health status

(Fischbach & Herbert 1997). An important study in this area was the WHO Multi-Country Study on Women's Health and Domestic Violence (World Health Organization 2005). This study demonstrated significant correlation between lifetime experiences of male partners' physical or sexual abuse with a spectrum of physical and mental problems.

Menopause

This can be a major transition phase for some women. From a clinical perspective, risk factors in this phase include infertility, hysterectomy, family discord, and divorce, amongst others. Some women may experience physical symptoms such as hot flashes and psychological symptoms such as irritability and dysphoria. During this period their physical condition includes cardiovascular disorders, degenerative diseases, and cancers. The comorbidities of these conditions, together with depression during this period, may be responsible in the United States for the explosion in the use of opiates and benzodiazepines. This in turn has led to an increase in overdoses and deaths in older women.

Old age (post-menopause)

Social isolation and physical impairment can influence the psychic distress during this phase of a women's life. In this age group in the USA, suicide is disproportionate to the size of the group (Dubin 2011). The physical correlate of the above stage is increased in the post-menopausal stage. There is an increase in cardiovascular disorders, degenerative disorders, bladder and other gynecological disorders, as well as cancers. From a clinical point of view a phenomenon sometimes overlooked is the abuse by elderly and dementing men of their spouses. The female victims may be reluctant to report this to either family members or the authorities because of loyalty or shame.

Maternal health and mental health

From a public health perspective, the perinatal period can be seen as a "crisis" that when well managed can lead to good outcomes and when ignored or unmanaged may lead to poorer outcomes. It represents a risky or significant life event with potential consequences for the pregnant woman, her infant, her other children, and the family. It is known for example that mood disorders, schizophrenia, and specific anxiety disorders contribute 3.3% of the total global burden of disease and 7% of the global burden for women of all ages. Mental health problems during pregnancy can lead to more obstetric complications, more visits to physicians, and more hospital visits. Psychosis during pregnancy can increase mortality and result in greater hospitalization of children (Department of Health 2002). As indicated elsewhere in this volume (Chapter 2), depression is likely to increase in the coming decades. The perinatal period is a particularly risky period for women. Several investigators have found that pregnant women experience depression and commit suicide at a higher rate than non-pregnant women. They have reported rates varying from 10% to 40% in low- and middle-income countries. Although figures for the developing world are harder to come by, it is to be assumed that the corresponding figures are likely to be higher. For example, a study in Maputo General Hospital, Mozambique, found that 9 (33%) of 27 pregnancy-related deaths were cases of suicide (World Health Organization 2008). While the specific reasons for increased psychopathology in the perinatal period are not fully known, suffice it to say that during this period there are significant biological and psychosocial factors in operation. Some of the risk factors include adolescent pregnancy, being unmarried, lack of social support, poverty, past psychiatric illness, family problems and discord.

As previously mentioned, there are also consequences of impaired maternal mental health on the infants. Some of these include deficits in physical and psychosocial developments as well as lack of compliance with immunization schedules. There are consequences for older children, including impaired social skills and educational attainment. Therefore, a primary preventive approach to recognize and identify individuals at risk is paramount.

Microfinancing, education, and family planning

All of the eight Millennium Development Goals have relevance for the individual woman, her family, and her communities. This is reflected in an emphasis on the intersectional nature of strategies to improve the status and quality of life of women. One strategy that has been used is "microfinancing." This is "the supply of loans, savings and other financial services to the poor."

There are several models of microfinance. Amongst the successful ones are the Bangladesh Rural Advancement Committee, Freedom from Hunger, and the Grameen Bank. Naturally the outcomes for various models at different sites are likely to vary. Nevertheless, two cautionary observations have been made (Outlook 2011):

(1) Standalone microfinance schemes appear to be less successful than those that integrate into their plans women's health needs from a health-sector perspective. Some of these needs include health education and promotion, support groups, and case management to assist with linkages and health and social service providers.

(2) There is a potential for the exploitation of already vulnerable and poor individuals and their families.

Developing gender-sensitive mental health care

A recent and welcome trend is the inclusion of users and survivors in the planning of services and research. This orientation should also be extended to women. Women individually and in groups should have the opportunity to express their specific needs. Advocacy should go beyond feminism. Culturally sensitive, woman-friendly, and woman-centered approaches are likely to enhance compliance and improve the care provided to women. In planning service delivery, women's limited resources of time, money, and mobility should be taken into consideration. The relative lack of autonomy of women in traditional marriages is likely to influence the health and help-seeking behavior of female patients. The low self-esteem of some women may hinder these individuals from freely communicating their needs. Additionally, appropriate healthcare decisions may be compromised. There can be no substitute for self-determination in planning women's service-delivery systems. Various agencies and institutions have attempted best practices. Usually these include the opportunity for the women to express their preferences, the need to respect culture and religious practices, and the availability of a safe environment that respects the needs of individual categories of women, such as traumatized women who have suffered from rape or other experiences (Johnson & Stewart 2010).

From a research point of view, there is a need for further studies to explore the interactions of sex/gender and the factors that may impinge on the mental health and quality of life of women and girls. For health promotion and service delivery, proven public health approaches including the provision of reliable information, early detection, referral treatment, and follow-ups can be useful, as well as interagency case management. Policy-wise, partnerships between behavioral service providers, administrators, policy makers, and users and survivors need to be expanded.

Summary and conclusions

In summary, it has become more widely believed that when women are given the appropriate opportunities, and access to education, family planning, and job training, they can make significant contributions to their communities. One illustration of this is the Goldman Sachs 10 000 Women Project. This is an empowerment program that provides women with the means and resources to start their own businesses. Rasha, an Egyptian entrepreneur and participant in this initiative, stated, "a woman can be a mother, wife, and a business woman." Dina Powell, head of global corporate engagement with Goldman Sachs, emphasized the connection between the empowerment of women and economic growth, saying, "when women are economically empowered, there is a direct benefit to their societies" (Goldman Sachs 2012, undated). All in all, elimination of inequality, access to appropriate education and training, and access to family planning can in concert unleash the potential of women worldwide and improve their quality of life.

In this chapter we have tried to highlight the protean issues that relate to any attempt to reduce mental illness in women and girls. Women have specific sex and gender needs that have to do with the reproductive years, their social roles, and inequalities in contemporary society.

The Millennium Development Goals have been described as holding "a promise" to unleash the potential in women and girls and help to provide economic and social inclusion. For women and girls the issues go beyond just diagnosis and services. The issues include cultural, economic, and psychosocial factors. A public health approach that identifies vulnerable populations from a chronological and developmental perspective can be a starting point for service delivery and interagency collaboration. From a policy perspective there are local, national, regional, and international perspectives. These perspectives should be interagency and intersectoral. From a global perspective, the UN, WHO, World Bank, the IMF, and related agencies can continue to use the Millennium Development Goals as a road map. NGOs and foundations can continue to play a role. An example of this is the commitment of the European Union to assist in the elimination of violence against women and girls by sharing experiences and resources with agencies from developing countries. Sometimes child bearing, child rearing, and work outside the home are challenging tasks even for the average woman.

References

Ahlstrom C (1991) *Casualties of Conflict: Report for the World Campaign for the Protection of Victims of War.* Uppsala: Uppsala University.

American Psychiatric Association (1994) *Diagnostic and Statistical Manual of Mental Disorders, Fourth Edition (DSM-IV).* Washington, DC: APA.

Astbury J (1999) Gender and mental health. http://people.stfx.ca/accamero/gender%20and%20health/mental%20health/gender%20and%20mental%20health.pdf (accessed September 2013).

Cheng W (2009) Families of origin as agents determining women's mental health. In PS Chandra, H Herrman, JE Fisher, *et al.*, eds., *Contemporary Topics in Women's Mental Health: Global Perspectives in a Changing Society.* Chichester: Wiley; pp. 517–24.

Counts DA, Brown JK, Campbell JC (1992) *Sanctions and Sanctuary: Cultural Perspectives on the Beating of Wives.* Boulder, CO: Westview Press.

Department of Health (2002) *Women's Mental Health: Into the Mainstream. Strategic Development of Mental Health Care for Women.* London: DOH. http://www.nmhdu.org.uk/silo/files/into-the-mainstream-full-document.pdf (accessed September 2013).

Dubin JW (2011) Suicide spike among middle-aged women: experts speculate that depression, substance abuse and sleep issues may all play a part. *NBS News: Today Health.* http://www.today.com/id/43714272/ns/today-today_health/t/suicide-spikes-among-middle-aged-women/#.UjiBoKgo59A (accessed September 2013).

Fischbach RL, Herbert B (1997) Domestic violence and mental health: correlates and conundrums within and across cultures. *Social Science and Medicine* 45: 1161–76.

Fulu E, Warner X, Miedema S, *et al.* (2013) *Why Do Some Men Use Violence Against Women and How Can We Prevent It? Quantitative Findings from the United Nations Multi-country Study on Men and Violence in Asia and the Pacific.* Bangkok: UNDP, UNFPA, UN Women and UNV.

Goldman Sachs (2012) 10,000 women in the growth markets. [Video.] Focus on Investing in Women: Empowering Women. http://www.goldmansachs.com/our-thinking/focus-on-investing-in-women/empowering-women/index.html (accessed September 2013).

Goldman Sachs (undated) 10,000 women. http://www.goldmansachs.com/s/gs-10k-womens-voice (accessed September 2013).

Harway M (undated) Intimate partner abuse and relationship violence. Intimate Partner Abuse and Relationship Violence Working Group. http://www.apa.org/about/awards/partner-violence.pdf (accessed September 2013).

Hulme D (2009) *The Millennium Development Goals (MDGs): A Short History of the World's Biggest Promise.* BWPI Working Paper 100. Manchester: Brooks World Poverty Institute. http://www.bwpi.manchester.ac.uk/resources/Working-Papers/bwpi-wp-10009.pdf (accessed September 2013).

Jeyaseelan L, Kumar S, Neelakantan N, *et al.* (2007) Physical spousal violence against women in India: some risk factors. *Journal of Biosocial Science* 39: 657–70.

Johnson J, Stewart DE (2010) DSM-V: toward a gender sensitive approach to psychiatric diagnosis. *Archives of Women's Mental Health* 13: 17–19.

Kallon R (2003) The third leading cause of death amongst teenagers: suicide. *Serendip.* http://serendip.brynmawr.edu/biology/b103/f03/web3/r2kallon.html (accessed September 2013).

Kristof ND, WuDunn S (2009) *Half the Sky: Turning Oppression into Opportunity for Women Worldwide.* New York, NY: Knopf.

Kruger DJ, Nesse RM (2004) Sexual selection and the male:female mortality ratio. *Evolutionary Psychology* 2: 66–85.

McDonough P, Walters V (2001) Gender and health: reassessing patterns and explanations. *Social Science and Medicine* 52: 547–59.

Mead M (1935) *Sex and Temperament in Three Primitive Societies.* New York, NY: Morrow.

Moffitt TE, Robins RW, Caspi A (2001) A couples analysis of partner abuse with implications for abuse prevention policy. *Criminal Public Policy* 1: 5–36.

Mullen PE, Martin JL, Anderson JC, Romans SE, Herbison GP (1996) The long-term impact of the physical, emotional, and sexual abuse of children: a community study. *Child Abuse and Neglect* 20: 7–21.

Narrow WE, First MB, Sirovatka PJ, Regier DA (2007) *Age and Gender Considerations in Psychiatric*

Diagnosis: a Research Agenda for DSM-V. Arlington, VA: American Psychiatric Publishing.

Outlook (2011) Microfinance and women's health: what do we know? *Outlook* **28** (1). http://www.gbchealth.org/system/documents/category_1/367/Microfinance_and_womens_health.pdf?1345234137 (accessed September 2013).

Patel V, Araya R, de Lima M, Ludermir A, Todd C (1999) Women, poverty and common mental disorders in four restructuring societies. *Social Science and Medicine* **49**: 1461–71.

Seedat S, Scott KM, Angermeyer MC, *et al.* (2009) Cross-national associations between gender and mental disorders in the World Health Organization World Mental Health Surveys. *Archives of General Psychiatry* **66**: 785–95.

Stewart DE (2006) The International Consensus Statement on Women's Mental Health and the WPA Consensus Statement on Interpersonal Violence against Women. *World Psychiatry* **5**: 61–4.

United Nations (1996) *Report of the Fourth World Conference on Women, Beijing, September 4–5, 1995.* New York, NY: UN. http://www.un.org/womenwatch/daw/beijing/pdf/Beijing%20full%20report%20E.pdf (accessed September 2013).

United Nations (undated) The United Nations Millennium Development Goals. http://www.un.org/millenniumgoals (accessed September 2013).

Washington University (1998) Why women are less likely than men to commit suicide. *ScienceDaily.* http://www.sciencedaily.com/releases/1998/11/981112075159.htm (accessed September 2013).

World Health Organization (2000) *Women's Mental Health: an Evidence-based Review. Mental Health Determinants and Populations.* Geneva: WHO.

World Health Organization (2005) *WHO Multi-Country Study on Women's Health and Domestic Violence Against Women: Initial Results on Prevalence, Health Outcomes and Women's Responses.* Geneva: WHO.

World Health Organization (2008) *Maternal mental health and child health and development in low and middle income countries: report of the WHO-UNFPA meeting held in Geneva, Switzerland, 30 January – 1 February, 2008.* Geneva: WHO.

Violence against women

Erminia Colucci and Reima Pryor

Introduction

Violence against women is now widely recognized as a significant global problem, a major public health concern, and one of the most widespread violations of human rights (World Health Organization 2005, Eng *et al.* 2010). The United Nations Declaration on the Elimination of Violence against Women (1993) defines *violence against women* as any act of gender-based violence that results in, or is likely to result in, physical, sexual, or psychological harm or suffering to women, including threats of such acts, coercion, or arbitrary deprivation of liberty, whether occurring in public or private life. This declaration further distinguishes between violence occurring in the family, violence occurring within the broader community, and "structural violence" perpetrated or condoned by the state. Unicef (2000) focused on *domestic violence* (DV) as one of the most prevalent and yet hidden and ignored forms of violence against women and girls globally, and defined this as comprising violence by an intimate partner or other family members, including violence occurring beyond the confines of the home, and across all ages from pregnancy to old age. The World Health Organization (2010) distinguished *intimate-partner violence* (IPV) and *sexual violence* (SV), while recognizing significant overlap between these.

Violence against women is a universal phenomenon that persists in all countries and societies of the world (World Health Organization 2005), affecting all communities irrespective of race, gender, class, religion, cultural background, or ethnicity (Bannenberg & Rossner 2003). Even a country such as Norway, characterized by welfare and gender equality, is not immune to violence against women, as was strongly captured by a recent campaign by

Amnesty International (http://www.imow.org/wpp/stories/viewstory?storyid=178). The WHO's Multi-Country Study on Women's Health and Domestic Violence Against Women (2005) provides a comprehensive picture of the prevalence and nature of IPV and SV within high-income countries (HICs) and low- and middle-income countries (LMICs), and demonstrates significant variations in prevalence rates between and within countries. However, this study shows that higher rates tend to occur in lower-income countries. In particular, a higher risk of violence is found in societies with traditional gender norms and roles, unequal distribution of power and resources between men and women, a normative use of violence to resolve conflicts, and cultural approval of (or weak sanctions against) violence against women (VicHealth 2011, World Health Organization 2011).

Unicef (2000) recognizes that specific groups of women are more vulnerable, including minority groups, indigenous and migrant women, refugee women and those in situations of armed conflict, women in institutions and detention, women with disabilities, female children, and elderly women.

Violence against women, mental health, and suicide

Violence against women is not only a serious breach of human rights, but has major health, social, and economic consequences for women, their families, and communities. Several studies have highlighted the impact of violence against women, particularly domestic/family violence, on physical and mental health (e.g., Coker *et al.* 2000, World Health Organization 2005, Ellsberg *et al.* 2008), including suicidal behavior (Chowdhary & Patel 2008, Davar 2003,

Essentials of Global Mental Health, ed. Samuel O. Okpaku. Published by Cambridge University Press. © Cambridge University Press 2014.

World Health Organization 2005, Ellsberg *et al.* 2008, Devries *et al.* 2011, Colucci & Heredia Montesinos 2013). In regard to this latter impact, a significant correlation between DV and suicidal ideation has been found in population-based studies in many developing countries: 48% in Brazil, 61% in Egypt, 64% in India, 11% in Indonesia, and 28% in the Philippines (Vijayakumar *et al.* 2004). Devries *et al.* (2011) highlighted discussion in the literature about the role of having a dowry/bride price, control over choosing one's husband, and being childless in marriage in increasing suicide risk; however, the authors noted that only a few studies have explored the contributing role of DV to suicidal behavior. Each of these factors, the authors observed, may result in poor mental health status directly and suicide, but also may be associated with restricted autonomy and loss of control, which can in turn lead to poor mental health status and suicide.

Waters (1999) indicated a strong link between suicide and violence against women and argued that among Indian women (as for many other women) suicide is the endpoint of suffering and that abetment to suicide is considered so ubiquitous and powerful that many social activists have claimed that "every suicide is a murder" (p. 526). High prevalence of violence against women, particularly family/domestic violence, and the influence of this on suicidal behavior, has been also demonstrated among women from South/East Asia and other low-income countries who migrated to high-income countries (e.g., Hicks & Bhugra 2003, van Bergen *et al.* 2011). A study of South Asian women by Chantler and colleagues (2010) showed that for the women who self-harmed, self-harm was seen both as a coping mechanism – a way to experience a sense of power and control normally not available to them – and also as a way of punishing themselves, as they blamed themselves for being "bad." Thus, the authors concluded that for those women "suicide attempts and self-harming appear to be a 'rational' response to such violence and brutality, rather than a mental 'illness'" (p. 86). This conclusion is supported by a WHO study of 13 worldwide sites, which showed that IPV, non-partner physical violence, and having a mother who was exposed to IPV were the most consistent risk factors for suicide attempts after adjusting for common mental health problems (Devries *et al.* 2011). As violence against women has been shown to have a strong impact on a person's mental health and a direct or indirect impact on suicidal behavior, it is essential for anybody working in the mental health and/or suicide prevention sectors, in low-income and middle-income as well as high-income countries, to familiarize themselves with the topic and become involved in the prevention of violence against women and the defence of women's rights (see also Colucci & Heredia Montesinos 2013, Colucci & Lester 2013). As strongly stated by Vijayakumar (2004) in India – although this also applies to several other countries – "suicide prevention is more of a social and public health objective than a traditional exercise in the mental health sector."

As observed by Mercy and collaborators (2003), "it is clear that the consequences of violence extend far beyond death and physical injury. Violence prevention, therefore, is an essential component of improving the mental health of people throughout the world."

On top of the "costs" of violence against women on the personal and community levels, such violence represents a financial loss to government. The annual cost of providing public services (including health, legal, and social services) to victims, and the lost economic output of women in the UK alone, amounts to approximately £36 billion (Home Office 2012a). In Australia it has been estimated that domestic violence and sexual assault perpetrated against women cost the nation $13.6 billion each year, and that by 2021 the figure is likely to rise to $15.6 billion if extra steps are not taken for its prevention (Council of Australian Governments 2012).

What is prevention?

In considering *prevention* of violence against women, the WHO (2010) applies a public health approach to this health risk issue, and classifies prevention strategies into three types (Dahlberg & Krug 2002):

(1) *primary prevention* (aiming to prevent violence before it occurs)
(2) *secondary prevention* (immediate responses once violence has occurred)
(3) *tertiary prevention* (efforts to reduce the impacts of the violence)

The WHO (2010) highlights that primary prevention has been neglected within the field of violence against women, in comparison to secondary and tertiary-level interventions, in terms of resource allocation. The

WHO report provides a strong conceptual framework and initial international evidence base as a foundation or starting point for primary prevention practices.

A public health approach to prevention

The WHO (2010) draws on the *public health approach* to prevention, as used by the *World Report on Violence and Health* (Krug *et al.* 2002), as a "science-driven, population-based, interdisciplinary, inter-sectoral approach and based on the ecological model which emphasizes primary prevention" (p. 6). A population health approach uses population-based data to describe the problem, its impact, and the associated risk and protective factors, in order to derive directions for intervention, test such intervention, and, eventually, implement it (Mercy *et al.* 1993). A complex array of risk (and protective) factors have been identified through research as the underlying determinants or causes of violence against women, which increase (or reduce) the likelihood of violence occurring in the first place, and some of which are modifiable via interventions. The "ecological model" (Dahlberg & Krug 2002) organizes risk and protective factors into four levels of a nested hierarchy:

- individual level
- relationship/family level
- community level
- societal level

At the core of the ecological model is its emphasis on multiple and dynamic interactions among risk factors within and between its levels, and its promotion of the importance of cross-sectoral prevention policies and programs.

In terms of the risk and protective factors theorized to be causally related to IPV and SV, a comprehensive review of the literature of risk and protective factors identified over 50 risk factors, with most being at the *individual* and *relationship/family* levels of the ecological model, and with some being modifiable and others not (World Health Organization 2010). The low numbers of factors identified for *community* and *societal* levels is put down to lack of research at these levels rather than a lack of risk factors as such, and likewise for protective factors.

Strong risk factors identified for both IPV and SV across the four levels of influence were as follows: low education for men and women (no simple explanation, yet the most consistent factor associated with perpetration and experience of violence); young age of women; sexual abuse of men; intraparental violence for women (present although less strong association for men); antisocial personality for men (and related characteristics of impulsivity and lack of empathy); harmful use of alcohol for men and women (including in LMICs, with the nature of its role unclear); acceptance of violence by men and women (in conjunction with patriarchal views of women as inferior); and multiple partners/infidelity for men (also associated with unprotected sex). Exposure to child maltreatment, in particular exposure to parental IPV, is one factor consistently cited across countries (including in LMICs) as a risk factor for both perpetration and victimization of/by violence.

It is interesting to note that, in relation to community-level factors, it was observed that community sanctions (legal or social prohibitions) against violence and availability of community sanctuaries (refuges) for victims were associated with lower levels of IPV and SV. It was further hypothesized that IPV would be higher in communities where women's status was in a state of transition from low status towards higher status, when men's authority would be perceived to be under threat, as is the case in several LMICs, and as may be expected in the case of some migrant and refugee communities.

It was noted that gender-based power is one of the most common theories to explain IPV and SV, and yet gender inequality as a societal-level factor is significantly under-researched in terms of the nature of its risk and protective associations, within different sociocultural contexts, and is a priority for research.

A WHO (2010) finding in relation to societal-level factors (of particular relevance to the research data that we present later in this chapter) was that IPV is more common in communities in which males have economic and decision-making power, where there is not easy access to divorce, and where violence is used to resolve conflicts. The availability of women's workgroups was also found to reduce risk for women, presumably through the provision of stable social support and economic independence. The maintenance of patriarchal values or male dominance norms within a society reflects gender inequality, and may legitimize violence against women, with gender-based power as one of the most common theories to explain IPV and SV. This may also mean that women who are not submissive or who are independent are considered less attractive, or disliked within society. At the societal level, this issue of gender-based power influences access to health resources available to women, and it also plays out across the levels of community, relationship/family, and individual. In this way, macro-level interventions to address structural inequities as well as those targeting gender inequality at the other levels may serve to reduce IPV. Also, at the community level, increasing educational attainment, urbanization, access to media, and joint decision making were associated with decreased levels of IPV in most countries (while the strength of these factors requires further validation).

Protective factors for IPV and SV are less well researched, with initial associations found as follows: higher education for women and men; experience of healthy parenting as a child; availability of own supportive family; living within an extended family structure; belonging to an association; and women's ability to recognize risk. More research is urged to understand protective factors towards violence against women.

Developmental prevention

Farrington (1996) identified four approaches to the related field of crime prevention, namely: *criminal justice* (e.g., deterrence, incarceration, and rehabilitation); *situational* (e.g., making changes to the physical or psychological environment to make crime more difficult or to strengthen moral condemnation); *community or social* (e.g., changes at the local level to empower residents, to provide opportunities for young people, and to strengthen social infrastructure); and *developmental* (e.g., interventions designed to inhibit the development of criminal potential in individuals).

Australia's National Crime Prevention initiative (1999) provides a comprehensive analysis of the developmental approach to (crime) prevention. This approach sees the series of transitions or points of change across the life course (towards offending) as being points at which there is increased stress, and a fork in the pathway with more than one possible outcome, as well as being points at which there is increased malleability, with associated opportunity for effective intervention. In this way, *developmental prevention* is an attempt to put risk and protective factors into a "phase-related path," and sees past

transitions as having created a pattern of cumulative risk or protection. The importance of social context is highlighted within this theoretical framework for its impact on skills, strategies, and identity as well as on the support available to an individual at a given transition point. This "pathways to prevention" approach considers "early intervention" as meaning an intervention early in the pathway of development of a behavior, which may or may not mean early in life.

Primary prevention interventions

The WHO (2010) conducted a comprehensive and rigorous international review of primary prevention programs, and identified programs that were (1) effective in primary prevention according to robust scientific trials, and (2) not yet systematically implemented or evaluated but which showed promise (based on early limited evidence or on sound theoretical presuppositions such as targeting of known risk factors). Most of the high-quality research studies were found to come from HICs, and in particular the United States; the point was made that generalizability from HICs to LMICs cannot be assumed. Promising practice for LMICs, however, was also identified. Again, individual and relationship levels of the ecological model were found to have been targeted for programs and evaluation more frequently than the community and societal levels. At times when societal-level strategies have been implemented (for example, policies to promote gender equality), evaluation of their impacts on the level or nature of IPV or SV has not been undertaken.

The WHO report (2010) classified outcomes of those rigorously evaluated primary prevention strategies as follows: effective; emerging/promising; unclear; emerging/ineffective; ineffective; and harmful. Of note, evidence of the deterrent effects of criminal justice system responses was found to be lacking, with some studies showing equivalent effects of arrest and police "warnings," some studies showing no effect of arrests for some subgroups, and other studies showing increased violence effect with arrests. Only one strategy was identified to be effective based on a robust evaluation design, and that was the use of school-based programs to prevent violence in dating relationships, with outcomes of reduced experience of and perpetration of physical, sexual, and emotional abuse during subsequent dates (e.g., Youth Relationship Project: Wolfe *et al.* 2003). This was the most evaluated of all IPV prevention programs, with 12 evaluations, of which five were randomized controlled trials (RCTs). A link between dating violence and later IPV/SV has been found, with dating violence found to be a risk factor for IPV later in life (along with other health-compromising behaviors of injuries, unsafe sex, substance abuse, and suicide attempts). It was noted that the relevance of these programs for other cultures, however, such as within LMICs, is questionable.

Given the low numbers of rigorously evaluated programs available, the report also summarized primary prevention programs and strategies showing promise, worthy of future evaluation. "Strategy" (e.g., home visiting) was distinguished from "program" (e.g., Nurse Family Partnership Program: Olds *et al* 2007), as while this particular program was found to be highly effective according to RCTs, not all programs utilizing the given strategy of "home visiting" were found to be effective. Strategies were grouped according to life stage (infancy/childhood/ early adolescence, adolescence/early adulthood, adulthood, all life stages). The report also drew on research from the child maltreatment and youth violence fields, with extrapolations acknowledged to be speculative.

In regards to the life stages of infancy/childhood and early adolescence, the authors cite research indicating that the most promising strategies for preventing child maltreatment (and its related intergenerational transmission of violence and abuse: WHO & ISPCAN 2006) include home visitation and parent education programs, and improving maternal mental health (including depression), which can interfere with bonding and attachment and increase the risk of conduct disorders, a key risk for later perpetration of violence. Other promising IPV and SV prevention strategies for childhood/early adolescence include: early identification and treatment of child conduct and emotional disorders; psychological treatment for children who have been maltreated; school-based programs targeting various risks or skills (e.g., precursors for antisocial personality disorder, sexual violence, sexually protective behaviors, bullying prevention), including multicomponent programs such as peer, parent, and teacher education.

Promising prevention strategies for adults include empowering and participatory approaches to reduce gender inequality. Comprehensive approaches engage a whole community or subgroups of a community, use several components, and create an environment supportive of changing individual and community attitudes and behaviors. Such approaches may include education and skills training, public awareness-raising campaigns, and community action (e.g. Lankester 1992). The WHO (2010) identified two examples of this strategy, one that incorporates microfinance with gender equality training, and one that promotes communication and relationship skills to separate gender groups within communities, with both intended to increase the economic and social power of women. The latter program has been evaluated in 40 LMICs, including an RCT in South Africa for 15–26-year-olds, which found reduced IPV in the two years following the program, and a program in Gambia which found that after one year couples showed improved communication and reduced conflict. An RCT is currently under way in a Uganda regarding an activist kit for mobilizing communities to prevent violence against women, focusing on its link with HIV/AIDS. Thus, there is emerging evidence of the effectiveness of these empowering strategies within LMICs. It was noted that interventions resulting in the empowerment of women, as for communities experiencing transition of women from low to higher status, may also have an unintended outcome of increased risk of violence for participants or communities, and it was indicated that efforts to engage men within the second intervention appeared to mitigate this risk.

A further strategy thought to show promise is counseling for couples, focusing on violence, substance abuse, and/or relationship skills for those who have not yet used violence but who may be at risk. One un-evaluated IPV prevention program in Ecuador used friends or relatives to monitor newly-weds and intervene should conflict arise.

Some programs intended to target other issues are being found to show promise in terms of impacts on IPV. For example, home-visitation programs for parents with infants/young children, found to be effective in reducing child maltreatment, are also showing promise and being trialled in relation to IPV with mothers at risk; a suicide prevention initiative within the United States, incorporating a multidisciplinary health team, had unintended benefits of reduced IPV (World Health Organization 2005).

While the nature of the relationship between substance abuse and IPV, for example, as cause or mediating factor, is unclear, beliefs about its role in violence are supported by the fact that it has been found to be associated with violent behavior, and there is some emerging evidence of the impacts of reducing alcohol consumption on IPV, so this is also an area worthy of continued scrutiny. The unregulated nature of the alcohol industry in LMICs makes it hard to implement societal-level consumption reduction interventions within these countries, and the lack of access to specialist services may likewise be a barrier; however, training of primary health workers and general practitioners may be an alternative intervention to reduce alcohol consumption and possibly IPV in LMICs. The social acceptability of excessive drinking, and beliefs about masculinity and heavy drinking, should be included in efforts to prevent alcohol-related IPV and SV.

Unspoken social and cultural norms dictate social approval, disapproval, social punishments, guilt, or shame. Strategies to change social norms that support IPV and SV (including misperceptions about norms) and media awareness campaigns to break the silence that often surrounds IPV and SV, including working with men and boys, are thought to be key in primary prevention (including for LMICs). While such strategies have been adopted, they have rarely been evaluated, however.

In Australia, The Victorian Health Promotion Foundation (VicHealth) has over the last eight years overseen extensive program and policy activity in relation to preventing violence against women in the state of Victoria. This effort arose out of a broader focus on addressing preventable causes of poor mental health and well-being, and their groundbreaking study demonstrating that IPV was the largest known contributor to the total disease burden of Victorian women aged 15–44 years (VicHealth 2004). VicHealth (2006) has also provided a major study on community attitudes to violence against women, and other publications relating to the prevention of violence against women including in migrant and refugee communities, and within the Australian Rules football sector, as well as providing new funding streams to develop policy and practice in preventing violence against women (VicHealth 2012). Further, in conjunction with the Victorian government, VicHealth (2006) has developed a framework to guide whole-of-government policy and activity on preventing violence against women. This framework is consistent with WHO's framework in its use of the ecological model in organizing identified risk and protective factors, and levels for action. VicHealth further identified three key themes for action: (1) promoting equal and respectful relationships between men and women; (2) promoting non-violent social norms and reducing the effects of prior exposure to violence; and (3) improving access to resources and systems of support. VicHealth specifically recognizes opportunities for violence prevention at the family life stages of relationship formation, pregnancy and transition to parenthood, and relationship separation.

Within the Victorian community, another promising prevention intervention within the Indian Australian migrant community of Melbourne involved a partnership between four agencies (E. Colucci, M. O'Connor, K. Field, *et al.*, submitted). The Indian Australian community may be seen as a community "in transition," with migration offering women the potential to gain empowerment,

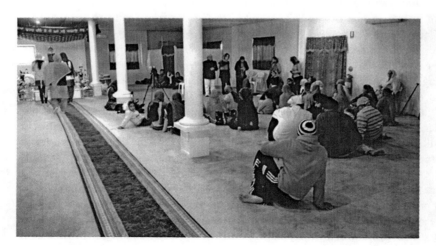

Figure 27.1 Performance in Sikh temple (photo by E. Colucci, 2011).

Table 27.1 Summary of themes and sub-themes about the nature of domestic violence, as revealed by the participatory action research project

Nature of domestic violence	Participant's quotations
Emotional/psychological abuse	
Also described as one of the most common forms of violence	"The worst one" "The one that takes longer to heal"
Excessive control, being dominated, lack of freedom in decision making	"Initially my own parents try to command me, then my husband, my in-laws and later my own children" Imposition, also from the in-laws, on how to behave, what to wear ("touch the feet, cover the head"), which work to do
Verbal abuse, insults or/and verbal threats (including deportation or visa cancellation)	"If a man is violent and the woman leaves him, he can get another wife in India and bring her here without a sponsor or PR, so that if she complains he sends her back"
Silence that is expected to be maintained	"The silence kills . . . I'm listening since three generations"
Be blamed, humiliated, and put down in one's self-esteem; not treated with dignity and equality (used as a way of controlling)	"For everything happening in their lives the woman is blamed, whether they can't find a home, whether the woman does not have a job, or whether he has had a car accident. And eventually she becomes convinced of that and genuinely believes that it is her fault" "He said that he married her so he can have a hot chapatti cooker"
Unrealistic expectations	"Expectations get to a point where they are unrealistic, and when these expectations became unrealistic they became social abuse, emotional abuse"
Social abuse	
Described as the biggest abuse within the Indian community.	"The fears of the society never make you change the things that are happening in your life"
Isolated or not allowed to talk to anybody (including having phone and email use "tapped")	"He used to go and tell my friends how bad I am like, you know, he used to give a wrong opinion about me and then slowly people stopped coming to me"
Pressure to be submissive and quiet	"Men keep saying: talk softly"
Physical abuse	
Beating, hitting, punching	"I'm going to punch her because she doesn't listen, but she's going to listen this [the punch]"
Sexual abuse	
Particularly difficult to identify and to disclose	"It's my husband, he can do it" "The girl cannot go and tell to her parents like my husband is demanding me to do oral sex"
No consensual sex, or kind of sexual demands (including being forced sex during their period, when pregnant or unwell)	"He asks me to do bad stuff which I really don't want to do"
Financial abuse	
Control of money and/or other of her possessions	"If the wife is earning, the husband wants to monitor her money and even control the financial resources"

Table 27.1 (cont.)

Nature of domestic violence	Participant's quotations
Non-acceptance of woman's financial independency	"Since the day you have got a job, it seems you have started talking a lot"
Dowry and other economic pressures	"My son is in Australia, he has a PR, drives a BMW, you pay this much money to get your daughter there in Australia and your daughter will have to do this for my son" "Expectation that all the money they might need to move in Australia and get settled with visa, tickets, etc. should be given by the girl's family because it's for her betterment. But the girl's family might not be capable of giving that much money and then the emotional abuse starts"
Spiritual/religious abuse	
Not letting her go to the temple, not letting her pray, not letting her cook food to offer to God	"She is coming from a very religious family and he would not let her go to the temple because of the controlling behavior" "He does not let me cook good food to offer to God because he has adapted too much to the Western culture"

autonomy, and financial independence, and therefore a threat to the traditional patriarchal structure, with an associated potential for an increase in family violence. This project used a participatory action research model based on community interactive theatre methods (particularly forum theatre) to explore the nature of family violence and barriers to help-seeking within the Indian community. The method comprised three stages: (1) information/focus group sessions, (2) theatre workshops, and (3) community theatre performances. A total of 54 women took part in phase 1, 12 in phase 2, and a further 111 participants (mainly women; one performance was open to a mixed audience) in phase 3. Figure 27.1 shows an example of one of the community performances (in this instance, in a Sikh temple in the outskirts of Melbourne).

Outcomes for this project included contribution to knowledge and the evidence base in relation to its two aims, as well as additional individual-level impacts on participants' knowledge and attitudes, and strengthening of women's support networks. The project also had community-level impacts of building awareness of the community-level factors, which silence the issue and prevent support for victims, raising of community cohesion and activism around the issue, and the identification of culturally appropriate interventions across the spectrum from prevention, early intervention, treatment, and recovery. The key findings regarding the nature of domestic/family violence in the Indian Australian

community sample are summarized in Table 27.1, and findings related to barriers to help-seeking are summarized in Table 27.2.

Where to from here?

While promising practice is occurring across the world, the need for rigorous evaluations of primary prevention programs, integrated at the outset, and incorporating existing theoretical frameworks and models of behavior change, is a strong advocacy message within the WHO report (2010). The authors of this report suggest that outcome measures of prevention effectiveness should include changes in knowledge, attitudes, and beliefs regarding violence against women (while recognizing that changes in these do not equate to changes in behaviors), in conjunction with reductions in perpetration or experiencing of vidence, in their different forms (using consistent operational definitions for these). Other outcomes required for program efficacy include evidence of sustained effects, and the independent replication of outcomes. Significant government and other philanthropic funding, as well as strong partnerships between research and practice (that is, between academic institutions with strong research and evaluation expertise and community organizations creating innovative service delivery solutions to the problem of violence against women) are required as a matter of urgency, to progress this

Table 27.2 Barriers to seeking help

Barriers to help	Participants' quotations	Participants' suggestions
Generic barriers		
Acceptance of inequality and violence against women	"When a girl child is born in India, the man is head of the family and she is always told that girls should be submissive and not argue" "Even a father when you are getting married says you should manage to fit in wherever you go into"	Empower the community to break the silence and assist the woman in seeking help, and providing "good role models in Indian women" able to challenge the
Expectation that a woman will **maintain silence** in such situations	"The best strategy in any situation for an Indian woman is to keep quiet and maintain the silence and suffer" "It is considered not right to tell people that you're having violence in the house"	expectation of silence and submission "So the need of the hour is to start this new idea to propagate that your daughters are not supposed to submit
Social stigma towards a woman victim of violence Fear of the possible consequences of disclosure: • be blamed • be re-victimized • regretting the effects • consequences for their immigration status/ deportation • consequences to others of their immigration status/ deportation • not to be believed and find understanding in others • fear of being isolated	"People don't want to be associated with a woman who has put herself in that situation" "Women are getting abused physically and emotionally and the whole blame is put on them. And the lady can't go anywhere, they are so scared" "People say there must be something wrong with her, that is why the husband is beating her" "If a woman asks for help, the police get involved and they ask her to leave the house, but leaving the house is not necessarily the solution she wants" "You don't tell much to your family because you don't want to hurt them" "If you choose to leave what will become of children" "When people come to Australia they are so isolated so they keep in everything until it blows up. Then they can look for extreme solutions, like killing themselves" "People don't want to be associated with a woman who has put herself in the situation"	to whatever has been told to them" "It is not considered healthy to ask for help in Indian society [. . .] if you are going and seeking help means you are sick. So it needs to be changed" "All we can do is empowering them by telling them that they are good and by giving them positive feedback but eventually the decision has to be hers" "The first step is that we say as a community that it is okay
Lack of freedom and dependency	"My phone was tapped, each conversation I took and each email I sent was tapped" "I couldn't talk with anyone, I never was given money to talk to anyone"	to talk about it. If my husband hits me it's not my fault"
Lack of evidence	"In Australia the domestic violence is only called when you are physically beaten up but that didn't happen to me, so I couldn't prove it was domestic violence"	Give migrant women, especially on arrival, the correct information about their rights and laws available in the host country.
Lack of violence **awareness**, lack of **information** and **knowledge** about laws and their rights	"You don't realize you have been affected [. . .] you haven't been brought up that [emotional abuse] is domestic violence. It's just that these are not clearly defined" "Women need to be aware that if they do seek an intervention, it is generally the perpetrator of the violence who is asked to leave the home"	"If the community is given awareness then they can advise the victim to see a GP, a psychologist or a counselor" "Freedom will come with knowledge, education, know what's fair and not fair, what is your right"

Table 27.2 (cont.)

Barriers to help	Participants' quotations	Participants' suggestions
Barriers specific to services		
Cultural background of the professional	"If it took me 5 minutes to explain my name, how long is this person (talking about service providers) going to take even with my first problem?"	Professionals from Indian background would be better equipped because of the shared understanding of the culture, easiness to establish a relationship and knowledge of the language: "she can surely better understand rather than an Australian counselor because Australian culture is different from our culture" In some instances, advantages were highlighted also in regard to workers who do not belong to the same cultural communities, but are culturally responsive
Cultural sensitiveness of the intervention provided by services	"Go too fast", expect them to do "too big steps" Leaving the husband is not a culturally appropriate answer to domedtic violence. Although this is a "solution" that Australian people or services can propose, that's not possible for an Indian as it "is not the Indian way"	
Lack of knowledge about services: what, where, and how to access them	"The biggest barrier to seeking help is that people don't know who to tell" "They [migrant women] feel very isolated and don't know who to go to and what help is available"	Educating community members about services and access to services: "People go to services when they are really desperate, before that the help must come from the community. Even just one person in the community who knows where to go, will at least give some hope"
Kind of help provided	"[Leaving the husband] is not the Indian way [. . .], they would cut you out if you did that"	Some typologies of help were seen positively, such as violence prevention and outreach programs, activities aimed to women's empowerment, helplines and community groups such as self-help groups: "If information was disseminated at prominent point, like you did not have to go and ask someone but the information was just there like at the GP's, community organizations and you could just pick up the leaflets and keep it, I think that would be helpful."

Table 27.2 (cont.)

Barriers to help	Participants' quotations	Participants' suggestions
		"Having someone in the community who is trained to help those people"
Confidentiality, privacy, and trust in the services	"She has fear to disclose anything on the paper because she thinks that this might go to her husband"	Assure confidentiality and build trust: "She has to know that there is someone she can talk to where confidentiality will be maintained"
Bureaucratic barriers such as lengthy waiting lists, assessment and consent forms	"Signing forms is frightening especially if you are a migrant" "The paperwork came in between and she just wanted to speak to a human being without all these paperworks on the table"	Explain the use of the information collected and the circumstances where the confidentiality might be broken, and do so only when the person has established some engagement with the worker: "After the victim is engaged and gains confidence that is when you say okay by the way we need to sign this form. But you need to gain that trust first"
Social stigma towards mental health service	"The immediate answer is, 'Why do you want to go to Dr. X, I know her, she is a psychiatrist, what is wrong with you?'"	Challenge the stigma: "Counselors are not a big deal, they are not a disease, and rather they are just people with whom you can share your problems, open your heart out. It is very important to spread out this information to the community"
Migration-related barriers (see also fear of deportation)	"He was so violent [. . .] he took me back to India and cancelled my visa [. . .]. I wrote to immigration about all [that] happened to me and they revoked the cancellation [. . .] but I have no clues about Australian laws"	Education, awareness about migration laws and rights

crucial and fertile field of primary prevention of violence against women. The building of prevention partnerships between different sectors is a key theme also in Mercy *et al.* (2003).

Furthermore, the need for international support in decreasing violence against women is well established, and it is the responsibility of every HIC to raise awareness and to tackle violence not only in its own country (including among migrant and refugee communities) but also overseas, especially in low-resourced countries (see Home Office 2012b for a list of actions).

Acknowledgments

We thank Alice Baroni for her contribution to this manuscript.

References

Bannenberg B, Rossner D (2003) New developments in restorative justice to handle family violence. In EGM Weitekamp, HJ Kerner, eds., *Restorative Justice in Context: International Practice and Directions.* Cullompton: Willan; pp. 51–79.

Chantler K, Burman E, Batsleer J, Bashir C (2010) *Attempted Suicide and Self-Harm (South Asian Women).* Manchester: Salford and Trafford Health Action Zone.

Chowdhary N, Patel V (2008) The effect of spousal violence on women's health: Findings from the Stree Arogya Shodh in Goa, India. *Journal of Postgraduate Medicine* 54: 306–12.

Coker AL, Smith PH, Bethea L, King M, McKeown R (2000) Physical health consequences of physical and psychological intimate partner violence. *Archives of Family Medicine* 9: 451–7.

Colucci E, Heredia Montesinos A (2013) Violence against women and suicide in the context of migration. *Suicidology Online* 4: 81–91. www. suicidology-online.com/pdf/SOL-2013-4-81-91.pdf (accessed December 2013).

Colucci E, Lester D (2013) *Suicide and Culture: Understanding the Context.* Cambridge, MA: Hogrefe.

Council of Australian Governments (2012) *National Plan to Reduce Violence Against Women and their Children 2010–2022.* http://www. fahcsia.gov.au/sites/default/files/ documents/05_2012/national_plan. pdf (accessed July 2013).

Dahlberg LL, Krug EG (2002) Violence: a global public health problem. In Krug EG, Dahlberg LL, Mercy JA, Zwi AB, Lozano R, eds. *World Report on Violence and Health.* Geneva: World Health Organization; pp. 3–21.

Davar BV (2003) Mental health in the women's health agenda. *National Medical Journal of India,* 16 (Suppl 2): 39–41.

Devries K, Watts C, Yoshihama M, *et al.* (2011) Violence against women is strongly associated with suicide attempts: evidence from the WHO multi-country study on women's health and domestic violence against women. *Social Science and Medicine* 73: 79–86.

Ellsberg M, Jansen HA, Heise L, Watts CH, Garcia-Moreno C (2008) Intimate partner violence and women's physical and mental health in the WHO multi-country study on women's health and domestic violence: an observational study. *Lancet* 371: 1165–72.

Eng S, Li Y, Mulsow M, Fischer J (2010) Domestic violence against women in Cambodia: husband's control, frequency of spousal discussion, and domestic violence reported by Cambodian women. *Journal of Family Violence* 25: 237–46.

Farrington DP (1996) *Understanding and Preventing Youth Crime.* York: Joseph Rowntree Foundation.

Hicks MHR, Bhugra D (2003) Perceived causes of suicide attempts by UK South Asian women. *American Journal of Orthopsychiatry* 27: 455–62.

Home Office (2012a) 100 actions to tackle violence against women, http://www.homeoffice.gov.uk/ crime/violence-against-women-girls/strategic-vision (accessed July 2013).

Home Office (2012b) *Call to End Violence against Women and Girls.* London: The Stationery Office.

Krug EG, Dahlberg LL, Mercy JA, Zwi AB, Lozano R, eds. (2002) *World Report on Violence and Health.* Geneva: World Health Organization.

Lankester T (1992) *Setting up Community Health Programmes: a Practical Manual for Use in Developing Countries.* London: Macmillan.

Mercy JA, Rosenberg ML, Powell KE, Broome CV, Roper WL (1993) Public health policy for preventing violence. *Health Affairs* 12 (4): 7–29.

Mercy JA, Butchart A, Dahlberg LL, Zwi AB, Krug EG (2003) Violence and mental health: perspectives from the World Health Organization's World Report on Violence and Health. *International Journal of Mental Health* 32: 20–35.

National Crime Prevention (1999) *Pathways to Prevention: Developmental and Early Intervention Approaches to Crime in Australia.* Canberra: National Crime Prevention, Attorney-General's Department.

Olds DL, Sadler L, Kitzman H (2007) Programs for parents of infants and toddlers: recent evidence from randomized trials. *Journal of Child Psychology and Psychiatry* 48: 355–91.

Unicef (2000) Domestic violence against women and girls. *Innocenti Digesti* 6. Florence: Unicef. www. unicef-irc.org/publications/pdf/ digest6e.pdf (accessed July 2013).

United Nations (1993) Declaration on the Elimination of Violence against Women. http://www.un-documents.net/a48r104.htm (accessed July 2013).

van Bergen D, van Balkom AJLM, Smit JH, Saharso S (2011) "I felt so hurt and lonely": suicidal behavior in South Asian-Surinamese, Turkish, and Moroccan women in the Netherlands. *Transcultural Psychiatry* 49 (1): 69–86.

VicHealth (2004) *The Health Costs of Violence: Measuring the Burden of Disease caused by Intimate Partner Violence. A Summary of Findings.* Melbourne: Victorian Health Promotion Foundation.

VicHealth (2006) *Two Steps Forward, One Step Back: Community*

Attitudes to Violence Against Women. Progress and Challenged in Creating Safe and Healthy Environments for Victorian Women. A Summary of Findings. Melbourne: Victorian Health Promotion Foundation.

VicHealth (2011) *Preventing Violence Against Women in Australia Melbourne.* Australia: Victorian Health Promotion Foundation.

VicHealth (2012) *The Respect, Responsibility and Equality program. A summary report on five projects that build new knowledge to prevent violence against women.* Melbourne: Victorian Health Promotion Foundation.

Vijayakumar L (2004) Suicide prevention: the urgent need in developing countries. *World Psychiatry* **3**: 158–9.

Vijayakumar L, Nagaraj K, John S (2004) *Suicide and Suicide Prevention in Developing Countries.* Working Paper No. 27. Disease Control Priorities Project.

Waters AB (1999) Domestic dangers approaches to women's suicide in contemporary Maharashtra, India. *Violence Against Women* **5** (5): 525–47.

Wolfe DA, Wekerle C, Scott K, *et al.* (2003) Dating violence prevention with at-risk youth: a controlled outcome evaluation. *Journal of Consulting and Clinical Psychology* **71**: 279–91.

World Health Organization (2005) *WHO Multi-Country Study on Women's Health and Domestic Violence Against Women: Initial Results on Prevalence, Health Outcomes and Women's Responses.* Geneva: WHO.

World Health Organization (2010) *Preventing Intimate Partner and Sexual Violence Against Women: Taking Action and Generating Evidence.* Geneva: WHO. http://whqlibdoc.who.int/publications/2010/9789241564007_eng.pdf (accessed July 2013).

World Health Organization (2011) Violence against women. Fact sheet 239. Geneva: WHO. http://www.who.int/mediacentre/factsheets/fs239/en (accessed January 2012).

World Health Organization (WHO), International Society for Prevention of Child Abuse and Neglect (ISPCAN) (2006) *Preventing Child Maltreatment: a Guide to Taking Action and Generating Evidence.* www.who.int/violence_injury_prevention/violence/activities/child_maltreatment/en (accessed July 2013).

263

Chapter

28

Women and global mental health: vulnerability and empowerment

Janis H. Jenkins and Mary-Jo DelVecchio Good

Introduction

This chapter takes an anthropological approach to the study of global mental health among women. We begin by framing our review broadly with the prolegomenon that "there is no health without mental health" (Prince *et al.* 2007). This declaration is welcome not only to researchers and clinicians dedicated to understanding mental illness but also to persons, families, and caregivers whose daily lives are much affected. Yet illness experience, cultural interpretation, and social response are not uniformly patterned. The realities of the social, cultural, and political dimensions of mental illness are not the same for women and men across diverse sociocultural settings. Research over the past three decades has empirically established the vital roles of culture and gender across a range of illness-related features such as etiology, vulnerability factors, illness onset, formation, social and occupational functioning, psychotherapeutic and medication experience, resilience, and course and outcome (Goldstein *et al.* 1989, McGlashan & Bardenstein 1990, Jenkins 2007, 2010).

These issues could hardly be of greater significance insofar as substantial bodies of research have demonstrated that gender and social response are significant for who becomes ill and who recovers (Jenkins & Karno 1992). A precise anthropological definition of global health is as:

an area of research and practice that endeavours to link health, broadly conceived as a dynamic state that is an essential resource for life and well-being, to assemblages of global processes, recognizing that these assemblages are complex, diverse, temporally unstable, contingent, and often contested or resisted at different social scales.

(Janes & Corbett 2010, pp. 406–7)

Taking up the challenge to integrate mental health into the global health agenda specific to women will require development of innovative programs of transnational research and intervention (Kermode *et al.* 2007, Alegria *et al.* 2008). In this chapter we explore the cultural, economic, and political determinants of women's mental health in an effort to identify directions for future research on pathways to improve women's well-being, emphasizing the role of empowerment.

In charting the course for a wide-ranging research agenda to expand the study of women's mental health, it is useful to bear in mind two impediments to such research in the form of paradigmatic bias within the health and social sciences. First is the enduring problem of dichotomous thinking about illness as "physical" or "mental," with the latter often non-existent or a secondary concern. The need for recognition of the tangible indivisibility of mental and physical illness holds particular relevance for women's mental health. Consider, for example, mental and infectious diseases. Research shows that regardless of race or ethnicity, HIV-positive women have more severe histories of abuse than do women who are HIV-negative (Wyatt *et al.* 2002). The significant risk for HIV among women with histories of physical and sexual abuse is related to the mental health risks of adverse social conditions, such as depression, psychological trauma, and psychosis (Breslau *et al.* 1997, Tolin & Foa 2006, Fisher *et al.* 2009). For instance, when girls and women who have been abused become depressed or traumatized, they may not feel motivated or entitled to insist on condom use that would reduce their risk of infection (Abt 2008). Such a situation illustrates not only the interrelation of infectious disease and mental illness but also the nexus of gender and power as a social determinant of illness.

Essentials of Global Mental Health, ed. Samuel O. Okpaku. Published by Cambridge University Press. © Cambridge University Press 2014.

Second, it is only within the last two decades that women have not been largely excluded from research protocols, based in part upon the presumption that disease processes among women are similar to those among men, typically European or North American men. Empirical studies have shown otherwise. There are distinctive features of illness among women that do not apply to men (Jenkins & Schumacher 1999, Nasser *et al.* 2002). For example, meta-analyses by Tolin and Foa (2006) demonstrate a significant relationship between child abuse and post-traumatic stress disorder (PTSD) for females but not for males. For psychotic-related disorders, childhood sexual and/or physical abuse is a major risk factor in the onset of psychosis for women, but not for men (Fisher *et al.* 2009). Symptoms of PTSD as developed by the DSM-IV for male American war veterans do not fully apply to Central American women who have experienced warfare and political violence (Jenkins 1996).

Taken together, these observations point to the need for research that takes into account features of culture and gender for investigation of women's mental health in a globalizing world. As an initial step toward this objective, we turn first to epidemiological data regarding the prevalence and economic burden of mental illness worldwide.

Epidemiology

In an extensive report on *The Global Burden of Disease*, the World Health Organization (WHO) has compared calculations for the total number of years of potential life lost due to premature mortality and the years of productive life lost to disability (disability-adjusted life years: DALYs). Globally, neuropsychiatric disorders among non-communicable diseases rank number one in global burden of disease (Figure 28.1). This is especially striking considering that non-communicable diseases account for nearly half of the global burden of disease (Figure 28.2). However, as Table 28.1 shows, there is some cross-national and gendered variation. For men and women in the six most populous countries (USA, Japan, China, Indonesia, Brazil, and India) as well as in Pakistan and Iran, neuropsychiatric disorders have the highest burden among non-communicable diseases, followed by cardiovascular illness. In Afghanistan, both men and women have a greater cardiovascular disease burden, followed by neuropsychiatric illness, and in Turkey, Iraq, and Saudi Arabia this pattern only holds for men (World Health Organization 2008). Considering the dramatic burden caused by neuropsychiatric illness, it is all the more

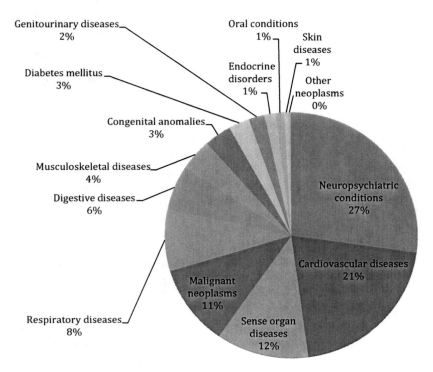

Figure 28.1 Distribution of global DALYs among non-communicable conditions. Source: Mortality and Burden of Disease Estimates for WHO Member States in 2004. February 2009 Update. Compiled by Seth Hannah.

Table 28.1 Leading sources of DALYs among non-communicable disease in selected countries

	Men		Women	
	Neuropsychiatric conditions	Cardiovascular conditions	Neuropsychiatric conditions	Cardiovascular conditions
	Rank	Rank	Rank	Rank
USA	1	2	1	2
Japan	1	2	1	2
China	1	2	1	2
Indonesia	1	2	1	2
Brazil	1	2	1	2
India	1	2	1	2
Pakistan	1	2	1	2
Iran	1	2	1	2
Afghanistan	2	1	2	1
Turkey	2	1	1	2
Iraq	2	1	1	2
Saudi Arabia	2	1	1	2

Source: Mortality and Burden of Disease Estimates for WHO Member States in 2004. February 2009 Update. Compiled by Seth Hannah.

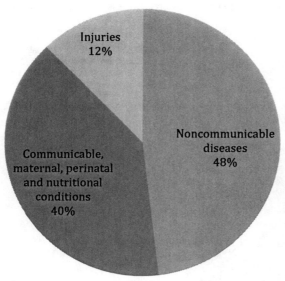

Figure 28.2 Distribution of global DALYs by type of condition. Source: Mortality and Burden of Disease Estimates for WHO Member States in 2004. February 2009 Update. Compiled by Seth Hannah.

remarkable that mental health care receives such low priority in global health. In many countries, there is scant attention from policy makers and little funding allocated to provide basic care.

For this chapter, we elaborate upon the WHO analyses, utilizing the 2009 updates on the DALYS and global burden of disease to consider comparisons between women and men in the context of selected countries (World Health Organization 2008, 2009). We present global trends as well as a comparison across the world's five most populous countries (China, India, USA, Indonesia, Brazil) and six quite diverse predominantly Muslim countries of high, medium, and low income, three of which have been highly affected by war (Turkey, Saudi Arabia, Iran, Iraq, Pakistan, and Afghanistan).

In agreement with decades of research on gender differences in the rate of depression (Good & Ware 1995), the WHO reported that "the burden of depression is 50% higher for females than for males," and that "the burden of alcohol and drug use disorders is nearly seven times higher" for males than for females in all countries, even if categorized by low, middle, and high income (World Health Organization 2008; p. 36), as illustrated by Figure 28.3.

Women's mental health across the lifespan is characterized not only by a higher burden of depression, but also by higher prevalence of anxiety

(A)

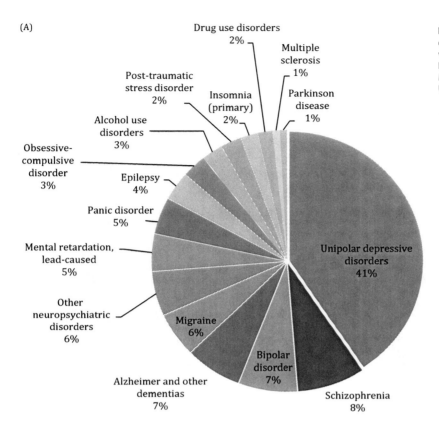

Figure 28.3 Distribution of global DALYs due to neuropsychiatric conditions: (A) women; (B) men. Source: Mortality and Burden of Disease Estimates for WHO Member States in 2004. February 2009 Update. Compiled by Seth Hannah.

disorders, and, given greater longevity, dementias (World Health Organization 2008; p. 36). The gendered experience of neuropsychiatric disorders is born out by the number of DALYs experienced by men and women across the globe. Figure 28.4 documents gender differences by country for the burden of unipolar depression, with women consistently showing higher DALYs than men, with the exception of Iran. Although women have a greater burden of disease across all countries from unipolar depression, the six Middle Eastern countries have a higher percentage of DALY burden from unipolar depression than the six largest countries, including Indonesia, also a Muslim-majority country.

Figure 28.5 illustrates the burden of alcohol and drug abuse for each of the six countries. Men suffer more disability from alcoholism or drug use, in contrast to women, who suffer depression. Cross-national variations are notable, with Japan, Turkey, and Saudi Arabia showing men with the least burden of either alcohol or drug dependence.

In contrast to depression and alcohol and drug disorders, there are few gender differences in the burden of bipolar disorder and schizophrenia across the 12 countries we examined. Figure 28.6 shows little difference in the DALYS per 100 000 population between males and females, yet differences are notable across the selected countries, with USA and Japan standing out with much lower burdens. One might ask, is this notable difference due to lack of effective treatment coverage?

Based on a comparison of data from Middle Eastern countries with the statistics for the six largest countries, one might hypothesize that the gender gap for depression is likely to be lower in countries with state ideologies that value and invest in women's health and promote female education to achieve equality and parity with men. However, the diverse sources of DALYs due to neuropsychiatric conditions make it difficult to evaluate this claim. As Figure 28.7 shows, while there is a consistent gender gap across all 12 countries in neuropsychiatric disorders, in China, Turkey, Iraq, and Afghanistan it is actually men who suffer a greater burden than women. What is more, the size of the gender gap is not larger in the Muslim countries than in the

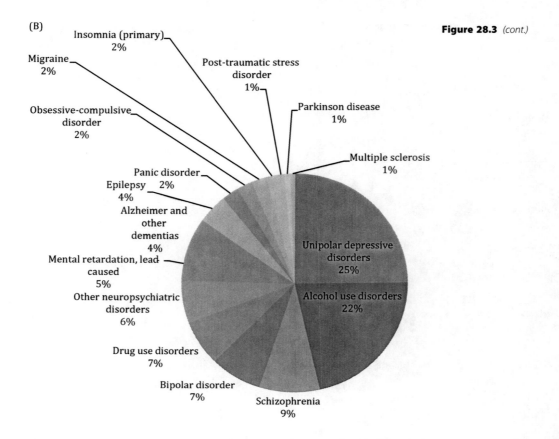

(B)

Figure 28.3 *(cont.)*

non-Muslim countries. Despite these inconsistent findings, when examining individual neuropsychiatric disorders as we do here, interesting gender differences do emerge. As shown in Figure 28.4a, there is substantial gendered variation across countries, with Muslim countries suffering greater depression burden than non-Muslim countries and with women in Muslim countries suffering from a greater gender gap in depression burden than women in non-Muslim countries. Additionally, as shown in Figure 28.5a, the gendered pattern of alcohol and drug use disorder implicates state-level policy differences regarding the availability of drugs and alcohol, with women's access to these substances severely restricted in some countries, and more general availability in others. This raises the possibility that in countries where drugs and alcohol are less available, as in the many Muslim countries, depression levels may be elevated due to the inability to "self-medicate" with other substances. As Figure 28.4a shows, depression is highest in countries where alcohol abuse is the lowest.

Another potential factor driving the gendered burden of neuropsychiatric illness across countries is the experience of violence and war. Table 28.2 illustrates the burden of disease from intentional injuries (self-inflicted injuries/suicides, war and violence). Afghanistan, Iraq, and Pakistan have suffered disproportionately from the burden of war, which has particularly impacted the men in those countries. Although war, violence, murder, and suicide affect low percentages of a population, insecure societies are highly related to mental distress and illness.

Anthropological concepts as foundation

Because we are convinced that meaningful appreciation of these epidemiological data is usefully guided by enriching the theoretical models from which we work, we briefly review anthropological concepts that we believe can refine and guide research on mental health and illness among women. While there have been important strides in obtaining

(A)

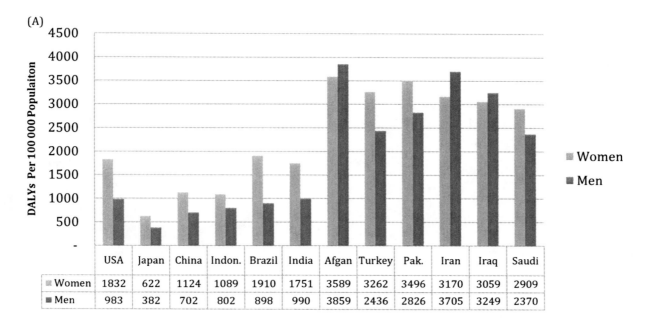

	USA	Japan	China	Indon.	Brazil	India	Afgan	Turkey	Pak.	Iran	Iraq	Saudi
Women	1832	622	1124	1089	1910	1751	3589	3262	3496	3170	3059	2909
Men	983	382	702	802	898	990	3859	2436	2826	3705	3249	2370

(B)

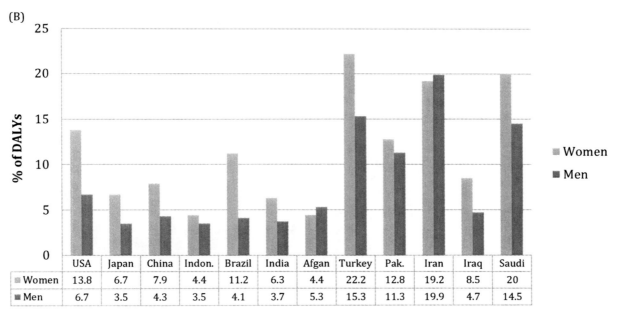

	USA	Japan	China	Indon.	Brazil	India	Afgan	Turkey	Pak.	Iran	Iraq	Saudi
Women	13.8	6.7	7.9	4.4	11.2	6.3	4.4	22.2	12.8	19.2	8.5	20
Men	6.7	3.5	4.3	3.5	4.1	3.7	5.3	15.3	11.3	19.9	4.7	14.5

Figure 28.4 Distribution by gender of DALYs due to unipolar depressive disorders in selected countries: (A) DALYs per 100 000 population; (B) DALYs due to unipolar depressive disorders as a percentage of DALYs due to non-communicable disease. Source: Mortality and Burden of Disease Estimates for WHO Member States in 2004. February 2009 Update. Compiled by Seth Hannah.

fundamental empirical data for this burgeoning field, there is a critical need for well-formulated theoretical frameworks that can advance our understandings of cultural, social, and political processes that affect health and illness. To that end, we provide brief discussion of three central organizing concepts that can guide research: culture, gender, and power.

(A)

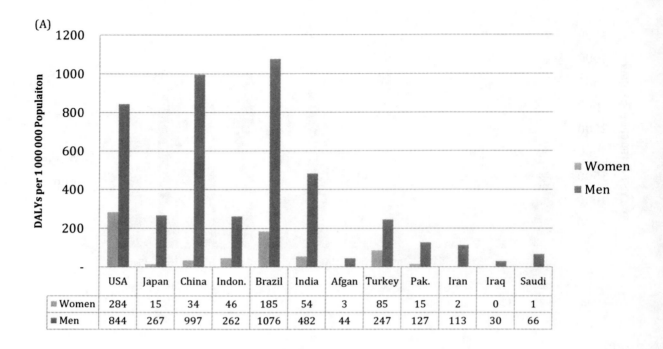

	USA	Japan	China	Indon.	Brazil	India	Afgan	Turkey	Pak.	Iran	Iraq	Saudi
▪ Women	284	15	34	46	185	54	3	85	15	2	0	1
▪ Men	844	267	997	262	1076	482	44	247	127	113	30	66

(B)

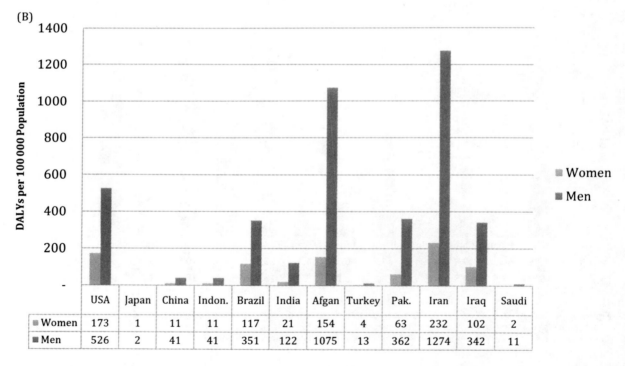

	USA	Japan	China	Indon.	Brazil	India	Afgan	Turkey	Pak.	Iran	Iraq	Saudi
▪ Women	173	1	11	11	117	21	154	4	63	232	102	2
▪ Men	526	2	41	41	351	122	1075	13	362	1274	342	11

Figure 28.5 Distribution by gender of DALYs due to (A) alcohol disorders and (B) drug disorders, in selected countries. Source: Mortality and Burden of Disease Estimates for WHO Member States in 2004. February 2009 Update. Compiled by Seth Hannah.

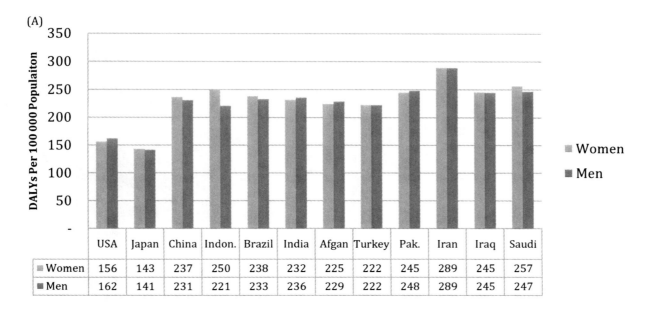

(A)

	USA	Japan	China	Indon.	Brazil	India	Afgan	Turkey	Pak.	Iran	Iraq	Saudi
Women	156	143	237	250	238	232	225	222	245	289	245	257
Men	162	141	231	221	233	236	229	222	248	289	245	247

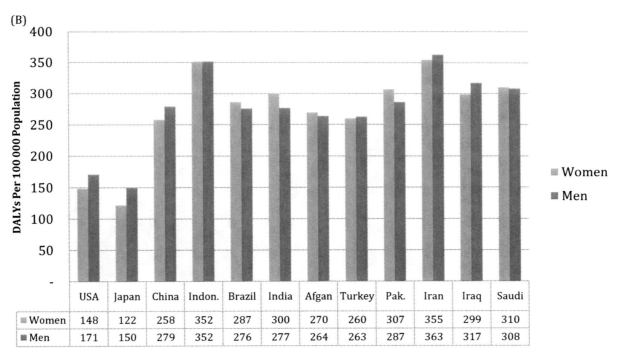

(B)

	USA	Japan	China	Indon.	Brazil	India	Afgan	Turkey	Pak.	Iran	Iraq	Saudi
Women	148	122	258	352	287	300	270	260	307	355	299	310
Men	171	150	279	352	276	277	264	263	287	363	317	308

Figure 28.6 Distribution by gender of DALYs due to (A) bipolar disorder and (B) schizophrenia, in selected countries. Source: Mortality and Burden of Disease Estimates for WHO Member States in 2004. February 2009 Update. Compiled by Seth Hannah.

Culture can be conceptualized as an emergent property of context-bound human interaction, and cannot be operationalized as a variable. In its broadest dimensions, "culture can be conceived as shared symbols and meanings that people create and recreate in the process of social interaction. Culture shapes experience, interpretation, and action. It thereby orients people in their ways of feeling, thinking, and

Table 28.2 The distribution of DALYs due to intentional injuries: suicide, violence, and war. Selected countries, per 100 000 population

	Total for all categories		Self-inflicted injuries		Violence		War	
	M	F	M	F	M	F	M	F
Afghanistan	21.5	12.2	3.9	8.8	5.6	0.9	10.6	2.2
Brazil	66.8	7.4	8.5	2.3	57.7	5.1	–	–
China	18.3	20.3	15.1	18.9	2.9	1.3	–	–
India	28.7	17.4	20.2	13.3	7.1	3.8	0.8	0.1
Indonesia	29.4	13.1	12.4	9.1	14.4	3.6	2.2	0.3
Iran	11.3	6.6	6.7	5.5	3.9	1.1	–	–
Iraq	404.5	46.6	22.8	7.6	13.1	1.5	364.2	37.4
Japan	37.4	13.9	36.8	13.4	0.6	0.5	–	–
Pakistan	19.6	15.1	9.6	11.1	4.0	3.1	5.7	0.8
Saudi Arabia	16.0	4.0	10.1	1.6	4.2	2.0	1.0	0.2
Turkey	9.2	3.9	4.4	2.9	4.8	1.0	–	–
USA	28.1	7.4	17.8	4.8	9.4	2.6	0.6	0.0

Source: Mortality and Burden of Disease Estimates for WHO Member States in 2004. February 2009 Update. Compiled by Seth Hannah.

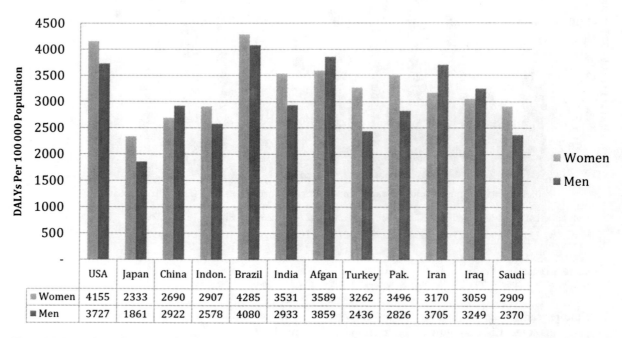

	USA	Japan	China	Indon.	Brazil	India	Afgan	Turkey	Pak.	Iran	Iraq	Saudi
■ Women	4155	2333	2690	2907	4285	3531	3589	3262	3496	3170	3059	2909
■ Men	3727	1861	2922	2578	4080	2933	3859	2436	2826	3705	3249	2370

Figure 28.7 Distribution by gender of DALYs due to neuropsychiatric disorders in selected countries. Source: Mortality and Burden of Disease Estimates for WHO Member States in 2004. February 2009 Update. Compiled by Seth Hannah.

being in the world" (Jenkins & Barrett 2004, p. 5). Fully understood, culture affects all aspects of mental illness. Traditionally, there have been two anthropological directions from which to understand culture: from multiple perspectives of actors who are the subject of study (*emic perspective*) and from conceptual and analytic perspectives of the anthropologist (*etic perspective*). The value of the latter is contingent on the validity and depth of understanding of the former.

Mental health and illness cannot be adequately understood without specific attention to sex and gender (Lewine 2004, Keyes & Goodman 2006, Chandra & Satyanarayana 2010, Kohen 2010). Typically in the health sciences the term *gender* is used when what is really under discussion is a dichotomous distinction of biological sex assignment of women or men. Gender, however, is a construct better conceived on a continuum as diverse assemblies of masculine and feminine cultural orientations. As a dimension of culture, gender pervades social life and experience (Rosaldo & Lamphere 1974, Rosaldo 1980). This cultural pervasion notably includes illness experience (Jenkins 2004), with gender role and identity as domains of particular relevance (Nasser *et al.* 2002). What is critical in the arena of health is the identification not only of gender difference but also of inequity. Comparatively, there are significant differences in preferences and moral injunctions for what women and men can or cannot do. Fairly consistent across cultures is a distinct difference between women's and men's access to economic resources and decision-making authority. Analysis of the cross-cultural record led Rosaldo (1980) to comment as follows on male dominance in these areas:

> Male dominance, in short, does not inhere in any isolated and measurable set of omnipresent facts. Rather, it seems to be an aspect of the organization of collective life, a patterning of expectations and beliefs which gives rise to imbalance in the ways people interpret, evaluate, and respond to particular forms of male and female action. We see it not in physical constraints on things that men or women can or cannot do but, rather, in the ways they think about their lives, the kinds of opportunities they enjoy, and in their ways of making claims.
>
> (Rosaldo 1980, p. 394)

However, as noted by Scheper-Hughes (1983, p. 30), "this 'gendering' of social life is situational and contextual, not meaningful in all spheres of behavior and activity, and variable, too, throughout the life cycle."

There is no absolute fixity of female subordination, and indeed there is considerable social and cultural movement across place and over time. As Ortner (2006, p. 7) has argued, it is important to recognize that "male dominance always coexists with other patterns of gender relations; what is important is the mix, and the relations between them."

Sociocultural definitions of power take into account the relationship between institutional and structural arrangements and the agency of persons living under such arrangements. The cultural process of shaping varies not only in relation to broad dimensions of subjectivity but also in relation to historic regimes of power. While it is essential to conceive this relationship as an active process that is subject to dynamic change, the construction of individual and collective agency directed toward social change is contingent on access to vital economic and educational resources largely controlled by elites, the state, and other governmental and non-governmental organizations. Drawing on practice theorists such as Bourdieu, Ortner (2006, pp. 6–9) frames the question of power in relation to the extent of pervasiveness and invasiveness, internal dynamics (local relations) and external forces (such as capitalism and colonialism) over time. In this view, it is necessary to conceive of power as structures external to individuals and as lived social process that can be modified, resisted, and challenged. From this perspective, there exists a broad spectrum of the psychological "depth" of power as deeply internalized or resisted (Ortner 2006).

Women and depression: gender vulnerability

Because depression looms large for women and girls and the condition is common across populations, we examine this illness in relation to factors of vulnerability. To expand upon the epidemiological data we presented above, there now exists a great volume of research demonstrating that depression affects women at a rate at least twice that of men, posing the question of how to account for this variance. Investigation has been carried out concluding that the etiology of depression among girls and women is multidimensional, to include biological, psychological, economic, and social factors (Nolen-Hoeksema *et al.* 1999). The classic work by Brown and Harris (1978) demonstrated the significance of a constellation of factors that shape the lives of working-class London women: unemployment, poor housing conditions, three or more small children in the house, loss of mother before the age of 11, and the lack of a confiding relationship. The etiological significance of these interlocking conditions may point to thinking about depression in this case as a diagnosis of a situation rather than of an individual woman.

Another situational factor for the development of depression among women is workload. Abbott and Klein (1979) have identified depression among rural Kenyan women who have increased workload in the context of patrilineal determination of property rights and migratory flight of husbands seeking employment. The presence of strain in a domestic environment characterized by scarcity of economic resources, male dominance, overwhelming workload, familial demands in the absence of support, along with a tendency for ruminative worry and perceived lack of control or mastery over the conditions of one's life, are strongly correlated with depression in women (Ullrich 1987, Scheper-Hughes 1993, Nolen-Hoeksema *et al.* 1999). Taken together, the body of empirical research on depression suggests that depression among women can be conceived less as a psychological or individual ailment but more broadly as a diagnosis of the social situation, not only among working-class women in London but for many women the world over. This is not to deny or minimize the experience of intense distress and personal pain that defines depression in a woman's life, but rather to emphasize the structural conditions under which depression is produced. The intractability of these conditions parallels the severity of the disorder insofar as "depression appears to affect women more seriously than men, as manifested by an earlier age of onset, greater family history of affective disorders, greater symptom reporting, poorer social adjustment and poorer quality of life" (Kornstein *et al.* 2000, p. 1).

Review of a particular case study provides illustration. In a classic work entitled *Search for Security: an Ethno-Psychiatric Study of Rural Ghana* (Field 1960), anthropologist–psychiatrist M. J. Field provides the basis for comparing recent historical and contemporary conditions among women. Field found depression to be common among women. Locally the problem is conceived as witchcraft, for which "nearly all such patients come to the [healing] shrines with spontaneous self-

accusations of witchcraft – that is, of having caused harm without concrete act or conscious will." A woman "is taken at her word when she says she has done harm" (Field 1960, p. 149). For example, one woman conveyed that she knew she was "no good and had become a witch. I have done so much evil that I ought to be killed" (Field 1960, p. 150). Among middle-aged and elderly women, Field observed depression with agitation to be "one of the commonest and most clearly defined of mental illnesses." The majority of these women spent their lives laboring to provide income for children's schooling through trading, market gardening, or cocoa farming (Field 1960, p. 149).

As common as these women's misery and self-accusations of witchcraft is their experience of "seeing their husband take on an extra and younger wife so that he may continue to beget children" and in so doing allocating funds for the young woman that are "the fruits of his older wife's years of labor" (Field 1960, p. 152). The cultural value of middle-aged women and their right to economic and psychological well-being is undermined by the gendered inequality of male social privilege and opportunity.

To bring the issue into more contemporary focus, the problem has worsened dramatically as older women suspected of witchcraft are not infrequently assaulted and sometimes killed (Adinkrah 2004). In Ghana, witchcraft-related femicide is rooted in "patriarchal attitudes, misogynistic beliefs, and ageist values [that] mediate witch beliefs in Akan society" (Adinkrah 2004, p. 335). At risk are poor and elderly women with little formal education who may be "threatened, drugged, beaten, forced to submit to humiliating ordeals, or coerced into confessing to imaginary witch activities" (p. 337). In certain cases, the accused are abandoned by their families and communities and banished to remote camps with threats of violence should they return. The camps are abject sites for the containment of witches (predominantly women) and the mentally ill (Van Dijk 1997, Palmer 2010). Only recently has there been political will to abolish these camps through meetings of civil leaders and the chief psychiatrist of Ghana's Health Services, who has argued for public awareness of psychological disorders and behavior associated with witchcraft.

As we have seen above, depression takes root in the lives of girls and women living under conditions of social adversity and cultural degradation. As also noted, psychotic-related illnesses, eating disorders, and PTSD are more likely to develop in females than in males after exposure to sexual, physical, or psychological assault. Gendered dimensions of the illness are likely multifactorial, and include biological as well as psychological and sociocultural processes (Bird & Rieker 1999). Nevertheless, the overall vulnerability of girls and women to mental illness must be accounted for in part by women's greater likelihood of occupying socially subordinate status and being subject to unequal power relations. This state of affairs has sparked governmental and non-governmental agencies to undertake an array of initiatives under the banner of female "empowerment," to which we now turn.

Empowerment

Bearing in mind the above sociocultural conceptualization of power as a relationship between institutional and structural arrangements and the agency of persons living under such social arrangements, we turn now to what currently has become a global movement. Since the 1980s there has been an ever-increasing attention to the global reach of the notion of women's "empowerment" as central to development programs. The UN Program on Population and Development and Inter-Agency Task Force has advanced "guidelines on women's empowerment" (United Nations 2001), defining the concept as follows:

> Women's empowerment has five components: women's sense of self-worth; their right to have and to determine choices; their right to have access to opportunities and resources; their right to have the power to control their own lives both within and outside the home; and their ability to influence the direction of social change to create a more just social and economic order, nationally and internationally.

In this formulation, it is critical to conceive of the notion of empowerment in culturally substantive terms. This applies with equal force to projects intended to foster empowerment. These must be generated in light of local preferences and priorities. The extent to which the numerous governmental and non-governmental agencies dedicated to the task of empowerment of women are likely to succeed is directly proportional to the extent to which the implementation of programs is carried out in partnerships that contribute to infrastructure that local residents regard as useful.

Of interest for mental health in relation to the UN definition of empowerment is the explicit concern for cultural and psychological "self-worth."

Anthropologists have established cultural and gender differences in the orientation of the self (e.g., egocentric or sociocentric) that while not entirely different from European or North American selves may nonetheless differ in non-trivial ways (Shweder & Bourne 1984). With this in mind, the task force set up by the UN has usefully moved beyond a prior emphasis on reproductive health and toward health understood as "complete physical, mental, and social well-being." Actions and attitudes that can improve self-regard, countering institutional misogyny, sexism, and violence against women, are sorely needed. We emphasize that these need to be pursued in socially and culturally meaningful ways that are non-hegemonic.

Another recent document that targets the empowerment of women was produced by the World Psychiatry Association (WPA) (Stewart 2006). As for the UN Task Force, the focus on the improvement of women's mental health is grounded in the discourse of human rights and equal access to employment, health care, adequate food, water, and shelter. The WPA has also called for the "elimination of violence and discrimination based on sex, age, income, race, ethnic background, sexual orientation, or religious beliefs" (Stewart 2006, p. 62).

Challenges to the implementation of principles designed by organizations dedicated to the empowerment of women are daunting, given widespread and longstanding conditions for women. Principal among these are sexism and poverty. Sexism, defined as institutional and cultural devaluation of girls and women, runs the gamut from legal codification to subtle and near-invisible hostility and constraint on the lives of women. Sexism as cultural devaluation is evident in poor countries through the denial of educational opportunities to girls, and in more affluent countries in the form of unequal pay and representation in the political arena. Sexism as hostility is evident in the harassment and sexual assault of women, for example among the small contingent of Afghan women carrying out their duties as policewomen (Gutcher 2011) or among American female troops sexually assaulted by their fellow soldiers (Myers 2009). Institutional sexism leading to a preference for males in Asia prompted Amartya Sen (1990) to famously inquire about the more than 100 million girls who are "missing" as evidence of abnormal sex ratios in India, China, and elsewhere in the developing world. While many factors account for this disparity, perhaps the most notable is what has been termed "gendercide" (Economist 2010a, 2010b), whether through selective abortion, infanticide, or neglect (Scheper-Hughes 1993).

From a global perspective, the mental health of women is greatly affected by poverty, violence, and scarcity of basic resources such as food and water (Scheper-Hughes 1993, Desjarlais *et al.* 1995, Das *et al.* 2000, Farmer 2004, Janes & Corbett 2010). In a review of studies in low- and middle-income communities, however, Patel and Kleinman (2003) found that while most studies showed an association between indicators of poverty and the risk of mental disorder, the most consistent association was with low levels of education, with lesser evidence to support a specific correlation with income levels. Instead, "factors such as the experience of insecurity and hopelessness, rapid social change and the risks of violence and physical ill-health may explain the greater vulnerability of the poor to common mental disorders" (Patel & Kleinman 2003, p. 609). Low income was noted to have direct and indirect costs associated with mental illness through exacerbation of adverse economic conditions that create a vicious cycle of poverty and mental disorder.

In the face of these conditions, it is important to identify sources of strength and resilience displayed by women under such circumstances (Jenkins 1996, Scheper-Hughes 2008). Women are adept at maintaining relations that are strategic for emotional support and social capital (Almedom 2005). In times of crisis or warfare, women often intensify their labor and go to great lengths to protect their kin and community (Jenkins 1996). Currently, there is a pressing need for better understanding of the qualities and conditions of resilience among women. In this chapter, we feel the most compelling way to explore this is through presentation of a case study of women exercising power to safeguard the security of families and community under siege.

Mental health in a post-conflict zone: women as protectors in Aceh

The following is an ethnographic example of women in the position of powerful protectors in post-conflict Aceh, Indonesia. This provides an example of the impact of localized armed conflict on women's mental health, exemplified by a generational conflict between the national military of Indonesia and the

Free Aceh Movement (GAM) seeking provincial autonomy and ultimately independence. Following the Indian Ocean tsunami of December 25, 2004, a lasting peace in August 2005 granted local political autonomy and greater control over the province's wealth (Good 2010). Women and men described sustained violence by the military in their

---

Box 28.1: Case study 1

In July 2008 I reviewed the work of the International Organization for Migration (IOM) medical mental health outreach team. Villagers praised the IOM clinicians, and stories of appreciation for the medications as well as the attention seemed truly genuine, especially given the Acehnese tendency to be straightforward and critical. However, even if biased, stories of therapeutic benefit and "awakenings" (Jenkins & Carpenter-Song 2005) were impressive. An elderly village woman described herself as an activist and explained how, after two months of IOM pharmacological therapy for anxiety, depression, and PTSD due to conflict-related chronic trauma, she awoke one day suddenly able to see her surroundings in a new way. For years she said everything seemed to be behind a screen, nothing was bright, everything was fuzzy and dark. Now she could see people clearly, colors were bright, as was the sky, the ribs on the deep green leaves of the plants visible. She laughed as she described her experience of this change, delightful and vivid. She told us her trauma story too. She described her life before the peace memorandum of understanding (MOU): always tense, always worried about the soldiers searching for her sons, and having to buffer her sons from the military. Her husband, who was much older than her, "did not leave the house much." Her eldest son was shot on his motorcycle while trying to escape soldiers who were harassing young men in the village. He later died in the hospital from his wounds. She told how women were exhausted by buffering the men. She told how she had to teach her grandchildren – and all the village's young children from the time they were toddlers – to protect the men, their fathers, grandfathers, uncles. "We taught them," she said, "when you see the sipahi, run, hide ... if they ask you a question, say nothing ... if they show you a gun and ask if your daddy has one of these, say no ... if there is a gun in the house, say no ... run, hide, do not speak to them." In twentieth-century Aceh, "sipahi" were Javanese or Batak from the Dutch colonial military viewed as "those who do evil." (excerpted with rephrasing from Good 2010, p. 61).

Box 28.2: Case study 2

A woman in her forties suffered from a long depression in response to losing her son, who fled to the capital city to escape the conflict only to be seriously injured in a traffic accident. Although near death, he recovered. During our visit, the woman told how after two months of antidepressants, she felt her normal self. She could cook and farm again. Her husband confirmed how she was deeply depressed and was now herself. Her husband was excited and voluble, wanting to talk about more than just his wife's depression and recovery. He laughed as a small group of men and women gathered round, talking about how excited they were that they could directly vote for their own choices and display the paper flag of the *Partai Aceh*, the newly formed political party formally representing much of the old GAM structure. In the past he said one could be killed for displaying this flag. "Now, we celebrate it!" The once-depressed wife smiled gently as her husband expressed how he and she felt "inside," about being able to vote for their party, and psychologically free to support those he trusted. Certainly the politics of peace provided succor to those who suffered "trauma" from years of conflict. The peace pill combined with psychopharmaceutical treatment appears to have significant efficacy in reducing remainders of violence (Good 2010).

communities, with houses and schools razed or burned, and villagers beaten, tortured, or killed, often in retaliation for attacks by GAM on the Indonesian military. Women told us of being forced to watch spouses killed and sons taken to the forest to be executed, and of their own beatings and humiliation. They complained of waking up with vivid images of what happened and being unable to return to sleep (Good *et al.* 2006, 2007, Grayman *et al.* 2009, Good 2010, in press). Constant fear and sadness made daily activities difficult, and anger made them unable to forget humiliating and traumatic events. Women's experiences were unique in that their anxiety and traumatic experiences often arose from their roles as buffers and protectors of men from military aggression. Post-conflict mental health treatment even three years after the peace was declared was needed by many; it proved to be helpful in addressing the mental health symptoms associated with remainders of violence. The Aceh experience of women as activists and protectors of men and not as

merely victims is common in many conflict situations, and thus generalizable to larger post-conflict mental health issues (Fassin & Rechtman 2009, Siapno 2009, Good in press Hinton & Hinton in press). The interviews presented in Boxes 28.1 and 28.2 illustrate post-conflict experiences with therapeutic interventions as part of a mental health intervention.

Future directions

We conclude with suggestions for future research on women's mental health and issues of empowerment. Efforts to measure empowerment among women paint a picture of inequality that, while uneven, is nonetheless pervasive. Women account for two-thirds of the world's poor and illiterate, with a fraction (less than 16%) of representation as elected officials. Outside of the agricultural sector, in wealthy and poor nations alike, women average 78% of the wages given to men for the same work. Furthermore, the obstacle of cultural attitudes that favor males is found to persist (Lopez-Claros & Zahidi 2005, p. 3). The overall picture of the status of women worldwide has been and continues to be unacceptable.

To remedy this state of affairs, Sen has made a compelling case for governments and agencies (governmental and non-governmental alike) to view women not as passive recipients of assistance but instead as dynamic engines for social transformation (Sen 1999, Lopez-Claros & Zahidi 2005, p. 3). For such to occur requires education, economic opportunity, and ownership rights. This is critical insofar as it may be that when women have decision-making control over economic issues, there is a greater likelihood of resources being spent on such basic needs as food, education, and health. While such efforts (including microfinancing) are worthwhile, their effect on women's mental health has not invariably been found to be salubrious (Fernald *et al.* 2008). Thus there remains a critical need for social change with the capacity to go beyond assistance to individuals and communities. Collaborative efforts by local actors must be pursued in tandem with the political will of institutional structures.

Drawing on a survey by the World Psychiatric Association and the Berlin Congress of Women's Mental Health, Stewart and colleagues (2001) emphasize the importance of health promotion (rather than services) and on further interventions to address determinants of health (poverty, illiteracy, discrimination, and violence against women). For improvement of mental health, they argue that education is essential not only for knowledge acquisition but also for "gender consciousness (that is, the awareness that the inequities she suffers are not caused by her own short-comings, but are the result of discrimination and injustice) and should provide her with assertiveness and decision-taking capacity; in short, it should be empowering" (Stewart *et al.* 2001, p. 14). These educational goals should include critical gender thinking undertaken in light of local women's conceptualizations and perceived need (Niaz 2004; Douki *et al.* 2007). That is, empowerment must hold culturally experiential meaning to effect change. Furthermore, while "empowerment" is central in the literature on battered women, the manner and definition of finding one's own strength may be distinctive across persons and places. The intricacies of such processes must go hand in hand with cultural change of attitudes and practice surrounding violence against women, to target men to include not only physical violence but also the unrecognized but serious psychological damage of verbal abuse (Orava *et al.* 1996).

Future research on global mental health of women should be grounded in the lived experience of mental illness in an inexorably entangled nexus of relations of culture, power, gender, and meaning. Further study of the relation between lived experience and social forces in a globalizing world holds the potential to be incorporated into health policy and action that are key to addressing the mental health and well-being of girls and women worldwide (Cosgrove 2000, Doyal 2000, Nicki 2001, Biehl & Moran-Thomas 2009, Kostick *et al.* 2011). This task will help to improve the quality of research on women's experience of distress over the lifespan.

Acknowledgments

We wish to acknowledge our appreciation for research assistance and bibliographic preparation from Charlotte van den Hout of the University of California at San Diego, and Seth Hannah of Harvard Medical School.

References

Abbott S, Klein R (1979) Depression and anxiety among rural Kikuyu in Kenya. *Ethos* 7: 161–88.

Abt E (2008) *All of Us* [film, directed by Emily Abt]. Brooklyn, NY: Pureland Pictures.

Adinkrah M (2004) Witchcraft accusations and female homicide victimization in contemporary Ghana. *Violence Against Women* 10: 325–56.

Alegria M, Polo A, Gao S, *et al.* (2008) Evaluation of a patient activation and empowerment intervention in mental health care. *Medical Care* 46: 247–56.

Almedom AM (2005) Social capital and mental health: an interdisciplinary review of primary evidence. *Social Science and Medicine* 61: 943–64.

Biehl J , Moran-Thomas A (2009) Symptom: subjectivities, social ills, technologies. *Annual Review of Anthropology* 38: 267–88.

Bird CE , Rieker PP (1999) Gender matters: an integrated model for understanding men's and women's health. *Social Science and Medicine* 48: 745–55.

Breslau N, Davis GC, Andreski P, Peterson EL, Schultz LR (1997) Sex differences in posttraumatic stress disorder. *Archives of General Psychiatry* 54: 1044–8.

Brown GW, Harris T (1978) *Social Origins of Depression*. New York, NY: Free Press.

Chandra PS, Satyanarayana VA (2010) Gender disadvantage and common mental disorders in women. *International Review of Psychiatry* 22: 513–24.

Cosgrove L (2000) Crying out loud: understanding women's emotional distress as both lived experience and social construction. *Feminism and Psychology* 10: 247–67.

Das V, Kleinman A, Ramphele M, Reynolds P, eds. (2000) *Violence and Subjectivity*. Berkeley, CA: University of California Press.

Desjarlais R, Eisenberg L, Good B, Kleinman A, eds. (1995) *World Mental Health: Problems and Priorities in Low-Income Countries*. New York, NY: Oxford University Press.

Douki S, Ben Zineb S, Nacef F, Halbreich U (2007) Women's mental health in the Muslim world: cultural, religious, and social issues. *Journal of Affective Disorders* 102: 177–89.

Doyal L (2000) Gender equity in health: debates and dilemmas. *Social Science and Medicine* 51, 931–9.

Economist (2010a) Gendercide: killed, aborted, or neglected, at least 100m girls have disappeared – and the number is rising. *The Economist* [online] March 4, 2010. http://www.economist.com/node/15606229 (accessed July 2013).

Economist (2010b) Gendercide: the worldwide war on baby girls. *The Economist* [online]. March 4, 2010. http://www.economist.com/node/15636231 (accessed July 2013).

Farmer P (2004) *Pathologies of Power: Health, Human Rights, and the New War on the Poor.* Berkeley, CA: University of California Press.

Fassin D, Rechtman R (2009) *The Empire of Trauma: an Inquiry into the Condition of Victimhood.* Translated by Rachel Gomme. Princeton, NJ: Princeton University Press.

Fernald LCH, Hamad R, Karlan D, Ozer EJ, Zinman J (2008) Small individual loans and mental health: a randomized controlled trial among South African adults. *BMC Public Health* 8: 409.

Field MJ (1960) *Search for Security: an Ethno-Psychiatric Study of Rural Ghana.* New York, NY: WW Norton.

Fisher H, Morgan C, Dazzan P, *et al.* (2009) Gender differences in the association between childhood abuse and psychosis. *British Journal of Psychiatry* 194: 319–25.

Goldstein JM, Tsuang MT, Faraone SV (1989) Gender and schizophrenia: implications for understanding the heterogeneity of the illness. *Psychiatry Research* 28: 243–53.

Good B, Good MJD, Grayman J, Lakoma M (2006) *Psychosocial Needs Assessment of Communities Affected by the Conflict in the Districts of Pidie, Bireuen and Aceh Utara.* Jakarta: International Organization for Migration.

Good MJD (2010) Trauma in postconflict Aceh and psychopharmaceuticals as a medium of exchange. In JH Jenkins, ed., *Pharmaceutical Self: the Global Shaping of Experience in an Age of Psychopharmacology.* Santa Fe, NM:

School for Advanced Research Press; pp. 41–66.

Good MJD (in press) Acehnese women's narratives of traumatic experience, resilience and recovery. In A Hinton, D Hinton, eds., *Mass Violence: Memory, Symptoms, and Response.* Durham, NC: Duke University Press.

Good MJD, Ware N (1995) Women. In R Desjarlais, L Eisenberg, B Good, A Kleinman, eds., *World Mental Health: Problems and Priorities in Low-Income Countries.* New York, NY: Oxford University Press.

Good MJD, Good B, Grayman J, Lakoma M (2007) *A Psychosocial Needs Assessment in 14 Conflict-Affected Districts in Aceh.* Jakarta: International Organization for Migration.

Grayman J, Good MJD, Good B (2009) Conflict nightmares and trauma in Aceh. *Culture, Medicine and Psychiatry* 33: 290–312.

Gutcher L (2011) Fighting is cultural, criminal for Afghan policewomen. *USA Today Online* September 19, 2011. http://usatoday30.usatoday.com/news/world/story/2011-09-19/Afghan-National-Police-force-women-Islam/50471816/1 (accessed July 2013).

Hinton D, Hinton A, eds. (in press) Mass Violence: Memory, Symptoms, and Response. Durham, NC: Duke University Press.

Janes CR, Corbett KK (2010) Anthropology and global health. In BJ Good, MMJ Fischer, SS Willen, MJD Good, eds., *A Reader in Medical Anthropology: Theoretical Trajectories, Emergent Realities.* Chichester: Wiley-Blackwell; pp. 405–21.

Jenkins JH (1996) The impress of extremity: women's experience of trauma and political violence. In C Sargent, C Brettel, eds., *Gender and Health: an International Perspective.* Upper Saddle River, NJ: Prentice Hall; pp. 278–91.

Jenkins JH (2004) Schizophrenia as a paradigm case for understanding fundamental human processes. In JH Jenkins, RJ Barrett, eds., *Schizophrenia, Culture, and Subjectivity: the Edge of Experience.* Cambridge: Cambridge University Press; pp. 29–61.

Jenkins JH (2007) Anthropology and psychiatry: the contemporary convergence. In D Bhugra, K Bhui, eds., *Textbook of Cultural Psychiatry.* Cambridge: Cambridge University Press; pp. 20–32.

Jenkins JH, ed. (2010) *Pharmaceutical Self: the Global Shaping of Experience in an Age of Psychopharmacology.* Santa Fe, NM: School for Advanced Research Press.

Jenkins JH, Barrett RJ (2004) Introduction. In JH Jenkins, RJ Barrett, eds., *Schizophrenia, Culture, and Subjectivity: the Edge of Experience.* Cambridge: Cambridge University Press; pp. 1–25.

Jenkins JH, Carpenter-Song E (2005) The new paradigm of recovery from schizophrenia: cultural conundrums of improvement without cure. culture. *Medicine and Psychiatry* 29: 379–413.

Jenkins JH, Karno M (1992) The meaning of "expressed emotion": theoretical issues raised by cross-cultural research. *American Journal of Psychiatry* 149: 9–21.

Jenkins JH, Schumacher J (1999) Family burden of schizophrenia and depressive illness: specifying the effects of ethnicity, gender and social ecology. *British Journal of Psychiatry* 174: 31–8.

Kermode M, Herrman H, Arole R, *et al.* (2007) Empowerment of women and mental health promotion: a qualitative study in rural Maharashtra, India. *BMC Public Health* 7: 225.

Keyes CLM, Goodman SH (2006) *Women and Depression: a Handbook for the Social, Behavioral, and Biomedical Sciences.*

Cambridge: Cambridge University Press.

Kohen D (2010) *Oxford Textbook of Women and Mental Health.* Oxford: Oxford University Press.

Kornstein SG, Schatzberg AF, Thase ME, *et al.* (2000) Gender differences in chronic major and double depression. *Journal of Affective Disorders* **60**: 1–11.

Kostick KM, Schensul SL, Singh R, Pelto P, Saggurti N (2011) A methodology for building culture and gender norms into intervention: an example from Mumbai, India. *Social Science and Medicine* **72**: 1630–8.

Lewine R (2004) At issue: sex and gender in schizophrenia. *Schizophrenia Bulletin* **30**: 755–62.

Lopez-Claros A, Zahidi S (2005) *Women's Empowerment: Measuring the Global Gender Gap.* Geneva: World Economic Forum.

McGlashan TH, Bardenstein KK (1990) Gender differences in affective, schizoaffective, and schizophrenic disorders. *Schizophrenia Bulletin* **16**: 319–29.

Myers SL (2009) A peril in war zones: sexual abuse by fellow G.I.'s. *New York Times* December 27, 2009. http://www.nytimes.com/2009/12/ 28/us/28women.html? ref=womenatarms (accessed July 2013).

Nasser EH, Walders N, Jenkins JH (2002) The experience of schizophrenia: what's gender got to do with it? A critical review of the current status of research on schizophrenia. *Schizophrenia Bulletin* **28**: 351–62.

Niaz U (2004) Women's mental health in Pakistan. *Journal of World Psychiatry* **3**: 60–2.

Nicki A (2001) The abused mind: feminist theory, psychiatric disability, and trauma. *Hypatia* **16** (4): 80–104.

Nolen Hoeksema S, Larson J, Grayson C (1999) Explaining the gender difference in depressive symptoms. *Journal of Personality and Social Psychology* **77**: 1061–72.

Orava TA, McLeod PJ, Sharpe D (1996) Perceptions of control, depressive symptomatology, and self-esteem of women in transition from abusive relationships. *Journal of Family Violence* **11**: 167–86.

Ortner S (2006) *Anthropology and Social Theory: Culture, Power, and the Acting Subject.* Durham, NC: Duke University Press.

Palmer K (2010) *Spellbound: Inside West Africa's Witch Camps.* New York, NY: Free Press.

Patel V, Kleinman A (2003) Poverty and common mental disorders in developing countries. *Bulletin of the World Health Organization* **81**: 609–15.

Prince M, Patel V, Saxena S, *et al.* (2007) No health without mental health. *Lancet* **370**: 859–77.

Rosaldo MZ (1980) The use and abuse of anthropology: reflections on feminism and cross-cultural understanding. *Signs: Journal of Women in Culture and Society* **5**: 389–417.

Rosaldo MZ, Lamphere L (1974) Introduction. In MZ Rosaldo, L Lamphere, eds., *Woman, Culture, and Society.* Stanford, CA: Stanford University Press.

Scheper-Hughes N (1983) Vernacular sexism: an anthropological response to Ivan Illich. *Gender Issues* **3** (1): 8–37.

Scheper-Hughes N (1993) *Death Without Weeping: the Violence of Everyday Life in Brazil.* Berkeley, CA: University of California Press.

Scheper-Hughes N (2008) A talent for life: reflections on human vulnerability and resilience. *Ethnos* **73** (1), 25–56.

Shweder RA, Bourne EJ (1984) Does the concept of the person vary cross- culturally? In RA Shweder, RA LeVine, eds., *Culture Theory: Essays on Mind, Self, and Emotion.* Cambridge: Cambridge University Press; pp. 158–99.

Sen A (1990) More than 100 million women are missing. *New York Times Review of Books* **37** (20) [online], December 20, 1990. http://ucatlas.ucsc.edu/gender/ Sen100M.html (accessed July 2013).

Sen A (1999) *Development as Freedom.* Oxford: Oxford University Press.

Siapno JA (2009) Living through terror: everyday resilience in East Timor and Aceh. *Social Identities: Journal for the Study of Race, Nation and Culture* **15** (1), 43–64.

Stewart DE (2006) The International Consensus Statement on women's mental health and the WPA Consensus Statement on interpersonal violence against women. *World Psychiatry* **5**: 61–4.

Stewart DE, Rondon M, Damiani G, Honikman J (2001) International psychosocial and systemic issues in women's mental health. *Archives of Women's Mental Health* **4** (1), 13–17.

Tolin DF, Foa EB (2006) Sex differences in trauma and posttraumatic stress disorder: a quantitative review of 25 years of research. *Psychological Bulletin* **132**: 959–92.

Ullrich H (1987) A study of change and depression among Havik Brahmin women in a south Indian village. *Culture, Medicine and Psychiatry* **11**: 261–87.

United Nations (2001) Guidelines on Women's Empowerment. UN Inter-Agency Task Force on the Implementation of the ICPD Programme of Action. http://www. un.org/popin/unfpa/taskforce/

guide/iatfwemp.gdl.html (accessed July 2013).

Van Dijk R (1997) From camp to encompassment: discourses of transsubjectivity in the Ghanaian Pentecostal diaspora. *Journal of Religion in Africa* **27**: 135–59.

World Health Organization (2008) *The Global Burden of Disease: 2004 Update.* Geneva: WHO.

World Health Organization (2009) *Global Health Risks: Mortality and Burden of Disease Attributable to Selected Major Risks.* Geneva: WHO.

Wyatt GE, Myers HF, Williams JK, *et al.* (2002) Does a history of trauma contribute to HIV risk for women of color? Implications for prevention and policy. *American Journal of Public Health* **92**: 660–5.

Chapter

29

Trafficking in persons

Atsuro Tsutsumi and Takashi Izutsu

Introduction

Human trafficking and sex work are key issues in global mental health. There are no reliable statistics regarding human trafficking, because of the nature of the issue (International Organization for Migration *et al.* 2009). However, according to the International Labour Organization (ILO), it was estimated that at least 2.45 million trafficked victims were living under exploitative conditions (International Labour Organization 2005).

In 2007 a new initiative, the United Nations Global Initiative to Fight Human Trafficking (UN.GIFT), was established through ILO, the Office of the United Nations High Commissioner for Human Rights (OHCHR), the United Nations Children's Fund (Unicef), the United Nations Office on Drugs and Crime (UNODC), the International Organization for Migration (IOM), and the Organization for Security and Cooperation in Europe (OSCE) joining forces, and began implementing various programs to fight human trafficking, in collaboration with other stakeholders such as the United Nations Population Fund (UNFPA).

Sex work is another largely neglected area which needs increased focus and attention. While some may freely choose sex work as their occupation, many people are coerced through violence, trafficking, debt-bondage, and other powerful influences (UNAIDS 2006). Among the 10 UN agencies that co-sponsor the Joint United Nations Programme on HIV and AIDS (UNAIDS), UNFPA is the focal point for HIV and sex work, and as a result has been working on numerous programs.

In many cases, one of the major purposes of human trafficking is sexual exploitation, including forced participation in sex work. In this sense, human trafficking and sex work are often closely related.

Both human trafficking and sex work have a strong impact on the mental health and psychological well-being of the victims involved. Common factors include sexual and reproductive health, poverty, violence, stigma, and other human rights violations. However, mental health and psychological aspects of both human trafficking and sex work have been largely neglected.

In this chapter we review the definitions and backgrounds of human trafficking and sex work, and their relationship with mental health and psychological well-being, and conclude with a discussion on the way forward.

Human trafficking
Definition of human trafficking

Trafficking in persons or *human trafficking* is defined in the Protocol to Prevent, Suppress and Punish Trafficking in Persons, Especially Women and Children (one of the three Palermo Protocols) (United Nations 2001) as follows:

(a) "Trafficking in persons" shall mean the recruitment, transportation, transfer, harbouring or receipt of persons, by means of the threat or use of force or other forms of coercion, of abduction, of fraud, of deception, of the abuse of power or of a position of vulnerability or of the giving or receiving of payments or benefits to achieve the consent of a person having control over another person, for the purpose of exploitation. Exploitation shall include, at a minimum, the exploitation of the prostitution of others or other forms of sexual exploitation, forced labour or services, slavery or practices similar to slavery, servitude or the removal of organs;

(b) The consent of a victim of trafficking in persons to the intended exploitation set forth in subparagraph (a) of this article shall be irrelevant where any of the means set forth in subparagraph (a) have been used;

(c) The recruitment, transportation, transfer, harbouring or receipt of a child for the purpose of exploitation shall be considered "trafficking in persons" even if this does not involve any of the means set forth in subparagraph (a) of this article;

(d) "Child" shall mean any person under eighteen years of age.

Background to human trafficking

As described above, human trafficking is the exploitation of human beings by means of sexual exploitation, forms of forced labour, slavery, servitude, or the removal of human organs through threat or use of force, coercion, abduction, fraud, deception, abuse of positions of power or vulnerability (United Nations 2001). Though there are no global statistics, as stated above, the US Department of State (2006) estimates that, annually, approximately 600 000–800 000 people are trafficked across national borders worldwide; among them, 80% are women and girls. Not only has international trafficking been increasing in several countries, but there has also been an increase in domestic trafficking (UNIAP 2010).

Human trafficking is estimated to generate approximately US$9.5 billion annually in revenue, and is linked to other organized crime such as human smuggling, drug trafficking, and money laundering (US Department of State 2006). The ILO estimates that the average profit generated from trafficked forced labour is as high as US$32 billion a year (International Labour Organization 2005).

One of the major purposes of human trafficking is sex trafficking. Even in the case where the primary purpose is not for sex work, victims of other forced or bonded labour, especially women and girls in domestic servitude, are also often sexually exploited (US Department of State 2006, 2011, UNODC 2006).

To tackle human trafficking, which is one of the most devastating human rights violations, there are international legal frameworks including the Optional Protocol to the Convention on the Rights of the Child on the Sale of Children, Child Prostitution and Child Pornography (United Nations 2000); and the Protocol to Prevent, Suppress and Punish Trafficking in Persons, Especially Women and Children (United Nations 2001). These conventions have laid down intensive countermeasures for the issue in terms of prevention, including constructing legal frameworks and interventions.

These conventions explicitly require the ratifying states to provide survivors of human trafficking with psychological care and assistance with their psychological recovery, while training the individuals working with survivors (United Nations 2000, 2001). However, mental health and psychological aspects of survivors/victims are often more neglected than the physical and social aspects, despite the former's huge impact on their personal quality of life and beyond.

Research on human trafficking and mental health

There are few studies on mental health focusing on survivors/victims of human trafficking who have not been involved in sex work (research on mental health aspects of sex-trafficking is discussed below, under *Research on sex trafficking and mental health*).

Among them, a study in Nepal demonstrated that approximately 88% of female survivors/victims of non-sex trafficking marked over the cut-off point of a standardized scale for symptoms of anxiety, 81% for symptoms of depression, and 8% for symptoms of post-traumatic stress disorder (PTSD) (Tsutsumi *et al.* 2008). In Europe, Zimmerman and colleagues (2006) reported a similar outcome, in that female survivors/victims of human trafficking showed anxiety, depression, and PTSD symptoms (some of the participants may have engaged in sex work). A study conducted in Moldova found that 54% of its participants met criteria for at least one psychiatric diagnosis: PTSD only (15%); mood, other anxiety, or substance use disorder comorbid with PTSD (21%); anxiety and/or mood disorder (10%); mood or anxiety disorder comorbid with substance use disorder or others (8%) (Ostrovschi *et al.* 2011).

Sex work
Definition of sex work

The term *sex work* covers a broad range of transactions, and sex workers include men and women, young and old.

According to UNAIDS (2002), sex workers are defined as:

female, male and transgender adults and young people who receive money or goods in exchange for sexual services, either regularly or occasionally, and who may or may not consciously define those activities as income-generating.

Sex work varies between and within countries and communities. Sex work also varies in the degree to which it is organized or informal. Self-employed sex workers usually find their clients through independent means, increasingly through mobile phones and the internet. Individuals may sell sex as a full-time occupation, part-time, or occasionally to meet specific economic needs such as education costs, or in a family financial crisis. Others are trafficked or coerced into selling sex.

The settings in which sex work may occur range from brothels to roadsides, markets, parks, hotels, bars, and private homes, and may be recognizable or hidden. Sex workers may be victimized by stigma, discriminatory gender-based attitudes, violence, and sexual exploitation. In many countries, laws, policies, discriminatory practices, and stigmatizing social attitudes drive sex work underground, impeding efforts to reach sex workers and their clients for support. Sex workers frequently have insufficient access to adequate health services, protection from violence or abuse, and social and legal support. Inadequate service access could be compounded by abuse from law enforcement officers.

Background to sex work

Although there are no global statistics on the number of sex workers, this issue has been drawing increased attention in terms of their physical health, including issues related to HIV, and human rights. Physical health and safety risks of sex work have been shown in several studies. These include a high risk of sexually transmitted infections (STIs) (Gossop et al. 1995), and exposure to violence (Farley & Barkan 1998, Church et al. 2001, Harcourt et al. 2001, Kurtz et al. 2004, McCauley et al. 2010). UNAIDS (2008) reports that sex workers experience a higher rate of HIV infection than other population groups in various countries.

Research on sex work and mental health

Among sex workers in general (as opposed to survivors/victims of human trafficking who engage in sex work), a significantly higher rate of depressive

symptoms has been reported, regardless of HIV status (Alegria et al. 1994). Other studies have also consistently shown the burden of mental health problems among sex workers (El-Bassel et al. 1997, Farley & Barkan 1998, Gilchrist et al. 2005, Roxburgh et al. 2006). A higher rate of PTSD symptoms was also observed in several studies (Farley & Barkan 1998, Roxburgh et al. 2006). Female drug users with lifetime involvement in sex work had a significantly higher prevalence of suicidal attempts and depressive ideas (Gilchrist et al. 2005). Another study observed drug dependence and poor mental health among female drug users who had engaged in sex work in the preceding 30 days (El-Bassel et al. 1997). These results indicate the profound impact of sex work on mental health and psychological well-being.

Research on sex trafficking and mental health

As stated above, sex work can happen as a result of human trafficking. Trafficking into sex work is a profound human rights violation that demands effective and comprehensive international action.

Studies have shown high rates of HIV infection (Silverman et al. 2006, 2007, Tsutsumi et al. 2008) and STIs (Gossop et al. 1995, Bal Kumar et al. 2001, Beyrer 2001, Silverman et al. 2006, 2008, Dharmadhikari et al. 2009, Falb et al. 2011) among sex-trafficked survivors/victims. One study reported that the longer duration of forced sex work increased the risk for HIV (Silverman et al. 2007). In addition, experience of sexual violence was associated with lower rates of condom use and higher rates of HIV infection (Sarkar et al. 2008) among sex-trafficked survivors/victims.

Several research studies have shown an elevated risk of tuberculosis as well (Silverman et al. 2007, Dharmadhikari et al. 2009).

In Thailand, risk to sexual and reproductive health issues was reported: survivors/victims of sex trafficking were twice as likely to be exposed to sexual violence, and they were significantly vulnerable to workplace violence or mistreatment, non-condom use, and abortion compared to non-trafficked counterparts (Decker et al. 2011). In addition, they are at high risk of other forms of violence (Decker et al. 2011, Gupta et al. 2011, Sarkar et al. 2008).

Regarding the mental health problems of sex trafficking victims/survivors, the number of available studies is limited. Crawford and Kaufman (2008) reported that all the survivors suffered from somatic and behavioral sequelae in Nepal. Eller and Mahat (2003) indicated similar outcomes, also in Nepal. A study on trafficked survivors in Israel reported that about 19% satisfied criteria for depression and 17% for PTSD (Chudakov *et al.* 2002). Another study in India indicated that female teenage survivors of sex trafficking showed a higher rate of aggression compared to those who had not been trafficked (Deb *et al.* 2011). A study in Moldova documented that survivors of sex trafficking suffer from PTSD, depression, and anxiety, and that a longer duration of sex trafficking was associated with higher levels of depression and anxiety (Hossain *et al.* 2010). In addition, high rates of sexual risk behaviors have also been documented among victims of sex trafficking (Gupta *et al.* 2011).

Box 29.1 summarizes the results of a study on survivors of sex trafficking in Nepal.

The way forward

Issues related to human trafficking and sex work are one of the biggest priorities of the current world in terms of health, including sexual and reproductive health and HIV prevention, and the promotion of human rights and gender equality. As seen above, there is emerging evidence showing the various impacts of human trafficking and sex work on mental health and psychological well-being. There are encouraging initiatives on integrating mental health and psychological well-being as part of the effort to address issues related to human trafficking and sex work, as evidenced by the work of UNAIDS, UN.GIFT, UNFPA, and other stakeholders including governments, non-governmental organizations (NGOs), and local health, legal, and social services.

Now is the time to reiterate that providing survivors of human trafficking with mental health and psychological care, and assistance with their psychological recovery, while also training the individuals who work with survivors, is a global obligation set up by international conventions. In particular, states parties of these conventions are legally bound to provide mental health and psychological support systems in their countries. The monitoring bodies of these protocols are great mechanisms to make sure that the mental health and psychological well-being of people affected by human trafficking and sex work are protected and promoted.

Box 29.1: Case study

One of the studies conducted by the authors illustrated a higher prevalence of anxiety, depression, and PTSD symptoms among female survivors of sex trafficking in Nepal (Tsutsumi *et al.* 2008).

Background: In Nepal, an estimated 12 000 women and children are trafficked annually for sexual work beyond the national borders of Nepal. The study aims at exploring the mental health status, including anxiety, depression and PTSD, of female survivors of human trafficking in Nepal. The mental health status of survivors of sex trafficking was compared with that of those who were trafficked and forced to work in non-sexual work.

Methods: Participants were female survivors of human trafficking in Nepal. One hundred sixty-four participated in the study. Trafficking survivors who had been forced to work as sex workers were categorized in the sex worker (SW) group, and those who worked in different areas were categorized in the Non-SW group. The questionnaire included the Hopkins Symptoms Checklist-25 (HSCL-25) to evaluate their anxiety and depression status. In addition, the PTSD Checklist Civilian Version (PCL-C) was employed to screen for past-month symptoms of PTSD.

Results: As for depression, all the constituents of the SW group were over the cut-off point, compared to 80.8% of the Non-SW group, indicating a significant difference ($p < 0.01$). A significantly higher proportion of the SW group (29.6%) screened positively for PSTD symptoms in the past month than the Non-SW group (7.5%) ($p < 0.01$).

Discussion: The mental health status of female survivors of human trafficking was explored, showing their vulnerability to anxiety, depression, and PTSD, especially the higher vulnerability of the SW group. The findings also suggest that measures to address this situation should include interventions to improve survivors' mental health status, paying attention to the category of work performed during the trafficking period. It would also be an effective intervention to provide community/mass education on human rights, on the increasing risk of physical and mental disorders among the general public, and on how to prevent females from being trafficked.

In addition, poor mental health and poor psychological well-being are important factors that increase vulnerability to risky sexual behaviors. Prevention and intervention for human trafficking and issues related to sex work still require that more attention is paid to mental health and psychological aspects as a key factor.

There are still big gaps in the areas of human trafficking and sex work, and mental health and psychological well-being. Further research on human trafficking and sex work and mental health and psychological well-being, awareness raising among the general public, capacity building of health workers, policy development at global, national, and municipality levels, and program implementation on the ground are paramount. Mainstreaming mental health and psychological well-being is the key to addressing the devastating human rights violations of human trafficking and sex work.

References

Alegria M, Vera M, Freeman DH, *et al.* (1994) HIV infection, risk behaviors, and depressive symptoms among Puerto Rican sex workers. *American Journal of Public Health* **84**: 2000–2.

Bal Kumar K, Subedi G, Gurung Y, Adhikari K (2001) *Nepal Trafficking in Girls with Special Reference to Prostitution: a Rapid Assessment.* Geneva: International Labour Organization.

Beyrer C (2001) Shan women and girls and the sex industry in Southeast Asia; political causes and human rights implications. *Social Science and Medicine* **53**: 543–50.

Chudakov B, Ilan K, Belmaker RH, Cwikel J (2002) The motivation and mental health of sex workers. *Journal of Sex and Marital Therapy* **28**: 305–15.

Church S, Henderson M, Barnard M, Hart G (2001) Violence by clients towards female prostitutes in different work settings: questionnaire survey. *BMJ* **322**: 524–5.

Crawford M, Kaufman MR (2008) Sex trafficking in Nepal: survivor characteristics and long-term outcomes. *Violence Against Women* **14**: 905–16.

Deb S, Mukherjee A, Mathews B (2011) Aggression in sexually abused trafficked girls and efficacy of intervention. *Journal of Interpersonal Violence* **26**: 745–68.

Decker MR, Mccauley HL, Phuengsamran D, Janyam S, Silverman JG (2011) Sex trafficking, sexual risk, sexually transmitted infection and reproductive health among female sex workers in Thailand. *Journal of Epidemiology and Community Health* **65**: 334–9.

Dharmadhikari AS, Gupta J, Decker MR, Raj A, Silverman JG (2009) Tuberculosis and HIV: a global menace exacerbated via sex trafficking. *International Journal of Infectious Diseases* **13**: 543–6.

El-Bassel N, Schilling RF, Irwin KL, *et al.* (1997) Sex trading and psychological distress among women recruited from the streets of Harlem. *American Journal of Public Health* **87**: 66–70.

Eller LS, Mahat G (2003) Psychological factors in Nepali former commercial sex workers with HIV. *Journal of Nursing Scholarship* **35**: 53–60.

Falb KL, McCauley HL, Decker MR, *et al.* (2011) Trafficking mechanisms and HIV status among sex-trafficking survivors in Calcutta, India. *International Journal of Gynaecology and Obstetrics* **113**: 86–7.

Farley M, Barkan H (1998) Prostitution, violence, and posttraumatic stress disorder. *Women and Health* **27**: 37–49.

Gilchrist G, Gruer L, Atkinson J (2005) Comparison of drug use and psychiatric morbidity between prostitute and non-prostitute female drug users in Glasgow, Scotland. *Addictive Behaviors* **30**: 1019–23.

Gossop M, Powis B, Griffiths P, Strang J (1995) Female prostitutes in south London: use of heroin, cocaine and alcohol, and their relationship to health risk behaviours. *AIDS Care* **7**: 253–60.

Gupta J, Reed E, Kershaw T, Blankenship KM (2011) History of sex trafficking, recent experiences of violence, and HIV vulnerability among female sex workers in coastal Andhra Pradesh, India. *International Journal of Gynaecology and Obstetrics* **114**: 101–5.

Harcourt C, Van Beek I, Heslop J, McMahon M, Donovan B (2001) The health and welfare needs of female and transgender street sex workers in New South Wales. *Australian and New Zealand Journal of Public Health* **25**: 84–9.

Hossain M, Zimmerman C, Abas M, Light M, Watts C (2010) The relationship of trauma to mental disorders among trafficked and sexually exploited girls and women. *American Journal of Public Health* **100**: 2442–9.

International Labour Organization (2005) *A Global Alliance Against Forced Labour.* Geneva: ILO.

International Organization for Migration, London School for Hygiene and Tropical Medicine, United Nations Global Initiative to Fight Trafficking in Persons (UN.GIFT) (2009) *Caring for Trafficked Persons: Guidance for Health Providers.* Geneva: IOM.

Kurtz S, Suratt H, Inciardi J, Kiley M (2004) Sex work and "date" violence. *Violence Against Women* **10**: 357–85.

McCauley HL, Decker MR, Silverman JG (2010) Trafficking experiences and violence victimization of sex-trafficked young women in Cambodia. *International Journal of Gynaecology and Obstetrics* **110**: 266–7.

Ostrovschi NV, Prince MJ, Zimmerman C, et al. (2011) Women in post-trafficking services in Moldova: diagnostic interviews over two time periods to assess returning women's mental health. *BMC Public Health* **11**: 232.

Roxburgh A, Degenhardt L, Copeland J (2006) Posttraumatic stress disorder among female street-based sex workers In the greater Sydney area, Australia. *BMC Psychiatry* **6**: 24.

Sarkar K, Bal B, Mukherjee R, et al. (2008) Sex-trafficking, violence, negotiating skill, and HIV infection in brothel-based sex workers of eastern India, adjoining Nepal, Bhutan, and Bangladesh. *Journal of Health, Population and Nutrition* **26**: 223–31.

Silverman JG, Decker MR, Gupta J, et al. (2008) Syphilis and hepatitis B co-infection among HIV-infected, sex-trafficked women and girls, Nepal. *Emerging Infectious Diseases* **14**: 932–4.

Silverman JG, Decker MR, Gupta J, et al. (2006) HIV prevalence and predictors among rescued sex-trafficked women and girls in Mumbai, India. *Journal of Acquired Immune Deficiency Syndromes* **43**: 588–93.

Silverman JG, Decker MR, Gupta J, et al. (2007) HIV prevalence and predictors of infection in sex-trafficked Nepalese girls and women. *JAMA* **298**: 536–42.

Tsutsumi A, Izutsu T, Poudyal AK, Kato S, Marui E (2008) Mental health of female survivors of human trafficking in Nepal. *Social Science and Medicine* **66**: 1841–7.

UNAIDS (2002) *Sex Work and HIV/AIDS Technical Update*. Geneva: UNAIDS.

UNAIDS (2006) *Resource Pack on Gender and HIV/AIDS; A Rights-Based Approach*. Geneva: UNAIDS.

UNAIDS (2008) *2008 Report on the Global AIDS Epidemic*. Geneva: UNAIDS.

UNIAP (2010) *The Mekong Region Human Country Datasheets on Human Trafficking 2010*. Bangkok: UNIAP.

United Nations (2000) *Optional Protocols to the Convention on the Right of the Child on the Involvement of Children in Armed Conflict and on the Sale of Children, Child Prostitution and Child Pornography*. New York, NY: UN.

United Nations (2001) *Protocol to Prevent, Suppress and Punish Trafficking in Persons, Especially Women and Children, Supplementing the United Nations Convention Against Transnational Organized Crime*. New York, NY: UN.

UNODC (2006) *Trafficking in Human Beings*. Vienna: United Nations Office on Drugs and Crime.

US Department Of State (2006) *Trafficking in Persons Report 2008*. Washington, DC: US Department of State.

US Department Of State (2011) *Trafficking in Persons Report 2011*. Washington, DC: US Department of State.

Zimmerman C, Hossain M, Yun K, et al. (2006) A summary report on the physical and psychological health consequences of women and adolescents trafficked in Europe. London: London School of Hygiene & Tropical Medicine, European Union's Daphne Programme, International Organization for Migration.

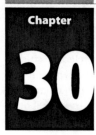

Chapter

30

Capacity building

Rachel Jenkins, Florence Baingana, David McDaid, and Rifat Atun

Introduction

Considerable advocacy in recent years to raise the importance of mental health in the global development agenda has yielded little success, despite the high prevalence of mental disorders in high-, middle-, and low-income countries, contributing up to 13% of the global disability burden. Mental and neurological disorders are highly disabling to individuals affected, impacting on both human and social capital. The economic costs of mental disorders are significant, not only for individuals with disorders and their families, but also for the wider community and for national economies. Therefore, there is a considerable need to build capacity to address these challenges at the levels of policy, strategic planning, implementation, quality assurance, and research. Multiple factors have prevented prioritization of mental health, including: the lack of appreciation of the impact of mental disorders on the risk of all-cause mortality and morbidity; competition for limited resources; the perceived complexity of mental health and its ensuing marginalization within health-sector reform agendas; limited research evidence on the economic impact of tackling mental illness and benefits of interventions in low- and middle-income countries; the erroneous presumption that mental health services can only be delivered by specialists; the lack of collaborative working with non-health sectors; a discontinuity with the work on psychological trauma following conflict and disasters; a lack of public health skills in mental health professionals; and a lack of integrated human resource strategies.

Capacity building needs to enable integration of mental health into general health policy and its inclusion in the essential healthcare services; expansion of economic research on resource use, costs, and effectiveness of essential mental health care services in different countries; better identification and use of levers and entry points for improved care delivery and policy development; greater participation in health-sector reforms; strengthening of links between mental health and public health; and more effective resource mobilization.

Issues and obstacles
Advocacy for mental health services has failed to raise the profile

There has been considerable advocacy for expanding mental health services globally (Murray & Lopez 1996, Jenkins 1997, 2001, Jenkins *et al.* 1997, Institute of Medicine 2001, World Health Organization 2002, Gureje *et al.* 2006, Chisholm *et al.* 2007a, Des Jarlais *et al.* 2007), and further epidemiological studies to demonstrate the growing burden of mental illness and the significant public health problems they cause right across the world (Jenkins *et al.* 2009, 2010a, 2010b, Kessler *et al.* 2009, Mbatia *et al.* 2009). Yet, in spite of the burden and advocacy, mental health is not included – even indirectly – in the Millennium Development Goals (United Nations 2007), and is rarely mentioned in generic policy statements, operational plans, and reports of the World Bank and the World Health Organization, either at country or at global level, or in the discourse of senior staff. The low profile of mental health within key international agencies suggests that the receptive audience for international mental health advocacy is restricted to the mental health community and not extended to international and national health policy makers and other advocates for international health. Furthermore, the links between policies, plans, and budgets in health

---

Essentials of Global Mental Health, ed. Samuel O. Okpaku. Published by Cambridge University Press. © Cambridge University Press 2014.

and non-health sectors for mental health in low- and middle-income countries remain very weak, so that even where mental health policies exist, there is very limited resource with which to implement them.

The contribution of mental disorders to global all-cause mortality and morbidity has not been appreciated

International health organizations have focused on financing prevention and control of major communicable diseases, thanks to the prominence given to HIV, malaria, and tuberculosis (TB) in the Millennium Development Goals. Even when the profile of non-communicable diseases (NCDs) has been discussed, as at the UN's high-level conference on NCDs in New York in September 2011, the focus has been restricted largely to discussion of cancer, cardiovascular disease, chronic obstructive pulmonary disorder, and diabetes. It is worth noting, however, that the final political declaration subsequently adopted by the UN General Assembly recognized that "mental and neurological disorders, including Alzheimer's disease, are an important cause of morbidity and contribute to the global non-communicable disease burden, for which there is a need to provide equitable access to effective programs and healthcare interventions" (United Nations 2012).

One reason for the limited attention given to mental illness has been that health policy makers are faced with many conflicting demands and find it easier to prioritize a few disorders rather than take a comprehensive public health approach. Disease priorities have historically been heavily influenced by consideration of mortality data. Even if policy decisions are to be based on mortality alone, mental illnesses should be considered a priority, because the mortality burden caused by mortality from both suicide (Moshiro *et al.* 2001, Jenkins 2002) and premature death from physical disease in those with mental illnesses (Harris & Barraclough 1998) is similar to the global mortality associated with malaria and HIV (Murray & Lopez 1996). However, despite these data, mental illness is still not perceived by most health policy makers as a major cause of mortality.

Policy decisions about the prioritization of healthcare financing and services should not of course be based on mortality alone, but also on morbidity, disability, and linkages between health conditions.

People with untreated mental illness are less likely to be productive (Patel *et al.* 1997, Baingana & Bos 2006, Friedman & Thomas 2007), and these economic losses to society have been found in selected studies to be considerable (Shah & Jenkins 2000), with mental illness being a major contributor to the overall ill-health burden in many countries (Murray & Lopez 1996, Institute of Medicine 2001, Chisholm *et al.* 2007a, Des Jarlais *et al.* 2007).

Limited economic research evidence

Estimated high burdens of disease or correlations between mental illness and poor socioeconomic outcomes (Patel *et al.* 1997, Baingana & Bos 2006, Friedman & Thomas 2007, Mbatia *et al.* 2009, Jenkins *et al.* 2010a, 2010b) are not sufficient to convince many policy makers of the possible channels of causation that run from mental health to economic behavior, or that scarce public funds are best utilized for mental health issues as opposed to other priorities. Outside of high-income countries, research is lacking on such key topics as costing, cost-effectiveness, financing, and intervention efficiency. The low priority afforded to mental health means it is very difficult to get funding for such critical work (Shah & Jenkins 2000).

Competition within health reforms for limited resources

Health reforms were initiated in the 1990s following recognition that existing health systems were over-centralized, inefficient, ineffective, donor-driven, and unresponsive. A sector-wide approach (SWAp) to reforms was adopted in many countries and often included a form of decentralization, along with development of a framework for policy and planning that emphasized a limited set of cost-effective prioritized health interventions and the integration of a number of vertical programs (externally funded public health programs with separate "vertical" logistics, supervisory, monitoring, and distribution systems from the center to the periphery) within mainstream health-system functions.

The SWAp framework provides both challenges and opportunities regarding the inclusion of mental health in sector policy and plans and in accessing generic funds. Despite the rationale for prioritization of mental health in 2011, only 71% of 184 countries who provided mental-health-related information to the WHO Atlas project had a mental health plan (World Health Organization 2011). Countries without such a plan are much less likely to have a budget line for mental health in health-sector budgets. This is crucial, as without a specific budget line mental health departments cannot easily attract new government-managed funds.

Scarce resources elicit counterproductive competition rather than collaboration between organizations and among personnel working on communicable and non-communicable disease. Mental health, for example, is a key influence on child health, reproductive health, and immunity, as well as on susceptibility to and prognosis of communicable diseases including malaria and HIV; yet it is unusual to find these specialties collaborating with mental health within the health system.

Lack of core indicators leads to invisibility and marginalization

Mental health indicators do not feature among the commonly agreed indicators of health needs, progress, and outcomes in countries or globally. Resource allocation and development priorities are increasingly driven to meet health indicator targets that only reinforce the lack of attention given to mental health, as mental health is usually not captured by the restricted set of national health indicators. The lack of investment in mental health infrastructure, information systems, and research, in low- and middle-income countries in particular, hampers the ability of ministries of health to make an effective case to ministries of finance.

Poor distribution of interventions

Mental disorders generally respond to psychological and social interventions and medications. There are issues with medication procurement and distribution which hamper ready availability of psychotropic medications at district and primary care levels. This is aggravated by a lack of resources, poor advance planning, and stigma about the need for mental health interventions from those involved in the distribution process. Basic psychosocial support is readily deliverable at primary care level if teams are given appropriate general training. The more complex psychotherapies, such as cognitive behavioral

therapy (CBT) and interpersonal therapy, require more extensive training and sustained supervision. Hence, in low-income countries much time and investment will be needed before adequate human resources are developed to provide these treatments on a national basis.

Mental illness is not perceived as amenable to quick solutions

The mental health field is not perceived by policy makers as amenable to defined, easily costed, readily understood, and easily implemented solutions, in contrast to the use of medications for AIDS, tuberculosis, and malaria. However, it is not just communicable disease where outcomes per dollar spent on medication have been computed; data on the cost-effectiveness of medications to treat mental disorders have been published by the World Health Organization (Chisholm et al. 2007b). Medications are a key part of a package of interventions designed to address severe mental disorders, while psychotropic medicines on essential medicine lists of low-income countries are inexpensive, affordable, and effective.

Nonetheless, enhanced outcomes are achieved where interventions are biopsychosocial, rather than just with medications. This complexity deters health-sector reformers, who are accustomed to working with what they see as more straightforward medical solutions for AIDS, tuberculosis, and malaria. In practice, however, such complexity also exists in these disease areas, where interventions also need to be multiaxial and multisectoral, including interventions for behavior changes.

Lack of a strategic approach to human resource planning

Donors and mental health specialists often share a presumption that mental health services can only be delivered by specialists. If senior psychiatrists in low-income countries advocate for mental health services in terms of increased expenditure on specialist services, rather than first ensuring that mental health is well integrated into primary care services, this antagonizes the decision makers, who see this request as special pleading for an unaffordable luxury. However, given the high prevalence of mental disorders in all countries (Kessler et al. 2007), not even high-income countries could afford specialty care for most people with mental disorders.

Assessment and treatment in primary care is essential, and this rationale is even more prominent in low-income countries, where there may be only one psychiatrist per 1–3 million people instead of the one psychiatrist per 10 000–25 000 people in high-income countries.

The supply of mental health providers is highly problematic, as the numbers of both primary care and specialist mental health staff are dwindling rather than increasing, due to increased training costs, as well as emigration from rural areas to urban areas, from the public sector to the higher-paying non-governmental organization (NGO) and private sectors, and from low-income to higher-income countries (Jenkins *et al.* 2010c). Negative attitudes towards mental health have also been observed in medical students and healthcare workers in low- and middle-income countries, which again has a negative impact on staff willing to provide mental health care (Kakuma *et al.* 2011).

Mental health has not been linked well to the social development sector

Research on the etiology, epidemiology, and impact of mental disorders has demonstrated the multiaxial nature of causation, consequences, and effective interventions for mental disorders, but the perception that the practice of psychiatry is still based on a predominantly "medical" model alienates social development experts who would otherwise be natural partners for those wishing to improve the mental health of populations. The contribution of better mental health to social development goes beyond reduction of clinical symptoms and disability, greater workplace productivity, and restoring the lost productivity of informal carers. For example, research in Kenya and Cambodia shows links between economic, institutional, social, gender, and psychological dimensions of social change (Baingana *et al.* 2004, Das *et al.* 2007, World Bank 2007, Francis & Amuyunzu-Nyamongo 2008). However, it is unusual to find comprehensive approaches to social change which incorporate attention to mental health. Such social efforts are rarely developed in collaboration with developments in national mental health policy.

The so-called "psychosocial" domain (understood by international agencies and NGOs as the psychological and social issues surrounding major stresses such as conflict or HIV) has recently gained attention and funding from international donors in relation to post-conflict and HIV-affected populations. Such donors find it more acceptable to talk about psychosocial issues than about mental health issues, and this can lead to a narrowed policy perspective, with a donor focus on post-traumatic stress disorders (PTSD) rather than on the spectrum of disorders found in general and vulnerable populations (World Health Organization 2002). This narrow focus also leads to small-scale NGO-led psychosocial interventions rather than comprehensive integration of mental health policy, planning, and delivery into national health and non-health sector developments and civil society building. Standards, guidelines, and indicators for mental health in social development work are not well developed, and mental health promotion evidence, which is relevant for social action, has not been extensively used (Barry & Jenkins 2006).

Senior mental health professionals do not always have the requisite public health skills for effective national advocacy

There is often a lack of policy, planning, or financing knowledge or skills in mental health professionals who advise or work within ministries of health. They often find it difficult to address the broader public development agenda of problem definition, implementation and defining appropriate outcomes. This lack of key skills impedes their capacity to take advantage of policy and implementation opportunities that may occur, while funding that is allocated is often used inefficiently.

Priorities for capacity building
Capacity building for economic research

There is already some evidence for the costs and impact of inadequately addressed poor mental health on already overburdened health systems (Shah & Jenkins 2000, Chisholm 2007, Chisholm *et al.* 2007b). For instance, data showing that poor mental health leads to inefficiencies in economic productivity in sub-Saharan Africa (SSA) could persuade funders that providing public funds for mental health interventions is justified, and that good mental health policy is good economic development policy. Such research, aimed at estimating benefits of mental health interventions, will need to be largely funded by richer countries' health research and development organizations, as it is unlikely that the SSA countries will be able to afford it. However, health research institutions in SSA should ensure that mental health is a core part of their remit, health economists in SSA need to be oriented to mental health research questions, and mental health researchers need to be trained in the methods of economic research.

Other important areas for further economic research and dissemination in low-income countries include awareness and attention to the increased use of healthcare services by those in poor mental health, costly misdiagnosis of somatic symptoms that are actually symptoms of unrecognized mental disorders, and the contribution of comorbid mental health problems to the prognosis of physical health problems. If mental disorders are not diagnosed and treated effectively, there is a high rate of repeat consultations, placing an additional burden on already stretched health systems (Ustun & Sartorius 1995, Kiima *et al.* 2004). Therefore much of the significant health investments already made by developing countries may be wasted if mental health is not appropriately addressed. For example, treatment adherence for TB, HIV, and stroke is improved when comorbid depression is treated (Trenton & Currier 2001, Ramasubbu & Patten 2003).

Capacity building for policy and strategic planning

As well as the development of specific mental health policies (World Health Organization 2001, Jenkins 2002, Jenkins *et al.* 2002), mental health should be a part of all health sector reform plans (national strategic plans prepared by governments covering a 5–10-year period), the essential packages of health care (an agreed set of prioritized cost effective priority health care interventions), medium-term expenditure frameworks (government national budgets for 3–5 years within which health spending is integrated), and district annual operational plans, as well as in the sector reforms and spending plans of prisons, schools, social welfare, and police at national and district levels. Donors need to back the implementation of whole-country plans through a range of aid instruments, as is already happening through the International Health Partnership. This means clear

targets and effective health management information systems so that national policy makers and district health management teams will be able to monitor needs, use of services, interventions, and outcomes. Mental health advocates need to link with other sectors, and with programs funded by global health initiatives such as the Global Fund. There is a need to understand the broad principles of resource allocation and expenditure frameworks set by ministries of finance and to recognize the increased link between resource allocations and results, in terms of both expenditure and outcomes. This can help with the necessity of making full and effective use of funds within annual operational plans. There is, therefore, a need to include policy and strategic planning skills in the training of mental health professionals, at the levels of post-basic training and continuing professional development, sharing experience between countries.

Capacity building for participation in health sector reforms

Country-level SWAps and health-sector reforms generally focus on developing common systems and on decentralization of decision making and budgets. Health programs such as those dealing with malaria, tuberculosis, and HIV have sources of support and investment which help them to respond to the changes in health system structures and operations brought about by sector reforms. However, the mental health specialty sector does not have the sources of political support and financial investment enjoyed by HIV and malaria. Hence, it is extremely difficult to mobilize decision makers involved in mental health collectively to incorporate mental health issues within new reforms.

Nevertheless, national mental health leaders must vigorously engage in health-sector reform, understand the bureaucratic and political mechanisms and the potential points of influence, and be proactive in understanding the reform implications so as to minimize threats and maximize opportunities for promoting sound mental health policies. To do so, they need to present a strong evidence base to strategically influence policy and resource allocation, and promote the integration of mental health into essential services.

Regional partnerships among mental health policy makers would be a useful platform to share experience of prioritizing mental health and of methods of integration with health and social-sector reforms, especially with long-term mentors from multiple countries to support the process (Beddington *et al.* 2008, Kiima & Jenkins 2010). For example, in the case of SSA, recognition from international donors and the African Union of the importance of mental health to the region would crucially help stimulate pooling of resources for this underfunded area.

Capacity building for public health skills

Mental health professionals would benefit from public health training and education on principles of policy development, health-sector reform, non-health-sector reform, epidemiology, health economics, and research. Similarly, public health professionals would benefit from education on mental health, addressing the epidemiology, risk factors, and consequences of disorders, as well as on opportunities for intervention in the health and relevant non-health sectors.

Capacity building for those engaged in development, to strengthen the linkage of mental health to social development

The contribution of better health goes well beyond the important reduction of clinical symptoms and disability, toward greater workplace productivity and reduction of the lost productivity of carers. While, as argued above, a renewed approach to mental health in the context of the health sector is crucial, this needs to be complemented by a multisectoral and multilevel perspective on mental health, with an appreciation of factors which influence mental well-being, and its relationship to physical well-being, empowerment at family and community levels, livelihoods, productivity, human security, and the development of human, social, and economic capital. Such multisectoral analyses have recently been undertaken for the UK in the Foresight Mental Capital and Wellbeing Project (2008).

A societal perspective is not just an analytical point of view, but needs to be reflected in structures for planning and financing that realize an integrative and synergistic role for mental health capacity and expertise across sectors. Mental health needs to access existing financing mechanisms such as the Global Fund (as has been successfully done in Zambia), to link in to the activities and plans funded by foundations (e.g., the mental health training program for

Kenya primary care staff funded by the Nuffield Foundation: Jenkins *et al.* 2010d), and to develop a coordinated resource mobilization campaign, to put mental health onto an integrated global agenda. Finally, developed nations and donors need also to understand that the benefits of robust community-based approaches, and working through of cross-sector relevance of mental health in development, is relevant and beneficial to all countries (Ustun & Sartorius 1995, Jenkins 2002).

Capacity building for resource mobilization

It is important to learn lessons from vertical communicable disease programs, which have often fragmented care. Resources will be better used if applied in an integrated way which strengthens rather than weakens front-line primary health care. For example, the mental health continuing professional development of 3000 primary care workers in Kenya funded by the Nuffield Foundation is being delivered through the Kenya Medical Training College and the Ministry of Health to strengthen primary care. The training has a health and social systems approach and includes modules integrating the understanding of mental health and child health, reproductive health, malaria, and HIV, as well as addressing issues such as health information systems, working with community health workers and traditional healers, and annual operational planning.

Other examples can also be identified. Zambia has successfully integrated mental health into Global Fund proposals for training of health staff, while Tanzania, Kenya, and Malawi have integrated mental health into general health service delivery, utilizing general health service budgets as set out in national health-sector strategic plans and annual operational plans. All these provide excellent examples of the systematic implementation of mental health service delivery within highly resource-constrained environments.

Conclusions

Capacity building for mental health is an urgent priority because of the significant contribution which mental health makes to global health, social, educational, and economic development. The issues discussed above need to be incorporated into core and post-core training of health and social care professionals and their continuing professional development. There is a need to build capacity for policy, strategic planning, and implementation in mental health and its wider ramifications among politicians, civil servants, directors of mental health, researchers, economists, development experts, specialist professionals, primary care professionals, and other sectors. Addressing mental health issues is crucial for global health, as well as for economic and social development. Training of mental health professionals, public health professionals, research economists, and development experts needs to pay particular attention to the skills discussed in this chapter.

References

Baingana FK, Bos ER (2006) Changing patterns of disease and mortality in sub-Saharan Africa: an overview. In DT Jamison, RG Feachem, MW Makogoba, *et al.*, eds., *Disease and Mortality in Sub-Saharan Africa*, 2nd edn. Washington, DC: World Bank.

Baingana F, Dabalen A, Menye E, Prywes M, Rosholm M (2004) *Mental Health and Socio-Economic Outcomes in Burundi*. Washington, DC: World Bank.

Barry M, Jenkins R (2006) *Implementing Mental Health Promotion*. London: Elsevier.

Beddington J, Cooper CL, Field J, *et al.* (2008) The mental wealth of nations. *Nature* **455**: 1057–60.

Chisholm D (2007) Mental health system financing in developing countries: policy questions and research responses. *Epidemiolica e Psichiatria Sociale* **16**: 282–8.

Chisholm D, Flisher AJ, Lund C, *et al.* (2007a) Scale up services for mental disorders: a call for action. *Lancet* **370**: 1241–52.

Chisholm D, Lund C, Saxena S (2007b) Cost of scaling up mental healthcare in low- and middle-income countries. *British Journal of Psychiatry* **191**: 528–35.

Das J, Do QT, Friedman J, McKenzie D, Scott K (2007) Mental health and poverty in developing countries: revisiting the relationship. *Social Science and Medicine* **65**: 467–80.

Des Jarlais DC, Arasteh K, Perlis T, *et al.* (2007) Convergence of HIV seroprevalence among injecting and non-injecting drug users in New York City. *AIDS* **21**: 231–5.

Foresight Mental Capital and Wellbeing Project (2008) *Final Project Report: Executive Summary*. London: Government Office for Science.

Francis P, Amuyunzu-Nyamongo M (2008) Bitter harvest: the social costs of state failure in rural Kenya. In C Moser, AA Dani, eds., *Assets, Livelihoods, and Social Policy*. Washington DC: World Bank Publications; pp. 217–35.

Friedman J, Thomas D (2007) Psychological health before, during and after an economic crisis: results from Indonesia, 1993–2000. *World Bank Economic Review* 23 (1).

Gureje O, Lasebikan VO, Kola L, Makanjuola VA (2006) Lifetime and 12-month prevalence of mental disorders in the Nigerian Survey of Mental Health and Well-Being. *British Journal of Psychiatry* **188**: 465–71.

Harris EC, Barraclough B (1998) Excess mortality of mental disorder. *British Journal of Psychiatry* **173**: 11–53.

Institute of Medicine (2001) *Neurological, Psychiatric, and Developmental Disorders: Meeting the Challenge in the Developing World*. Washington DC: National Academy Press.

Jenkins R (1997) Reducing the burden of mental illness. *Lancet* **349**: 1340.

Jenkins R (2001) World Health Day 2001: minding the world's mental health. *Social Psychiatry and Psychiatric Epidemiology* 36: 165–8.

Jenkins R (2002) Addressing suicide as a public-health problem. *Lancet* **359**: 813–14.

Jenkins R, de Vries M, Eisenberg L, Kleinman A (1997) WHO: where

there is no vision the people perish. *Lancet* **350**: 1480–1.

Jenkins R, Meltzer H, Bebbington P, *et al.* (2009) The British Mental Health Survey Programme: achievements and latest findings. *Social Psychiatry and Psychiatric Epidemiology*; **44**: 899–904.

Jenkins R, McCulloch A, Friedli L, Parker C (2002) *Developing a National Mental Health Policy*. Hove: Psychology Press.

Jenkins R, Mbatia J, Singleton N, White B (2010a) Prevalence of psychotic symptoms and their risk factors in urban Tanzania. *International Journal of Environmental Research and Public Health* 7: 2514–25.

Jenkins R, Mbatia J, Singleton N, White B (2010b) Common mental disorders and risk factors in urban Tanzania. *International Journal of Environmental Research and Public Health* 7: 2543–58.

Jenkins R, Kydd R, Mullen P, *et al.* (2010c) International migration of doctors, and its impact on availability of psychiatrists in low and middle income countries. *PLoS ONE* 5 (2): e9049.

Jenkins R, Kiima D, Okonji M, *et al.* (2010d) Integration of mental health in primary care and community health workers in Kenya-context, rationale, coverage and sustainability. *Mental Health in Family Medicine* 7: 37–47.

Kakuma R, Minas H, van Ginneken N, *et al.* (2011) Human resources for mental health care: current situation and strategies for action. *Lancet* **378**: 1654–63.

Kessler RC, Angermeyer M, Anthony JC, *et al.* (2007) Lifetime prevalence and age-of-onset distributions of mental disorders in the World Health Organization's World Mental Health Survey Initiative. *World Psychiatry* **6**: 168–76.

Kessler RC, Aguilar-Gaxiola S, Alonso J, *et al.* (2009) The global burden of mental disorders: an update from the WHO World Mental Health (WMH) surveys. *Epidemiologia e Psichiatria Sociale* **18**: 23–33.

Kiima DM, Njenga FG, Okonji MM, Kigamwa PA (2004) Kenya mental health country profile. *International Review of Psychiatry* **16**: 48–53.

Kiima D, Jenkins R (2010) Mental health policy in Kenya: an integrated approach to scaling up equitable care for poor populations. *International Journal of Mental Health Systems* **4**: 19.

Mbatia J, Jenkins R, Singleton N, White B (2009) Prevalence of alcohol consumption and hazardous drinking, tobacco and drug use in urban Tanzania, and their associated risk factors. *International Journal of Environmental Research and Public Health* **6**: 1991–2006.

Moshiro C, Mswiia R, Alberti KG, *et al.* (2001) The importance of injury as a cause of death in sub-Saharan Africa: results of a community based study in Tanzania. *Public Health* **115**: 96–102.

Murray CJL, Lopez AD (1996) *The Global Burden of Disease: a Comprehensive Assessment of Mortality and Disability from Diseases, Injuries, and Risk Factors in 1990 and Projected to 2020.* Cambridge, MA: Harvard University Press.

Patel V, Todd C, Winston M, *et al.* (1997) Common mental disorders in primary care in Harare, Zimbabwe: associations and risk factors. *British Journal of Psychiatry* **171**: 60–4.

Ramasubbu R, Patten SB (2003) Effect of depression on stroke morbidity and mortality. *Canadian Journal of Psychiatry* **48**: 250–7.

Shah A, Jenkins R (2000) Mental health economic studies from developing countries reviewed in the context of those from developed countries. *Acta Psychiatrica Scandinavica* **101**: 87–103.

Trenton AJ, Currier GW (2001) Treatment of comorbid tuberculosis and depression. *Primary Care Companion to the Journal of Clinical Psychiatry* **3**: 236–43.

United Nations (2007) *The Millennium Development Goals Report.* New York, NY: United Nations.

United Nations (2012) *Resolution 66/2. Adoption of Political Declaration of the High-level Meeting of the General Assembly on the Prevention and Control of Non-communicable Diseases.* New York, NY: United Nations.

Ustun TB, Sartorius N (1995) *Mental Illness in General Health Care: an International Study.* Chichester: Wiley.

World Bank (2007) *Country Social Analysis, Kenya.* World Bank Conflict and Social Development Unit, Africa Region.

World Health Organization (2001) *The World Health Report 2001. Mental Health: New Understanding, New Hope.* Geneva: WHO.

World Health Organization (2002) *The World Health Report 2002. Reducing Risks, Promoting Healthy Life.* Geneva: WHO.

World Health Organization (2011) *Mental Health Atlas 2011.* Geneva: WHO.

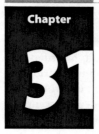

Chapter

31

Child mental health services in Liberia: human resources implications

Janice L. Cooper and Rodney D. Presley

Introduction

This chapter discusses the challenges and opportunities associated with building a practice for child mental health services in Liberia. This can serve as an example of a low-income country with a dire need for systems and services to address the mental health and well-being of children and adolescents. It synthesizes the research on child and adolescent mental health prevalence and the treatment gap for children and youth. It outlines what is at stake if the status quo is maintained, discusses the policy and practice tasks associated with developing services and systems de novo, and provides a case example of a post-conflict country. Finally, the chapter examines the policy implementation considerations needed to move forward.

Child mental health services in Liberia: the background

Services and supports for children and youth with neuropsychiatric disorders fall short across the world. Children and adolescents with mental health problems and their parents often struggle to get the services they need, irrespective of whether they live in high-, middle-, or low-income countries (Patel *et al.* 2007). The situation for children and youth living in sub-Saharan Africa is dire. For children and youth in post-conflict settings such as Liberia, mental health services are almost non-existent, despite the greater need (World Health Organization 2011).

Extant research shows a high prevalence of mental health disorders in low- and middle-income countries (LMICs) in general, ranging from 10% to 20% (Kieling *et al.* 2011). In sub-Saharan Africa, the range was 15–18% (Patel *et al.* 2007). In Liberia, over 53% of

the population is below 18 years old (Ministry of Health and Social Welfare 2011a). While no child-specific national prevalence studies have been carried out, indications are that children and adolescents have high rates of mental health disorders. Liberia's history of civil strife, in conjunction with large income-based disparities, has resulted in a poor healthcare infrastructure. These factors have contributed to the high prevalence of mental health disorders and substance use conditions seen among the general population.

Several county-level epidemiological studies show high rates of major depression (40%), exposure to sexual violence (42–73%), post-traumatic stress disorder (44%), and high rates of substance abuse (12–44%) (Johnson *et al.* 2008, CPC Learning Network 2010). Other multi-county studies showed rates of behavioral health problems among the general public that ranged from 43% with psychological distress, to 10–29% with substance abuse issues, to 14.5% with a history of attempted suicide (Isis-WICCE 2008). Moreover, exposure to some form of physical or psychological torture was almost universal. Nearly 63% of women reported having experienced sexual trauma, with many having physical injuries resulting from that experience (Isis-WICCE 2008). Rape was the predominant form of sexual violence, accounting for 74% of the sexual violence perpetrated during the conflict, with nearly 50% of such acts involving children under age 18 (Isis-WICCE 2008). Epilepsy is epidemic, with over 45% of visits for neuropsychiatry attributed to epilepsy (Ministry of Health and Social Welfare 2011a). This high prevalence of epilepsy contributes to the estimated burden of neuropsychiatric disorders in Liberia, which includes depression (33%), epilepsy (12%), anxiety (including post-traumatic stress disorder, PTSD) (12%), psychosis (11%), bipolar disorder (11%), and substance abuse disorder (8%)

(World Health Organization 2008). Child-specific data on the burden of disease is unavailable, but global statistics, including data specific to Africa, indicate that young people disproportionally bear the burden of disease, especially for neuropsychiatric disorders (Gore *et al.* 2011).

Research implicates poverty as a risk factor for mental health problems (Patel 2007). In Liberia, an estimated 64% of the population lives in poverty, with 48% living in extreme poverty (Ministry of Planning and Economic Affairs 2008). The rate of unemployment is extremely high at 85%. One study found that nearly 70% of respondents reported that their psychological problems negatively impacted their ability to work (Isis-WICCE 2008).

While compelling, this evidence is not specific to children and adolescents. What we know is that the mental health of children and adolescents is strongly associated with their parents' or caregivers' emotional well-being (Nicholson *et al.* 2008). The evidence on the prevalence of mental health disorders for children, adolescents, and young adults is scanty. A key-informant study on the needs of children and adolescents in Liberia indicated that young Liberians had high rates of exposure to war-related stress, poverty, sexual violence, fear, witnessing atrocities, and poor education (Ministry of Health and Social Welfare *et al.* undated). Younger children (5–12) were more likely to exhibit problems of poor concentration, delinquent behaviors, low motivation, early onset of sexual activity, and bullying. Among older youth and young adults (13–22) high rates of unprotected sex, alcohol and drug abuse, disrespect for the law, delinquent behavior, and gang activity were primary problems. Respondents cited trouble sleeping and nightmares, physical body complaints, feeling hopeless about the future, and experiencing suicidal thoughts as signs and symptoms of these problems. High rates of depression, suicidality, and PTSD were also documented among participants in a study of children and adolescents with prior affiliation with the fighting forces (Behrendt 2008). All children reported high rates of symptoms of depression (48%), PTSD (73%), and suicidality (20%). Over two-fifths of youth in the exposure group had difficulty with social interactions and social skills. Both those who had been affiliated with the fighting forces and the control group had high rates of related mental health problems, but the former experienced greater problems, with 90% experiencing PTSD compared to

60% in the control group, and 70% with symptoms of major depression compared to 30% of children and youth who had not associated with fighters.

Indicators of high mental health disorders are matched by a large treatment gap, thus contributing to the burden of disease. One review put estimates of the treatment gap for children and adolescents in LMICs at between 10% and 90% (Kieling *et al.* 2011). These conditions are alarming for several reasons. First, children and adolescents with untreated neuropsychiatric disorders endure unnecessary suffering, morbidity, and in some cases mortality. Parents of children with these conditions bear significant caregiver burden and are less likely to contribute their optimal potential to society (Nuhu *et al.* 2010, Dada *et al.* 2011). Finally, children and adolescents with untreated mental health conditions are less likely to perform well in other domains such as at home, in school, and in their community (Stagman & Cooper 2010). Lack of access to treatment then becomes an impediment to development.

Formal mental health treatment in Liberia is concentrated in a few locations where trained mental health clinicians work. One inpatient psychiatric facility at Grant Hospital serves the country and operates as a brief-stay hospital. It also provides outpatient services. In the community, outpatient mental health services are provided in clinics and hospitals with wide variation in quality and distribution. The paucity of trained providers only partially explains poor penetration rates for mental health services. Service delivery is compromised by another factor: the lack of psychotropic and antiepileptic medications to treat individuals with mental health conditions. Over 80% of facilities report that they lack the staff trained to provide appropriate interventions for mental health. Overwhelmingly there is inferior quality in many places where services are purportedly provided. One large primary care development initiative reported that only 28 of their 100 facilities provided any mental health services (RBHS 2010). Less than 20% of clinicians in the facilities providing services had any mental health training, and only 20 of the facilities had any psychotropic medications available. For example, 79% of referral hospitals *did not* have antidepressants on hand, 37% *did not* have antiepileptic drugs, and 42% *did not* have antipsychotic drugs in stock (Ministry of Health and Social Welfare 2011b).

Liberia's health agenda includes a priority for maternal and child health, yet there is only scant evidence that the mental health needs of mothers, children, and adolescents are being met. In the face of empirical evidence of the consequences of poor maternal mental health on birth outcomes, attachment and later child mental health, and health management skills of mothers, little appears to be happening on the ground (Prince *et al.* 2007). For example, mothers of young children with untreated mental health conditions are less likely to adhere to immunization schedules and well-child visits, and are more likely to have suboptimal nursing experiences, but most of the development programs in the country reflect little interest in addressing these root causes (National Research Council & Institute of Medicine 2009, Watkins *et al.* 2011). Similarly, the focus on services for children and adolescents fails to reflect the need to address the social and emotional well-being of young people. Recent research indicates that intervening early can interrupt or at least slow down the course and intensity of some mental illnesses (Masi & Cooper 2009). Early childhood is a critical period for the onset of emotional and behavioral impairments (Sameroff & Fiese 2000). Without intervention, child and adolescent disorders frequently continue into adulthood (Kessler *et al.* 2005).

There are very few places in Liberia where a young person can access mental health services. For a child, only outpatient services exist irrespective of the severity of the disorder or any extenuating home situation. At Grant Hospital, while 33% of its outpatient cases are children and adolescents, children under 12 are not seen on an inpatient basis. A system of 16 mental health clinics run by Médecins du Monde in Bong County reported that children and adolescents comprise 31% of its approximately 1000 patients under active treatment (van Hofslot 2011).

The empirical evidence on effective treatments is mounting. The concept that we must simultaneously tackle the need for individual services for children and adolescents with the most severe emotional and behavioral problems, provide services and supports for those at risk of development problems, and promote mental health and well-being through universal promotion, prevention, and intervention strategies is being applied across the world. Critical components of this way of building a children's system include rooting it in a context that is not pathological, that optimizes the leveraging of community and individual resilience, that is family- and community-centered and youth-driven, and that uses existing structures including

schools and health clinics. It also seeks to meet children and adolescents where they are, engages youth, and prioritizes stigma reduction (Jordans *et al.* 2010).

Developing a vision for children's mental health

The policy response

The 2009 National Mental Health Policy provided a framework for children's mental health policy and practice (Ministry of Health and Social Welfare 2009). It was informed by prior research and a needs assessment that revealed problems by developmental stage. It also drew upon recommendations to make children a priority and spelled out policy and practice prescriptions for child mental health service delivery. The framework centered on a developmentally or contextually appropriate model of services and supports, using four specific developmental stages: young children (infants and toddlers), children, adolescents, and young adults.

The National Mental Health Policy outlines three broad goals: (1) to develop a quality mental health system, alcohol, and substance abuse prevention and intervention system; (2) to focus on mental health promotion and destigmatization, school-based mental health, and the development of guidelines for treatment for children and adolescents in community and outpatient settings; and (3) to develop a continuum of mental health care for children, adolescents, and young adults and their families based on the concept of least restrictive care and community-based hospital settings as a last resort. To achieve these goals, the framers of the policy proposed that the Ministry of Health and Social Welfare (MOHSW) focus on the following six areas:

- child and adolescent mental health promotion, primarily through schools
- integration of child and adolescent mental health into primary care
- capacity for inpatient mental health services, largely at regional hospitals and with the opening of wellness units
- availability of mental health services for specialized populations
- research and evaluation that support policy and practice decision making
- human rights of children, adolescents, young adults, and their families

The policy is prescriptive in charging the MOHSW with duties to address stigma through public campaigns aimed at mental health and substance abuse prevention; to use prevention approaches focused on primary, secondary, and tertiary levels of intervention; and to require that the MOHSW develop the human resources and technological capacity for case-finding, treatment, and aftercare. The policy unusually also has a heavy focus on financing child and adolescent mental health services. It calls for the guarantee of targeted funding for children's mental health services. Such a framework has been endorsed in the literature as best practice in global child mental health system development (Jordans et al. 2010). It remains, however, largely "aspirational," with small steps toward implementation for children and youth. Liberia is one of 31% of the countries in the world that lacks a specific budget for mental health and spends less than 1% of its health budget on mental health (Saxena et al. 2007).

Highlights of strategies in pursuit of this vision for children's mental health that have been implemented or are under way are shown in Box 31.1.

Box 31.1: Examples of strategies that have been implemented or are under way

- Drafting mental health legislation to provide for the care and support of individuals with mental health conditions and to ensure their protection and human rights, which is a key strategy in advancing a system of care (Eaton et al. 2011)
- Ensuring that the national essential medical list (EML) meets or exceeds WHO EML and is implemented to foster importation of necessary medications
- Creation of a Center for Outcomes Research in Mental Health, consistent with global calls to generate information in low-income settings that contributes to addressing the demand for mental health services, supports practice improvement, informs evidence-based decision making, and sets research priorities (Yasamy et al. 2011)
- Adoption of a 10-year plan with quantifiable benchmarks in mental health (Ministry of Health and Social Welfare 2011c), and a commitment to prison health and mental health

The role of allied professionals

Consistent with the global call to expand access and improve quality of treatment, and to address the treatment gap, the MOHSW in collaboration with an international non-governmental organization (NGO), the Carter Center, committed to train 150 nurses and physician assistants to provide mental health care in the primary care setting (Collins et al. 2011). To date, 100 have been trained. A lack of mental health specialists, especially psychiatrists, propelled the MOHSW to use a task-shifting model to train non-specialist primary care workers. Central to the training is knowledge and skill development in the use of standardized assessment tools and empirically supported interventions, including cognitive behavioral therapy (CBT) and motivational interviewing, and prescribing and management of medications. Using a curriculum developed jointly by practitioners and nurse educators, the program implementers incorporate local policy makers and service providers (both those who specialize in Western biomedical practices and those who focus on traditional practices) in the classroom. International and local faculty use the mhGAP Intervention Guide (mhGAP-IG) in the six months of training as a base on which they build. Students, graduates, and faculty participate in an online professional community where they share information and provide support to one another. Certified mental health clinicians undergo continuing education throughout the year, receiving needed refresher courses as well as new knowledge. Two of these clinicians form the core staff to the specialized mental health services for women and children discussed later.

Putting the evidence into practice in Liberia

John F. Kennedy Medical Center and Grant Mental Health Hospital

John F. Kennedy Medical Center (JFKMC) is the only tertiary care referral hospital in Liberia. It is government-run. Four institutions fall under its auspices: Grant Mental Health Hospital, Liberian Japanese Friendship Maternity Hospital, Memorial Hospital, and Tubman National Institute of Medical Arts. During the 14-year civil war the Catherine Mills Rehabilitation Hospital was destroyed. It was the only tertiary inpatient mental health facility in the country. Following its destruction, the Liberian government asked Dr. Grant, a Liberian psychiatrist, to temporarily turn over his private psychiatric hospital which provided short- and long-term inpatient services to individuals in the Paynesville area and surrounding communities in Monrovia. Grant Mental Health Hospital would serve as the national tertiary mental health facility. It was later sequentially run and operated by two international NGOs. In 2010, JFKMC took over operation of Grant. It remains the only inpatient mental health facility in the country. The following paragraphs outline how services for children are currently organized at Grant Hospital, with outpatient services at JFKMC.

Grant Mental Health Hospital (Grant), Paynesville, Liberia

Services are accessed by walk-in or appointment. Enrolled patients are seen in an outpatient clinic six days a week. They are generally seen once a month for follow-up consultation services and medication refills. Inpatient admission screening takes place six days a week. People not meeting criteria for admission will be seen on an outpatient basis. Individuals are referred to Grant from other hospitals and community mental health clinics throughout Liberia. Emergency mental health services are also available 24 hours a day. Children and adolescents seen at Grant are usually always accompanied by a parent or a family member.

Only adults are admitted for inpatient services at Grant. Teenagers over the age of 15 can be admitted for inpatient services on a case-by-case basis. Children are seen only through the outpatient clinic. Since there is a relatively small number of children seen at Grant, they are treated alongside the adults in the outpatient clinic.

Characteristics of service users

Children and adolescents make up one-third or 300 outpatient visits at Grant per month. Grant sees as many males as females between the ages of 4 and 16. On average there are 250 patient visits per month made by individuals between the ages 4 and 16. For 2012 the total of inpatient and outpatient visits at Grant was over 10 000.

Most of the children seen by Grant come from Montserrado County, with 14% of the individuals seen between the ages of 4 and 16 coming from other counties. Most of the patients from outside of Montserrado come from neighboring counties, including Margibi, Grand Bassa, Grand Cape Mount, and Bong. However, there are patients who come from Nimba and Maryland counties. Maryland is the southernmost county in Liberia, bordering Côte d'Ivoire (Figure 31.1).

Major conditions experienced by service users

At Grant children and adolescents are seen for general psychiatry problems and epilepsy. Half of all visits for

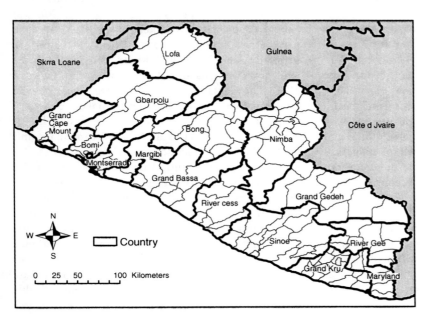

Figure 31.1 Liberia.

Table 31.1 The breakdown, by diagnosis, of patient visits in the psychiatry category seen at Grant Mental Health Hospital

Diagnosis	% of visits
Psychosis	30
Drug-induced psychosis	25
Attention-deficit/hyperactivity disorder (ADHD)	20
Mental retardation/developmental disorder	15
Autism	10

children and adolescents fall in the general psychiatry category. Table 31.1 shows a breakdown, by diagnosis, of patient visits in the latter category for individuals between the ages of 4 and 16.

Patients seen for psychotic-related disorders are between the ages of 13 and 15. Fifty percent of the adolescents and young adults (16–25 years of age) are hospitalized for drug-induced psychosis. Substance abuse among teenagers and young adults in Liberia is a serious problem. These individuals are the least compliant, and rarely return for follow-up appointments once discharged from inpatient care.

Epilepsy at Grant

Epilepsy is the most common serious neurological disorder worldwide, affecting about 50 million people. In most people with epilepsy, the disorder is clinically benign. However, because of the stigma associated with having epilepsy, which is common to many cultures, there can be a negative effect on the social identity of people with the disorder, particularly for those living in resource-poor countries (Jacoby *et al.* 2005). At Grant and in most of the other mental health facilities in Liberia, patients with epilepsy are seen because of the associated stigma. Of all children and adolescents seen at Grant, 50% are seen for epilepsy.

In 2011, Grant held a special child mental health clinic with a team of visiting psychiatrists from Mount Sinai Medical School Global Health Center. In this specialty children's clinic the children seen had either epilepsy or a behavioral diagnosis. Clinic data showed that among all the patients seen, their families had reported that an elevated fever with malaria preceded the child's problem. A correlation or connection had not been made before the clinic. This finding reinforces a recent study that showed that children

with cerebral malaria are at risk of developing several adverse neurological outcomes including epilepsy, disruptive behavior disorders, and disabilities characterized by motor, sensory, or language deficits (Birbeck *et al.* 2010).

Gaps in service delivery, including staffing and quality of care

There is a shortage of psychiatrists and other mental health professionals in Liberia. Currently, there is only one Liberian psychiatrist in the country. During the war, mental health services were primarily provided by international NGOs and directly connected to war-related trauma and the humanitarian crises. Most were in the form of psychosocial interventions. The NGO-supported mental health services were mostly provided by nurses and other health workers. The NGOs provided administrative and clinical oversight for the programs and trained professional medical staff and lay personnel to provide the services.

Mental health service provision today in Liberia is shaped by the war, but also reflects the scarcity of psychiatrists and other mental health professionals. The global scarcity of psychiatrists and the inequity in the global distribution of these specialists has been vividly illustrated by recent reports on mental health resources (World Health Organization 2011).

Presently, at Grant, there is a part-time staff psychiatrist. In January 2012 Mt. Sinai Medical School Global Health Center, in the USA, began a psychiatry rotation at Grant. Patients at Grant are primarily seen by mental health clinicians (nurses and physician assistants) trained by an international NGO. The mental health clinicians are licensed by the Liberian Board of Nursing and the Liberian Association of Physician Assistants. These mental health clinicians use the WHO mhGAP-IG to manage and treat children and adolescents at Grant.

Grant Mental Health Hospital is a catalyst for children's mental health in Liberia. It sees the majority of children's mental health patients in the country. While there are no child-specific services at Grant, it has the most experience with this population. Thus, three main factors led to the development of an integrated service delivery model for mothers, children, and adolescents. First, administrators at Grant saw the need to fill a gap in children's mental health services. Second, they recognized the experience and knowledge gained from working with children at Grant. Third, current leaders at Grant possessed child mental health expertise.

Implementation of a psychiatry consult service spanning maternal and child health

A second source of specialty mental health in the JFKMC system is housed in its main ambulatory service. In conjunction with partners, JFKMC launched a child and maternal mental health consultation service in early 2012. The major goals of the mental health service are:

- To staff JFKMC with a child psychiatrist or a psychiatrist for as much of the year as possible, providing clinical care.
- To train and supervise the identified mental health clinicians providing services in the absence of the Mount Sinai child psychiatrist.
- To focus on the mental health needs of children and mothers.
- To provide consultation services and training to Grant Mental Health Hospital and its staff.
- To establish a successful program within JFKMC/ Grant and build on this in the future to work more directly on proposed projects within the Liberian MOHSW and the Liberian Ministry of Education.

The structure and service of the psychiatry consult service

The Child and Maternal Mental Health Consultation Service is located within the Pediatric Department at JFKMC. The service provides consultation to pediatric patients and their families on both an inpatient and an outpatient basis. Mothers are also seen for services in the Liberian Japanese Friendship Maternity Hospital located in a neighboring building on the JFKMC campus.

The consultation service is provided weekly during pediatric outpatient clinic sessions. The mental health team participates in grand rounds on the pediatric ward and in the maternity hospital. The services provided are as follows:

- mental health screening and assessment
- emergency psychiatric evaluation
- psychoeducation
- psychotherapy treatment modalities, which may include individual, family, or group therapy
- psychiatric evaluation

- medication evaluation and consultation
- referral for inpatient mental health services

The focus of this project is on children, adolescents, and mothers, due to the fact that Liberia has such a young population.

Mental health services for children are extremely limited. It appears that the only children seen are those with behaviors that are unable to be controlled in the home. Grant Mental Health Hospital is able to provide services for children and adolescents, but because of limited resources, including limited funding, lack of trained mental health professionals, and lack of an adequate supply of psychotropic medication, it is difficult to provide high-quality mental health services.

The way forward

The child and adolescent services system for children's mental health as it is being developed reflects the wider international community's consensus of priorities for system building (Patel *et al.* 2010). Increasing mental health specialists and integrating mental health capacity in primary care, introducing and making available evidence-based psychosocial interventions and greater involvement of consumers and carers are all central to the MOHSW's plan of mental health delivery in Liberia. In partnership with the Carter Center in Atlanta, Georgia, USA, 150 mental health clinicians are being trained to integrate specialist mental health care into their primary care practices. Several challenges lie ahead. They include the need for: (1) congruity and education on child development and child rearing; (2) caution on replication of models; (3) building infrastructural capacity across sectors; and (4) sufficient financing to match the plans.

(1) **Child development and child rearing** – Child development theory and principles of best practices in parenting underlie much of the effective practices of mental health promotion, mental ill-health prevention, and early-childhood mental health. This knowledge is not widely available among professionals in the field, whether program designers or service providers. Closely linked is the impact of this knowledge on parenting practices which differ across countries,

resource settings, and religious and ethnic groups. One recent study of violence directed at children and adolescents in South Africa documented significant abuse by carers (Seedat *et al.* 2009). Other considerations related to child development include home environments as proxy indicators for early childcare and education. It is important to develop proxy indicators that are culturally appropriate for individuals in LMICs, and especially Liberia. Research amplifies the difficulty of using home observations as indicators for childhood development in developing countries where preschool programs and other resources may be scarce or lacking (Iltus 2007). For effective strategies to take hold, information on child development and child rearing must be widely available, supportive, applicable to the context, and adaptable.

(2) **Model replication** – It is tempting to create a system of care that duplicates one already created. Africa has a history of copying models from abroad, with mixed results. Large mental health institutions, providing little more than congregate care, keep people with mental illness in deplorable and inhumane conditions around the world. It is important to avoid the historical mis-steps that characterize much of Western mental health, where systems are separate and siloed and lead to iatrogenic outcomes. As Liberia tries to emulate best practices in other countries, the challenge will be to avoid repeating the mistakes of others. Starting de novo provides the opportunity to ground a new system in the cultural and economic underpinnings of its own society, while holding true to the values and principles of specific approaches.

(3) **Support for infrastructural capacity across sectors** – The guiding framework for system development lays a heavy emphasis on collaboration between education and health. Both sectors are struggling in their recovery from years of damage, with poor or no investment, and competing for limited resources. Proven vehicles for service delivery in some post-conflict settings, such as classroom-based intervention models, may be difficult to replicate in a place where the infrastructure for such integration and trust in the capacity of the workforce is lacking (Diallo & Castle 2008). Basics such as physical classroom space,

school environments, adequately trained and paid teachers and healthcare providers cannot be taken for granted. Lack of attention to these factors can undermine the most modest collaborative agenda and derail the most evidence-informed program (Ager *et al.* 2011). There is also the problem of discrimination associated with mental illness. The stigma attached to mental illness transcends throughout the country and in institutions involved with children and adolescents, primarily schools and primary healthcare settings. Some believe that children do not have mental health problems, while others believe that children with behavioral problems simply require firm discipline. While stigma is a national problem, schools and health care must rid their institutions of stigma. Children with neuropsychiatric conditions must not be excluded from their right to education or access to health services. The integration of mental health services into primary care settings and schools can help both to destigmatize mental illness and to identify and treat early. However, it will take an intentional and sustained effort to eradicate stigma.

(4) **Financing** – Funding remains the greatest challenge, despite evidence that development programs could be more effective if they incorporated mental health strategically into specific programs targeting child survival, maternal mortality, malaria, HIV/AIDS, and tuberculosis, for example. These and other vertically funded control programs fail to support a broad systems-strengthening approach (Eisenberg & Belfer 2009). They ignore the data on improved outcomes and linkages between epilepsy and malaria, HIV/AIDS and depression, maternal well-being and maternal depression and psychosis, to name a few (United Nations & World Health Organization 2010). In Liberia, where funding for mental health is limited, there is a move to ignite a movement for children's mental health services with a focus on early intervention and prevention in children. Its success will depend on whether the case can be made politically for investing development dollars in a smarter manner.

Given the dire lack of mental health services and supports for children, adolescents, and young adults, the approach to organizing services becomes vitally important. Liberia's MOHSW has committed to improving its citizens' mental health. Its leader, Africa's first elected female president, oversees peace in a fragile post-conflict state and has pledged to channel resources to support youth. Liberia has a rare opportunity to develop an evidence-informed system of care for its young citizens. It has a unique chance to address the challenges and seize the opportunities to get it right in the provision of services for children and adolescents. Choosing the right path will not simply take expertise, but will require courage and determination.

References

Ager A, Akesson B, Stark L, *et al.* (2011) The impact of the school-based Psychosocial Structured Activities (PSSA) program on conflict-affected children in northern Uganda. *Journal of Child Psychology and Psychiatry* **52**: 1124–33.

Behrendt A (2008) *Mental Health of Children Formerly Associated with the Fighting Forces in Liberia: a Cross Section Study in Lofa.* Dakar, Senegal: Plan International.

Birbeck G, Molyneux ME, Kaplan P, *et al.* (2010) Blantyre Malaria Project Epilepsy Study (BMPES) of neurological outcomes in retinopathy-positive paediatric cerebral malaria survivors: a prospective study. *Lancet Neurology* **9**: 1173–81.

Collins PY, Patel V, Joestl SS, *et al.* (2011) Grand challenges in global mental health. *Nature* **475**: 27–30.

CPC Learning Network (2010) *Rethinking Gender-Based Violence.* CPC Learning Network Policy Change Brief. New York, NY: CPC Learning Network, Mailman School of Public Health, Columbia University.

Dada MU, Okewole NO, Ogun OC, Bello-Mojeed MA (2011) Factors associated with caregiver burden in a child and adolescent psychiatric facility in Lagos, Nigeria: a descriptive cross-sectional study. *BMC Pediatrics* **11**: 110–15.

Diallo V, Castle S (2008) *Desk Review of Evidence About Violence in Educational Settings in West and Central Africa.* Plan West Africa,

Save the Children Sweden, Action Aid, and Unicef.

Eaton J, McCay L, Semrau M, *et al.* (2011) Scale up of services for mental health in low-income and middle-income countries. *Lancet* **278**: 1592–603.

Eisenberg L, Belfer M (2009) Prerequisites for global child and adolescent mental health. *Child Psychology and Psychiatry* **50**: 26–35.

Gore FM, Bloem PJN, Patton G, *et al.* (2011) Global burden of disease in young people aged 10–24 years: a systematic analysis. *Lancet* **377**: 293–301.

Iltus S (2007) The significance of home environments as proxy indicators for early childhood care and education. Background paper prepared for the *Education for All Global Monitoring Report 2007. Strong Foundations: Early Childhood Care and Education.* New York, NY: Graduate Center of the City University of New York.

Isis-WICCE (2008) *A Situation Analysis of the Women Survivors of the 1989–2003 Armed Conflict in Liberia.* An Isis-WICCE Research Report. Kampala, Uganda: Isis-WICCE, Ministry of Gender and Development Liberia, and WANEP/WIPNET, Liberia.

Jacoby ADS, Baker GA (2005) Epilepsy and social identity: the stigma of a chronic neurological disorder. *Lancet Neurology* **4**: 171–8.

Johnson K, Asher J, Rosborough S, Raja A, Panjabi R (2008) Association of combatant status and sexual violence with health and mental health outcomes in

postconflict Liberia. *JAMA* **300**: 676–90.

Jordans M, Wietse TA, Komproe IH, *et al.* (2010) Development of a multi-layered psychosocial care system for children in areas of political violence. *International Journal of Mental Health Systems,* **4**: 15.

Kessler RC, Beglund P, Demler O, Jin R, Walters EE (2005) Life-time prevalence and the age of onset distribution of DSM-IV disorders in the National Co-morbidity Survey Replication *Archives of General Psychiatry* **62**: 593–602.

Kieling C, Baker-Henningham H, Belfer M, *et al.* (2011) Child and adolescent mental health worldwide: Evidence for action. *Lancet* **378**: 1515–25.

Masi R, Cooper JL (2009) *Social-Emotional Development in Early Childhood: What Every Policymaker Should Know.* New York, NY: National Center for Children in Poverty.

Ministry of Health and Social Welfare (2009) *National Mental Health Policy.* Monrovia, Liberia: Ministry of Health and Social Welfare.

Ministry of Health and Social Welfare (2011a) *Country Situational Analysis Report.* Monrovia, Liberia: Ministry of Health and Social Welfare.

Ministry of Health and Social Wefare (2011b) *National Health and Social Welfare Policy and Plan: Final Draft for Validation.* Monrovia, Liberia: Ministry of Health and Social Welfare.

Ministry of Health and Social Welfare (2011c) *January 2011 BPHS Accreditation Final Results Report.*

Monrovia, Liberia: Ministry of Health and Social Welfare.

Ministry of Health and Social Welfare, Massachusetts General Hospital, Harvard Program on Refugee Trauma & Mother Patern College of Health Sciences (undated) *Mental Health Needs Assessment of Liberian Children, Adolescents and Young Adults: Summary of Initial Findings.* Monrovia, Liberia: Ministry of Health and Social Welfare.

Ministry of Planning and Economic Affairs (2008) *Poverty Reduction Strategy.* Monrovia, Liberia: Ministry of Planning and Economic Affairs.

National Research Council, Institute Of Medicine (2009) *Depression in Parents, Parenting, and Children: Opportunities to Improve Identification, Treatment, and Prevention. Committee on Depression, Parenting Practices, and the Healthy Development of Children, Board on Children, Youth and Families, Division on Behavioral and Social Sciences and Education.* Washington, DC: National Academies Press.

Nicholson J, Cooper JL, Freed R, Isaacs MR (2008) Children of parents with mental illness. In TP Gullota, GM Blau, eds., *Family Influences on Childhood Behavior and Development, Evidence-Based Prevention and Treatment Approaches.* New York, NY: Routledge.

Nuhu FT, Yusuf AJ, Akinbiyi A, *et al.* (2010) The burden experiences by family caregivers of patients with epilepsy attending the Government Psychiatric Hospital, Kaduna, Nigeria. *Pan African Medical Journal* 5: 16–26.

Patel V (2007) Mental health in low- and middle-income countries. *British Medical Bulletin* 81 & 82: 81–96.

Patel V, Fisher AJ, Hetrick S, McGarry P (2007) Mental health of young people: a global public health challenge. *Lancet* 369: 1302–13.

Patel V, Maj M, Flisher AJ, *et al.* (2010) Reducing the treatment gap for mental disorders: a WPA survey. *World Psychiatry* 9: 169–76.

Prince M, Patel V, Saxena S, *et al.* (2007) No health without mental health. *Lancet* 370: 859–77.

RBHS (2010) *RBHS Facility Mental Health Survey, 2010.* Monrovia, Liberia: RBHS, JPEIGO.

Sameroff AJ, Fiese BH (2000) Models of development and developmental risk. In C Zeanah, ed., *Handbook on Infant Mental Health.* New York, NY: Guilford Press.

Saxena S, Lora A, Van Ommeren M, *et al.* (2007) WHO's assessment instrument for mental health systems: collecting essential information for policy and service delivery. *Psychiatric Services* 58: 816–21.

Seedat M, Van Niekerk AV, Jewkes R, Suffla S, Ratele K (2009) Violence and injuries in South Africa: prioritizing an agenda for prevention. *Lancet* 374: 1011–22.

Stagman S, Cooper JL (2010) *Children's Mental Health: What Every Policymaker Should Know.* New York, NY: National Center for Children in Poverty.

United Nations, World Health Organization (2010) *United Nations (DESA)-WHO Policy Analysis: Mental Health and Development: Integrating Mental Health into All Development Efforts including MDGs.* New York, NY: UN.

van Hofslot S (2011) MDM Mental Health Program: Bong County. Presentation to Second Cohort of Mental Health Clinicians: Carter Center Mental Health Program, Suakoko, Bong County.

Watkins S, Meltzer-Brody S, Zolnoun D, Stuebe A (2011) Early breastfeeding experiences and postpartum depression. *Obstetrics and Gynecology* 118: 214–21.

World Health Organization (2008) *The Global Burden of Disease: 2004 Update.* Geneva: WHO.

World Health Organization (2011) *Mental Health Atlas 2011.* Geneva: WHO.

Yasamy MT, Maulik PK, Tomlinson M, *et al.* (2011) Responsible governance for mental health research in low resource countries. *PLoS Medicine* 8 (11): e1001126.

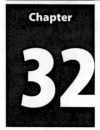

Chapter

32 Mental health and illness outcomes in civilian populations exposed to armed conflict and war

Duncan Pedersen and Hanna Kienzler

Introduction

It is estimated that since the end of World War II, a total of 240 armed conflicts have been active in 151 locations throughout the world (Harbom & Wallensteen 2009). While the number of *interstate* wars has been declining since the early 1990s, the number of *intrastate* wars, most often fought between ethnic groups or loosely connected networks challenging both poor and underdeveloped states and powerful nation states, has increased both in frequency and in levels of organized violence, inflicted atrocities, and psychological warfare. The largest increase of active intrastate conflicts is being reported in Africa, from nine in 2003 and seven in 2005, to twelve in 2008.

If we limit the review to the last two centuries only, wars with a long-lasting – so-called "transformational" – effect on the course of world history, leading to important changes in the global order, represent an estimated total of 42 years of conflicts with a conservative estimate of about 95 million deaths, including both combatants and civilians (Smil 2008). The megawars with the largest number of fatalities (over 10 million) were the Taiping War (1851–64), the Second Sino-Japanese War (1937–41), World War I (1914–18), and World War II (1939–45). Contemporary wars and changes in war strategic targets and warfare styles and technologies (e.g., aerial bombing) have led to a significant increase in the number of civilian casualties, now making up approximately 90% of all war-related deaths (Pedersen & Kienzler 2008). In Africa, the style of warfare has shifted dramatically in recent years. Emerging rebel movements are mushrooming, and the continent is now plagued by countless small-scale "dirty wars" with no front lines, no battlefields, and no distinctions between combatants and civilians. Many of the recruits are children and young adolescents who are engaged in a vicious circle of gang-rape, pillage, and crime, leaving behind a trail of mutilation and murder, trauma, despair, and suffering (Reno 2012). The Arab countries have a distinct experience of revolt and rebellion against authoritarian regimes and a recent history of violent military repression, with a high death toll among civilians engaged in massive demonstrations and exposed to different forms of organized violence, including jail, torture, and summary executions. Psychological warfare is a devastatingly effective central feature in these contemporary wars, where terror and atrocities, murder and mass executions, disappearances, torture, and rape are the norm (Summerfield 1995, Pedersen 2002).

In addition to the mounting number of casualties, these conflicts have resulted in large flows of refugees and internally displaced persons (IDPs). For example, the 2010 United Nations Refugee Agency's *Global Trends* report (UNHCR 2011) shows that there were 43.7 million forcibly displaced people worldwide at the end of 2010, the highest number since the mid-1990s. Of these, 15.4 million were refugees, 27.5 million were IDPs, and 850 000 were asylum seekers, of whom 15 500 were unaccompanied or separated children. Although demographic information on displaced populations is not always available for all countries, some recent estimates indicate that women represent half of most populations falling under UNHCR's responsibility. In all, a significant proportion of the forcibly displaced populations and victims of genocide and armed conflict in the world involve mostly the poor and politically marginal, so called "Fourth World" peoples (Pedersen 2002).

But what are the consequences and main health outcomes experienced among civilian populations affected by endemic conflict, protracted violence,

Essentials of Global Mental Health, ed. Samuel O. Okpaku. Published by Cambridge University Press. © Cambridge University Press 2014.

and contemporary wars? We posit as a unique challenge in the years to come to better understand not only what are the most obvious direct consequences and health outcomes of conflict and war, but also (1) *which* political, social, and environmental factors are of relevance to explain mental health outcomes, including traumatic stress disorders; (2) *how* these factors interact and *what* links, paths, or mechanisms might explain their impact or influence on the health of populations around the globe; and (3) *how* does this web of causes, linkages, and pathways determine the level of suffering, disease, disability, and death in a given population? The future research agenda should be focusing not only on the short-term, but also on the longer-term impact in those exposed to violence and traumatic events. Moreover, we need to continue searching for new ways of preventing violence and conflict, to reduce its sequelae and impact in affected populations, and to develop innovations for effective treatment and improved recovery strategies, at both the individual and the collective levels.

In the following, we will attempt to answer some of these questions by focusing on (1) structural consequences of organized violence, armed conflict, and war; (2) trauma-related disorders: psychological trauma and post-traumatic stress disorder (PTSD); and (3) treatment and intervention strategies for PTSD and trauma-related disorders in local and global contexts. We will finish with some concluding remarks discussing implications for further work on the subject of mental health in war and conflict areas.

Structural consequences of organized violence, armed conflict, and war

There is a growing body of evidence suggesting that the short- and long-term consequences of organized violence, endemic conflict, and war on civilian populations are more complex than initially thought. In the strict sense, the impact of a war cannot be solely examined by the sheer number of casualties, the numbers of refugees and forcibly displaced populations, or the material losses and breakdown of social services resulting from it. There are significant effects expressed in the lingering additional burden of disease, disability, and death and other less evident but more pervasive ecological, social, and economic consequences, such as family disintegration and attrition of social networks, environmental degradation, dislocation of food production systems, disruption of the

local economies, and exodus of the work force, all of which have profound implications for the health and well-being of survivors (Pedersen *et al.* 2008).

Evidence from studies conducted in the aftermath of World War II, the Indochina wars, and more recently in central Asia (Afghanistan) and some countries of the African, Latin American, and Caribbean regions, has consistently shown that exposure to multiple physiological stressors, including famine-induced malnutrition, occurring in utero or early infancy, may lead to chronic diseases later in life, ranging from osteoporosis to cardiovascular disease and diabetes (Markowitz 1955, Toole & Waldman 1997, Gluckman & Hanson 2005). Sharp declines of childhood growth have been shown in many European countries during World War II. For example, a study by Bruntland *et al.* (1980) conducted in Oslo, Norway, revealed a decline in height of school children in the mid-1940s, as a direct consequence of food shortages and adversities experienced during the German occupation. In Guatemala, stunting has been reported among Mayan and Ladino children from 1974 to 1984, a period where extreme violence and massacres were inflicted in the civilian population along with increased levels of poverty, ethnic conflict, nutritional deprivation, and rising social inequalities (Bogin & Keep 1999).

Another spill-over effect of armed conflict and war is the increase of interpersonal violence, armed assaults, homicides, and other drug-related crimes. The "dirty wars" often result in a breakdown of the state, creating territories controlled by local war lords who provide safe haven for the illegal production and trade of drugs. It is estimated that some 95% of the production of hard drugs, mainly opium and coca, is concentrated in countries undergoing conflict and civil war or in post-conflict environments (Collier *et al.* 2009). The drug trade, in turn, has worldwide rippling effects and creates multiple niches of endemic violence with significant negative repercussions in population health.

More recently, researchers have begun to explore how trauma is both a marker and a product of social inequality and exclusion. Studies on narratives of distress have emphasized the taxonomies of stress, pain, and suffering, but have not sufficiently contributed to our understanding of the many interrelations between poverty and exposure to violence as health determinants. This is so, despite the recognition that the effects of war cannot be separated from those of other forces such as structural violence and social injustice, unemployment, falling commodity prices, unbridled environmental exploitation, and landlessness. Moreover, a wealth of data are available that show that imposed structural adjustment packages reflecting Western neoliberal economic models most often result in slashed budgets for health, education, and social welfare on which the poorest are most dependent. This may undermine the social fabric no less effectively than armed conflicts and wars (Summerfield 1998). In short, when trying to explain disease occurrence, distress, trauma, and social suffering in relation to collective violence and contemporary wars, the issues of poverty and social inequalities cannot be ignored.

Trauma-related disorders: psychological trauma and PTSD

In this section, we focus on the mental health outcomes of conflict, war, and other forms of intentional violence in civilian populations, with particular attention to trauma-related disorders, such as psychological trauma and PTSD. More specifically, we discuss first the metamorphosis of PTSD as a trauma construct over time, including issues pertaining to the heterogeneity and universality of PTSD. Second, we examine the relation of causality between exposure to traumatic events and psychological trauma, followed by a brief discussion of the dose–response relations. Third, we address the question of what constitutes a normal and a pathological reaction among civilians to life-threatening circumstances, as happens in endemic violence, armed conflict, and war.

The metamorphosis of PTSD

Over the last few decades, the language of violence, terror, and dislocation has often been conflated with the discourse of trauma. In Western popular and professional discourses, "trauma" has undergone a metamorphosis, and has become a dominant category to explain not only the origins or cause of other health-related problems, but also the consequence of exposure to violence. It has become an emblematic category that is invasive in everyday life and has reached epidemic proportions: the media, the lay public and the scientists, the sports and the arts, are all claiming the universality of trauma as a unique and unavoidable outcome of exposure to violence. In this context, trauma has almost become synonymous with PTSD in both popular and scientific thought.

It was in 1980 that PTSD was adopted as a diagnostic category by the American Psychiatric Association and included in the third edition of the *Diagnostic and Statistical Manual* (DSM-III). The early versions (DSM-III) described PTSD as being an issue restricted to those victims directly affected by events "outside the range of ordinary human experience," while in more recent versions (DSM-IV: American Psychiatric Association 1994) the trauma construct is applied to everyday occurrences, such as a road accident, a difficult birth, a mugging, or hearing the news that a significant other has died (Summerfield 1999).

The diagnostic criteria for PTSD include, next to a history of exposure to a traumatic event (criterion A), two criteria and symptoms from each of three symptom clusters: intrusive recollections (criterion B), avoidant/numbing symptoms (criterion C), and hyperarousal symptoms (criterion D). A fifth criterion, concerning the duration of symptoms (criterion E), and a sixth, assessing the functioning (criterion F), were added in later versions (American Psychiatric Association 2000). The symptom clusters constituting PTSD have grown and vanished in importance across time. These variations in symptom clusters reflect advances of medical theories as much as new knowledge and changes in medical diagnosis and treatment. Interestingly, criterion A, the traumatic event creating the distressful memory, has remained so far untouched in more recent versions of the DSM. Epidemiological studies have confirmed previous DSM revisions and shown that exposure to extreme stress sometimes precedes severe and long-lasting psychopathology. While the concept of trauma appears to be universal, it has, in fact, been described in many different ways throughout the past three decades. The ever expanding and inclusive definition of trauma has made the objective assessment of its existence problematic, and one should exercise caution when trying to measure it.

The etiology of PTSD

The current formulation of PTSD (American Psychiatric Association 1994) implies a causal link between the triggering traumatic event (criterion A) and the other clusters that follow. In other words, the symptoms composing the syndrome are connected by a simple logic: criterion A causes B, and criterion B causes C and possibly D (physiological arousal). In other words, a traumatic event may generate distressful memories, and the individual adapts to recurrent memories and arousal through avoidance behavior and numbing (Young & Breslau in press). This causal link (ABC) is most often invoked in the survivors' narratives, as well as in the descriptions made by external observers or clinicians (Shalev 2008).

However, epidemiologic studies in the general population show that PTSD does not occur in everyone who has experienced traumatic events, and that the traumatic event itself does not sufficiently explain why PTSD develops or persists over time (Yehuda 2002). It is acknowledged that war exposure typically accounts for less than 25% of the variance of PTSD symptoms, and often much less than that (Miller & Rasmussen 2010). Moreover, PTSD prevalence in the general population has been estimated to be low, which may be explained by the differences in the sensitivity of instruments used to measure the presence of PTSD, but may also reflect the presence of other "hidden" factors involved (Shalev & Yehuda 1998). Thus we may conclude, with other researchers, that the traumatic event per se is a necessary but not sufficient cause of PTSD.

Presumed risk factors are currently divided into two categories: (1) those pertinent to the traumatic event (e.g., severity and duration of the type of trauma) and (2) those relevant to individuals who experience the event (e.g., gender, prior traumatic experiences, personality characteristics). Studies have found that higher rates of PTSD symptoms are associated with the degree of direct war exposure and higher numbers of traumatic experiences (Scholte et al. 2004). This characteristic is called dose–response, and it is argued that individuals could possibly develop PTSD "regardless of other risk factors once the trauma load reaches a certain threshold" (Neuner et al. 2004, p. 1).

Empirical studies among war-affected populations have shown that the experience of repeated traumatic stress renders a person increasingly vulnerable to develop PTSD in a cumulative manner (Kolassa et al. 2010). Marshall et al. (2005) assessed the prevalence, comorbidity, and correlates of psychiatric disorder in the US-Cambodian refugee community by conducting cross-sectional, face-to-face interviews on a random sample of households. The analysis of 490 interviews revealed that all study participants had been exposed to severe trauma before immigration and consequently suffered from PTSD (62%), major depression (51%), and alcohol use disorder (4%). PTSD and depression were comorbid findings in the population, and each showed a strong dose–response relationship with measures of traumatic exposure. Similarly, the cumulative effect of traumatic events on the rate of PTSD appeared crucial in the surveys of both Cardozo et al. (2000) and Eytan et al. (2004) concerned with Kosovar Albanian populations. That is, a linear decline in mental health status and social functioning with increasing amounts of traumatic events was discerned. In addition, post-traumatic reactions persist as such beyond the presence of the stressor, and as time goes by the intensity of the initial reaction tends to decrease in the days, weeks, or months following exposure, although at different rates according to the nature of the stressor.

Biological and biographical factors

Other factors most likely to be involved in the causality of PTSD are, apart from individual differences in vulnerability, a combination of biological and biographical factors, such as family history, gender, race, age at time of exposure, previous history of childhood adversity, child abuse, low socioeconomic status, education, and lack of social support (Brewin et al. 2000). For example, Breslau et al. (1997) conducted a study on sex differences in PTSD. Their data reveal that lifetime prevalence of exposure to traumatic events and the number of traumatic events do not vary by gender. However, the risk for PTSD after exposure to traumatic events is more than twice as high among women as among men; and sex differences in PTSD are markedly wider if the exposure occurs in childhood than after the age of 15 years. Alonzo (2000), on the other hand, focuses on the relation of the concept to chronic disease and other life-course events. He concludes that there is evidence to suggest that chronic disease, in addition to sudden and unexpected onsets, and the traumatogenic changes in life circumstances, may produce maladaptive illness coping over the life course. Therefore, attention needs to be paid to the additive effects of comorbidity and the traumatic potential of ineffective therapies.

Besides vulnerability, epidemiologists consider resilience a crucial construct within the traumatic stress response (Paton & Volati 2006). Research that emphasizes coping and resilience among survivors includes, for instance, investigations that document the psychosocial adjustment of young Cambodian refugees in Canada. Rousseau *et al.* (2003) argue that the trauma a family suffered before leaving their homeland and prior to the teenager's birth seems to play a protective role at various times in adolescence with regard to externalized symptoms, risk behavior, and school failure in boys, and fosters positive social adjustment in girls. Similar findings are reported by Beiser *et al.* (1989), who studied 1348 adults who fled from Vietnam and Laos to Canada after having lived in refugee camps for a period of time. They argue that in the case of the Southeast Asian refugees, the impact on depressive mood proved significant but short-lived as it was moderated by social support provided by family, neighbors, and other community members. Thus, it is presumed that personal and social resources cannot only help overcome the traumas of the refugee experience, but also reduce the risk of PTSD. Overall, these studies also recognize that trauma-related mental illness seems to reduce steadily over time, but that a subgroup of people with a high degree of exposure to traumatic experiences has long-term psychiatric morbidity which would in turn exert a higher demand for mental health services and programs.

Normal versus pathological reactions

Finally, it is important to distinguish between what constitutes a normal and what a pathological reaction among civilians exposed to life-threatening circumstances. Critics argue that it cannot be presumed that people globally understand their suffering through the "prism of psychology" (Pupavac 2004). For example, Weine *et al.* (1995) state that Bosnian teenagers who survived ethnic cleansing and immigrated to the USA had, in fact, intrusive memories, yet "they did not view having these memories as being abnormal or pathological but as understandable response to tragic occurrences." They did not see themselves as victims of a horrific singular event but understood their experiences as a collective assault on their people. Nevertheless, they enjoyed their lives in the USA, considered their new teachers supportive, and did outstandingly well in school.

Several researchers reveal that it would be simplistic to regard survivors as passive receptacles of negative psychological effects. On the contrary, they show that survivors act actively and in a problem-solving way attuned with their environment by negotiating disrupted life courses, loss of status, culture shock, and the attitude of the host society, thereby shaping themselves, their communities, and ultimately the legacy of war itself (Summerfield 1998, Almendom & Summerfield 2004, Jones 2004). According to the critics, new questions have to be asked in order to conduct adequate research that does not follow a medicalized model of care, offering psychiatric counseling and psychological support. Humanitarian interventions should be built on the basis of (1) avoiding the misconception of defining resilience only in terms of absence of diagnosable psychopathology, and focusing instead on resilient trajectories of adjustment and adaptation over time (Bonanno 2012); and (2) on retaining and fostering social support and social rehabilitation frameworks, starting with the strengthening of damaged local capacities in line with local needs and priorities.

Treatment and intervention strategies for PTSD and trauma-related disorders in local and global contexts

In this section, we discuss some of the existing paradigms for helping individuals, families, and communities to manage and cope with the aftermath of organized violence, armed conflict, and war-related adversities. The aftermath of atrocities and contemporary wars is partly characterized by the overall re-ordering of post-conflict post-war politics and the emergence of a "therapeutic moral order" that is largely driven by the premise that not only combatants but entire civilian populations exposed to the adversities of endemic violence and armed conflict are traumatized and require therapeutic management of one kind or another (Moon 2009). That is, psychiatric teams or trauma counselors are mobilized under the assumption that trauma-related disorders will necessarily affect most, if not all, of the exposed.

At the same time, it is acknowledged that states recently emerging from armed conflict or under endemic and protracted organized violence have inadequate mental health resources because of a lack of funding, reduced health budgets, and a shortage and inequitable distribution of mental health professionals (Allden *et al.* 2009, Al-Obaidi *et al.* 2010). In order to ameliorate this situation, the funding and delivery of humanitarian aid is increasingly organized by international and local non-governmental organizations (NGOs), and most current therapeutic interventions are exported with little adaptation from Western countries to war-torn societies worldwide.

Miller and Rasmussen (2010) have made an important distinction based on a cleavage existing between trauma-focused approaches and psychosocial frameworks to understanding and addressing mental health needs of populations affected by armed conflict and war. They further state that underlying these two main approaches there are fundamentally different assumptions regarding the causality, among other factors, that most influences mental health outcomes in conflict and post-conflict settings. For those so-called trauma-focused advocates, the critical factor involved in the causality chain is direct exposure to a traumatic event, which is in turn fueled by the growing clinical field of traumatology. In contrast, for those grouped as supportive of a psychosocial approach, the attribution of causality focuses primarily on the overall "stressful social and material conditions caused or worsened by armed conflict" (Miller & Rasmussen 2010, p. 7), including other coexisting conditions such as extreme poverty and malnutrition, or derived from internal displacement and refugee status resulting in loss of social and material support.

Practitioners and scholars in the field of humanitarian assistance largely agree that despite the plethora of available treatment options, including both pharmacotherapy and psychotherapy, there remains an absence of a solid evidence base for mental health and psychosocial support interventions (Allden et al. 2009). In 2008, the Institute of Medicine published a report with a systematic review of the scientific evidence on treatment modalities for PTSD. The report states that for all drug classes and specific drugs reviewed in each of the classes the evidence is inadequate to determine efficacy in the treatment of PTSD. With regard to psychotherapies the committee states that only for exposure therapies is the evidence sufficient to support its efficacy in the treatment of PTSD.

A prior report, entitled the *World Disaster Report* (International Committee of the Red Cross 2000), sharply criticized international mental health initiatives for their lack of evidence and standardization, and issued the call for standards so as to better structure relief efforts. It was partly in response to this report that several standards were developed,

such as the *Sphere Handbook*, which was revised in 2004 to include international guidelines for treating psychological trauma (Sphere Project 2004). According to the handbook, access to psychological first aid should be guaranteed to individuals experiencing acute mental distress after exposure to traumatizing experiences. It is further argued that acute distress following exposure to psychological trauma is best managed following the principles of "psychosocial first aid," which include "basic, non-intrusive pragmatic care with a focus on listening but not forcing talk; assessing needs and ensuring that basic needs are met; encouraging but not forcing company from significant others; and protecting from further harm" (Sphere Project 2004, p. 293). Similar reports have been published by the World Health Organization (2003) on *Mental Health in Emergencies* and the Inter-Agency Standing Committee (2007), stating that it is crucial to protect and improve people's mental health and psychosocial well-being in the midst of an emergency through well-organized psychosocial intervention strategies.

There is a growing consensus that mental health interventions for conflict-affected populations must address the broad impact of armed conflict, promoting a sense of safety, self- and collective efficacy, feelings of connectedness and hope (Kirmayer et al. 2010). However, translating these general goals into specific interventions requires an ecosocial perspective, with a fair knowledge of individual and community psychology at the local level, and awareness of prevailing social, economic, and political constraints, as well as a solid understanding of cultural meaning systems. Although there seems to be awareness of the importance of culture in most of the guidelines, there are few, if any, specific recommendations with regards to how to articulate cultural data (i.e., local idioms of distress) with the professional discourses of trauma and suffering. As a consequence, mainstream approaches to diagnosis and treatment of trauma-related disorders overlook the extent to which the trauma experience is culture-specific in that personal, political, social, and cultural factors mediate the experience of war or other forms of violence (Bracken et al. 1995, Kienzler 2008).

Thus, we would argue that in order to provide meaningful psychosocial assistance to civilian populations exposed to armed conflict and war, we must learn more about mental health problems and psychosocial stressors locally identified as most important, and about the impact that other forms of violence, such as structural violence and gender-based discrimination, may have on the mental health of populations. To live up to the complexities involved, humanitarian interventions should combine both *emic* and *etic* approaches by taking existing healing strategies, endogenous initiatives and programs into consideration "in a participatory, empowering and ownership manner" (Aro *et al.* 2008, p. 548).

Concluding remarks

In this chapter we have reviewed both short- and long-term consequences of protracted violence, endemic conflict, and war on civilian populations and their relationships, which turn out to be more complex than initially thought. The impact of a war cannot be solely examined by the sheer number of casualties, physically wounded, and displaced; there are many indirect effects expressed in the additional burden of disease and death, suffering and disability, and other less evident but more pervasive consequences (Pedersen 2002, Pedersen *et al.* 2008).

In discussing specific mental health outcomes of war and violence in civilian populations, we focused on psychological trauma and PTSD as a trauma construct and its changes over time, including issues pertaining to the heterogeneity and universality of the disorder. We further critically examined the relation of causality between exposure to traumatic events and psychological trauma, and the limited explanatory power of the linear model of trauma in which exposure to traumatic events invariably leads to PTSD as a single outcome. We addressed the question of what constitutes the sequencing of events in the progression between the initial acute reaction and the chronic stage among civilians exposed to life-threatening circumstances.

The interconnection between higher rates of PTSD symptoms and the degree of direct exposure and higher numbers of traumatic experiences was presented, and it was concluded that greater exposure to traumatic events was predictive of more abundant PTSD symptomatology. In concluding this section, we considered the many limitations of the PTSD model, arguing that mental illness is not the single consequence of trauma, but closely associated with social inequalities, gender disparities, poor nutrition, and overall poor physical health. Thus, the usefulness and applicability of PTSD as a category in diverse social and cultural contexts would depend on previous research conducted in the particular contexts in which is utilized (Kirmayer *et al.* 2007).

There seems to be consensus that despite the abundance and variety of available treatment options, there remains a lack of a solid evidence base for psychosocial interventions aimed at improving mental health outcomes for populations in need. The guidelines reviewed in this chapter are serious attempts to standardize the various approaches to mental health care for populations affected by conflict and war, but they tend to be mostly based on expert opinion, literature reviews, or single case studies. It would therefore be essential to rigorously field-test the guidelines before putting them to use in culturally and socially diverse settings.

The study of traumatic stress disorders emerges as one critical area of enquiry to assess the effects of the environment on the central nervous system, and this turns out to be crucial, as it may lead to significant changes in the existing healthcare paradigms and ultimately improve current clinical practices and humanitarian interventions. We need to build solid research evidence that takes into account not only the opinion of experts but above all the social and cultural context for understanding trauma-related disorders, and, based on this new paradigm, we must develop effective clinical approaches addressing the needs and real concerns of people on the ground.

For interventions to be meaningful, they should reflect a macro perspective that recognizes the transnational impacts of globalization, war, and violence on mental health, as well as "the importance of addressing local and national health care issues within a global context" (Rylko-Bauer *et al.* 2009, p. 8), and, on the other hand, they must pay attention to how these multiple macro-level forces play out locally, in the lives of individuals, families, and communities. More specifically, current approaches discussing the need for community-based interventions aimed at civilian populations highlight the importance of (1) assessing the transnational and structural forces *and* the local sociocultural setting, (2) relating these complex, multilayered contexts to both the local formulation of problems and their endogenous solutions (i.e., resilience outcomes), and (3) identifying features of the culture and community that suggest local ways of coping as well as healing practices (see also Weiss *et al.* 2003). These are crucial steps required to build both individual and collective interventions, which may be more effective as well as socially relevant and culturally meaningful for civilian populations in need.

References

Allden K, Jones L, Weissbecker I, *et al.* (2009) Mental health and psychosocial support in crisis and conflict: Report of the mental health working group. *Prehospital and Disaster Medicine* 24 (Suppl 2): s217–27.

Al-Obaidi A, Budosan B, Jeffrey L (2010) Child and adolescent mental health in Iraq: current situation and scope of promotion of child and adolescent mental health policy. *Intervention* 8: 40–51.

Almendom A, Summerfield D (2004) Mental well-being in settings of complex emergency: an overview. *Journal of Biosocial Science* 36: 381–8.

Alonzo A (2000) The experience of chronic illness and post-traumatic stress disorder: The consequences of cumulative adversity. *Social Science and Medicine* 50: 1475–84.

American Psychiatric Association (1994) *Diagnostic and Statistical Manual of Mental Disorders, Fourth Edition (DSM-IV)*. Washington, DC: APA.

American Psychiatric Association (2000) *Diagnostic and Statistical Manual of Mental Disorders, Fourth Edition Revised (DSM-IV-TR)*. Washinghton, DC: APA.

Aro AR, Smith J, Dekker J (2008) Contextual evidence in clinical medicine and health promotion. *European Journal of Public Health* 18: 548–9.

Beiser M, Turner J, Ganesan S (1989) Catastrophic stress and factors affecting its consequences among Southeast Asian refugees. *Social Science and Medicine* 28: 183–95.

Bogin B, Keep R (1999) Eight thousand years of economic and political history in Latin America, revealed by anthropometry. *Annals of Human Biology* 19: 631–42.

Bonanno GA (2012) Uses and abuses of the resilience construct: loss, trauma, and health-related adversities. *Social Science and Medicine* 74: 753–6.

Bracken P, Giller J, Summerfield D (1995) Psychological responses to war and atrocity: The limitations of current concepts. *Social Science and Medicine* 40: 1073–82.

Breslau N, Davis G, Andreski P, Schultz L (1997) Sex differences in posttraumatic stress disorder. *Archives of General Psychiatry* 54: 1044–8.

Brewin CR, Andrew B, Valentine JD (2000) Meta-analysis of risk factors for posttraumatic stress disorder in trauma-exposed adults. *Journal of Consulting and Clinical Psychology* 68: 748–66.

Bruntland GH, Liestol K, Walloe L (1980) Height, weight and menarcheal age of Oslo schoolchildren during the last 60 years. *Annals of Human Biology* 7: 307–22.

Cardozo B, Vergara A, Agani F, *et al.* (2000) Mental health, social functioning, and attitudes of Kosovar Albanians following the war in Kosovo. *JAMA* 284: 569–77.

Collier P, Chauvet L, Hegre H (2009) The security challenge in conflict-prone countries. In B Lomborg, ed., *Global Crises, Global Solutions*. Cambridge: Cambridge University Press; pp. 58–103.

Eytan A, Gex-Fabry M, Toscani L, *et al.* (2004) Determinants of postconflict symptoms in Albanian Kosovars. *Journal of Nervous and Mental Disease* 192: 664–71.

Gluckman PD, Hanson MA (2005) *The Fetal Matrix: Evolution, Development and Disease*. Cambridge: Cambridge University Press.

Harbom L, Wallensteen P (2009) Armed conflicts, 1946–2008. *Journal of Peace Research* 46: 577–87.

Institute of Medicine (2008) *Treatment of Posttraumatic Stress Disorder: an Assessment of the Evidence*. Washington: National Academies Press.

Inter-Agency Standing Committee (2007) *IASC Guidelines on Mental Health and Psychological Support in Emergency Settings*. Geneva: IASC.

International Committee of the Red Cross (2000) *World Disaster Report 2000*. Geneva: International Federation of Red Cross and Red Crescent Societies.

Jones L (2004) *Then They Started Shooting: Growing Up in Wartime Bosnia*. Cambridge, MA: Harvard University Press.

Kienzler H (2008) Debating war-trauma and post-traumatic stress disorder (PTSD) in an interdisciplinary arena. *Social Science and Medicine* 67: 218–27.

Kirmayer LK, Lemelson R, Barad M (2007) *Understanding Trauma: Integrating Biological, Clinical and Cultural Perspectives*. Cambridge: Cambridge University Press

Kirmayer L, Kienzler H, Afana H, *et al.* (2010) Trauma and disasters in social and cultural context. In D Bhugra and C Morgan, eds., *Principles of Social Psychiatry*. New York, NY: Wiley-Blackwell; pp. 155–77.

Kolassa I, Ertl V, Eckart C, *et al.* (2010) Spontaneous remission from PTSD depends on the number of traumatic event types experienced. *Psychological Trauma: Theory, Research, Practice, and Policy* 2: 169–74.

Markowitz SD (1955) Retardation in growth of children in Europe and Asia during World War II. *Human Biology* 27: 258–73.

Marshall GN, Schell TL, Elliott MN, *et al.* (2005) Mental health of Cambodian refugees two decades after resettlement in the United States. *JAMA* 294: 571–9.

Miller KE, Rasmussen A (2010) War exposure, daily stressors, and mental health in conflict and post-conflict settings: bridging the divide between trauma-focused and psychosocial frameworks. *Social Science and Medicine* 70: 7–16.

Moon C (2009) Healing past violence: traumatic assumptions and therapeutic interventions in war and reconciliation. *Journal of Human Rights* **8**: 71–91.

Neuner F, Schauer M, Karunakara U, *et al.* (2004) Psychological trauma and evidence for enhanced vulnerability for posttraumatic stress disorder through previous trauma among West Nile refugees. *BMC Psychiatry* **4**: 34.

Paton D, Volati J (2006) Vulnerability to traumatic stress: personal, organizational and contextual influences. In J Volati, D Paton, eds., *Who Gets PTSD? Issues of Posttraumatic Stress Vulnerability*. Springfield, IL: Charles C. Thomas.

Pedersen D (2002) Political violence, ethnic conflict and contemporary wars: broad implications for health and social well-being. *Social Science and Medicine* **55**: 175–90.

Pedersen D, Kienzler H (2008) Ethnic conflict and public health. In HK Heggenhougen, SR Quah, eds., *International Encyclopedia of Public Health*, Vol. 2. San Diego, CA: Academic Press; pp. 508–18.

Pedersen D, Tremblay J, Errazuriz C *et al.* (2008) The sequelae of political violence: assessing trauma, suffering and dislocation in the Peruvian highlands. *Social Science and Medicine* **67**: 205–17.

Pupavac V (2004) War on the couch: the emotionology of the new international security paradigm. *European Journal of Social Theory* **7**: 149–70.

Reno W (2012) *Warfare in Independent Africa*. Cambridge: Cambridge University Press.

Rousseau C, Drapeau A, Rahimi S (2003) The complexity of trauma response: a four year follow-up of adolescent Cambodian refugees. *Child Abuse and Neglect* **27**: 1277–90.

Rylko-Bauer B, Whiteford L, Farmer P (2009) Prologue: Coming to terms with global violence and health. In B Rylko-Bauer, L Whiteford, P Farmer, eds., *Global Health in Times of Violence*. Santa Fe, NM: School for Advanced Research Press; pp. 3–16.

Scholte WF, Olff M, Ventevogel P, *et al.* (2004) Mental health symptoms following war and repression in eastern Afghanistan. *JAMA* **292**: 585–93.

Shalev AY (2008) PTSD: a disorder of recovery? In LJ Kirmayer, R Lemelson, M Barad, eds., *Understanding Trauma: Integrating Biological, Clinical and Cultural Perspectives*. Cambridge: Cambridge University Press; pp. 207–23.

Shalev AY, Yehuda R (1998) Longitudinal development of traumatic stress disorders. In R Yehuda, ed., *Psychological Trauma*. Washington, DC: American Psychiatric Press; pp. 31–66.

Smil V (2008) *Global Catastrophes and Trends: the Next 50 Years*. Cambridge, MA: MIT Press.

Sphere Project (2004) *Humanitarian Charter and Minimum Standards in Disaster Response*. Oxford: Oxfam.

Summerfield D (1995) Addressing human response to war and atrocity. In RJ Kleber, CR Figley, BPR Gersons, eds., *Beyond Trauma: Cultural and Societal Dynamics*. New York, NY: Plenum Press; pp. 17–29.

Summerfield D (1998) The social experience of war and some issues for the humanitarian field. In P Bracken, C Petty eds., *Rethinking the Trauma of War*. New York, NY: Free Association Books; pp. 9–37.

Summerfield D (1999) A critique of seven assumptions behind psychological trauma programs in war affected areas. *Social Science and Medicine* **48**: 1449–62.

Toole MJ, Waldman RJ (1997) The public health aspects of complex emergencies and refugee situations. *Annual Review of Public Health* **18**: 283–312.

UNHCR (2011) *UNHCR Global Trends 2010*. Geneva: UNHCR.

Weine S, Becker D, McGlashan T, *et al.* (1995) Adolescent survivors of "ethnic cleansing": observations on the first year in America. *Journal of the American Academy of Child and Adolescent Psychiatry* **34**: 1153–8.

Weiss MG, Saraceno B, Saxena S, *et al.* (2003) Mental health in the aftermath of disasters: consensus and controversy. *Journal of Nervous and Mental Disease* **191**: 611–15.

World Health Organization (2003) *Mental Health in Emergencies. Mental Health and Social Aspects of Health of Populations Exposed to Extreme Stressors*. Geneva: WHO.

Yehuda R (2002) Post-traumatic stress disorder. *New England Journal of Medicine* **346**: 108–14.

Young A, Breslau N (in press). Is PTSD a single disorder? In D Hinton, B Good, eds., *Culture and PTSD*. Ithaca, NY: Cornell University Press.

Chapter

33

Implications of disasters for global mental health

Sabrina Hermosilla and Sandro Galea

Disasters and global health

Both the number of disasters and the number of people affected by them have been increasing over the past two decades. In 2011, there was a total of 302 natural disasters reported to the United Nations International Strategy for Disaster Reduction (UNISDR), with over 205 million people affected (UNISDR 2012). While many of these natural disasters and their impact have been concentrated in Asia, every region across the world reported humanitarian emergencies in 2011 (Office for the Coordination of Humanitarian Affairs 2011, UNISDR 2012).

There are several potential definitions of "disasters" (Thywissen 2006). The Centre for Research on the Epidemiology of Disasters (CRED) defines a disaster as "a situation or event which overwhelms local capacity, necessitating a request to a national or international level for external assistance; an unforeseen and often sudden event that causes great damage, destruction, and human suffering" (Steenland et al. 2010). The main criteria for disaster-level event include: "10 or more people reported killed, 100 or more people reported affected, declaration of a state of emergency, or a call for international assistance" (Steenland et al. 2010). The UNISDR defines a disaster as "a serious disruption of the functioning of a community or a society involving widespread human, material, economic or environmental losses and impacts, which exceeds the ability of the affected community or society to cope using its own resources" (UNISDR 2009).

These definitions suggest that disasters are less importantly classified by their precipitating cause, but rather by their relative impact on society. It is thus possible that a disaster in one community would not be a disaster in a different community, or the same community under different circumstances. While the original cause of the disaster event, natural, human-made, technological, is important, in this chapter we will focus on the response component of the disaster definition, understanding that response to disasters is often understood best when causal agency is explicit.

This chapter will review how disasters affect mental health globally, examine some key concepts for understanding the psychological impact of disasters, and conclude with a discussion of implications for policy, research, and field practitioners.

Effect of disasters on mental health
Psychological health in disasters

The burden of mental illness on individuals, families, and communities following a disaster is substantial (Abrahams 2011a). In the immediate aftermath of a disaster, distress and health risk behaviors manifest as increased substance use, sleep disruption, stress-related psychosomatic and psychological symptoms, and non-specific distress (Neria et al. 2009). Psychopathology is typically elevated in the immediate aftermath of a disaster and can persist for months or years after the event. Anxiety disorders including post-traumatic stress disorder (PTSD), substance abuse, depression, and grief all have been documented at higher rates after disasters than in pre-disaster periods (McFarlane et al. 2009, Neria et al. 2009).

Research on anxiety disorders in disasters has focused primarily around PTSD (McFarlane et al. 2009, Neria et al. 2009). Prevalence of PTSD within 1–6 months following a human-made disaster event has been reported as low as 2.3% (Miguel-Tobal et al. 2006, Neria et al. 2008) and as high as 17.0% (Silver

Essentials of Global Mental Health, ed. Samuel O. Okpaku. Published by Cambridge University Press. © Cambridge University Press 2014.

et al. 2002, Neria *et al.* 2008). Comparable prevalence ranges in technological and natural disasters are 0.4–44% (Havenaar *et al.* 1997, Godeau *et al.* 2005) and 3.0–40% (Carr *et al.* 1997, van Griensven *et al.* 2006, Neria *et al.* 2008), respectively. As time after the event increases, the prevalence of PTSD decreases (Carr *et al.* 1997, Galea *et al.* 2003, van Griensven *et al.* 2006), although longitudinal research in this area is limited (Neria *et al.* 2008).

Disaster-related substance abuse is largely limited to pre-disaster users (Neria *et al.* 2009, Van der Velden & Kleber 2009). Consistent with dominant literature findings, exemplar studies exploring disasters in populations of natural-disaster survivors in 1988 Florida, technological disaster survivors in 1972 West Virginia, and terrorism-related disaster survivors in 2001 New York have reported the overall prevalence of substance dependency and abuse in post-disaster periods to be comparable to pre-disaster population prevalence (Van der Velden & Kleber 2009). However, stability in population-based measurements does not always imply a lack of change. An examination of cigarette smoking after the 2003 Australian fires found that smokers who had quit before the fires had a higher prevalence of smoking after the natural disaster event as compared to those who had never smoked (Parslow & Jorm 2006, Van der Velden & Kleber 2009). Comorbidity of substance abuse and other disaster-related psychopathology can be as high as 30–40% (Van der Velden and Kleber 2009). In the aftermath of natural disasters, significant increases in substance abuse, as might be expected from the literature on individual trauma (Morissette *et al.* 2007), have not been observed (Van der Velden & Kleber 2009). Data comparing post-disaster prevalence to pre-disaster levels is often non-existent or is derived from post-disaster self-report. A comprehensive understanding of the impact of disasters on substance abuse is limited by availability of comparable studies, especially with respect to study design, exposure and outcome measurement, inadequate follow-up periods, and Western-country population focus. Further rigorous longitudinal studies are required to disentangle the independent effects of disaster exposure on incident substance abuse and a disaster's synergistic effects with pre-existing substance abuse on post-disaster prevalence of substance abuse.

Prolonged grief and depression are probably the most prevalent disaster-related mental health disorders (Maguen *et al.* 2009; Neria *et al.* 2009). The burden of these affective disorders follows a continuum, from those who display transient symptoms, to those who are suffering prolonged grief (PGD) and/or major depressive disorder (MDD) with sustained long-term functional impairment (Maguen *et al.* 2009, Neria *et al.* 2009). Baseline pre-disaster population burden of PGD and MDD, type of disaster, nature of disaster exposure, symptom trajectories, and PGD and MDD measurement realities differ by context and study (Maguen *et al.* 2009). Over two years after the September 11 terrorist attack, 44% of bereaved study respondents screened positive for PGD (Neria *et al.* 2007, Maguen *et al.* 2009), while 16% of those exposed to the epicenter of an earthquake, interviewed over a year after the 1999 Turkey earthquake, met MDD criteria (Basoglu *et al.* 2004, Maguen *et al.* 2009). While the current research is insufficient to draw parallels across all disaster types and populations, predictors of PGD and MDD consistently fall into pre-event, peri-event, and post-event predictor categories (Maguen *et al.* 2009, Neria *et al.* 2009). Higher PGD and MDD prevalence estimates have been shown in settings with higher pre-disaster background PGD and MDD population prevalence, disasters involving agency or perceived agency of the surviving population, and relative proximity – physical or psychological – to the disaster event (Maguen *et al.* 2009). Inconsistent PGD and MDD prevalence estimates in disaster settings may be the result of unique study design and methodological considerations, such as PGD and MDD measurements and definitions (Maguen *et al.* 2009). Treatment outcomes for PGD and MDD have been inconsistently documented and require further research to make recommendations to practitioners responding to disasters (Maguen *et al.* 2009, Neria *et al.* 2009).

Mental health response to physical health insults in disasters

Disasters affect all aspects of population health. The year 2011 saw over 29 000 individuals lose their lives in natural disasters worldwide (UNISDR 2012). Disasters have been shown to increase the incidence of physical injury (Iezzoni & Ronan 2010) and resultant exposure-related conditions (diarrheal diseases, malaria, typhoid, measles, extreme temperatures, intimate partner violence, violence), aggravate existing chronic health conditions (Chan & Griffiths 2009), and compromise reproductive health (Abrahams 2011b).

These physical health consequences of disasters in turn are associated with adverse mental health consequences of these events. Excess mortality affects communities through both personal, individual mourning and community mourning (Bhugra *et al.* 2010). Physical injury is associated with substantially increased risk of psychopathology among both the persons injured and their caretakers (Bhugra *et al.* 2010). Chronic health conditions that are poorly managed because of disaster-related disruptions, such as diabetes or cardiovascular disease, similarly strain not only the patients suffering from the disruption in care, but also their direct caretakers and at times the entire healthcare system.

On average, one out of five women of childbearing age in a disaster is pregnant (Abrahams 2011b). Compromised reproductive health care is known to affect the mental health of expecting and new mothers, their children (born and unborn) (Talge *et al.* 2007, Harville *et al.* 2010), and caretakers of the children within the community (Harville *et al.* 2010, Kilic *et al.* 2011). Increased experience of sexual and gender-based violence has been extensively documented during the acute phase of disasters and immediately after, especially in conflict-related disaster settings (Amowitz *et al.* 2002, Marsh *et al.* 2006). Consistent with consequences of experiencing violence in other settings, women who experience or witness sexual violence in disasters report higher rates of psychopathology including anxiety, post-traumatic stress, and depression (Amowitz *et al.* 2002, Marsh *et al.* 2006).

The 2010 earthquake in Haiti provides an example of the impact of a large-scale disaster on physical disease and injury and in turn of these on mental health. Official reports show 5% of the population injured or killed in the earthquake and its aftermath, with a total of 19% of the population internally displaced (Shultz *et al.* 2011b). Physical injuries required emergency surgeries (often amputations) and rehabilitation (Iezzoni & Ronan 2010), services that overwhelmed the already limited healthcare provisions available in Haiti before the earthquake. International support both aided in the recovery process (Shultz 2011b) and caused delays (Tappero & Tauxe 2011). Debilitating psychopathology, pervasive traumatic grief, and psychological distress, in response to the scale of direct and indirect physical injury and mortality, were projected to increase in the interim period directly after the earthquake, on a population level (Shultz *et al.* 2011b), but insufficient follow-up studies have been conducted to see if the projected increase was realized or ameliorated through targeted interventions.

Particular considerations
Vulnerable groups

It is well documented that communities and subpopulations that are underserved and most vulnerable before a disaster are disproportionately harmed by the disaster (Laditka *et al.* 2010, Callaway *et al.* 2012). While vulnerable groups are by definition context-specific, general categories that require additional and specialized support during and after a disaster include children, elderly, women, first responders, and pre-disaster culturally, ethnically, economically, and socially marginalized populations (White *et al.* 2002, Jones *et al.* 2009, Cloyd & Dyer 2010, Laditka *et al.* 2010, Peek & Stough 2010, Xu & Wu 2011).

Individuals belonging to vulnerable groups have diverse needs during and after disasters. First responders and rescue personnel are consistently shown to be at higher risk of psychopathology after disasters than are other groups. For example, uniformed first responders and cleanup personnel in the September 11, 2001, attacks on the World Trade Center (WTC) in New York demonstrated higher acute stress reactions and other PTSD symptomology than the average for the affected community (DiMaggio & Madrid 2009, McCaslin *et al.* 2009, Neria *et al.* 2009). In the Oklahoma City terrorist bombing in 1995 first responders were found to suffer higher rates of PTSD than the general population, but lower than non-responder primary survivors (Neria *et al.* 2009, Pfefferbaum *et al.* 2009). The symptomology experienced by responders is chronic, compared to the symptomatology associated with acute exposures of affected non-responders (McCaslin *et al.* 2009, Neria *et al.* 2009). In addition to differential symptomology, the mental health services required by this group are also unique, characterized by their occupational nature, the need to translate healthy anxiety management and coping skills into field settings, and the stigma associated with seeking care (McCaslin *et al.* 2009, Neria *et al.* 2009).

Across contexts, disaster types, and studies, women consistently suffer higher disaster-related negative mental health outcomes, such as depression, grief, and PTSD, as compared to men (Breslau *et al.* 1999, Punamaki *et al.* 2005, Kimerling *et al.* 2009).

For example, women in a representative study of the same September 11, 2001, attacks on the WTC in New York reported 17.4% peri-event panic attack, compared to 7.3% reported by men (Pulcino *et al.* 2003, Kimerling *et al.* 2009). Women in the study, consistent with the literature, were more likely to report other factors that are known to increase vulnerability to PTSD, such as prior mental health diagnosis, experience of sexual assault, and low socioeconomic status (Kimerling *et al.* 2009). Health interventions must be designed to address the unique needs of vulnerable populations while not neglecting the greater disaster-affected population.

Access to health and relief services

Pre-disaster marginalized groups have limited access to health and relief services in the peri- and post-disaster time periods (Sphere Project 2011). Access to relief services can facilitate the return to normal mental health functioning. The relationship between access to health services and mental health is complex. For example, women who required and lacked access to reproductive health services after the October 2005 earthquake in Pakistan were found to suffer from higher levels of clinical depression and anxiety (Anwar *et al.* 2011). Many studies focus on health-seeking behaviors for mental health services based on symptom severity. After the 2000 Miyake Island volcanic eruption, increased health-seeking behavior was associated with PTSD and depression symptomatology severity (Goto *et al.* 2002).

How disasters affect public mental health

Several theoretical models have been proposed to help explain how disasters affect population mental health. One such model proposes that we can consider stressors in the aftermath of a disaster. This model proposes that an intermittent stressor, one that is not always present but is during the specific disaster event, is a vulnerability in response to a disaster situation that, had the disaster not occurred how and when it did, would not have evolved into a vulnerability (Rudenstine & Galea 2012). A disaster during the 2000 Italian floods illustrates how an intermittent stressor, disabled occupants of a campground, combined with heavy rains and resulting mudslide to drastically increase the disaster-related mortality

(Rudenstine & Galea 2012). Had aid responders been prepared to evacuate disabled occupants ahead of time, they could have minimized the extent of the disaster. The impact of intermittent stressors on mental health functioning is well established in animal models (Lu *et al.* 2003) but has as yet not been fully documented in post-disaster human settings.

An intermittent protector is a capacity in response to a disaster situation that, had the disaster not occurred how and when it did, would not necessarily have been viewed as a capacity (Rudenstine & Galea 2012). The May 21, 1950, earthquake in Cuzco, Peru, with an epicenter close to the city's heart, had a significantly lower impact because of the intermittent protector of a concurrent soccer game, with almost a third of the city's residents in attendance (Rudenstine & Galea 2012). Had these residents not been safely protected at the stadium, or had the stadium not withstood the quake as effectively as it did, the impact of the disaster would have been greatly increased.

Ongoing stressors and trauma after a disaster also provide detail to the experience of psychopathology in post-disaster populations. The impact of Hurricane Katrina, which made landfall in the southeastern United States in August of 2005, is one example of how ongoing stressors and trauma shape the impact of the disaster on a community. Forced migration and financial hardship are two key ongoing stressors that were still operative seven months after the initial disaster event (Kessler *et al.* 2009, Neria *et al.* 2009). Kessler *et al.* (2008) found a statistically significant increase in percentage of the population impacted by Hurricane Katrina (both living within the New Orleans metropolitan region and outside) who reported suicidal ideation, suicidal plan, and PTSD symptoms (non-New Orleans metropolitan region only) at 17–19 months after the disaster event as compared to 5–7 months after the event. A context-specific and temporally sensitive understanding of the ongoing stressors for the survivors of this disaster, coupled with a targeted intervention (Wolmer *et al.* 2011), could have ameliorated the increase in mental health psychopathology years after the disaster event.

Mediating and modifying the mental health impact of disasters

Not all hazards experienced by a community escalate to a disaster. Understanding why and how a disaster develops requires a detailed understanding of the environmental, historical, demographic and political, community wealth, and social factors that are operative at the time of the event.

The physical environment is the most central and obvious factor modifying the impact of a disaster on the affected community. Immediate emergency response is directly related to the accessibility of the affected community. Earthquakes of similar magnitude in the mountains of Pakistan and the foothills of California will elicit very different response times. Communities that are harder to access will also require more resources to deliver emergency aid, further increasing the burden of the event on the community. While communication developments of the past 20 years have greatly improved our knowledge of affected communities, when a disaster hits a community, knowing that people are affected is not the same as accessing and helping the affected.

The built environment of the affected area is also important. A key difference between the impact of the 2010 Haiti and Chile earthquakes was the quality of the built environment. While Chile experienced an earthquake 500 times the magnitude of that in Haiti only weeks earlier, the destruction on the physical environment was more extensive in Haiti (Kirsch et al. 2010). The quality of the existing structures, especially the key hospital and healthcare facilities central to local early disaster response, enabled the Chilean responders to provide care immediately to a large portion of the affected community, while responders in Haiti required immediate massive international assistance (Kirsch et al. 2010, Vanholder et al. 2011). The impact on the mental health of these two communities has not been sufficiently investigated to date. Through this mobilization and reliance on local resources, Chilean responders were able to provide, by definition, a context-specific, locally salient response. Local capacity was supported, thus providing protective mental assistance to both victims of the earthquake and first responders (Raphael & Stevens 2006, McCaslin et al. 2009, Neria et al. 2009, Vanholder et al. 2011).

The historical context of a region is essential to understanding the impact of disaster on mental health. Colonial histories are still present in many former colonial regions, both in how governments and local societies view international aid and in the frameworks through which they operate. In acute emergency situations, having access to international aid responders who speak the local language – because it is a shared colonial language such as English, Portuguese, or French – greatly facilitates early response efforts and meaningful coordination between local and international responders. Countries have responded to emergencies where they have a historical connection. In the 2005 Pakistan earthquake, the majority of aid came from countries with historical colonial connections with Pakistan, regional neighbors, and the United States, which has a historical relation with Pakistan of trying, through economic and military aid, to support the stabilization of the region (Wilder 2010).

Pre-existing demographic and political structures within the disaster-affected area play a key role in modifying the impact of a disaster. In the 2011 Japanese earthquake and tsunami, the relative demographic homogeneity of the affected population, coupled with a highly functioning government, facilitated the rapid deployment of response teams, including specialized psychosocial teams (Shultz et al. 2011a). While it is impossible to measure what the impact would have been on the mental health of the population had they not acted so swiftly and coherently, an informative comparison can be draw with the 2010 Haiti earthquake, where a poorly functioning political system and language and cultural differences between the affected population and aid responders may have exacerbated the negative mental health outcomes (Vanholder et al. 2011).

Pre-existing community and individual wealth mediates the impact of a disaster on mental health. Individual wealth and family status has been associated with faster and improved receipt of aid packages in India following the 2004 Southeast Asian tsunami (Aldrich 2010). Beyond receipt of aid, individuals with greater pre-existing wealth have greater access to pre-disaster emergency preparedness precautions, such as voluntary pre-evacuation, which would modify the mental health impact of a disaster, since increased proximity to a disaster event has been repeatedly shown to be associated with increased negative mental health outcomes (Basoglu et al. 2004, Maguen et al. 2009). On a community level, community wealth enables infrastructure investments in the form of physical preparedness, first-responder personnel and training, and communications networks that act synergistically to mediate the negative impact of a disaster on the affected community.

Pre-existing and developing social factors are essential in mediating the impact of a disaster on mental health. Social support is a construct that is challenging to evaluate across different cultural realities. Received and perceived social support can both exacerbate the mental health consequences of a disaster (when received support is greater than perceived support or dissipates too quickly over time) and ameliorate them (when perceived social support is great) (Kaniasty & Norris 2009, Neria *et al.* 2009). Different types of social support and social resource networks might modify the negative mental health impact of a disaster. When comparing the impact of terrorist bombings in Nairobi, Kenya, in 1998 and Oklahoma City in 1995 on the psychopathology of affected populations, North *et al.* (2005) found that the Kenyan community relied more heavily on religious networks while the United States community turned to formal psychological medical clinicians after the bombing.

By its very nature, social support must be understood in a local context, and responders to disasters must ensure that they do not deteriorate, diminish, or replace pre-existing social support networks through the delivery of aid, as this could have negative long-term consequences on the psychopathology burden of affected populations. This ability that disaster responders can have, to support or erode existing local social structures, has been codified in the Inter-Agency Standing Committee *Guidelines on Mental Health and Psychosocial Support in Emergency Settings* (Inter-Agency Standing Committee 2007). The IASC recommends that baseline social support structures be understood and supported by exploring if they existed during the pre-disaster period, if they are disaster-induced, or if they can be classified as induced by humanitarian aid or response. While the classification of social support and networks is challenging, it is central in understanding local context and the role that the support and networks play in modifying deleterious mental health outcomes of disasters.

Ongoing topics for mental health in disaster responses

Research implications

Commiserate with the experiences of those affected by disasters; there is a growing body of literature exploring the impact of disasters on population health. We suggest that further disaster-related

mental health research is needed on the following topics: development of context-specific measures, responsive methodological advances, increased geographic representation, and improved research funding policies.

Clinical manifestations of mental health symptoms are by definition culturally specific. However, measurement methodologies and instruments have not been developed, and perhaps will never be developed, for every context. While some disaster-related health measurements, such as access to a clean water supply, are universal and only need slight cultural and linguistic adaptations, mental health constructs must be validated before an instrument is used. This will lead both to improved baseline estimates and to better understanding of disaster-related mental health burden (Jones 2008).

Unique logistical, methodological, analytic, and ethical challenges exist when conducting mental health research in disasters. New recruitment, follow-up, and population enumeration methods are required to increase representativeness and size of samples. Stigma, migration, and constrained resources challenge research in all settings, and disaster-affected populations can be even more vulnerable to their pressures and eventual effect on research findings. Advancement in study design and data collection methods should focus on accessing understudied populations, such as the vulnerable groups previously discussed. Intervention research has demonstrated repeatedly that an enhanced understanding of local context and community-level research provides improved quality in research (Norris *et al.* 2002).

Geographic representation in the current literature is limited. Translation by policy makers and practitioners of research findings is limited by the dearth of context-relevant available findings. The shortage of published disaster mental health studies in the African context is only one extreme example of this imbalance.

Existing funding cycles and priorities challenge disaster mental health research initiatives. Longitudinal studies are needed to understand the trajectory of key disaster-related psychopathologies. These studies are expensive to conduct and must be initiated close to the disaster event, as many instruments rely on self-report for exposure measurements. Funding agencies interested in public mental health that encourages rigorous geographically non-specific proposals and expedited review processes will improve the dissemination of quality mental health research.

Implications for practitioners

Recent research indicates that mental health practitioners are knowledgeable about different underlying constructs associated with the development of positive and deleterious mental health conditions (Ager *et al.* 2010). More work is needed to include non-mental-health practitioners. In 2005, during the post-Hurricane Katrina response, the colocation of services, physical and mental health, was able to address this knowledge gap while overcoming stigma and other deterrents to accessing care (Madrid *et al.* 2008). While more work can be done here, practitioners are key allies in supporting positive mental health outcomes for communities, as they are the front line of disaster survivors' interaction with the public health system.

Local and international responders to disasters, regardless of their specialty, need to have a basic understanding of the impact of disasters and response on the mental health of affected populations. Disasters must be recognized as an ongoing component of the environment within which public health practitioners operate, and as such should be considered essential in training and preparation, not outlier, extreme events or situations. Trained responders are better able to both help the affected population and prevent personal adverse mental health outcomes through strengthening coping skills and decreasing uncertainty (McCaslin *et al.* 2009). As articulated by Shultz *et al* (2011a) in their review of the mental health response to the March 11, 2011, Japanese earthquake and resultant tsunami, key components of a successful response that incorporates the importance of mental health awareness include: increased prioritization of disaster victims' and responders' mental health requirements; locally validated mental health evaluation tool development and dissemination; evidence-based, timely, and locally relevant response models; contextually appropriate interventions focused on survivors with significant psychopathology; continual monitoring and evaluation of mental health needs and services, with special attention to adverse events of responding activities; and increased support of pre-existing social support networks and other factors that support and promote community resilience (Shultz *et al.* 2011a).

Policy implications

Addressing the mental health needs of post-disaster communities is a public health policy priority. Increased exposure to multiple, consecutive disaster events has been shown to increase distress (Shultz *et al.* 2011a), and therefore policies to protect and foster positive mental health environments before, during, and after a disaster are required. Disasters are often acute and short-term in nature, but the resultant shift in the distribution of mental health conditions in a population leads to long-term and often chronic mental health needs. Disaster events are not unique and unexpected, nor are their resultant mental health consequences inevitable. Policies that support improved health and building codes and conducting of disaster response drills will significantly reduce the negative mental health impact of a disaster, perhaps ameliorating the impact enough so that a disaster event never causes sufficient damage to be categorized as a disaster. Only through coordinated, informed, and locally derived policy can the formulation of the disaster public mental health burden be mitigated.

References

Abrahams J (2011a) Disaster risk management for health: mental health and psychosocial support. Disaster Risk Management for Health Fact Sheets. WHO. http://www.who.int/hac/events/drm_fact_sheet_mental_health.pdf (accessed July 2013).

Abrahams J (2011b) Disaster risk management for health: sexual and reproductive health. Disaster Risk Management for Health Fact Sheets. WHO. http://www.who.int/hac/events/drm_fact_sheet_sexual_and_reproductive_health.pdf (accessed July 2013).

Ager A, Stark L, Akesson B, Boothby N (2010) Defining best practice in care and protection of children in crisis-affected settings: a Delphi study. *Child Development* **81**: 1271–86.

Aldrich DP (2010) Separate and unequal: post-tsunami aid distribution in Southern India. *Social Science Quarterly* **91**: 1369–89.

Amowitz LL, Reis C, Lyons KH, *et al.* (2002) Prevalence of war-related sexual violence and other human rights abuses among internally displaced persons in Sierra Leone. *JAMA* **287**: 513–21.

Anwar J, Mpofu E, Matthews LR, Shadoul AF, Brock KE (2011) Reproductive health and access to healthcare facilities: risk factors for depression and anxiety in women with an earthquake experience. *BMC Public Health* **11**: 523.

Basoglu M, Kilic C, Salcioglu E, Livanou M (2004) Prevalence of posttraumatic stress disorder and comorbid depression in earthquake survivors in Turkey: an epidemiological study. *Journal of Traumatic Stress* **17**: 133–41.

Bhugra D, Craig T, Bhui K (2010) *Mental Health of Refugees and Asylum Seekers*. New York, NY: Oxford University Press.

Breslau N, Chilcoat HD, Kessler RC, Peterson EL , Lucia VC (1999) Vulnerability to assaultive violence: further specification of the sex difference in post-traumatic stress disorder. *Psychological Medicine* **29**: 813–21.

Callaway DW, Yim ES, Stack C, Burkle FM (2012) Integrating the disaster cycle model into traditional disaster diplomacy concepts. *Disaster Medicine and Public Health Preparedness* **6**: 53–9.

Carr VJ, Lewin TJ, Webster RA, *et al.* (1997) Psychosocial sequelae of the 1989 Newcastle earthquake: II. Exposure and morbidity profiles during the first 2 years post-disaster. *Psychological Medicine* **27**: 167–78.

Chan EY, Griffiths S (2009) Comparision of health needs of older people between affected rural and urban areas after the 2005 Kashmir, Pakistan earthquake. *Prehospital and Disaster Medicine* **24**: 365–71.

Cloyd E, Dyer CB (2010) Catastrophic events and older adults. *Critical Care Nursing Clinics of North America* **22**: 501–13.

DiMaggio C, Madrid PA (2009) The terrorist attacks of September 11, 2011, in New York City. In Y Neria, S Galea, FH Norris, eds., *Mental Health and Disasters*. New York,

NY: Cambridge University Press; pp. 522–37.

Galea S, Vlahov D, Resnick H, *et al.* (2003). Trends of probable post-traumatic stress disorder in New York City after the September 11 terrorist attacks. *American Journal of Epidemiology* **158**: 514–24.

Godeau E, Vignes C, Navarro F, *et al.* (2005) Effects of a large-scale industrial disaster on rates of symptoms consistent with posttraumatic stress disorders among schoolchildren in Toulouse. *Archives of Pediatrics and Adolescent Medicine* **159**: 579–84.

Goto T, Wilson JP, Kahana B, Slane S (2002) PTSD, depression and help-seeking patterns following the Miyake Island volcanic eruption. *International Journal of Emergency Mental Health* **4**: 157–71.

Harville E, Xiong X, Buekens P (2010) Disasters and perinatal health:a systematic review. *Obstetrical and Gynecological Survey* **65**: 713–28.

Havenaar JM, Rumyantzeva GM, van den Brink W, *et al.* (1997) Long-term mental health effects of the Chernobyl disaster: an epidemiologic survey in two former Soviet regions. *American Journal of Psychiatry* **154**: 1605–7.

Iezzoni LI, Ronan LJ (2010) Disability legacy of the Haitian earthquake. *Annals of Internal Medicine* **152**: 812–14.

Inter-Agency Standing Committee (2007). *IASC Guidelines on Mental Health and Psychosocial Support in Emergency Settings*. Geneva, IASC.

Jones L (2008) Responding to the needs of children in crisis. *International Review of Psychiatry* **20**: 291–303.

Jones L, Asare JB, El Masri M, *et al.* (2009) Severe mental disorders in complex emergencies. *Lancet* **374**: 654–61.

Kaniasty K, Norris FH (2009) Distinctions that matter: recieved social support, percieved social support, and social embeddedness after disasters. In Y Neria, S Galea,

FH Norris, eds., *Mental Health and Disasters*. New York, NY: Cambridge University Press; pp. 175–202.

Kessler RC, Galea S, Gruber MJ, *et al.* (2008) Trends in mental illness and suicidality after Hurricane Katrina. *Molecular Psychiatry* **13**: 374–84.

Kessler RC, Galea S, Gruber M, *et al.* (2009) Hurricane Katrina. In Y Neria, S Galea, FH Norris, eds., *Mental Health and Disasters*. New York, NY: Cambridge University Press; pp. 419–40.

Kilic C, Kilic EZ, Aydin IO (2011) Effect of relocation and parental psychopathology on earthquake survivor-children's mental health. *Journal of Nervous and Mental Disease* **199**: 335–41.

Kimerling R, Mack KP, Alvarez J (2009) Women and disasters. In Y Neria, S Galea, FH Norris, eds., *Mental Health and Disasters*. New York, NY: Cambridge University Press; pp. 203–17.

Kirsch TD, Mitrani-Reiser J, Bissell R, *et al.* (2010) Impact on hospital functions following the 2010 Chilean earthquake. *Disaster Medicine and Public Health Preparedness* **4**: 122–8.

Laditka SB, Murray LM, Laditka JN (2010). In the eye of the storm: resilience and vulnerability among African American women in the wake of Hurricane Katrina. *Health Care for Women International* **31**: 1013–27.

Lu L, Shepard JD, Hall FS, Shaham Y (2003) Effect of environmental stressors on opiate and psychostimulant reinforcement, reinstatement and discrimination in rats: a review. *Neuroscience and Biobehavioral Reviews* **27**: 457–91.

Madrid PA, Sinclair H, Bankston AQ, *et al.* (2008) Building integrated mental health and medical programs for vulnerable populations post-disaster: connecting children and families to a medical home. *Prehospital and Disaster Medicine* **23**: 314–21.

323

Maguen S, Neria Y, Conoscenti LM, Litz BT (2009) Depression and prolonged grief in the wake of disasters. In Y Neria, S Galea, FH Norris, eds., *Mental Health and Disasters*. New York, NY: Cambridge University Press; pp. 116–130.

Marsh M, Purdin S, Navani S (2006) Addressing sexual violence in humanitarian emergencies. *Global Public Health* 1: 133–46.

McCaslin SE, Inslicht SS, Henn-Haase C, *et al.* (2009) Uniformed rescue workers responding to disaster. In Y Neria, S Galea, FH Norris, eds., *Mental Health and Disasters*. New York, NY: Cambridge University Press; pp. 302–20.

McFarlane AC, Van Hooff M, Goodhew F (2009) Anxiety disorders and PTSD. In Y Neria, S Galea, FH Norris, eds., *Mental Health and Disasters*. New York, NY: Cambridge University Press; pp. 47–66.

Miguel-Tobal JJ, Cano-Vindel A, Gonzalez-Ordi H, *et al.* (2006) PTSD and depression after the Madrid March 11 train bombings. *Journal of Traumatic Stress* 19: 69–80.

Morissette SB, Tull MT, Gulliver SB, Kamholz BW, Zimering RT (2007). Anxiety, anxiety disorders, tobacco use, and nicotine: a critical review of interrelationships. *Psychological Bulletin* 133: 245–72.

Neria Y, Gross R, Litz B, *et al.* (2007) Prevalence and psychological correlates of complicated grief among bereaved adults 2.5–3.5 years after September 11th attacks. *Journal of Traumatic Stress* 20: 251–62.

Neria Y, Nandi A, Galea S (2008) Post-traumatic stress disorder following disasters: a systematic review. *Psychological Medicine* 38: 467–80.

Neria Y, Galea S, Norris FH, eds. (2009) *Mental Health and Disasters*. New York, NY: Cambridge University Press.

Norris FH, Friedman MJ, Watson PJ (2002) 60,000 disaster victims speak: Part II. Summary and implications of the disaster mental health research. *Psychiatry* 65: 240–60.

North CS, Pfefferbaum B, Narayanan P, *et al.* (2005) Comparison of post-disaster psychiatric disorders after terrorist bombings in Nairobi and Oklahoma City. *British Journal of Psychiatry* 186: 487–93.

Office for the Coordination of Humanitarian Affairs (2011) OCHA Annual Report 2010. Geneva: United Nations. http://ochanet.unocha.org/p/Documents/OCHA_2010AR.pdf (accessed July 2013).

Parslow RA, Jorm AF (2006) Tobacco use after experiencing a major natural disaster: analysis of a longitudinal study of 2063 young adults. *Addiction* 101: 1044–50.

Peek L, Stough LM (2010) Children with disabilities in the context of disaster: a social vulnerability perspective. *Child Development* 81: 1260–70.

Pfefferbaum B, Tucker P, North CS (2009) The Oklahoma City bombing. In Y Neria, S Galea, FH Norris, eds., *Mental Health and Disasters*. New York, NY: Cambridge University Press; pp. 508–21.

Pulcino T, Galea S, Ahern J, *et al.* (2003) Posttraumatic stress in women after the September 11 terrorist attacks in New York City. *Journal of Women's Health* 12: 809–20.

Punamaki RL, Komproe IH, Qouta S, Elmasri M, de Jong JT (2005) The role of peritraumatic dissociation and gender in the association between trauma and mental health in a Palestinian community sample. *American Journal of Psychiatry* 162: 545–51.

Raphael B, Stevens G (2006) Disaster and response:science, systems and realities. *Journal of Social Work in Disability and Rehabilitation* 5: 1–22.

Rudenstine S, Galea S (2012) *The Causes and Behavioral Consequences of Disasters: Models Informed by the Global Experience 1950–2005*. New York, NY: Springer.

Shultz JM, Kelly F, Forbes D, *et al.* (2011a) Triple threat trauma: evidence-based mental health response for the 2011 Japan disaster. *Prehospital and Disaster Medicine* 26: 141–5.

Shultz JM, Marcelin LH, Madanes SB, Espinel Z, Neria Y (2011b) The trauma signature: understanding the psychological consequences of the 2010 Haiti earthquake. *Prehospital and Disaster Medicine* 26: 353–66.

Silver RC, Holman EA, McIntosh DN, Poulin M, Gil-Rivas V (2002) Nationwide longitudinal study of psychological responses to September 11. *JAMA* 288: 1235–44.

Sphere Project (2011) The Sphere Project: humanitarian charter and minimum standards in humanitarian response. http://www.sphereproject.org (accessed July 2013).

Steenland M, Mbaruku G, Galea S (2010) A global perspective on disasters and their consequences in the urban environment. In D Vlahov, JI Boufford, P Pearson, eds., *Urban Health: Global Perspectives*. San Francisco, CA: Josey Bass; pp. 175–90.

Talge NM, Neal C, Glover V (2007) Antenatal maternal stress and long-term effects on child neurodevelopment: how and why? *Journal of Child Psychology and Psychiatry* 48: 245–61.

Tappero JW, Tauxe RV (2011) Lessons learned during public health response to cholera epidemic in Haiti and the Dominican Republic. *Emerging Infectious Diseases* 17: 2087–93.

Thywissen K (2006) *Components of Risk: a Comparative Glossary*. Bonn: United Nations University, Institute for Environment and Human Security (UNU-EHS).

UNISDR (2009) UNISDR terminology. http://www.unisdr.org/we/inform/terminology (accessed July 2013).

UNISDR (2012) 2011 Disasters in numbers. http://www.unisdr.org/files/24692_2011disasterstats.pdf (accessed July 2013).

Van der Velden PG, Kleber RJ (2009) Substance use and misuse after disasters: prevalence and correlates. In Y Neria, S Galea, FH Norris, eds., *Mental Health and Disasters.* New York, NY: Cambridge University Press; pp. 94–115.

van Griensven F, Chakkraband ML, Thienkrua W, *et al.* (2006) Mental health problems among adults in tsunami-affected areas in southern Thailand. *JAMA* **296**: 537–48.

Vanholder R, Borniche D, Claus S, *et al.* (2011) When the earth trembles in the Americas: the experience of Haiti and Chile 2010. *Nephron Clinical Practice* **117**: c184–97.

White SR, Henretig FM, Dukes RG (2002) Medical management of vulnerable populations and co-morbid conditions of victims of bioterrorism. *Emergency Medicine Clinics of North America* **20**: 365–92, xi.

Wilder A (2010) Aid and stability in Pakistan: lessons from the 2005 earthquake response. *Disasters* **34** (Suppl 3): S406–26.

Wolmer L, Hamiel D, Laor N (2011) Preventing children's posttraumatic stress after disaster with teacher-based intervention: a controlled study. *Journal of the American Academy of Child and Adolescent Psychiatry* **50**: 340–8.

Xu J, Wu Z (2011) One-year follow-up analysis of cognitive and psychological consequences among survivors of the Wenchuan earthquake. *International Journal of Psychology* **46**: 144–52.

Chapter 34

International response to natural and manmade disasters

Inka Weissbecker and Lynne Jones

Effects of humanitarian crises on mental health and psychosocial well-being

What is a humanitarian crisis?

There is not complete agreement on what constitutes a humanitarian crisis or what should be regarded as an emergency or disaster. Humanitarian emergencies have been defined as situations where the risks of ongoing excess deaths, diseases, and malnutrition justifies external assistance (Office for the Coordination of Humanitarian Affairs 1999). Acute humanitarian crises often turn into prolonged emergencies in geographical areas with difficulties arising from instability, mass migration, lack of accountability, and human rights abuses. Vulnerabilities interact. The Fund for Peace Failed States Index ranks the vulnerability of nations to collapse or conflict based on 12 social, economic, political, and military indicators (Fund for Peace 2013). The countries identified as being most at risk are mainly located in central and eastern Africa (Somalia, Sudan, Zimbabwe), Asia (Afghanistan, Pakistan), and Small Island States (Haiti). Many of these nations are the same areas that have been identified as being most likely to be affected by climate change and natural disasters, which already disproportionately affect lower-resource countries (Thow & de Blois 2008).

Stressors and stress reactions

Individuals affected by humanitarian crises frequently suffer various severe and interrelated stressors such as losing their home, livelihoods, material belongings, and community or social support systems. They may also witness horrific events and atrocities, lose loved ones, become separated from family members, and can be at risk for physical assault, gender-based violence, or malnutrition (Inter-Agency Standing Committee [IASC] 2007). Children and youth are especially vulnerable, as they are often dependent on caregivers and may become orphaned or separated.

As a result of exposure to these stressors, many survivors of humanitarian crises may experience some form of acute psychological distress such as anxiety, tearfulness, problems sleeping, fear, feelings of helplessness or hopelessness, guilt, anger, and somatic complaints. Children may display behavioral problems, aggression, bed wetting, or increased anxiety (Norris *et al.* 2002, IASC 2007). For most individuals, the psychological distress experienced in the initial days and weeks is a normal response to an abnormal event, and they will recover utilizing their own coping strategies, resources, and natural social support networks (IASC 2007). In situations where resources are lacking and such networks destroyed, the urgent primary interventions required are usually social. However, some individuals may experience enduring symptoms of psychological and functional impairments, which may require more specialized care (IASC 2007).

Mental disorders

It is difficult to estimate the impact of humanitarian crises on mental health, as many existing studies in this area suffer from methodological limitations that do not give due consideration to culturally shaped local expressions of distress. The World Health Organization (WHO) estimates that in humanitarian emergencies, the percentage of people with a severe mental disorder increases from a baseline of 2–3% to 3–4%, while mild or moderate mental disorders such as post-traumatic stress disorder (PTSD) or depression may increase to 15–20%, from an estimated baseline of 10% (WHO & UNHCR 2012).

Essentials of Global Mental Health, ed. Samuel O. Okpaku. Published by Cambridge University Press. © Cambridge University Press 2014.

Adjustment and common mental disorders

A recent comprehensive review estimates prevalences of 15.4% (30 studies) for PTSD and 17.3% (26 studies) for depression among populations affected by conflict (Tol *et al.* 2011) Those estimates are higher than general population prevalences reported in 17 populations participating in the World Mental Health Survey, which include 7.6% (any anxiety disorder, including PTSD) and 5.3% (any mood disorder, including major depressive disorder (Tol *et al.* 2011). The incidence of substance abuse and suicide rates may also increase following exposure to humanitarian crises and disasters (Norris *et al.* 2002). Somatic complaints such as headaches or muscle pain are common in many cultural contexts among individuals who have suffered from distressing events.

In the past there has been an overemphasis on addressing and treating PTSD, supported by citing high prevalence rates obtained through inappropriate survey methodology and instruments that had mainly been validated in Western settings (Rodin & van Ommeren 2009). As the above figures make clear, PTSD is only one of many possible crisis-induced mental health problems to be addressed. Complex PTSD is a more severe form of PTSD that is relevant because it is associated with exposure to multiple traumatic events. It is likely that complex PTSD will be part of the new and revised *International Classification of Diseases* (ICD-11) classification system for stress-related disorders.

Severe mental disorders

A recent study compiling data from community-based mental health services in five humanitarian settings found that complaints of reactions to extreme stress and adjustment disorders constituted only 0–19% of presenting problems, while other severe neuropsychiatric disorders (such as epilepsy and schizophrenia) made up 28–91% of complaints (Jones *et al.* 2009). Addressing chronic and severe mental disorders is an important but frequently overlooked need in humanitarian settings.

Risk and vulnerability

A number of factors have been identified in the literature as making an individual more vulnerable to mental health problems following humanitarian crises. Vulnerable groups include children, women, the elderly, the poor, racial and ethnic minorities, marginalized groups, and those with a previous history of severe stressors or mental disorder (Norris *et al.* 2002). Factors such as poverty, low education, political insecurity, poor overall health, and social exclusion have been associated with higher rates of mental health problems (Patel *et al.* 1999). It is important to note that the current environment can be more important than the severity of past distressing events. Indeed, one study in Afghanistan reported that not only war experiences but daily stressors such as family violence played a significant role in predicting lower functioning and mental health problems (Miller *et al.* 2006). In eastern Sri Lanka, poverty, child abuse, and witnessing parents fighting were just as likely to cause psychological distress and PTSD in youth as living through decades of civil war and experiencing the Southeast Asian tsunami of 2004 (Fernando *et al.* 2010). Providing social support in the form of humanitarian assistance also changes vulnerability. A study of two communities in China after an earthquake showed that the most exposed community, which had suffered more damage, had lower rates of PTSD than the less exposed community, which received less assistance (Wang *et al.* 2000).

Human rights issues

People with mental health problems have been recognized as a vulnerable population at a high risk for human rights violations, violence, poor health, and injuries (IASC 2007). They are often subject to social exclusion, marginalization, and discrimination within the community. They have limited access to employment opportunities and effective mental health and general health services, and they can suffer from physical and sexual abuse, financial exploitation, arbitrary detention, and denial of opportunities for founding a family. During humanitarian crises they may be left behind, or they may be outcast, tied to trees, or chained (Jones *et al.* 2009). This vulnerability is compounded by the fact that mental health and psychosocial programs that are set up during humanitarian crises are often narrowly focused on "trauma" and PTSD, leaving other mental health problems untreated. Jones *et al.* (2009) have argued that "protection and care of people with severe mental disorders in complex emergencies is a humanitarian responsibility."

Mental health service gaps

Several countries that currently have a high burden of mental, neurological, and substance use disorders, few mental health professionals, and a low GDP (World Health Organization 2008) are also at high risk for natural disasters. These include Africa (e.g., Burundi, DRC, Ethiopia, Nigeria, Djibouti), Asia (e.g., Afghanistan, Bangladesh, India, Indonesia), the Americas (e.g., Haiti), and eastern Europe and western Asia (e.g., Azerbaijan). As a result, countries affected by humanitarian crises typically have the least human resources or appropriate infrastructures to address mental health. Low-income countries have 0.05 psychiatrists and 0.16 psychiatric nurses per 100 000 people, compared to 200 times more in high-income countries. The WHO estimates that 76–85% of serious mental health cases in less-developed countries have received no treatment in the previous 12 months (World Health Organization 2008).

Relevant global guidelines

Currently, best practices and guidelines are emerging that can assist governments and non-governmental organizations (NGOs) in addressing mental health issues from a public health perspective in low-resource settings affected by humanitarian crises. The *IASC Guidelines on Mental Health and Psychosocial Support in Emergency Settings* (2007) offer practical advice for protecting and promoting mental health and psychosocial well-being, and include aspects of coordination, monitoring and evaluation, human rights, human resources, community mobilization, health services, and education. Additional more specific IASC guidelines have been published for health and protection actors as well as for advocacy purposes, targeting various audiences. The *Sphere Handbook*, which reflects consensus among more than 200 major agencies, is consistent with IASC guidelines, and sets minimum standards for humanitarian aid, also has a section on mental health and social aspects of health, which covers topics such as psychological first aid, designing community-based psychological interventions, and considering the existing sociocultural context in all programmatic efforts (Sphere Project 2011). The guidelines promote the adoption of a public health framework in working with populations affected by crises and conflict. They focus on both the community and the individual by supporting preventive efforts and well-being as well as

treating psychopathology. This approach is potentially cost-effective and can be more sensitive to social, economic, and political issues.

Assessments to inform mental health programs in humanitarian crises

Mental health and psychosocial assessments in humanitarian contexts are still controversial. There is disagreement over what should be assessed, by whom, the cultural validity of the methods used, and the ethical approach to take (Allden *et al.* 2009). There are concerns that the preoccupation with individual psychopathological responses which characterizes many assessments ignores the sociopolitical context, does not account for culture-specific expressions of distress, ignores the priorities of the affected population, and does not translate into project planning (Summerfield 1999, Miller *et al.* 2006).

Measurement of prevalence of disorders

Assessing the prevalence of mental disorders in complex emergency situations goes beyond the minimum response and poses challenges (WHO & UNHCR 2012). Prevalence surveys in humanitarian settings have been unable to distinguish between normal stress reactions and mental disorders, leading to inflated estimates. They have often used symptom checklists that have only been validated in Western settings. Local "idioms of distress" and concepts or experiences of mental health in different cultures may vary considerably from Western diagnostic DSM or ICD categories (Kleinman 1995). The checklists have usually focused on psychopathology, with little attention paid to positive factors such as hope (Tol *et al.* 2011).

While such assessments may help with advocacy (e.g., for potential donors), they are of limited usefulness for program planning. General WHO estimations of prevalence already exist (see *Mental disorders*, earlier in this chapter). Any assessments of mental health problems among emergency-affected populations should be culturally validated for the local population and include severe mental health problems (e.g., impaired functioning, bizarre behavior, danger to self or others: WHO & UNHCR 2012). Some researchers have developed culturally and methodologically sound methods of assessing mental health problems in varying contexts, using mixed qualitative and quantitative methods to capture local idioms of distress, develop culturally relevant indicators of functioning, and validate measures (e.g., Eisenbruch *et al.* 2004, Bolton *et al.* 2007). Similar methods have been developed for rapid mental health and psychosocial support assessments and to map local community resources such as natural healers (Bolton 2001, De Jong & Van Ommeren 2002). Such methods address many of the criticisms mentioned above and actively engage affected communities in discussing their priorities and defining what constitutes well-being, distress, and functioning within their cultural and regional context.

Assessment tools and guidelines

WHO and UNHCR have recently released a toolkit for assessing mental health and psychosocial needs and resources in humanitarian crises (WHO & UNHCR 2012). This toolkit contains various assessment instruments, including:

- A 4W (who is doing what where and when) mental health and psychosocial support (MHPSS) mapping tool for identifying gaps and coordinating the MHPSS response, which has already been used in post-crisis contexts (e.g., Fitzgerald *et al.* 2012).
- The Humanitarian Emergency Settings PERceived Needs (HESPER) scale, which assesses the perceived physical, social, and psychological needs in representative samples of populations in humanitarian settings.
- A survey of Serious Symptoms in Humanitarian Settings (WASS), which is not meant to diagnose mental disorders but indicates the extent of mental-health-related problems and can be used for advocacy purposes.
- An institutional checklist to indicate to what extent mental health is integrated into primary health care, including staffing, referral points, availability of psychotropic medication and previous mental health training.
- A classification of seven mental disorder categories which should be part of a health information system (HIS).
- A participatory assessment about perceptions and impact among severely people.

Additionally, the IASC Reference Group, with support from WHO, has developed a brief draft assessment guide for MHPSS in humanitarian settings, which also includes tools from the toolkit (Inter-Agency Standing Committee 2012). This guide outlines key MHPSS questions relevant in humanitarian emergencies, which can be selected and adapted based on the specific context and available resources and needs. Information can be obtained from desk review as well as individual and group interviews with the affected population and key stakeholders. Questions cover the areas of (1) relevant contextual information (culture-specific beliefs and practices, practices around death and mourning, at-risk groups, attitudes toward severe mental disorder); (2) experience of the emergency (perceived causes and expected consequences); (3) mental health and psychosocial problems (culture-specific expressions of distress, priority mental-health-related problems, impairment of daily activities); and (4) existing sources of psychosocial well-being and mental health (coping methods, community sources of support and resources).

Ethics of assessment

MHPSS research in humanitarian settings requires careful consideration of ethical issues. Allden *et al.* (2009) recommend that research should:

- benefit the affected population
- use culturally valid assessment instruments and measures
- consider power dynamics and the relative social statuses of researchers and beneficiaries
- do no harm by protecting participants from potential negative effects of participation such as stigmatization, discrimination, and security threats
- minimize psychological risks such as raised expectations and labeling while ensuring review of research by affected communities
- protect confidentiality
- involve affected communities in selection of research topics
- obtain genuine informed consent (e.g., understandable explanations, avoiding inappropriate incentives, repeating consent as appropriate)
- share findings with affected communities and make reports accessible to relevant stakeholders and others in the field

The authors argue that it would be unethical not to conduct research and evaluations on MHPSS interventions in emergencies, given the need for more evidence in this field, while it would also be unethical to conduct such research without benefit to beneficiaries. These sentiments are summarized in the statement "no survey without service and no service without survey." It should be said that this aspiration is rarely achieved.

Mental-health-related interventions in humanitarian crises

Global guidelines and the intervention pyramid

Interventions focused on mental health needs in the context of humanitarian crises can be conceptualized as a pyramid or a continuum of care ranging from non-specialized and community services designed to meet basic needs of an entire population, to specialized services for select individuals needing more specialized psychiatric care. The most important interventions in the wake of a disaster are primarily social and community-based. Levels of "basic services and security, community and family supports, focused non-specialized supports (e.g. paraprofessionals), and specialized services" should be integrated and complement one another (IASC 2007).

Providing integrated mental health services

IASC guidelines recommend avoiding the creation of standalone programs that focus on specific groups or diagnoses such as PTSD. Such fragmented programs can play into dynamics of power and social exclusion, lead to the neglect of individuals who do not fit into the specified group, and increase the perception of unjustified privilege and tension in communities or to stigmatization and labeling. Services should be integrated into services with a broader outreach such as school health services or primary health care (IASC 2007).

Building on existing community support

Interventions should make use of "naturally occurring community resources." They should reinforce or rebuild social networks and recognize the value of local and indigenous community knowledge and perspectives (IASC 2007). Mental health interventions during humanitarian crises can undermine traditional family and community support mechanisms and local coping strategies (Summerfield 1999,

Bonnano *et al.* 2010). After the 2004 Indian Ocean tsunami, most individuals turned to family members, prayer, and religious leaders for support, and some reported being upset by counselors from different organizations that would come for brief periods of time and ask them to re-tell their story multiple times (Good *et al.* 2010). However, it should also be noted that not all local or cultural practices to address mental health problems may merit support. For example, individuals with severe mental disorders are often excluded from communities, are given potentially harmful substances, are subject to physical abuse such as cutting or whipping, or are kept outside the living facilities in inhumane conditions.

Using local knowledge and facilitating local participation

Good practices should be supported, and local professionals or community leaders can serve as culture brokers. They have important knowledge of expressions of distress and methods of coping. Furthermore, they can receive appropriate training to deliver basic interventions and provide referrals. They often have established relationships of trust in the community, and will remain in the country after outside funding for mental health or psychosocial programs has ended. Participation in recovery efforts and in shaping and implementing programming are important principles of IASC MHPSS and Sphere guidelines. It has been shown that people tend to fare better when they feel that they are in control of their own destiny, which can be undermined by humanitarian interventions that foster a sense of dependency and helplessness (Pupavac 2004). Participatory methods can involve communities in designing and shaping interventions that are acceptable and useful to them, and in monitoring and evaluating outcomes (Eisenbruch *et al.* 2004, IASC 2007).

Current interventions

A recent review of 160 mental health program reports showed that the five most commonly reported activities were "basic counseling for individuals (39%); facilitation of community support of vulnerable individuals (23%); provision of child-friendly spaces (21%); support of community-initiated social support (21%); and basic counseling for groups and families (20%)" (Tol *et al.* 2011). Psychoeducation, structured social activities, and counseling, which are frequently used in practice, were only included in few evaluation studies, often with mixed results. In spite of the guidelines advice above, most of the reviewed studies consisted of specialized, narrowly focused interventions for reducing symptoms of PTSD.

Suggested interventions

In this section we will look in detail at three approaches to intervention that provide examples of what can be done in both preventive and treatment approaches to mental health.

Psychological first aid (PFA)

There has been considerable discussion and controversy over how to provide an appropriate response to whole populations exposed to very distressing experiences and conditions over the past decade. Some organizations and agencies still conduct psychological "debriefing," which involves recounting details of distressing events in a group setting. A large meta-analysis of debriefing studies has concluded that debriefing is not effective in improving mental health or protecting against developing mental disorders, and that it can even be harmful and result in worsening of symptoms (Rose *et al.* 2009). It is therefore no longer recommended by IASC and WHO (IASC 2007). Individuals subjected to very distressing events should have access to psychological first aid (PFA) at health service facilities and in the community (IASC 2007, Sphere Project 2011). PFA is not a clinical intervention but involves listening in a supportive way, protecting those affected from further harm, mobilizing social support, encouraging positive coping strategies, and linking people to services, including specialized referral for those experiencing severe distress (World Health Organization *et al.* 2011). Most studies of the effectiveness of PFA have been conducted in Western settings. After the Haiti earthquake of 2010, Schafer *et al.* (2010) reported that staff found PFA to be a useful, empowering approach to providing psychosocial support to affected people, and that both a full version and a shorter generic PFA resource would be most helpful in humanitarian settings. PFA has also been shown to result in improve perceived competency among helpers after the 2011 Japan earthquake (Semlitz *et al.* in press)

Addressing low maternal mood and early childhood development (ECD)

Mothers who are displaced often have to face loss, separation from extended families, and the burden of childcare combined with poverty and harsh living situations. A recent review suggests high prevalence rates of depression of 11.3% during pregnancy and 18.3% after birth in various African countries (Sawyer *et al.* 2009). Mothers with mental health problems are at higher risk of poor health during pregnancy and may not seek prenatal care. They are also less likely to care adequately for their children and develop healthy attachments. Research has found that lack of infant stimulation, poor mother–child interaction, and maternal depression can inhibit feeding and growth even when food supplements are provided (Unicef & WHO 2012). Maternal depression is associated with poor child development and growth, poor social development, and lower educational achievements (Wachs *et al.* 2009). WHO and Unicef now advocate combined psychosocial early childhood development (ECD) and nutritional programming in food shortage situations in order to address the physical, emotional, and intellectual developmental needs of the child and to enhance maternal well-being (Unicef & WHO 2012). ECD mother and baby groups teach about infant stimulation, fostering child development, and the importance of play. Studies suggest that ECD and nutritional interventions together have a more positive effect on child cognitive and physical development than either intervention alone, and that both home visits to improve mother–child interaction and group interventions to support the mother can improve maternal mood (Wachs 2009, Unicef & WHO 2012). However, psychosocial support, infant stimulation and early childhood education are still rarely integrated into either nutritional programs or mother and child health programs.

Integration of mental health into primary health care

Integrating mental health into general health care has been recommended by IASC (2007), Sphere, and WHO guidelines. It is one of the most viable ways of closing the treatment gap for mental illnesses (World Health Organization 2008). Existing research and practice suggests that mental health services can be delivered effectively through primary health care, if there is appropriate training and on-the-job supervision of non-specialist health professionals as well as lay professionals such as community health workers (CHWs). Such integrated services are more sustainable, less stigmatizing, and more accessible to affected populations (World Health Organization 2008). In 2011, the WHO launched the *Mental Health Gap Action Programme Intervention Guide* (mhGAP-IG), which outlines how to assess and manage priority conditions (depression, schizophrenia and other psychotic disorders, suicide, epilepsy, dementia, disorders due to use of alcohol and illicit drugs, and mental disorders in children) and provides guidance on pharmacological and non-pharmacological interventions (World Health Organization 2010). It is for use by general health workers in low- and middle-income countries. The mhGAP-IG is currently being rolled out in several countries including Ethiopia, Uganda, Panama, and Jordan. An additional mhGAP guide for disorders specific to stress (SPE-STRESS, covering common stress reactions, acute stress, PTSD, hyperventilation, dissociation (conversion), insomnia, and bed wetting), which is especially relevant in humanitarian settings, was published in 2013 (WHO & UNHCR 2013).

Several articles describe programs integrating mental health and general health care in humanitarian settings including Iraq (Sadik *et al.* 2011), Haiti (Rose *et al.* 2011), Lebanon (Hijazi *et al.* 2011), and Sierra Leone (Asare & Jones 2005). It has been suggested that mental health integration is most successful when it is part of health policy and legislative frameworks accompanied by adequate resources (World Health Organization 2008). Building positive relationships between the formal health system and community leaders who are often the first point of contact for chronic and severe mental illness can facilitate effective care provision. It is also important to work with clinic management to integrate mental health through agreed-upon quality standards, supporting HIS data collection, and holding referral workshops to strengthen networks among service providers (Hijazi *et al.* 2011).

Making interventions sustainable

Disasters or crisis can also be opportunities for the development of mental health services, because of the increased donor funding and attention paid to the needs of affected populations (Patel *et al.* 2011). For example, in Aceh, Indonesia, the creation of an emergency training program to add community

psychiatric nurses to existing primary healthcare posts in the disaster-affected area became the seed for a more comprehensive program to train community psychiatric nurses and general practitioners to better address mental health at the community level (Jones *et al.* 2007). Similarly in Sri Lanka, funding provided after the 2004 tsunami provided the opportunity to increase the number of medical officers of mental health working at the community level (Budosan *et al.* 2007). Factors that promote or hinder the long-term sustainability of emergency mental health and psychosocial interventions have recently been identified across areas of government and policy, human resources and training, programming and services, research and monitoring, and finance (Patel *et al.* 2011).

Mental health research

There is broad agreement on the critical need to build the evidence base for mental health and psychosocial interventions in humanitarian and low-resource settings and to gain a better understanding of mental health within different cultural contexts (Tol *et al.* 2011). The majority of existing research has focused on describing the prevalence of mental health problems among populations affected by humanitarian crises rather than on effective interventions. Intervention research has focused on PTSD (Allden *et al.* 2009, Tol *et al.* 2011) rather than on other important problems such epilepsy, developmental disorders, learning disabilities, or severe mental disorders. Groups such as the elderly, men, and perpetrators of violence tend to be neglected in research and programming (Allden *et al.* 2009). Most studies focus on interventions that are infrequently implemented (e.g., more specialized interventions), while less research exists on commonly implemented programs (e.g., child-friendly spaces, counseling, promotion of community supports, preventing mental disorders, promoting psychosocial well-being) (Tol *et al.* 2011). Very few studies have actively involved the affected population, conducted a prior needs assessment, or developed psychometric measures of local idioms of distress (Batniji *et al.* 2006, Bolton *et al.* 2007).

Research in humanitarian settings poses numerous difficulties, such as instability and insecurity, needs for cultural validity and acceptability of psychometric instruments and interventions, and designing research that is ethical and can benefit affected communities (Allden *et al.* 2009). Agencies and organizations providing mental health services in crises settings often do not evaluate the outcomes of their work, and it is difficult to obtain funding for such evaluations (Allden *et al.* 2009).

Research is needed to evaluate the effectiveness of feasible, accessible, low-cost interventions that could be scaled up. An example and notable exception is the randomized trial conducted by Bolton and colleagues (2007) using locally validated instruments to assess the effectiveness of interpersonal therapy as a treatment for depression in northern Uganda.

Tol *et al.* (2011) suggest linking research and practice and assessing a broader range of outcomes (e.g., aside from PTSD); increasing collaboration between researchers and practitioners; prioritizing the most commonly implemented interventions; using randomized controlled trials or other innovative research designs; testing interventions for people with severe mental disorders; assessing sustainable interventions integrated with national and local health, education, and social systems; as well as tracking MHPSS funding.

Several authors agree that rigorous monitoring, evaluation, and assessment should be an integral part of humanitarian mental health programming (Allden *et al.* 2009, Tol *et al.* 2011). This will require adequate donor funding and awareness as well as training and skills and academic partnerships to ensure that ethical standards are followed and appropriate research methods are employed. Future research is clearly needed. It should follow existing guidelines and recommendations, assess local expressions of distress and well-being, build on existing strengths and capacities, and have potential for sustainability and scaling up. This will require collaboration and partnerships between researchers, practitioners, and affected communities.

Summary and conclusions

Mental health problems in the context of humanitarian crises require attention. They have been missing from the global health agenda and have been ignored by many relief and development agencies. Underlying vulnerabilities such as poverty and poor health can exacerbate mental health problems and be compounded by them. The provision of mental health and psychosocial programming in humanitarian settings has experienced a significant and appropriate critique because of its tendency to over-pathologize normal stress, neglect actual population needs, and ignore cultural contexts. However, guidelines and approaches are emerging which hold considerable promise for deepening understanding of the way mental health problems are expressed in non-Western settings, filling training and service gaps, improving local participation and ownership, forging links with other humanitarian areas and programs, and building the evidence base on best practices. Better services should be the result. Addressing mental health needs in a humanitarian crisis is challenging, but it can be a window of opportunity to develop and scale up mental health services and supports for a previously neglected population (Jones *et al.* 2009).

References

Asare J, Jones L (2005) Tackling mental health in Sierra Leone. *BMJ* 331: 720.

Allden K, Jones L, Weissbecker I, *et al.* (2009) Mental health and psychosocial support in crisis and conflict: Report of the mental health working group. *Prehospital and Disaster Medicine* 24 (Suppl 2): s217–27.

Batniji R, Van Ommeren M, Saraceno B (2006) Mental and social health in disasters: relating qualitative social science research and the Sphere standard. *Social Science and Medicine* 62: 1853–64.

Bolton P (2001) Cross-cultural validity and reliability testing of a standard psychiatric assessment instrument without a gold standard. *Journal of Nervous and Mental Diseases* 189: 238–42.

Bolton P, Bass J, Betancourt T, *et al.* (2007) Interventions for depression symptoms among adolescent survivors of war and displacement in northern Uganda: a randomized controlled trial. *JAMA* 298: 519–27.

Bonanno GA, Brewin CR, Kaniasty K, La Greca AM (2010) Weighing the costs of disaster: consequences, risks, and resilience in individuals, families, and communities. *Psychological Science in the Public Interest* 11: 1–49.

Budosan B, Jones L, Wickramasinghe WAL *et al.* (2007) After the wave: a pilot project to develop mental health services in Ampara district, Sri Lanka post-tsunami. *Journal of Humanitarian Assistance.* http://sites.tufts.edu/jha/archives/53 (accessed July 2013).

De Jong J, van Ommeren M (2002) Toward a culture-informed epidemiology: combining qualitative and quantitative research in transcultural contexts. *Transcultural Psychiatry* 39: 422–33.

Eisenbruch M, De Jong J, van de Put W (2004) Bringing order out of chaos: a culturally competent approach to managing the problems of refugees and victims of organized violence. *Journal of Traumatic Stress* **17**: 123–31.

Fernando G, Miller KE, Berger DE (2010) Growing pains: the impact of disaster-related and daily stressors on the psychological and psychosocial functioning of youth in Sri Lanka. *Child Development* **81**: 1192–210.

Fitzgerald C, Elkaied A, Weissbecker I (2012) Mapping of mental health and psychosocial support in post-conflict Libya. *Intervention* **10**: 188–200.

Fund for Peace (2013) Failed States Index. http://ffp.statesindex.org (accessed July 2013).

Good MJ, Good B, Grayman J (2010) Complex engagements: responding to violence in post-conflict Aceh. In D Fassin, M Pandolfi, eds., *Contemporary States of Emergency: The Politics of Military and Humanitarian Interventions*. New York, NY: Zone Books.

Hijazi Z, Weissbecker I, Chammay R (2011) The integration of mental health into primary health care in Lebanon. *Intervention* **9**: 265–78.

Inter-Agency Standing Committee (2007) *IASC Guidelines on Mental Health and Psychosocial Support in Emergency Settings*. Geneva: IASC.

Inter-Agency Standing Committee (2012) *IASC Reference Group Mental Health and Psychosocial Support Assessment Guide, IASC RG MHPSS*. Geneva: IASC.

Jones L, Ghni H, Mohanraj A, *et al.* (2007) Crisis into opportunity: setting up community mental health services in post tsunami Aceh. *Asia Pacific Journal of Public Health* **19**: 60–8.

Jones L, Asare JB, El Masri M, *et al.* (2009) Severe mental disorders in complex emergencies. *Lancet* **374**: 654–61.

Kleinman A (1995) *Writing at the Margin: Discourse between Anthropology and Medicine*. Berkeley, CA: University of California Press.

Miller KE, Kulkarni M, Kushner H (2006) Beyond trauma-focused psychiatric epidemiology: bridging research and practice with war-affected populations. *American Journal of Orthopsychiatry* **76**: 409–22.

Norris FH, Friedman MJ, Watson PJ, *et al.* (2002) 60,000 disaster victims speak: Part I. An empirical review of the empirical literature, 1981–2001. *Psychiatry* **65**: 207–39.

Office for the Coordination of Humanitarian Affairs (1999) *OCHA Orientation Handbook on Complex Emergencies*. United Nations.

Patel PP, Russell J, Allden K, *et al.* (2011) Transitioning mental health and psychosocial support: from short-term emergency to sustainable post-disaster development. Humanitarian Action Summit 2011. *Prehospital and Disaster Medicine* **26**: 470–81.

Patel V, Araya R, de Lima M, Ludermir A, Todd C (1999) Women, poverty and common mental disorders in four restructuring societies. *Social Science and Medicine* **49**: 1461–71.

Pupavac V (2004) Psychosocial interventions and the demoralization of humanitarianism. *Journal of Biosocial Science* **36**: 491–504.

Rodin D, van Ommeren M (2009) Commentary: Explaining enormous variations in rates of disorder in trauma-focused psychiatric epidemiology after major emergencies. *International Journal of Epidemiology* **38**: 1045–8.

Rose S, Bisson J, Churchill R, Wessely S (2009) Psychological debriefing for preventing post-traumatic stress disorder (PTSD). *Cochrane Database of Systematic Reviews* 2009 (1): CD000560.

Rose N, Hughes P, Ali S, Jones L (2011) Integrating mental health into primary health care settings after an emergency: lessons from Haiti. *Intervention* **9**: 211–24.

Sadik S, Abdulrahman S, Bradley M, Jenkins R (2011) Integrating mental health into primary health care in Iraq. *Mental Health in Family Medicine* **8**: 39–49.

Sawyer A, Ayers S, Smith H (2009) Pre- and postnatal psychological wellbeing in Africa: a systematic review. *Journal of Affective Disorders* **123**: 17–29.

Schafer A, Snider L, van Ommeren M (2010) Psychological first aid pilot: Haiti emergency response. *Intervention* **8**: 245–54.

Semlitz L, Ogiwara K, Weissbecker I, *et al.* (in press) Psychological first aid training after Japan's triple disaster: changes in perceived self competency. *International Journal of Emergency Mental Health*.

Sphere Project (2011) The Sphere Project: humanitarian charter and minimum standards in humanitarian response. http://www.sphereproject.org (accessed July 2013).

Summerfield D (1999) A critique of seven assumptions behind psychological trauma programs in war affected areas. *Social Science and Medicine* **48**: 1449–62.

Thow A, de Blois M (2008) Climate change and human vulnerability: Mapping emerging trends and risk hotspots for humanitarian actors. *Report to the UN Office for Coordination of Humanitarian Affairs*, Geneva: UN.

Tol WA, Barbui C, Galappatti A, *et al.* (2011) Mental health and psychosocial support in humanitarian settings: linking practice and research. *Lancet* **378**: 1581–91. doi: 10.1016/s0140-6736 (11)61094-5

Unicef, World Health Organization (2012) *Integrating Early Childhood Development (ECD) activities into Nutrition Programmes in*

Emergencies. Why, What and How. Guidance note for integrating ECD activities into nutrition programmes in emergencies. New York, NY: Unicef.

Wachs TD, Black M, Engle P (2009) Maternal depression: a global threat to children's health, development and behavior and to human rights. *Child Development Perspectives* **3**: 51–9.

Wang X, Gao L, Shinfuku N, *et al.* (2000) Longitudinal study of earthquake-related PTSD in a randomly selected community sample in north China. *American Journal of Psychiatry* **157**: 1260–6.

World Health Organization (2008) *mhGAP: Mental Health Gap Action Programme. Scaling up Care for Mental, Neurological, and Substance Use Disorders.* Geneva: WHO.

World Health Organization (2010) *mhGAP Intervention Guide for Mental, Neurological and Substance Use Disorders in Non-Specialized Health Settings.* Geneva: WHO.

World Health Organization, UNHCR (2012) *Assessing Mental Health and Psychosocial Needs and Resources: Toolkit for Major Humanitarian Settings.* Geneva: WHO.

World Health Organization, UNHCR (2013) *Assessment and Management of Conditions Specifically Related to Stress: mhGAP Intervention Guide Module (version 1.0).* Geneva: WHO.

World Health Organization, War Trauma Foundation, World Vision International (2011) *Psychological First Aid: Guide for Field Workers.* Geneva: WHO.

Chapter

35

Global health governance, international law, and mental health

Lance Gable

Introduction

The scope and direction of global health governance has changed in the early twenty-first century. As the interconnectedness of health status and health outcomes across countries and regions has become more evident, the political salience of global health has continued to increase. Growing attention to health as a global concern has led to the expansion of infrastructure impacting health at the global level, built upon both legal obligations and economic development initiatives. Simultaneously, these developments have prompted a proliferation of actors participating in global health governance, ranging from perennial international actors such as national governments and intergovernmental institutions to newer participants such as international non-governmental organizations (NGOs), philanthropic foundations, and multinational corporations. The expansion of participants in global health governance has in turn raised the political stakes of these endeavors and complicated global health governance and diplomacy. This upsurge in complexity and attention to global health has galvanized a renewed effort to interpret and explore the changing conceptual underpinnings of global health governance (Ruger 2007, Gostin 2008, Fidler 2010).

While mental health has not received as much attention as other areas of health governance at the global level, the changing architecture of global health governance has important implications for how mental health laws, policies, and practices are implemented at the global, national, and local levels. Two contemporary trends define this movement toward global solutions to improve mental health. First, mental health advocates, policy makers, and consumers of mental health services have realized that the norms, structures, and conceptual and rhetorical influence of international law can provide useful mechanisms to achieve better mental health at a population level, encourage national governments to implement more responsive health systems using rights-based models, and allow for individuals to benefit from legal protections to seek improved conditions more conducive to good mental health. Second, global mental health has followed the more general shift toward norm-driven global health policies grounded in common notions based on justice, ethics, and human rights (Meier 2012). Those engaged in mental health advocacy and policy making have recognized the value of using consistent norms – often contained in international human rights treaties and related documents – across jurisdictions and initiatives to govern mental health and its underlying determinants and to pursue universal minimum standards of mental health.

This chapter will explore the many ways that international law and global health governance strategies impact mental health. Further, it will identify the promise and shortcomings of global-level mental health strategies. Lastly, it suggests possible approaches for improving global mental health using mechanisms of global health governance grounded in international law. Legal and institutional frameworks at the global level can be influential on mental health. It is imperative that these frameworks be designed and applied in a way that is conducive to achieving good mental health, while protecting the human rights of persons with mental and intellectual disabilities.

The ongoing global burden of mental health problems

Mental health is a pervasive, global health concern. Mental-health-related illness and disability remain as some of the most prevalent and persistent health

Essentials of Global Mental Health, ed. Samuel O. Okpaku. Published by Cambridge University Press. © Cambridge University Press 2014.

conditions worldwide. The World Health Organization (WHO) estimates that mental, neurological, or behavioral health conditions affect approximately 450 million people globally (WHO 2001). Neuropsychiatric conditions cause approximately one-third of years lost due to disability among people over 15 years of age (WHO 2008). Mental health conditions occur along a continuum of severity ranging from schizophrenia to mild depression. Unipolar depressive disorders comprise the most common mental health conditions, affecting more than 150 million people worldwide (WHO 2003a). Due to their prevalence and ubiquity, mental health conditions thus have substantial effects on the overall health of individuals with these conditions, and systemic impacts on population health and society more generally.

The burdens of mental health conditions fall substantially and disproportionately on women, young adults, and those with low socioeconomic status. Depression leads all other causes of disease burden among women living in both high-income and low-income countries (WHO 2008). Further, in every region of the world, neuropsychiatric disorders result in more disability among people aged 10–24 years than any other cause (Gore *et al.* 2011). Studies have found links between lower socioeconomic status and higher prevalence of mental disabilities (Pickett & Wilkinson 2010).

Persons with mental disabilities also must contend with economic, social, and political factors that limit their ability to receive care and treatment, and constrain their full participation in society. Access to mental health services varies, as do the approaches used in providing services and the settings within which services are provided. Mental health services can be costly, and persons with mental and intellectual disabilities often lack effective political representation. The recent global economic crisis has exacerbated the challenges of providing access to mental healthcare services, as countries have cut budgets for existing programs and chosen not to implement new programs (WHO 2011a, p. 3). Stigma and ostracization against persons with mental disabilities persist around the world and contribute to their marginalization and social exclusion. These factors have an aggregative effect: stigma and discrimination lead to invisibility and political powerlessness of people with mental disabilities, which in turn inhibit efforts to overcome political antipathy toward funding mental health services (WHO 2011a, p. 6).

Historically, the legal landscape applicable to mental health at the national level around the world has been meager and outdated, with laws often relying on antiquated assumptions about persons with mental disabilities, punitive institutionalization, and overly medicalized approaches to treatment, if access to care was provided at all. However, the legislative and policy activity surrounding mental health has increased in recent years. The WHO has noted a recent upsurge in the passage of dedicated mental health legislation at the national level in many countries, with more than half of all existing mental health laws being passed since 2001, most of these since 2005. In addition, the number of countries with dedicated mental health policies and plans has increased substantially (WHO 2011b). These changes occurred across all regions, but were more pronounced in higher-income countries than in lower-income countries. Notably, many of these laws adopted rights-based models designed to protect persons with mental disabilities and to maximize their freedom, autonomy, and opportunities in society. These recent legislative changes at the national level may reflect the influence of global mental health initiatives and other factors related to global-level governance, as will be further discussed below.

The changing architecture of global mental health governance: an expansion of scope and complexity

International health governance as traditionally conceived involved national governments working together directly and through international institutions created by treaties enacted by these national governments to address common health objectives. Over the past decade, however, a broader concept of global health governance has emerged, encompassing "the use of formal and informal institutions, rules, and processes by states, intergovernmental organizations, and non-state actors to deal with challenges to health that require cross-border collective action to address effectively" (Fidler 2010, p.3). This shift marks a dissipation of the formerly rigid line between formal international actors – national governments and international institutions – and the other increasingly influential informal, non-governmental participants in global health. Efforts to pursue global health governance recognize that collective efforts to address health concerns often must occur at a global level with input from many participants.

Global health governance and mental health

Governance of mental health continues to occur primarily at the national and subnational level. National and local considerations, including legal infrastructure, access to mental health services, and economic and social factors, drive mental health outcomes at the population level. However, efforts to govern health at the global level have demonstrated that entities and systems situated beyond and across national borders can influence mental health. Moreover, global-level mechanisms for health governance generally and mental health governance in particular have become more numerous and robust.

The rise in prominence of global health governance has spurred a proliferation of interest, capacity, and participation in global mental health across three overlapping but distinct contexts. First, the *structural aspects* applicable to global health governance, including the legal and institutional infrastructure at the global level relevant for mental health, have been augmented (Gable 2007). Notably, both the formal and informal structures for governance have evolved. Second, the number of *participants* in global health governance has expanded and the relative influence of these participants has been recalibrated to some extent (Fidler 2010). While intergovernmental institutions and governmental entities remain central to mental health governance at the global level, the ascent in influence of non-governmental entities has been precipitous. Third, the *normative foundations* of global health have been developed even though the application and extent of adoption of global health norms varies across different fora (Ruger 2007, Meier 2012). In each of these contexts, global health governance has important implications for mental health, many of which have yet to be realized.

Structural proliferation in global mental health

Expanded structural mechanisms at the global level contribute to the increased prominence of global health governance. Structural enhancements incorporate new legal regimes, institutions, processes, and oversight and enforcement mechanisms that can be marshaled to govern health access and outcomes, or influence the underlying determinants of health. The structural developments most relevant to global mental health include the creation of new global mechanisms and institutions under international law relevant to mental health and the expansion of mental health capacity in existing institutions at the global level. The Convention on the Rights of Persons with Disabilities (CRPD) and its related institutional structures comprise the most significant new legal regime applicable to mental health (United Nations 2006). The CRPD establishes important human rights for persons with physical and mental disabilities, and creates a series of institutions and mechanisms to uphold these rights. Similarly, developments in international trade law related to patent protection of pharmaceuticals have implications for countries seeking to increase affordable access to psychotropic medications covered by patent (WHO 2005). The structural overlay of these international legal regimes and their corresponding institutions influences mental health systems at the national level.

Existing global institutions also have expanded their capacity to address mental health issues. The efforts of the WHO to develop programs to influence national mental health laws, policies, and systems have particular import for mental health as the WHO has developed global resources to help create infrastructure and expertise at the national level (WHO 2011b). However, ongoing funding and support for mental health programs within intergovernmental organizations, such as the WHO, remains tenuous (WHO 2011b). Further, the expansion of global infrastructure based in human rights and trade agreements has been mirrored in some countries at the national level. For example, the rise of national human rights institutions charged with monitoring and implementing international human rights law reflects the deepening of structural connections between the international and national levels. These institutions contribute to the diffusion of human rights norms into regional- and national-level law and practice (Simmons 2009, Goodman & Pegram 2012).

Proliferation of participants in global mental health governance

As the capacity for, and interest in, global-level health governance strategies have expanded, the number of participants actively involved in global health governance has similarly multiplied (D'Aspremont 2011, Fidler 2011). The expansion of the number and variety of participants involved in global health governance both builds on and contributes to the global structural changes mentioned above. These participants in global health governance can be roughly divided into formal participants – often long-standing institutional participants in international law and policy supported by legal authority under international law – and informal participants who work within and outside of these systems to influence law, policy, and health outcomes.

National governments and intergovernmental organizations – the primary formal participants in global mental health governance – continue to hold important and influential positions as participants in global health governance, even as their relationships have changed. Formal participants who govern mental health pursuant to their direct institutional mandate, such as the WHO and the oversight committees for international human rights conventions such as the International Covenant on Economic, Social and Cultural Rights (ICESCR) (United Nations 1966) and CRPD, have the greatest influence over global mental health given their prominence, capacity, and focus. Yet, other international institutions, including global financial, trade, and development institutions, often play consequential roles in affecting mental health outcomes. For instance, the World Bank impacts health through the implementation of development programs in low-income countries. The global trade system fosters the movement of goods and services internationally, often with negative impacts on health in some countries by restricting affordable access to needed medications. Further, other UN agencies, such as United Nation Children's Fund (Unicef), the United Nations Industrial Development Organization (UNIDO), and the Food and Agricultural Organization (FAO), frequently advance initiatives that have implications for health. The result has been the addition of new participants to existing international institutions that may address mental health issues, creating an increasingly complex framework of governance.

The informal participants in global health governance include international NGOs, philanthropic funders with an interest in global health, and multinational corporations who fulfill multiple roles as coordinators, supporters, funders, advocates, policy developers, and capacity builders, often in conjunction with national or local groups. Overall, these informal governance participants have expanded their influence at the expense of the more formal global health institutions. Global health funders, such as the Bill and Melinda Gates Foundation, Rockefeller Foundation, and Open Society Institute, have challenged the primacy of international organizations in setting priorities for global health due to their ability to advance their initiatives through significant economic resources and streamlined, non-bureaucratic processes. These large funders have not yet devoted substantial resources to mental health, but their impact on global health governance over the past decade has been profound. NGOs have been more directly involved in mental health. Organizations specializing in mental health advocacy and capacity-building, such as the Mental Disability Advocacy Center (MDAC) (2006), Mental Disability Rights International (MDRI) (2008), the NGO Committee on Mental Health, and the World Network of Users and Survivors of Psychiatry, have grown to take on more prominent roles in global mental health governance, but their influence on global mental health governance remains modest in comparison to governmental and intergovernmental institutions.

Normative proliferation in global mental health

The normative aspects of global mental health governance have developed in tandem with the proliferation of structural aspects and participants. A number of notable recent developments in human rights law have greatly expanded the understanding of norms related to the human right to health. The CRPD represents a significant recognition that core human rights norms apply specifically to people with mental disabilities. General Comment 14 to the ICESCR (United Nations 2000) explains in great detail the obligations that states must respect, protect, and fulfill to satisfy the right to health. Further, non-legal tools such as the WHO Mental Health Gap Action Program (mhGAP) (WHO 2010) and Mental Health Legislation Manual (WHO 2003b) have articulated best practices in mental health care and services grounded in human rights, influencing the decisions of law and policy makers at the national level.

Targeting improved global governance for mental health

The trajectory of global health governance suggests a set of interconnected systems that remain in flux. A multifaceted strategy that includes law must be considered to understand and target improvements in global governance of mental health to sufficiently address – or complement other efforts to address – the myriad systemic problems facing persons with mental disabilities.

Clarifying and expanding legal systems in global mental health governance

International and regional human rights systems exert considerable influence over global mental health governance, as do other systems of international law such as the international trade system. The WHO also has used its legal powers to broaden global health governance. These systems and institutions of international law currently exhibit some success in fulfilling infrastructure-building and norm-codifying roles with regard to mental health governance, but they often fail on measures of implementation, enforcement, and regulation of activity.

The World Health Organization as legal innovator

Since its inception in 1948, the WHO has gone through many phases as the premier international health institution. One of the more unexpected developments in global health governance in the past decade has been the embrace by the WHO of its treaty and regulatory powers. Drawing on popular global support for tobacco control, the WHO promulgated the Framework Convention on Tobacco Control in 2003, marking the first instance of the WHO using its treaty powers (Taylor & Bettcher 2000). Two years later, the WHO completed its revisions of the International Health Regulations, a legally binding set of regulations designed to limited the spread of infectious agents of international concern and to allow for rapid response to pandemic and other global health threats (Fidler & Gostin 2006). These developments demonstrate the willingness of the WHO to apply its legal authority to advance global health governance in some areas. WHO has not yet shown an inclination to use these powers to advance mental health initiatives, and such initiatives would surely be more complex and controversial than tobacco control.

Human rights systems in global mental health governance

The international human rights system forms the most significant and well-developed system of global health governance. Multiple international human rights documents form the legal basis for an internationally recognized right to health, including the Constitution of the WHO (1946), the Universal Declaration of Human Rights (United Nations 1948, art. 25), the ICESCR (United Nations 1966, art. 12), and the CRPD (United Nations 2006, art. 25), among others. These documents create substantial institutional mechanisms to advance mental health at the global and regional levels (Gable 2007). A strong foundation of human rights jurisprudence protecting the rights of persons with disabilities also exists at the regional levels within the European and Inter-American Human Rights Systems (Gostin & Gable 2004, Gable et al. 2005).

Human rights systems also advance normative development of the right to health (Meier 2012) and specifically affirm the right to mental health as a core component of the right to health. The attainment of the right to mental health additionally requires the fulfillment of other human rights. Mental health policies and practices often violate human rights. Persons with mental disabilities frequently face stigma, discrimination, deprivation of basic rights of citizenship, and limitations on access to services and opportunities, whether perpetrated by state or by private actors. Likewise, human rights violations may imperil mental health. Egregious human rights abuses such as torture, systematic rape, and inhuman and degrading treatment cause great harm to physical and mental health. Similarly, invasions of privacy, discrimination, and denials of opportunity can have negative effects on mental health. Therefore, mental health and human rights act synergistically and mutually reinforce each other. Mental health forms a foundation for political and social functioning and exercising human rights, just as the recognition and support for human rights allows a person's mental health to flourish. Mental health and human rights are thus inextricably linked (Gostin & Gable 2004).

Despite being grounded in foundational international agreements, the functional implementation of a right to mental health often fails to protect the rights and well-being of persons with mental disabilities. The former Special Rapporteur on the Right to Health recognized that mental health remains "among the most grossly neglected elements of the right to health" (Hunt 2005).

International trade law and global mental health governance

International trade law also plays a key role in the global governance of mental health. While a number of international treaties come under the enforcement authority of the World Trade Organization (WTO), perhaps the one most closely linked to mental health is the Agreement on Trade-Related Aspects of Intellectual Property Rights (TRIPS). TRIPS extends uniform patent protections for various types of intellectual property, including pharmaceuticals. Countries that fail to adequately protect patented medications for a minimum 20-year period can face economic sanctions, a provision that has raised the specter of greatly limited access to patented drugs in developing countries. The Doha Declaration permits developing countries to manufacture generic versions of patented medications if they claim a public health emergency and issue a compulsory license (Smith et al. 2009). Compulsory licensing of pharmaceuticals has not become widespread, but the threat of using this exception has helped in pressuring patent holders to sell their patented drugs to developing countries at lower cost. In the mental health context, TRIPS intellectual property protections may limit access to psychotropic medicines. While the compulsory licensing exception could be applied to psychotropic medicines, this approach to increase access to these medications has been infrequently considered and never pursued.

The rise of non-state participants in global mental health governance

The expansion of non-state participants in global health governance primarily falls outside of the formal legal infrastructures that typify international legal regimes. While these entities must operate within legal constraints (usually at the national level in whichever countries they operate), they often bring different sorts of legal issues to the forefront, including, in the case of funders and philanthropists, the imposition of contractual obligations on national and local governments to satisfy grant award allocations. Additionally, the lack of democratic input and accountability in many large NGOs has generated criticism and could be a significant drawback to their increased involvement in global mental health governance (Jordan & van Tuijl 2006).

Some recent international treaties have expanded the role of non-governmental entities in formal international institutions. The Protocol establishing the African Court on Human and Peoples' Rights grants NGOs standing to bring claims for human rights violations under the Charter (Organization of African Unity 1998, art. 5(3)). The CRPD provides for consultation and cooperation with civil society

organizations in its implementation (arts. 32–33). While these limited precedents do not yet represent a trend toward expansion in the inclusion of non-governmental entities as explicit participants in international treaties, non-state actors will continue to expand their role in influencing the evolution of international law and global health governance (D'Aspremont 2011).

The future of global mental health governance

While global mental health governance remains an evolving and largely piecemeal endeavor, the sections that follow suggest three areas conducive to better organizing and building on the potential for global-level mental health governance initiatives: augmenting global mental health governance capacity; harmonizing norms; and improving implementation and enforcement of global mental health governance efforts.

Augmenting global health governance capacity

A number of proposals in recent years suggest strengthening the capacity for global health governance through the reinforcement or refocusing of existing global institutions to better govern health. Proposals to increase the capacity and influence of the WHO (Silberschmidt et al. 2008) seek to overcome persistent limitations by restructuring the WHO. Likewise, calls to bolster the health focus of the WTO (Kimball 2006), the World Bank, and countries of the G8 (Kirton & Mannell 2007) conceive of these institutions playing a more direct and interventional role in global health governance beyond their traditionally circumscribed efforts. Others have proposed the establishment of new mechanisms to organize and focus global health governance, such as the creation of new treaty-based regimes championing health (Gostin 2008). At the national level, efforts to incorporate rights-based approaches into human rights systems remains an important, if underachieved, goal (Backman et al. 2008, Meier et al. 2010).

While it is unclear whether these specific proposals will advance, they advocate complementary strategies for multilevel reinforcement of the landscape of global governance in ways that could benefit mental health. For example, a renewed effort to advocate for mental health services capacity to be built into revamped national health systems would be consistent with the right to health (Backman *et al.* 2008). Likewise, independent capacity for addressing mental health at a global level could be advanced through a standalone entity, a Global Fund for Mental Health similar to the Global Fund to Fight AIDS, Tuberculosis, and Malaria. Moreover, actual mental health infrastructure – not just governance infrastructure – should be expanded through financial and technical support to build capacity for mental health services, increase access, and reduce economic and social barriers to mental health care. The World Bank and other non-state funders interested in development could be integral in this effort. The potential impact of such initiatives, however, will likely be constrained by political and economic realities that often undermine international initiatives designed to augment institutional capacity for health generally and mental health in particular. Whether the rise of non-state participants and new sources of funding support can counteract or supplement the formal institutional capacity presents an interesting possibility for future exploration.

Development and harmonization of norms

Effective global mental health governance should seek a level of normative consistency to assure minimum levels of legal protection, access to care, and medical and social support related to mental health. Nevertheless, global mental health governance has not yet coalesced to reflect consistency in norms at different levels of governance. In order to attain this goal, a common system of norms must be developed for mental health governance. The human rights model provides the most promising approach.

Mental health law and policy have followed a meaningful trajectory from the use of the medical model to treat and confine persons with mental and intellectual disabilities to the implementation of a patients-rights model, grounded on individual human rights, autonomy, and freedom from coercive institutionalization (Gostin 2007). Notably, the advent of more effective psychiatric medications and the success of civil rights movements spurred the closure of many institutions for psychiatric confinement and the release of thousands of people back to the community. In many cases, however, these people did not receive adequate mental health care, and the availability of services suffered from lack of funding, poor organization, and political marginalization and deprioritization (Gable & Gostin 2009).

At the international level, institutional actors involved in international governance of mental health have followed a similar path. The WHO has moved from a purely medical model focusing on technical assistance and curative interventions for mental health to a rights-based approach that has recognized the importance of sustaining the underlying determinants of health as well as the protection of human rights as essential preconditions for good mental health (Meier 2010). The embrace of human rights by the WHO represents a fundamental conceptual shift in global governance, even if the practical effects of this shift are more difficult to discern. The efforts of the WHO to both use the language of human rights in describing mental health goals and urge countries to adopt rights-based legislation at the national level affirm this shift (WHO 2003b).

The right-to-health approach has particular salience, since efforts to improve the underlying determinants of mental health support the attainment of rights-based goals (Gable 2010). Programs at the WHO and elsewhere to develop legal and ethical norms for protecting the social determinants of health should incorporate mental health determinants into their list of essential factors. This effort would be consistent with widespread understandings of human rights and social justice with respect to mental health. Unfortunately, mental health has been left off the agenda in many of the most high-profile efforts to establish substantive norms and outcome goals for health, including the Millennium Development Goals (MDGs) and the 2011 UN High-Level Meeting on the Prevention and Control of Non-communicable Diseases plan. As the MDGs are revised for the next decade and the United Nations begins to implement its non-communicable disease strategy, mental health should be a part of the discussion, planning, and implementation of these initiatives (Miranda & Patel 2005).

Improving implementation and enforcement

Implementation and enforcement of the norms and goals of global mental health remains the most challenging aspect of global-level governance efforts. As international governance participants increasingly apply norms or strive to achieve rights-based or outcome-based goals supported by international legal instruments, this global governance of health can guide and influence, and in some cases pressure, national and subnational institutions to adapt their laws and policies to comply with international norms. Even where international human rights regimes lack effective enforcement mechanisms, the underlying normative bases for human rights obligation can find their legal expression, and thus their practical enforcement, through the application of national or local laws that uphold human rights. This influence, and the resulting complementarity of results, provides a model of international influence as global governance. Indeed, international influence mediated through national laws comprises a much more common form of global governance than direct governance through binding international legal authority.

This approach to governance potentially has several advantages. First, it may expand the influence of international actors beyond the limited legal authority granted to them under international treaties, which in turn increases the likelihood of harmonization of mental health norms around the world. Second, by avoiding formalistic legal infrastructure, this approach expands the group of participants involved in governance to include NGOs, funders, civil society organizations, private entities, and other global-level organizations that are not operating pursuant to international legal sanction, but rather have entered the field to participate on their own initiatives. Third, it allows for a greater degree of aggregative effort on the part of these actors to achieve consistent goals, if they are willing and able to coordinate and coexist (Meier 2012).

Despite these compelling potential advantages, relying on normative and institutional influence as a means of governance has several substantial drawbacks when compared with legally enforceable governance approaches. First, the absence of legal enforcement undermines the ability to hold governments accountable for the failure to provide mental health services or protect rights. The history of government policies affecting persons with mental disabilities reflects the deficiencies of this approach, as rampant human rights abuses and marginalization have been persistent and enduring in relation to persons with mental disabilities (Gable & Gostin 2009). Second, opening up governance to multiple participants does not necessarily result in consistent or harmonious outcomes. Different actors and institutions may have disparate interests and priorities, resulting in duplicative and confounding results and undermining efforts to improve mental health. Third, the

successes of the governance of influence are easily reversed, either by retrenchment through law and policy revisions when a new government with different priorities becomes ascendant in a particular country, or by the jettisoning of voluntary implementation of mental health programs when they become too expensive or political winds shift. Often, reactionary tendencies and anecdotal circumstances rooted in stigma and social animus drive mental health laws and policies. Even when more humane, rights-based policies are in place, these policies can be quickly reversed if their support wanes (Gostin 2007).

In addition, the expanded influence of non-state participants in international and global settings creates both opportunities and challenges. The involvement of non-state participants could result in greater normative consistency (Meier 2012), an expanded capacity to address health problems, and flexibility and adaptability in efforts to govern health. Non-state participants can play multiple roles related to mental health: directly providing mental health services or research; advancing efforts to improve the underlying determinants of health, which can support population-level mental health benefits; and serving as advocates through oversight, investigative reporting, law reform, policy development, and litigation. However, a proliferation of participants in global health governance may lead to confusion, redundancy, and conflicting goals and strategies (Fidler 2007). Various participants in global health governance will seek differing outcomes and be animated by different motivations. In cases where motives, methodologies, and resources do not align, the expansion in the number of governance participants may effectively undermine efforts to achieve good health. Even with the best intentions, there is no guarantee that any of these efforts would necessarily benefit mental health without a concerted effort to ensure that mental health concerns are included within efforts to reform and expand global health governance. This coordinating role could conceivably be played by an institutional authority with global reach, such as WHO or another similarly situated institution created for this purpose.

Conclusion

Global mental health governance is still quite nascent. Consequently, the ultimate shape of the changing architecture of global health governance remains uncertain but ripe with possibility. The mechanisms of governance available within the new architecture of global health governance create potential opportunities for mental health improvement. However, the persistent hurdles of invisibility, apathy, and complexity that impede support for mental health must be overcome. The design and ongoing development of international law can form a foundation upon which good mental health governance can be built.

References

Backman G, Hunt P, Khosla R, *et al.* (2008) Health systems and the right to health: an assessment of 194 countries. *Lancet* **372**: 2047–85.

D'Aspremont J, ed. (2011) *Participants in the International Legal System: Multiple Perspectives on Non-State Actors in International Law*. New York, NY: Routledge.

Fidler DP (2007) Architecture amidst anarchy: global health's quest for governance. *Global Health Governance* **1**: 1–17.

Fidler DP (2010) *The Challenges of Global Health Governance*. Council of Foreign Relations Working Paper. New York, NY: Council on Foreign Relations.

Fidler DP (2011) Navigating the global health terrain: mapping global health diplomacy. *Asian Journal of WTO and International Health Law and Policy* **6**: 1–43.

Fidler DP, Gostin LO (2006) The new international health regulations: an historic development for international law and public health. *Journal of Law, Medicine and Ethics* **34**: 85–94.

Gable L (2007) The proliferation of human rights in global health governance. *Journal of Law, Medicine and Ethics* **35**: 534–44.

Gable L (2010) Reproductive health as a human right. *Case Western Reserve Law Review* **60**: 957–96.

Gable L, Gostin LO (2009) Mental health as a human right. In A Clapham, M Robinson, eds., *Realizing the Right to Health*. Zurich: Ruffer & Rub; pp. 249–61.

Gable L, Vásquez J, Gostin LO, *et al.* (2005) Mental health and due process in the Americas: protecting the human rights of persons involuntarily admitted to and detained in psychiatric institutions. *Pan American Journal of Public Health* **18**: 366–73.

Goodman R, Pegram T (2012) *Human Rights, State Compliance, and Social Change: Assessing National Human Rights Institutions*. New York, NY: Cambridge University Press; pp. 1–20.

Gore FM, Bloem PJN, Patton GC, *et al.* (2011) Global burden of disease in young people aged 10–24 years: a systematic analysis. *Lancet* **377**: 2093–102.

Gostin LO (2007) From a civil libertarian to a sanitarian. *Journal of Law and Society* **34**: 594–616.

Gostin LO (2008) Meeting basic survival needs of the world's least healthy people: toward a framework convention on global health. *Georgetown Law Journal* **96**: 331–92.

Gostin LO, Gable L (2004) The human rights of persons with mental disabilities: a global perspective on the application of human rights principles to mental health. *Maryland Law Review* **63**: 20–121.

Hunt P (2005) Report of the Special Rapporteur on the right of everyone to the enjoyment of the highest attainable standard of physical and mental health. UN Commission on Human Rights. Doc. E/CN.4/2005/51.

Jordan L, van Tuijl P (2006) *NGO Accountability: Politics, Principles and Innovations*. London: Earthscan.

Kimball AM (2006) The health of nations: happy birthday WTO. *Lancet* **367**: 188–90.

Kirton JJ, Mannell J (2007) The G8 and global health governance. In AF Cooper, JJ Kirton, T Schrecker, eds., *Governing Global Health: Challenge, Response, Innovation*. Aldershot: Ashgate.

Meier BM (2010) The World Health Organization, human rights, and the failure to achieve health for all. In J Harrington, M Stuttaford, eds., *Global Health and Human Rights*. London: Routledge.

Meier BM (2012) Global health takes a normative turn: the expanding purview of international health law and global health policy to meet the public health challenges of the 21st century. *Global Community: Yearbook of International Law and Jurisprudence* (2011).

Meier BM, Gable L, Getgen JE, London L (2010) Rights-based approches to public health systems. In E Beracochea, C Weinstein, D Evans, eds., *Rights-Based Approaches to Public Health*. New York, NY: Springer; pp. 19–30.

Mental Disability Advocacy Center (2006) *Advocacy Services for People with Mental Health Problems and Intellectual Disabilities: Guidance and Model Policies*. Commission of the European Union: Mental Disability Advocacy Center.

Mental Disability Rights International (2008) *Mental Disability Rights Initiative of Serbia*. Washington, DC: Mental Disability Rights International.

Miranda JJ, Patel V (2005) Achieving the Millennium Development Goals: does mental health play a role? *PLoS Medicine* **2** (11): e291.

Organization of African Unity (1998) *Protocol to the African Charter on Human and Peoples' Rights on the*

Establishment of an African Court on Human and Peoples' Rights.

Pickett KE, Wilkinson RG (2010) Inequality: an underacknowledged source of mental illness and distress. *British Journal of Psychiatry* **197**: 426–8.

Ruger JP (2007) Normative foundations of global health law. *Georgetown Law Journal* **96**: 423–43.

Simmons BA (2009) *Mobilizing for Human Rights: International Law in Domestic Politics.* New York, NY: Cambridge University Press.

Silberschmidt G, Matheson D, Kickbusch I (2008) Creating a committee C of the World Health Assembly. *Lancet* **371**: 1483–6.

Smith RD, Correa C, Oh C (2009) Trade, TRIPS, and pharmaceuticals. *Lancet* **373**: 684–91.

Taylor A, Bettcher D (2000) WHO Framework Convention on Tobacco Control: a global "good" for public health. *Bulletin of the World Health Organization* **78**: 920–9.

United Nations (1948) *Universal Declaration of Human Rights.* (G.A. Res. 217A (III), U.N. Doc A/810) New York, NY: UN.

United Nations (1966) *International Covenant on Economic, Social and Cultural Rights (A/RES/21/2200 (XXI)).* New York, NY: UN.

United Nations (2000) General Comment No. 14: The right to the highest attainable standard of health (article 12 of the International Covenant on Economic, Social and Cultural Rights). Geneva: UN.

United Nations (2006) *Convention on the Rights of Persons with Disabilities (A/RES/61/106).* New York, NY: UN.

World Health Organization (1946) *Constitution of the World Health Organization.* New York, NY: International Health Conference.

World Health Organization (2001) *The World Health Report 2001. Mental Health: New Understanding, New Hope.* Geneva: WHO.

World Health Organization (2003a) *Investing in Mental Health.* Geneva: WHO.

World Health Organization (2003b) *Mental Health Legislation and Human Rights.* Geneva: WHO.

World Health Organization (2005) *Improving Access and Use of Psychotropic Medicines.* Geneva: WHO.

World Health Organization (2008) *The Global Burden of Disease: 2004 Update.* Geneva: WHO.

World Health Organization (2010) *mhGAP Intervention Guide for Mental, Neurological and Substance Use Disorders in Non-Specialized Health Settings.* Geneva: WHO.

World Health Organization (2011a) *Impact of Economic Crises on Mental Health.* Geneva: WHO Regional Office for Europe.

World Health Organization (2011b) *Mental Health Atlas 2011.* Geneva: WHO.

Chapter

36

The role of non-governmental organizations

Robert van Voren and Rob Keukens

My interest is in the future because I am going to spend the rest of my life there.
(Charles Kettering 1948)

Introduction

Non-governmental organizations (NGOs) encompass different types of value-based organizations depending on donations and voluntary service. They include, among others, local and international charities, research institutes, and lobby groups. The United Nations defines the NGO as "non-profit, voluntary citizens' group which is organized on a local, national or international level. Task-oriented and driven by people with a common interest, NGOs perform a variety of services and humanitarian functions, bring citizens' concerns to governments, monitor policies and encourage political participation at the community level" (United Nations, undated). There are more than 40 000 international NGOs active, 90% of which were founded during the past 30 years (Edwards 2000). The number of national and local NGOs is incomparably higher, but no statistics exist. Statistics about the number of NGOs in mental health are also not available, yet it is known that there are not many *international* NGOs active in the field of mental health (World Health Organization 2010).

Throughout Europe, as well as in most of the "developed" world, the mental health system that prevailed was a highly institutional, biologically oriented psychiatry, in which persons with chronic mental illness and persons with intellectual disability, as well as social outcasts, were locked away in institutions usually placed outside urban areas – a repetition of the

leper houses of the Middle Ages. As Michel Foucault wrote in *Madness and Civilization,*

> What doubtless remained longer than leprosy, and would persist when the lazar houses had been empty for years, were the values and images attached to the figure of the leper as well as the meaning of his exclusion, the social importance of that insistent and fearful figure which was not driven off without first being inscribed within a sacred circle ... Leprosy disappeared, the leper vanished, or almost, from memory; these structures remained. Often, in the same places, the formulas of exclusion would be repeated, strangely similar two or three centuries later.
>
> (Foucault 1965, pp. 6–7)

Psychiatry very much repeated that model, ridding society of all the unproductive elements and isolating them from the rest of society. In the eighteenth century the French statesman Guillaume-Chrétien de Lamoignon de Malesherbes wrote, "it seems that the honor of family requires the disappearance from society of the individual who by vile and abject habits shames his relatives" (Foucault 1965, p. 67). Equally, in many countries the stigma of mental illness or mental disability became such that often patients were kept indoors all the time, out of sight, and having a person with mental illness or intellectual disability in the family was seen as a shame that should be kept hidden at all cost.

In France at the turn of the nineteenth century it was Philippe Pinel who brought about a change in the perception of mental illness when he concluded in his *Traité de la Manie* that insanity was curable. The fundamental element in this change was Pinel's belief that an acute illness manifests a spontaneous dynamism inclining it towards a cure, and that it tends to pass through "successive periods of graduated

Essentials of Global Mental Health, ed. Samuel O. Okpaku. Published by Cambridge University Press. © Cambridge University Press 2014.

development, stationary state, decline and convalescence" (Gauchet & Swain 1999). The consequence of this was, according to Pinel, that a patient had to be kept in a therapeutic environment, because it was impossible to predict when the illness would end, and recovery could never be completely ruled out.

Action against the flaws of psychiatry amongst people experiencing mental health problems is not new. In 1620 concerned patients of the Bethlem Hospital sent a *Petition of the Poor Distracted People in the House of Bedlam*, a complaint against inhumane treatment, to the House of Lords (Barnes & Bowl 2000). But at the time of the rise of the feminist, gay, and disability movements, it was the emergence of the patient movement in the 1960s and 1970s that brought about a real change in mental health service delivery. Suddenly consumers of mental health services found a voice, and although often considered to be (too) radical and (too) demanding, their activism – focusing on empowerment, recovery, better services, implementation of user-led initiatives, and rights protection – led to a wave of "democratization" in the field of mental health and a gradual change from often highly custodial and paternalistic psychiatry for psychiatric patients to a system of community-based and user-oriented mental health care services where all stakeholders have a say in how they are designed and managed. The service users movement is predominantly a Western phenomenon, and in many countries the situation is still far from ideal. The tension between what persons with mental illness want, what their carers want, and what professionals think is best will always exist, but there is no doubt that, at least in theory, and more and more often also in practice, mental health at the beginning of the twenty-first century looks fundamentally different from the revolutionary model that Philippe Pinel designed 200 years ago.

The low priority of mental health

Nobel Prize winner Amartya Sen writes in his book *The Idea of Justice*:

> The relevance of disability in the understanding of deprivation in the world is often underestimated. People with physical or mental disability are not only among the most deprived human beings in the world, they are also frequently enough the most neglected . . . If the demands of justice have to give priority to the removal of manifest injustice rather than concentrating on the long-distance search for the perfect society, then the prevention and alleviation of disability cannot be but

> fairly central in the enterprise of advancing justice . . .
> It's not the economical power of an individual that is an adequate indication of development, but to which extent a person can use his capacities in the system.
>
> (Sen 2009, p. 258)

In spite of Sen's words, a major problem for NGOs is the low priority that is globally assigned to mental health.

Across the world, on average only 2% of national health budgets is dedicated to mental health, and approximately one-third of countries have no specified mental health budget at all. In effect, it is a moral issue that lies hidden behind the statistics of the burden of mental disorders – measured in disability-adjusted life years (DALYs) – and the high levels of prevalence, but this does not seem to motivate authorities and civil servants to give the state of mental health services more prominence on their national political agendas. Progress in mental health service development has been slow in most of the low-income countries, and mental health is considered a secondary issue in many countries, as well as by virtually all development agencies. Playing the moral card does not seem to convince donors, and it is not clear whether global structures can emerge from social and moral principles regarding distributive justice that are able to rival constitutional states. Factors that influence the marginal position on the priority agenda are (Saraceno *et al.* 2007, McDaid 2008, Ventevogel 2008, Keukens & van Voren 2009):

- A divided lobby and fragmented advocacy by different stakeholders, including NGOs, resulting in an incoherent message that is easy for policy makers and politicians to ignore.
- The social perceptions of mental health problems are dominated by negative stereotypes, leading to stigma, discrimination, and social exclusion.
- The invisibility of mental health.
- The lack of scientific data on prevalence and outcomes, and on mental health indicators.
- Growing criticism of the functioning of NGOs themselves.

Putting mental health on the international agenda

Until the late 1990s, mental health care was not considered to be a priority by international development aid agencies.

A crucial factor has been the publication by the World Bank of *The Global Burden of Disease* (Murray & Lopez 1996), which for the first time showed that psychoneurological diseases had a very significant negative impact on the world economy, and that the economic costs of these diseases would continue to grow considerably in the years to come. The report emphasized the significant burden associated with mental disorders, with five of the ten leading causes of disability worldwide being neuropsychiatric disorders, accounting for a quarter of total disability and 10% of total burden in 1990. The burden was estimated at 11.5% in 1998 and was expected to rise to 15% by the year 2020, with the rise being particularly sharp in developing countries. These data resulted in a major shift, as suddenly the economic impact of mental illness became visible, and it became clear that investing in mental health also had an economic benefit. The World Bank, convinced by the report and several other approaches to them, decided in 1999 to hire a mental heath consultant, Professor Harvey Whiteford. Although his tenure was relatively short, he managed to bring about a major change in the World Bank's understanding of the problem.

The first decade of the twenty-first century saw a fundamental shift in attitudes towards mental health. In 2001, the World Health Organization (WHO) devoted its annual *World Health Report* entirely to the issue of mental health. The report gave a detailed overview of mental health services throughout the world, often with shocking data showing the lack of adequate services available. Following WHO's example, the European Commission continued its political discussions on mental health issues, which reached a temporary climax during the Finnish Presidency of 2006. In 2005 WHO and the EU together organized a European Ministerial Conference on Mental Health in Helsinki which led to the signing of two documents: a Mental Health Declaration for Europe and a Mental Health Action Plan for Europe. The documents emphasized the need to adopt a comprehensive approach to mental health covering the provision of promotion, prevention, treatment and care, and social inclusion. Also, and important in the context of this chapter, the meeting was a turnaround for NGOs, as for the first time they were officially invited to participate in the process of preparing the final documents and, subsequently, in implementing their goals.

The prioritization of mental health by (inter)governmental bodies continued, and led to many other initiatives and documents. A further boost to the NGO community in mental heath was the adoption and ratification of the Convention on the Rights of Persons with Disabilities (CRPD), which clearly stipulates the rights of persons with disability, and therefore also of people with a mental disability or mental illness (United Nations 2006). The CRPD and its Optional Protocol were adopted in December 2006 and opened for signature in March 2007. There were 82 signatories to the convention, 44 signatories to the optional protocol, and one formal ratification of the convention, the highest number of signatories of a UN Convention on its opening day ever. The convention entered into force on May 3, 2008. In particular, NGOs monitoring the implementation of the convention became important actors in the field, as well as those who foster the development of more humane and user-oriented services that are more in line with the CRPD's framework (United Nations 2010).

A decade after the 2001 *World Health Report*, the WHO published a new world mental health report, adding many more data and again emphasizing the need to invest in mental health care (World Health Organization 2011). Both in the preparation of the report and in the implementation programs of WHO such as the mhGAP program, NGOs play a crucial role in monitoring implementation and implementing policies at grassroots level. Later that year, a High-level Meeting of the United Nations General Assembly on Prevention and Control of Non-communicable Diseases (New York, September 19–20, 2011) recognized that mental and neurological disorders, including Alzheimer's disease, are an important cause of morbidity and contribute to the global non-communicable disease burden, necessitating provision of equitable access to effective programs and healthcare interventions.

And finally, on January 20, 2012, the Executive Board of WHO adopted a resolution, titled "Global burden of mental disorders and the need for a comprehensive, coordinated response from health and social sectors at the country level," which detailed the problems facing persons with mental health problems and their environment, and also promoted the "involvement of civil society organizations, persons with mental disorders, families and caregivers in voicing their opinions and contributing to decision-making processes" and the "participation of people with mental disorders in family and community life and civic affairs," and urged the Director-General of WHO "to collaborate with Member States, and as appropriate, with international, regional and national non-governmental organizations, international development partners and technical agency partners in the development of the mental health action plan" (World Health Organization 2012).

Unfortunately, in spite of the fact that mental health has reached the state of being acknowledged as a priority issue, and also that NGOs are considered an important partner in developing and implementing national and international mental health plans, the outlook for the coming years is not altogether a positive one. The 2008 economic crisis, which with ups and downs dragged on well into 2013, severely affected available budgets for reform, and in many cases mental health was the first item on the budget to suffer budgetary cuts. In addition, however, the outlook on development aid is gradually shifting in Europe, with more and more countries being affected by an "anti-globalist" political course resulting in more isolationist and self-centered policies. In addition, the overall tendency is to work through large (inter)governmental agencies, and much less through NGOs, as an answer to the need for more accountability, transparency, and large-scale initiatives. Consequently, mental health seems to have become a priority at the worst possible moment, while NGOs are in practice often sidetracked by large (inter)governmental agencies that tend to work through governments rather than through grassroots organizations.

The role of NGOs: examples

NGOs, or non-state actors (NSAs), can have both a constructive and a destructive influence on the development of mental health care in specific regions or countries, and sometimes their effect on the ground is a combination of both. It is often NGOs that initiate new approaches in care and other innovations; or in countries where care is virtually absent they provide services that would otherwise not be available (almost half of the world's population lives in a country where, on average, there is one psychiatrist or less to serve 200 000 people: World Health Organization 2011). Also, NGOs often have the leading role in social services at grassroot level. They are sometimes of an excellent quality but also, unfortunately,

sometimes of a very poor quality with a limited experience and scale, not coordinated, and not in communication with public services, sometimes even in competition with them.

As a result of this tension, their services often remain unsustainable or become an obstacle to the development of a more comprehensive mental health care program. The authors have observed the influence of NGOs in countries in transition over a period of two decades, and have often observed situations where NGOs provide good and necessary services, but are fully dependent on external donors (hence not sustainable) and available to only a small number of people (hence not replicable). In other cases, services provide a short-term answer to an existing problem, without investing in a long-term sustainable solution. NGOs need to establish long-term ($>$ 15 years) partnerships, have a strong (value-driven) vision on change, focus on constant cycles of learning, and frame reflection, as well as balance changing capacities and structures to induce paradigm shifts (Essink 2012).

The following sections provide two examples of the role of NGOs in mental healthcare development and provision.

Example 1. Sri Lanka following the tsunami: trauma care

Much of the foreign aid given to Sri Lanka in mental-health-related areas has been concentrated on initiatives connected to the war in the north, in which more than 70 000 persons were killed over a period of 26 years. The constant displacement of people, the disruption of social networks and services, as well as the violence, all these factors resulted in enormous levels of suffering and distress within the communities in these areas. The aid was primarily given to a multitude of NGOs that, often under adverse circumstances, worked with those affected and tried to create a support network. For many organizations foreign aid remained the primary or even only source of income.

Even while the war was in progress, a growing number of foreign donors started to scale down their support, and the tsunami disaster of December 2004 was pushed to the background as a result of other natural and manmade disasters elsewhere, with the result that many of the remaining NGOs struggled to survive and continue their operations. Decreased funding, lack of staff, burnout, and pessimism about the future of the armed conflict led to an ever-increasing difficult situation. Ironically, the situation was to some extent even aggravated by the "tsunami" of competing health volunteers who rushed to the island after the tsunami to spread the blessings of Western counseling techniques and (sometimes obsolete) post-traumatic stress disorder (PTSD) treatments among the victims, by doing so tearing the local social fabric apart (Watters 2010).

Although the tsunami resulted in a number of post-disaster trauma care initiatives developing into regular community-based mental healthcare services, most of the foreign donors did not follow this development and limited their funding strategies to supporting post-conflict or post-disaster initiatives, staying away from regular mental healthcare service delivery. This was the result of a combination of factors, with on the one hand a mistaken understanding of the nature of mental healthcare services in general (usually seen as purely medical and targeted at only a very small part of the population) and on the other a series of limitations arising from the origin of the funds, the criteria for rendering support, and the background of the donor organization itself. Often when a link was forged between existing mental health structures and services and activities and projects deployed by NGOs, it was an exception and not part of a consistent strategy.

The result is that mental health care development in Sri Lanka, even at this crucial and challenging time when a structural development towards community mental healthcare services can be brought about, is under-funded and not a priority for foreign donors. The long-term governmental policy (2015) is ambitious and aims at the development of accessible mental healthcare services delivered by an adequately trained staff, with an emphasis on prevention and rehabilitation and community-based services (Mental Health Directorate 2005). However, at the same time only 1.6% of the total health budget is spent on mental health, the staff-to-population ratio is inadequate, and a lot of the post-conflict/disaster NGOs are struggling to survive and are functioning often in isolation, without larger support mechanisms and under adverse circumstances.

A stronger link between structural mental health-care service development and post-conflict trauma care would be beneficial to both sides. Community mental healthcare services would provide a structural framework within which trauma care could maintain itself, and the specialized trauma care would give extra capacity and specialized services to mental healthcare services that are needed to deal with traumatizing situations. In more general terms, the existence of regular, sustainable, and nationwide community-based mental healthcare services would make a lasting response to trauma much more effective in future (World Health Organization 2011).

At the same time, it is important to note that there is now a growing understanding that post-trauma care following a natural or manmade disaster is often relatively useless, and in some cases even counterproductive (Young 1995, Ventevogel & Jong 2006, Summerfield 2008). As Watters notes in his analysis on the impact of psychosocial trauma help in Sri Lanka following the tsunami, "Western traumatologists have developed a set of beliefs about how best to heal from the psychological effects of trauma ... Against a growing body of evidence, traumatologists assume these ideas to be universally true" (Watters 2010, p. 31). People need to fall back on their own resilience and coping capacity, and the initial focus is on getting back to a sense of "normalcy" as quickly as possible. This includes ensuring that services and support networks are supported and that the disruptions of people's lives, as well as the medicalization of their needs (since perceived mental health problems may be a normal human response to living in a stressful context), are minimized as much as possible.

Example 2. GIP in post-totalitarian societies

Global Initiative on Psychiatry (GIP: www.gip-global.org) was founded as the International Association on the Political Use of Psychiatry (IAPUP) in December 1980; it later became the Geneva Initiative on Psychiatry, and in 2005 changed its name to Global Initiative on Psychiatry (van Voren 2009, 2010). After the collapse of the Soviet Union in 1991, GIP entered the field of mental health reform. Started as an international campaign against the political use of psychiatry, it answered the call from Soviet psychiatrists and dissidents alike to help develop humane, ethical, and user-oriented mental health care in the formerly communist countries. One of the first priorities was to develop an NGO sector, because no independent organizations previously existed. In the late 1980s and early 1990s the first new independent psychiatric associations were set up, the first one being the Independent Psychiatric Association (IPA), set up in Moscow with close involvement of GIP. In 1992 the first organizations for relatives were formed, as well as professional associations such as those of psychiatric nurses and, later, social workers. Because of the enormous stigma prevailing in post-totalitarian societies, only in the late 1990s the first user groups were set up.

The emergence of an active NGO sector had a profound impact on mental health care development in this part of the world. Most of the innovations in mental health were started by NGOs rather than by governments, and pressure from the NGO community helped to convince local and national governments that the existing services were not meeting the needs of the population. Very often, people from the NGO field later became key individuals within governmental circles, pushing for reform from within. Even though the governmental bureaucracies often resisted reform and sided with directors of major psychiatric hospitals, who viewed reform as a threat to their positions and influence, in the course of 10 years the outlook changed fundamentally and the need to develop community-based services was generally accepted in most of the countries, the main issue of debate remaining what community psychiatric services actually are and to what extent the old institutional system should be discarded.

For instance, in the Caucasian former Soviet Republic of Georgia, one of the essential elements in the reform process in mental health during the past two decades was the strong voice of the NGO sector. The activity of civil society organizations, professional societies, user groups, and family member organizations created the momentum that was essential for a movement towards a rights-based and humane mental health care. The sector often functioned as the conduit for international expertise and knowledge about best practices in other countries.

In searching for innovative, locally appropriate, and implementable models, new projects and activities were developed by NGOs. Many new community-based services, such as crisis intervention and home care, were rolled out through the approach of starting with small pilots that were followed by a national scale-up financed and implemented by state structures.

In challenging the old model of psychiatry and introducing contemporary approaches, capacity-building activities were promoted, such as the translation and publication of modern mental health literature into Georgian, the opening of a Resource Center on Mental Health at Ilia State University in Tbilisi, the organization of a wide range of intensive trainings, workshops, and conferences, as well as exchange visits and research activities.

At the national level, the main strategy of the NGO community was to influence the government and other mental health policy makers to adopt legislation and to abide by the new laws, to develop relevant mental health policies and plans, and to help create monitoring mechanisms to ensure the protection of human rights. For more information on the reform process in mental health in Georgia and the role of NGOs see Makhashvili & van Voren (2013).

Legitimacy of NGOs in mental health

NGOs have become increasingly influential in world. The World Bank estimates that over 15% of total overseas development aid is channeled through NGOs (although probably not much of this concerns the rather few NGOs working in the field of mental health). However, there are a number of important issues to consider. Their increasing (economic) influence with only limited checks and balances in place, their shift from lobbying activities on behalf of a specific target group to becoming involved in the work of intergovernmental institutions, policy implementation, and service provision (which in turn often results in becoming caught up with political and commercial interests) – all these factors raise questions with regard to the legitimacy of NGOs.

At the same time, this shift in the positioning of NGOs has to be seen against the backdrop of a process in which primacy lies more and more with, e.g., notions concerning human rights or distributive justice rather than the priorities of specific nation states.

We cannot expect NGOs to fill the vacuum created by failing nation states, for instance by calling attention to the fact that in many countries there is hardly any psychiatric care for the population and the only available services are concentrated in large, often deteriorated hospitals. Nor can we expect NGOs to be the ones who have to ask governments why persons with mental health problems are excluded from employment or education or decent housing. Yet it is legitimate to point out shortcomings, to give a voice to people with mental health problems who belong to the most vulnerable groups in society (World Health Organization 2010), and to put social and moral themes on the international agenda as a way to contribute to a transcending democracy.

However, if legitimacy is practicing power on behalf of citizens to whom you are accountable, nation states are in principle bound by democratic procedures. In contrast to nations, NGOs strive to realize specific ambitions and do not have to account for the potentially conflicting interests of all citizens. The activities of NGOs are often not based on or legitimized by democratic procedures, and they bear responsibility only to their financial donors.

The question to what extent the pretentions of NGOs are democratically verified is further problematized in the case when an NGO fails to practice what it preaches. Does respecting clients' rights and involving them in decision making mean in fact that they actually participate in designing project proposals, or does it mean that they are represented in the boards and staff of the relevant NGOs? Is giving voice to vulnerable persons with mental health problems a form of political correctness or is it based on consensus among the target group? Is this rhetoric system of thought with non-offending ideas about "human values" going to dominate the debate and transcend the global cultural diversity with its myriad notions on mental health?

NGOs in the modern age

Rapid changes in the global economic landscape will have profound effects on foreign aid and the role of NGOs. While Europe and the United States are plunged into an economic crisis, Brazil, the Russian Federation, India, and China (BRIC) have the potential to form a powerful economic bloc based on their roles as global suppliers of manufactured goods, services, and raw materials. By 2030 the four BRICs may account for 41% of the world's market capitalization (Moe *et al.* 2010). In the wake of economic growth, countries that once were on the receiving end of foreign aid now mount the international aid platform as donors. However, while over the past decade the wealthy traditional donor countries cleaned up their assistance programs under the umbrella of the Organisation for Economic Co-operation and Development (OECD), which set rules and norms with regard to foreign aid, the BRIC countries are not member states of the OECD and thus not bound by these rules.

China, for instance, has a broad and vague definition of what constitutes foreign aid but is becoming a major source of "development aid," although yet difficult to quantify. Some of Chinese assistance resembles foreign aid as defined by the OECD, but it also shares characteristics of foreign investment. The major drive behind the non-transparent Chinese programs, which often take the form of cut-rate loans, is to secure and transport natural resources and to establish diplomatic alliances. Lum and colleagues (2009) noted in a report on China's growing role in Africa, Latin America, and Southeast Asia that their offerings are well received, not only because many of the funded works are highly visible and provide short-term effects such as the construction of highways and railroads, but also because the Chinese support comes without the usual bureaucratic procedures and the focus on social, political and environmental conditions that Western donors and NGOs impose. Whereas Western NGOs operate within the framework of ethical guidelines, with their emphasis on human rights, China offers quick solutions, a mix of aid and business in secret government-to-government agreements (LaFraniere & Grobler 2009).

Moreover, in Western countries the economic recession can lead to a significant reduction in foreign aid. Past economic crises have led to trimming governmental foreign aid budgets and a substantial decrease in contributions by foundations and NGOs. Experience from the past showed that drastic cuts resulted in an increase of poverty and reduced the supply and quality of healthcare services (USAID 2009). At the same time, since mental health and poverty are closely linked, with those on low incomes more likely to suffer from poor mental health and poverty contributing to poor mental health (Jenkins *et al.* 2008), the demand on mental health services will increase.

The shifts in global economy are reflected in changes in priorities and ambitions in foreign aid. New players in the field are motivated by their national interests, while the traditional donors re-evaluate their strategies and policies in light of their economic recession.

The road ahead

Edwards and Zadek (2003) identified two, often contradictory, imperatives that need to be reconciled when non-state involvement in global governance complements governmental decision making. First of all, the diversity of non-state actors and the inequalities among them make rules and protocols essential. Secondly, these rules and standards should be non-bureaucratic to prevent undermining the beneficial characteristics of these organizations. Edwards and Zadek provide a list of general recommendations to strike the balance between the two directives. These "rules of the road for non-state actors" comprise suggestions to enhance the legitimacy of the NGOs (for instance by ensuring transparency with regard to their legal status and funding), and also how to strengthen their role in global governance (for instance by providing – financial – support to local actors with fewer resources).

One of the key barriers that has prevented improvement in mental health is fragmentation among mental health advocacy groups (Thornicroft & Tansella 2008). Too many global mental health initiatives targeting specific needs run in parallel and potentially add pressure to already weak health systems. From a broader perspective, setting aside differences and forming alliances and umbrella groups with a clear-cut message, as well as mainstreaming mental health into more general advocacy programs and overarching themes (e.g., poverty reduction within the framework of the Millennium Development Goals, human rights and service user empowerment), could strengthen the lobby for mental health. Key issues that can function as a common denominator are the implementation of the CRPD, advocating for (new or improved) mental health laws and national policies, anti-stigma and anti-discrimination arrangements, and the implementation of human rights.

To increase the efficacy of the advocacy efforts of NGOs, the development of lobby and training programs in the sphere of public relations, among others regarding the use of social media and networks, is key to address politicians and policy makers who have a limited understanding of the issues surrounding mental health and also have limited time to make informed decisions. Reduction in negative media portrayal may lead to mobilizing (financial) resources and a reduction of stigma.

NGOs are much criticized (e.g., De Waal 1997, Polman 2010). Serious questions are raised with regard to the issue to what extent their support affects economic development and how much good aid ultimately does. We know, for instance, remarkably little about the long-term effects of humanitarian activities in the field of mental health. NGOs should strive to improve the evidence base of mental health interventions, and to develop best practices and effective culturally adapted interventions – in terms of outcomes and cost-effectiveness – as well as consensus-based indicators to substantiate the rationale for including mental health on the national agenda. Such developments are necessary not only to compete more effectively with other and more general health needs, but also to legitimize international efforts and involvement. When competing for available funds with general health needs and priorities, mental health is in arrears on providing evidence of its effectiveness.

The problem in mental health is that, no matter how much our knowledge of genetic and physiological processes has progressed over the years, a nosology of psychiatry based entirely on neuroscience not only seems unrealistic for decades to come but is perhaps "impossible to achieve at all" (Greenberg 2010). Moreover, it is clear that mental health problems cannot be understood without taking into account the sociocultural context in which they occur; social conditions and experiences during the course of life play an important role in the etiology of mental health problems, limiting the applicability of interventions. A panacea for mood disorders similar to immunization for polio is unrealistic and utopian. Hence, NGOs should rather prioritize and advocate for patients' rights and improving the quality of care, and, in short, support the basic demands of the client movement in mental health, rather than rub against the "vigorous effort to remedicalize psychiatry" (Sabshin 1977).

NGOs must also build their legitimacy by practicing what they preach. Besides being transparent and accountable to donors and the general public, global NGOs must ensure that local partners are included in the debate, and must empower the "target group" to participate in reform and act and speak for themselves. NGOs in mental health should therefore involve people who have experienced mental health problems in their organization. These people have expertise and can build effective partnerships between client and family organizations, mental health providers, and other stakeholders to streamline advocacy and build a "critical mass."

References

Barnes M, Bowl R (2000) *Taking Over the Asylum: Empowerment and Mental Health*. London: Macmillan.

De Waal A (1997) *Famine Crimes: Politics and the Disaster Industry in Africa*. Oxford: James Currey.

Edwards E, Zadek S (2003) Governing the provision of global public goods: the role and legitimacy of nonstate actors. In I Kaul, P Conceição, K Le Goulven, RU Mendoza, eds., *Providing Global Public Goods: Managing Globalization*. New York, NY: Oxford University Press; pp. 200–24.

Edwards M (2000) *NGO Rights and Responsibilities: a New Deal for Global Governance*. London: Foreign Policy Centre.

Essink DR (2012) *Sustainable Health Systems: the Role of Change Agents in Health System Innovation*. 's-Hertogenbosch: BoxPress.

Foucault M (1965) *Madness and Civilization: a History of Insanity in the Age of Reason*. New York: Pantheon Books.

Gauchet M, Swain G (1999) *Madness and Democracy: the Modern Psychiatric Universe*. Princeton, NJ: Princeton University Press. p. 41.

Greenberg G (2010) Inside the battle to define mental illness. *Wired*, December 27, 2010. http://www. wired.com/magazine/2010/12/ ff_dsmv/5 (accessed July 2013).

Jenkins R, Bhugra D, Bebbington P, *et al.* (2008) Debt, income and mental disorder in the general population. *Psychological Medicine* **38**: 1485–93.

Kettering C (1948) Thoughts on the business of life. *Forbes* **62**, 34.

Keukens R, van Voren R (2009) *Prioritizing Mental Health*. Hilversum: Global Initiative on Psychiatry.

LaFraniere S, Grobler J (2009) China spreads aid in Africa, with a catch. *New York Times*, September 21, 2009.

Lum T, Fischer H, Gomez-Granger J, Leland A (2009) *China's Foreign Aid Activities in Africa, Latin America and South East Asia*. CRS Report for Congress 7–5700 R40361. Washington, DC: Congressional Research Service. http://www.fas. org/sgp/crs/row/R40361.pdf (accessed July 2013).

Makhashvili N, van Voren R (2013) Balancing community and hospital care: a case study of reforming mental health services in Georgia. *PLOS Medicine* **10** (1): e1001366.

McDaid D (2008) Countering the discrimination and stigmatization of people with mental health problems in Europe. EU Directorate-General for Health & Consumers.

Mental Health Directorate (2005) *The Mental Health Policy of Sri Lanka 2005–2015*. http://www.ccpsl.lk/wp-content/uploads/2012/05/mental-health-policy-sri-lanka.pdf (accessed July 2013).

Moe T, Maasry C, Tang R (2010) *EM Equity in Two Decades: a Changing Landscape*. Global Economics paper 204. Goldman Sachs Global Economics, Commodities and Strategy Research.

Murray CJL, Lopez AD (1996) *The Global Burden of Disease: a Comprehensive Assessment of Mortality and Disability from Diseases, Injuries, and Risk Factors in 1990 and Projected to 2020*. Cambridge, MA: Harvard University Press.

Polman L (2010) *The Crisis Caravan: What's Wrong With Humanitarian Aid?* New York, NY: Metropolitan Books.

Sabshin M (1977) On remedicalization and holism in psychiatry. *Psychosomatics* **18**: 7–8.

Saraceno B, van Ommeren M, Batniji R, *et al.* (2007) Barriers to improvement of mental health services in low-income and middle-income countries. *Lancet* **370**: 1164–74

Sen A (2009) *The Idea of Justice*. Cambridge, MA: Harvard University Press. p. 258.

Summerfield D (2008) How scientifically valid is the knowledge base of global mental health? *BMJ* **336**: 992–4.

Thornicroft G, Tansella M (2008) *Better Mental Health Care*. Cambridge: Cambridge University Press.

United Nations (undated) Department of Information: Non-Governmental Organizations. http://outreach.un. org/ngorelations/about-us (accessed July 2013).

United Nations (2006) *Convention on the Rights of Persons with Disabilities (A/RES/61/106)*. New York, NY: UN.

United Nations (2010) *Monitoring the Convention on the Rights of Persons With Disabilities: Guidance for Human Rights Monitors*. Professional Training Series 17. New York, NY: UN Office of the High Commissioner for Human Rights.

USAID (2009) How will the global economic crisis impact the health of the world's poor? Global Health Perspectives series. http://transition. usaid.gov/locations/asia/ documents/Health-and-Impact-of-Economic-Crisis-4-13-final-duproof0413.pdf (accessed Juky 2013).

van Voren R (2009) *On Dissidents and Madness*. Amsterdam: Rodopi.

van Voren R (2010) *Cold War in Psychiatry: Human Factors, Secret Actors*. Amsterdam: Rodopi.

Ventevogel P (2008) De effectiviteit van de geestelijke gezondheidszorg in ontwikkelingslanden. In B Geerling, D Oosterbaan, MJ Stender, eds., *Psychiatrie over de Grens*. Zoetermeer: Free Musketeers.

Ventevogel P, Jong JTVM de (2006) De effectiviteit van de geestelijke gezondheidszorg in ontwikkelingslanden. *Tijdschrift voor Psychiatrie* **48**: 283–93.

Watters E (2010) *Crazy Like Us: the Globalization of the American Psyche.* New York, NY: Free Press.

World Health Organization (2001) *The World Health Report 2001. Mental Health: New Understanding, New Hope.* Geneva: WHO.

World Health Organization (2010) *Mental Health and Development: Targeting People with Mental Health Conditions as a Vulnerable Group.* Geneva: WHO.

World Health Organization (2011) *Mental Health Atlas 2011.* Geneva: WHO.

World Health Organization (2012) Global burden of mental disorders and the need for a comprehensive, coordinated response from health and social sectors at the country level. Document EB130.R8, January 20, 2012, WHO Executive Board 130th Session.

Young A (1995) *The Harmony of Illusions: Inventing Post-Traumatic Stress Disorder.* Princeton, NJ: Princeton University Press.

Chapter

37

Mental health, mass communication, and media

Marten W. de Vries

Introduction

Traditional and social media have considerable potential to reach a broad audience and cover a wide range of topics. Hence, it has application for providing mental health information and educational services quickly to the target audiences. The application of social media to mental health services can contribute immensely, as the costs of mental health care for individuals and communities rises (*Lancet* 2011). Traditional mental health approaches are too limited a response to current predictions of the burden of mental illness and identified treatment gaps, and have been inadequate in the task of stemming this upswell. Yet, the target population for mental health information is vast and diverse. Three main areas of mental health promotion – mental health literacy, destigmatization, and prevention – have demonstrated a strong impact. Television, radio, telephony, and web formats specifically designed to promote mental health yield results with respect to informing the public, challenging current beliefs and attitudes, and potentially obviating the development of mental illness.

Media in the form of telemedicine and distance learning has a long history in rural and congested urban areas, but it can be most efficiently used today when incorporated into modern media. These internet and telephone-based approaches, using mobile phones and internet vehicles such as Twitter and Facebook, provide exciting developments for mental health and provide an area of fruitful investigation for mental health deployment (Muñoz *et al.* 2005, Smit *et al.* 2006). Their use can be enhanced with newer insights gained through interactive media with mental health content across a range of platforms.

The World Health Organization (2008a, 2008b) promotes the internet as a powerful tool for communicating and accessing health information for professionals, organizations, and the population at large. But there is greater use of media than just providing information. Because of the very nature of contemporary media in day-to-day life, audiences have become media-sophisticated. More than 30% are active on the web globally, and the disparity between developed and developing countries, 64% and 20%, is rapidly closing (WSIS 2010). This increasing interconnectivity in media and information and communications technology (ICT) use provides new opportunities for partnership between mental health professionals and citizens as well as stimulating self-help, social networks, and social support activities. The basis of the interaction is appropriate and relevant content that speaks to issues people actually experience. The inadequacy of recent scare campaigns against smoking brings this home, and shows that in our use of media we must address the audience in engaging understandable, interactive, and respectful formats (Ruiter *et al.* 2001).

The basis for a successful media mental health approach is storytelling. The ability to communicate with one another allows global communities to become co-producers of mental health content. Moreover, this allows mental health media content to be embedded in the public mental health concepts of empowerment and participation, which encourage citizens, communities, and health professionals to engage through media to improve well-being. This interaction is equally important for intervening when this media, traditional or new, has a negative impact on mental health (Wahl 1992, Klin & Lemish, 2008, Murray 2008).

Essentials of Global Mental Health, ed. Samuel O. Okpaku. Published by Cambridge University Press. © Cambridge University Press 2014.

Background

Mental health problems and mental disorders represent a serious and growing public health burden. The impact in terms of personal suffering, utilization of health and mental health care, risk of physical illness and mortality, economic costs and social participation (e.g., raising children, work, education) is great (*Lancet* 2011). The relation between these mental health problems and the social functioning of communities is bidirectional (Latkin & Curry 2003). On the one hand, incidence and prevalence of depression and anxiety, for example, are significantly influenced by exposure to community stressors such as poverty, unemployment, living in disadvantaged areas, domestic violence, social isolation, and lack of social cohesion (Flannery-Schroeder 2006). On the other hand, mental health (mental capital) is increasingly recognized as a vital prerequisite to citizenship and social participation as well as to the experience of general well-being and adequate social and economic functioning of communities (Stuckler *et al.* 2009). Yet, despite this knowledge and the recognized lifetime prevalence of mental disorders at 40% worldwide, with only 8% reaching any sort of care under the best of conditions, this challenge to persons, institutions, businesses, and governments needs to be confronted more adequately (Kessler *et al.* 2007, World Health Organization 2008b).

At the same time, there are international efforts to stem this tide from organizations such as the World Federation for Mental Health (WFMH), the World Health Organization (WHO), the *Lancet*, universities, and some governments. These training, advocacy, and policy efforts are supported by strong data showing that a small shift in a population's well-being (one point on the General Health Questionnaire, GHQ) is associated with a substantial reduction (6%) in the prevalence of common mental disorders. Huppert (2004) and Rose (2008) suggest that impacting the well-being of communities can have a direct effect on mental health morbidity. Moreover, national councils including Raad voor Volksgezondheid en Zorg (2010) in the Netherlands and the Substance Abuse and Mental Health Services Administration (2011) in the USA have projected that implementing general prevention strategies, including the use of social media, will create substantial savings, potentially reaching billions of euros, over the next 20 years.

Relatively little scientific work has been carried out toward strengthening mental health in the world's communities. Programs still generally focus on the individual. A population-based frame of reference and action plan is necessary to allow governments and institutions to confront this global problem directly. Today, the public is experiencing new mental health and lifestyle needs. Societies are thus primed for such interventions. In part inspired through social media communication, there is increasing public interest in dealing with mental health issues, and institutions can take advantage of this groundswell in the population. Economic and market analysts have highlighted a growing international demand in mental health know-how and lifestyle products, particularly in the media, ranging from print to broadcasting to web-based self-help information (PricewaterhouseCoopers 2011). The "duty to be healthy" is pushed by governments internationally to stem healthcare costs, and their efforts have become accepted by a large portion of the world's citizens. Health and mental health products have become a multi-billion-dollar industry (Merrill Lynch 2000), demonstrating the public will to take action on their own behalf. How can mental health professionals capitalize on this process and the growing awareness that people need to take health into their own hands? There is now an opening to address the shortcomings of the limited reach of traditional healthcare approaches, challenging us to develop innovative approaches in order to respond to this public interest and need.

A rationale for public mental health and media action

Over the last decade those in the field of mental health have been confronted by perplexing and challenging mental ill-health prevalence statistics from almost every corner of the world (World Health Organization 2008a). Kessler and colleagues (2007) have derived a set of drivers explaining these high prevalence rates: chronicity, high impairment, young onset, and low treatment rates. To this we add lifestyle issues, rapid social change, global communication, work–life stress, and most recently financial stress, debt (de Vries & Wilkerson 2004), and perhaps developmental changes such as the earlier occurrence of puberty (Saugstad 1989). Finally, one long-term contributor to dealing with mental health problems has been the global stigma surrounding these human experiences (Sartorius & Schulze 2005), which discourages treatment and leads to exclusion and discrimination.

Although we have not stood idle, the efforts of professional, non-governmental organization (NGO), patient/client, and global government systems to respond to this global epidemic-like process have been limited. However, we have had some success. There is a growing body of evidence in prevention research (Hosman 2004) as well as primary care interventions (Jenkins & Üstün 1998) that demonstrate efficacy. Health promotion efforts have also demonstrated an impact in the areas of sexual behavior, smoking, diet, and exercise. Most recently internet interventions have demonstrated an impact on depression (Smit *et al.* 2006) and smoking (Muñoz *et al.* 2005) for larger numbers than have been traditionally reached. The majority of these efforts, however, have focused on small "captured settings," secondary and tertiary prevention, with groups at risk and individuals indicated for treatment. There is much to be learned from these successful programs that could be applied in larger population-based interventions. In the meantime, we can work to improve global mental health using a readily available yet underutilized tool, the media.

Can media help with psychosocial adaptation in today's world?

Life has become more "liquid" (Bauman 2005). Today's youth often live far away from their natal environments; populations are more mobile, resulting in increased urbanization; and social strife has uprooted vast numbers. Traditional social and family structures have thus been altered, and with them the secure authority dictated by custom. The information age has accelerated this process and rendered traditional hierarchies topsy-turvy (for classic discussions of this topic, see Toffler 1970 and Mead 1978). All of this is occurring at a time of increasing autonomy and independence of the individual with its direct consequences for maintaining social and other supportive networks. A new culture mix has occurred, often referred to as globalization, that has challenged the existing social fabric – resulting in stress, alienation, and, often, popular reactionary politics. But, primarily, it points to the need for new skills, tools, and habits. New skills are needed to manage these profound and fundamental changes that have

remained largely outside the control and power of citizens to comprehend and grasp in the context of their daily lives.

Youth have it particularly difficult because of numerous issues including unemployment, substance abuse, and school failure, as demonstrated by the earlier age of onset of almost all mental disorders (Kessler *et al.* 2007). Yet schools play an increasingly minor role in developing attitudes and mindsets in a liquid environment of constant and rapid change. More and more information comes from peers and the internet instead of the classroom and family networks. Adults are also faced with new uncertainties. Relationships such as marriage have become less stable, with soaring divorce rates and split families, and work insecurity in fragile economic times often results in debt and long-term financial insecurity. The work–life conundrum (de Vries & Wilkerson 2004) creates stress through time-management issues and leads to decreased concentration on tasks, resulting in less "flow" and greater anxiety, boredom, and apathy (Csikcentmihalyi 1990).

This chapter proposes that media can play a role here in encouraging positive mental health and well-being, thereby impacting prevalence rates of common mental disorders. Today, multiple forms of media and creative broadcasts are available and can be coupled to social interventions for a positive effect on mental health at the community and individual level. It can help through opening the discourse for improving mental health and facilitating the reciprocal *exchange* of mental health knowledge between professionals and local experts by experience. A negotiated use of media between professional, citizens, broadcasters, and publishers can provide a place where people re-find themselves and interact, a place where security, not anxiety, is fostered, and a place of both renewable resources and sustained references to the past. Formats that link information from the "past" to the current swell of new information can facilitate knowledge building, decreasing anxiety and apathy while maintaining stimulating yet secure social interactions (Riva *et al.* 2012).

How can media help?

Daily community life is delicately interrelated with the experience of mass and social media communication. Media has become one of the cornerstones of modern life and has evolved into a potential ally for improving the mental health of a population. Because of its reach and interactive aspects media can increase well-being and mental health in communities, especially when anchored in broader community projects, as was done in the *The Team* drama series and related community interventions after the ethnic violence of 2007 in Kenya (Abdalla 2012, Media Focus on Africa 2012), described below. *The Team*, associated social media, and community interventions decreased trauma in affected communities and opened up a discourse on improving relations, resulting in sustained social initiatives at the grassroots level that continue to this day. In the field of mental health, we can build on such an effect by expecting that the use of media can decrease the current mental disorder lifetime prevalence of 35–40% back to the level found by Leighton (1956) in small-town USA in the 1950s of 15–20%, over the next 20–30 years. This is still a high prevalence, but potentially manageable within the current reach of our healthcare systems.

To that end, extensive data have already demonstrated that mixed-media formats can increase mental health literacy, decrease stigma, and function preventively (Whitehorn 1989). At the population level, they can stimulate social networks in a community and facilitate "boundary crossing" between the citizens, the community, professionals, and policy makers, thus empowering populations in proactive and self-efficacious ways. Until recently, however, media approaches in health promotion, like mass media campaigns, had not worked well. They were often deployed in isolation, insufficiently engaging, and "too top-down" (Ruiter *et al.* 2001). Today, media and the web offer fresh opportunities, as they are interactive, not solely orientated to "informing." In this approach, social media interventions become shaped in the interaction between citizens, scientists, mental health and media professionals. Local communities are then not necessarily the "object" of these media productions but co-producers. Embedding media in diverse community activities and developing programs in concert with citizen interests, as well as attempting to do so with engaging formats, adjusts the shortcomings of previous interventions. Moreover, community interactive media, with web links and social gatherings, accelerates the reach and tempo of information exchange and influences behavior relatively more quickly than traditional approaches, often stimulating a new sense of community as well (Horstman & Houtepen 2005).

Media and mental health: the evidence

Media is globally pervasive, with a wide reach and a potentially broad target population estimated at 60–90% of a total population (Fonnebo & Sogaard 1995, Highet *et al.* 2006). Its impact is felt everywhere and its formats are rapidly evolving in an ever-changing digital landscape. In order to understand it effectively over the ensuing years and adjust our mental health interventions to this changing scene, we will need to rely on studies from and work with a variety of interdisciplinary fields.

There is considerable literature on the potential impact of social media in mental health. A variety of social media approaches have been used worldwide. Successful examples come from North America, Africa, and Asia, but particularly in Australia, New Zealand, the United States, and the United Kingdom (Regier *et al.* 1988, Voelker 1996, Paykel *et al.* 1997, Jorm *et al.* 2006). Successful outcomes have been seen with depression, suicide, anxiety, alcohol, sexual abuse, and aggression. Dramatized "edutainment" covering a host of social issues has been demonstrated in Latin America, particularly in the form of *telanovelas*, related to gender disharmony and female roles (Singhal & Rogers 2004). These encouraging results have been supported by scientific evaluative studies.

In addition, mass media interventions have a proven impact on mental health literacy, destigmatization, and prevention, as demonstrated by a variety of research methods (Sanders *et al.* 2000, Highet *et al.* 2002, 2006, Lauber *et al.* 2003, Penn *et al.* 2003, Bartlett *et al.* 2006, Jorm *et al.* 2006, Stip *et al.* 2006, Castiello & Magliano 2007, Finkelstein & Lapshin 2007, Twardzicki 2008). These studies have explored the impacts of media on mental health agenda setting, targeting key problems related to mental health, and facilitating identification and early detection (Fonnebo & Sogaard 1995, Paykel *et al.* 1997, Kato *et al.* 1999). Moreover, numerous studies have measured changes in attitude, in clarifying misconceptions, and in raising empathy with and understanding of mental illness (Fonnebo & Sogaard 1995, Penn *et al.* 2003, Warner 2005, Ritterfeld & Jin 2006, Finkelstein & Lapshin 2007, Twardzicki 2008). These media interventions are effective in a variety of cultural contexts. Sanders' Triple P program (Sanders *et al.* 2000) is an excellent example of the impact of a mixed-media, multilevel intervention for families and parents, a process that rolls over from community universal to individual family-targeted preventive interventions. This approach has been widely applied and studied. In over 40 controlled trials across different cultures, positive outcomes were sustained over one year in interventions related to dysfunctional parenting strategies (e.g., coercive), stress and anger, depression, well-being, and parent's relationship quality, while it had a positive effect on children's conduct problems and the reduction of verified cases of child abuse in communities (De Graaf *et al.* 2008).

A prime historical example of a media intervention is *The San Francisco Mood Survey*, a pioneering TV intervention in San Francisco, a mood management mini-series broadcast during primetime in 1978 (Muñoz *et al.* 1982). The researchers took advantage of an existing TV format, Dr. Uline's medical advice program, a series of brief, five-minute episodes shown after the news each night. The *Mood Survey* was designed as a cognitive behavioral treatment approach for depression aimed at the entire urban population. Each episode provided information in a newsroom format with video vignettes highlighting and illustrating the content, with an emphasis on positive psychological approaches. Segments specifically and directly described how to deal with depressive feelings and positive thinking, with a focus on gaining control of activities that "make you feel better." The population of San Francisco thus received a short course in behavioral techniques with video examples modeling how to do it while emphasizing and demonstrating potential positive outcomes. The *Mood Survey* found that on the average 36 minutes of TV was watched by the participants over the 12 days. Even though the viewing exposure was minimal, *Mood Survey* results indicated that the program was positively received. People who had not reported depressive symptoms had begun to pay more attention to mood, positive thinking, and their selection of daily activities in response to the program, a striking population effect. Even more remarkable was that those who had reported depressive symptoms before the series reported significant symptom reduction thereafter.

The *San Francisco Mood Survey* is an example of how a directive and instructive approach may benefit the well-being of a population as well as the already ill. Such programs respond to the need people have for health-related information, particularly in populations that have not been bombarded with media messages, as was the case in the 1970s. The effective mood management techniques depicted in the series implied that individuals can help themselves, to find relief from depression and/or to prevent it from re-occurring.

Among the many types of interventions is *edutainment*: the process of designing media messages to both entertain and educate. Entertainment–education is not a new form of programming, and goes back to the beginning of mass media more than 60 years ago. For example, in the late 1960s *telenovelas*, Latin American soap operas, began featuring educational messages designed specifically to "teach" audiences certain desired behaviors. These have been followed globally in diverse health and social-issue campaigns (Singhal & Rogers 2004), most notably the successful HIV prevention television series *Soul City* in South Africa (Usdin *et al.* 2004), to name only one.

Edutainment soaps often derive their motivation from psychological and social research. Bandura's influential work on social learning theory (Bandura 1977) and self-efficacy, as well his later writings on the impact of media, is one such source. Bandura (2009) concludes that mass media not only creates personal attributes but can also alter existing ones based on exposure to other forms of behavior. Social learning theory then postulates that exposure to new forms of behavior and information is central. Simply stated, individuals learn behaviors by watching others, whether in person or in the media, and imitating them. Imitating the modeled behaviors further increases the individual's sense of self-worth and efficacy, thereby reinforcing the effect (Bandura 2001).

New social media can improve on this already strong effect. It can facilitate reflection and learning focused on themes of mental health and mental resilience. It can create the opportunity and maintain interactive communication for the user to destigmatize mental health problems, to deconstruct the taboo on mental health issues, to give words to mental health concerns, to identify problems as well as multiple ways to deal with them, varying from interpersonal support to community support and professional help. This is a movement away from "providing information" to creating an interactive platform for the communities, individuals, and professionals, thereby enabling a process of continuous, grassroots learning about mental health issues.

However, as decades of research on media effects show, mass media does not work in a vacuum, it is rather part of a larger ecosystem, including audience, message, and environment (Bratic 2006). Interaction, engagement, and dialog are critical factors in the outcome of any media intervention (Becker 2004). In order to have a substantial impact on the well-being of a population, a number of theoretical (health promotion, public mental health, social learning, etc.), environmental, social, and historical factors need to align with the media effort. A change in behavior depends on many variables other than the impact of the media programs. Only the true integration of media, ongoing social processes, and other population-based strategies can guarantee a significant move toward greater well-being. Enlisting the involvement of the local or virtual community is a key ingredient in a successful intervention. Participation can take a variety of forms, from contributing to the form, content, and production of the media intervention to engaging in community screenings or assisting with promotion and dissemination of the program to a wider audience. The lesson for a successful mental health media approach with populations is clear: it requires the integration of mixed-media products with ongoing community-based interventions and staying in dynamic tune and participatory interaction with the realities of day-to-day life in a population (Tully & Ekdale 2010).

From the above and with limited human capacities social media can contribute to scaling up mental health services. Social media can also contribute to globalization, with its opportunities for collaboration. As the saying goes, "Health is not what doctors do, health is what people do." We need to engage populations to do so. For this, we are fortunate today in having the full arsenal of media, from traditional to new and evolving forms, at our fingertips. The rapid growth of mobile and internet communication renders this possible for reaching many in the developing world as well. Through media the mental health movement can engage and interact with global populations, step out of the limitations of a purely pathological orientation, and enter a global conversation of mutual learning as to how to improve mental health and well-being.

Two examples of the use of mass and social media will now be described.

Example 1. *The Team*: lessons from a social value soap dealing with a national trauma

The first example is an integrated media and social effort in Kenya employing a wide range of mixed-media techniques and community involvement to assist with increasing national unity and healing a traumatized population after the 2007–08 ethnic violence. It is an exemplary effort of multiple forms of media embedded at the national and village levels, centered on a soap series, *The Team*, and a talk show, *Fist to Five for Change*. After the violence and during the production of the interventions a process of mutual learning took place both for the population in the use of social media and social gatherings and for the producers in the production of appropriate messages. The result was a noticeable contribution to national unity, political involvement, and social healing with the creation of positive social spin-offs still active to this day.

The Team is a Kenyan TV drama series that was co-produced by the Media Focus on Africa Foundation (MFoA), and The Search for Common Ground in response to the devastating violence in Kenya following the 2007 general election. As the post-election violence shook the entire Kenyan nation in 2008, unity and reconciliation seemed like a distant dream and the future looked bleak. However, in the period immediately following the violence, the country began a process of healing and reunification that is still under way in which a media response played an important role. In concert with this process MFoA developed two television programs, *The Team* and *Fist to Five for Change*, which opened discussion related to the experienced trauma of the ethnic violence by encouraging social healing and national unity. *The Team* is a drama series targeting all Kenyans, but particularly the youth, through a fictional Kenyan soccer team designed as a metaphor for contemporary Kenyan society. They sought to use a multimedia strategy as a tool to promote discussion and understanding between people of different ethnic backgrounds with the immediate goal of preventing future violence through changing attitudes and promoting national unity.

Program content and approach

The series content depicts recognizable locations and daily life themes, often focusing on traumatic issues such as corruption, ethnic differences, coping with emotions, rape, and drugs. While *The Team* adopts many elements of the traditional *telenovela* model, it goes further by incorporating a social networking component to allow for audience participation; holding mobile screenings in conflict zones for larger societal impact; and creating morally complex characters who must make decisions that do not always have clear "right" and "wrong" choices. *The Team*'s use of the metaphor of a football team helped avoid paternalism and larger didactic statements by presenting situations in which characters must decide how to deal with conflict situations themselves. Audience members were not told which decisions to make, but were rather encouraged to evaluate decisions made by the show's characters and to think about what they would do in similar circumstances (Tully & Ekdale 2010).

The Team used an entertainment–education approach combined with social media, social networking, and offline interaction through facilitated screenings and discussion groups. Social networking sites, particularly Facebook and Twitter, as well as short message services (SMS), were incorporated into *The Team*'s larger strategy, given the rapid growth of internet use in Kenya. A lively internet presence evolved, targeting different audiences with the different types of media and adapting the messaging strategy for each medium. This cross-media approach also included a radio program, large-scale mobile screenings, and distribution of DVDs for community screenings (Media Focus on Africa 2012). This approach reached thousands of people, particularly the young, allowing for a two-way flow of information as opposed to the traditional one-way, top-down message delivery to viewers, which is an often-criticized approach particularly in developing countries (Huesca 2003).

Mixed-media outreach and impact

First of all, *The Team* was watched or listened to. Standard media viewer ratings showed that viewer density overall was high, with 73% of the population watching 55% of the episodes and 24% having listened to at least 10 of the episodes. When the approach was connected to outreach mobile cinema units in eight severely affected areas of Kenya, extra benefit accrued, as episodes were re-shown in villages throughout the country. This was especially true when *The Team* was linked to the *Fist to Five for Change* talk show, which included a presence at the village level. This show was aired on national television during primetime to reach the largest possible audience. It was formatted as a focus-group talk show, in which afflicted citizens participated in confrontations and discussions. *Fist to Five* is a consensus activity that allows people to show

their agreement or disagreement with an opinion or statement. A fist (a zero) represents total disagreement, while an open hand (a five) represents total agreement. One, two, three, and four fingers represent different levels of agreement. In this way, the facilitator would ask participants to show how they felt about issues raised by other participants. The show thus encouraged open dialog by offering participants a safe space and method to discuss contentious and often unspoken issues. As *The Team* series began receiving national attention, the issues raised and discussed in *Fist to Five* proved therapeutic and highlighted emotions shared across the country (Tully & Ekdale 2010). In addition to the national broadcasts, a strategy of free mobile screenings and facilitated small-group workshops was developed to bring *Fist to Five* to communities with little access to television and to areas most deeply affected by the post-election violence. Having a chance not only to watch others engage in this process on the talk show, but actually to do it, provided an opportunity for healing and community reconciliation (Tully 2010). Overall, *Fist to Five* successfully incorporated mass media and interpersonal communication at the broadcast and village level to create a useful strategy for coping with the post-election violence. The use of mobile community-based screenings and the facilitated workshops were arguably the most successful part of the program.

The overall impact of the intervention has been as diverse as the Kenyans themselves, leading to many ongoing spin-off activities across the country (Media Focus on Africa 2012). A public survey, developed to measure specific changes in citizens' awareness, knowledge, and attitudes in a diverse sample was carried out over the entire country. *The Team* contributed to positive changes on all three indicators for those who watched the dramas. Positive changes in citizen participation, ethnic understanding, improved skills, and facilitating action where found (Abdalla 2012). Regular viewers of *The Team* demonstrated significantly more positive attitudes compared to respondents who saw fewer episodes. Whether *The Team* directly contributed to initiating and shaping social attitudes and actions remains an open question, but reports from the field indicate its positive influence. Youth formed football teams across tribal lines, following *The Team*'s model; a national commemoration day incorporated *The Team* model into its educational activities; community members formed reconciliation teams to help displaced citizens return back home; and in Nairobi, a governmental response, Kenya's Ministry of Education incorporated *The Team* outreach model into the extracurricular activities of some government-run schools. Individuals testified to forsaking alcoholic lives, and others capable of doing so created "Peace" football, business and development clubs, to highlight only a few. All of these directly linked the TV drama and its mobile outreach activities to their initiatives. Moreover, respondents mentioned their increased ability to collaborate and problem-solve around the themes dealt with in *The Team*. Many demonstrated a desire to improve tribal and local relations and experienced an increased level of knowledge and understanding of governance issues. In conclusion, *The Team*'s success was dose-related, and its most powerful input was its community outreach activity.

The drama-soap and talk show broadcasts coupled to the outreach mobile screenings and social media presence were a success and contributed to increased social harmony and awareness in a significant part of a population that still describes itself as traumatically affected by the ethnic violence. It serves as an example of a remarkably successful mixed-media population-based intervention with demonstrated impact on the well-being and empowerment of a population under difficult circumstances.

Example 2. *Fit4All* (*Bianca in de Buurt*): a docu-soap for low-income communities in the Netherlands

The second example is *Fit4All*, a docu-drama series produced for poor and isolated communities in the Netherlands. It was created as an adjunct and center-piece in the context of a public mental health project in the city of Maastricht in order to facilitate relationships between institutions and neighborhoods. *Fit4All* targets low-socioeconomic-status (LSES) and ethnically diverse communities, attempting to apply mental health know-how alongside local knowledge and idioms in relatively isolated communities that have been largely left out of, or have been resistant to, health-promotion input. The approach is similar to *The Team*'s in using interactive social media and thereby enabling a two-way interaction between local and professional ideas about health. By doing this, it was postulated that social media would stimulate mental health skills and competences, contribute to

empowering people with respect to mental health, and help to reduce the gap between LSES communities and professionals.

Fit4All is produced in a group format through the interaction between writers, actors, filmmakers, mental health and city professionals, neighborhood residents, and researchers. It features weekly episodes of 20 minutes developed around a local fitness center and its manager Bianca. It was broadcast locally under the title *Bianca in de Buurt* (Bianca in the Neighbourhood; www.biancaindebuurt.nl). Each of the episodes is targeted at a specific mental health or well-being issue, using a metaphorical edutainment approach. The series is drama-based and involves both local citizens as actors and professional actors. The depicted episodes occur within the context of the social reality of the city's neighborhoods. The TV program starts out in a local fitness center where people come ostensibly to work on their physical health, but it slowly focuses on the emergence of psychosocial issues. An interactive easy-access website linked to the series provides a place where citizens can interact on the issues addressed in the series, and where they can find relevant psycho-education and information on local preventive and social services, as well as linkages to other e-mental health websites. With blogs and web commentaries, continuity between the series content and ongoing community issues will be sought on the web. Promotional and short features have been shown in closed, narrowcasting formats and discussion groups including health professionals, neighborhood residents, and researchers, and useful criticism was later incorporated in the scripts, influencing the issues raised and the development of the characters.

Preliminary research findings show that the series plus the website and social media presence resulted in a positive impact on the community. For example, 20 000–33 000 people were reached via the RTV-Maastricht broadcasts, and 1800 video views on the internet were watched by a total of 7200 people. In narrowcastings with small community discussion groups a least 153 participants took part during the weeks of broadcasting. The research, under the title of Crossing Boundaries, Maastricht University (Horstman *et al.* 2013), will continue as the project goes into its second year in response to popular demand.

A number of community reactions and processes have been identified that seemed to reflect increased resilience and social cohesion: people could identify with the content of the series, and they were able to share their experiences and reactions and make easier contact with one another. The humorous format, while dealing with serious issues, facilitated communication and discussion. Modestly, it became the "talk of the town." Lastly, people began coming up with creative solutions in relation to the depicted dilemmas that seemed to generalize to discussions of other issues. Of importance is also that the broadcasters saw the value in the project within a media context and were prepared to provide airtime and support for further productions.

How to be a media and mental health expert

For mental health professionals the advice is clear:

- Include media personnel at the outset when planning programs and research.
- Add an interactive virtual component to all interventions.
- Add a mass-media/communication component to all projects.
- Learn media rules, find trusted "media-pros" and partners.
- Provide media partners with mental health information.
- Translate mental health data into mixed-media community-friendly formats.
- Include target groups in the creation of formats and messages.
- Develop a two-pronged approach for community impact: broad- and virtual-casting linked to active community involvement.
- Embed mental health in existing population processes, including ongoing interventions, concerns, and daily-life realities.

- Take action when necessary to curtail abuse by the media.
- Accept that journalists have the right to report as they see fit.
- Aim to improve lifestyle resilience and mental health throughout the life cycle primarily by informing and facilitating the ability to share and talk about psychological and emotional issues through the use of entertaining and engaging mixed-media formats on any available platform.

Based on the presented evidence and examples, the impact of diverse media on mental health literacy and awareness, destigmatization, and prevention is sufficiently strong for mental health personnel globally to attempt creative solutions in partnership with local communication and media experts.

In the light of this, novel TV formats such as *The San Francisco Mood Survey*, *The Team*, and *Fit4All–Bianca in de Buurt* provide just a few examples of how media may contribute to improving the public's mental health globally. There are other examples, from Brazilian *telenovelas* to Sri Lanka's YATV (Young Asia Television) to the many interactive mental health formats being developed, that have had an impact on social behavior and health. The new world of social media and its capacity to facilitate interaction and promote health is at our doorstep. Linked to traditional mass media, these new approaches have the potential to provide global mental health with the tools it needs. The data and examples presented in this chapter provide models and encouragement to use the media and the range of digital tools that are becoming increasingly available for the improvement of mental health for everyone.

References

Abdalla A (2012) *The Team, Kenya: Final Evaluation Report*. Nairobi: University for Peace.

Bandura A (1977) *Social Learning Theory*. Englewood Cliffs, NJ: Prentice-Hall.

Bandura A (2001) Social cognitive theory of mass communication. *Media Psychology* 3: 265–98.

Bandura A (2009) Social cognitive theory of mass communication. In J Bryant, MB Oliver, eds., *Media Effects: Advances in Theory and Research*, 2nd edn. Mahwah, NJ: Lawrence Erlbaum; pp. 94–124.

Bartlett H, Travers C, Cartwright C, Smith N (2006) Mental health literacy in rural Queensland: results of a community survey. *Australian and New Zealand Journal of Psychiatry* 40: 783–9.

Bauman Z (2005) *Liquid Life*. Cambridge: Polity Press.

Becker J (2004) Contributions by the media to crisis prevention and conflict settlement. *Conflict and Communication Online* 3: 1–17. http://www.cco.regener-online.de/2004/pdf_2004/becker.pdf (accessed July 2013).

Bratic W (2006) Media effects during violent conflict: evaluating media contributions to peace building.

Conflict and Communication Online 5(1): 1–11. http://www.cco.regener-online.de/2006_1/pdf_2006-1/bratic.pdf (accessed July 2013).

Castiello G, Magliano L (2007) Beliefs about psychosocial consequences of schizophrenia and depression: a comparative study in a sample of secondary school students. *Epidemiologia e Psichiatria Sociale* 16: 163–71.

Csikszentmihalyi M (1990) *Flow: the Psychology of Optimal Experience.* New York, NY: Harper & Row.

De Graaf I, Speetjens P, Smit F, de Wolff M, Tavecchio L (2008) Effectiveness of the Triple P Positive Parenting Program on parenting: a meta-analysis. *Family Relations* 57: 553–66.

de Vries MW, Wilkerson B (2004) Retooling for mental health. Presentation: International Business Roundtable for Mental Health and Addiction, Toronto.

Finkelstein J, Lapshin O (2007) Reducing depression stigma using a web-based program. *International Journal of Medical Informatics* 76: 726–34.

Flannery-Schroeder EC (2006) Reducing anxiety to prevent depression. *American Journal of Preventive Medicine* 31: S136–42.

Fonnebo V, Sogaard AJ (1995) The Norwegian mental-health campaign in 1992. Population penetration. *Health Education Research* 10: 257–66.

Highet NJ, Hickie IB, Davenport TA (2002) Monitoring awareness of and attitudes to depression in Australia. *Medical Journal of Australia* 176: S63–8.

Highet NJ, Luscombe GM, Davenport TA, Burns JM, Hickie IB (2006) Positive relationships between public awareness activity and recognition of the impacts of depression in Australia. *Australian and New Zealand Journal of Psychiatry* 40: 55–8.

Hosman CMH, Jane-Llopis E, Saxena S, eds. (2004) *Prevention of Mental Disorders: Effective interventions and policyoptions. WHO Summary Report.* Geneva: World Health Organization.

Horstman K, Houtepen R (2005) *Worstelen met Gezond Leven.* Amsterdam: Het Spinhuis.

Horstman K, Knibbe M, deVries MW (2013) *Bianca in de Buurt*: De praktijk van een participatief project in de publieke geestelijke gezondheidszorg, in Participatie: ZON–MW, den Haag, NL.

Huppert FA (2004 A population approach to positive psychology: the potential for population interventions to promote well-being and prevent disorder. In PA Linley, S Joseph, eds., *Positive Psychology in Practice.* Hoboken, NJ: Wiley; pp. 693–712.

Huesca R (2003) Participatory approaches to communication for development. In B Mody, ed., *International and Development Communication: a 21st-Century Perspective.* Thousand Oaks, CA: Sage; pp. 209–26.

Jenkins R, Üstün TB (1998) *Preventing Mental Illness: Mental Health Promotion in Primary Care.* Chichester: Wiley.

Jorm AF, Christensen H, Griffiths KM (2006) Changes in depression awareness and attitudes in Australia: the impact of beyondblue: the national depression initiative. *Australian and New Zealand Journal of Psychiatry* 40: 42–6.

Kato T, Yamanaka G, Kaiya H (1999) Efficacy of media in motivating patients with panic disorder to visit specialists. *Psychiatry and Clinical Neurosciences* 53: 523–6.

Kessler RC, Angermeyer M, Anthony JC, *et al.* (2007) Lifetime prevalence and age-of-onset distributions of mental disorders in the World Health Organization's World Mental Health Survey *Initiative World Psychiatry* 6: 168–76.

Klin A, Lemish D (2008) Mental disorders stigma in the media: review of studies on production, content, and influences. *Journal of Health Communication* 13: 434–49.

Lancet (2011) Global Mental Health Series. *Lancet*, October 17, 2011. http://www.thelancet.com/series/global-mental-health-2011 (accessed July 2013).

Lauber C, Nordt C, Falcato L, Rossler W (2003) Do people recognise mental illness? Factors influencing mental health literacy. *European Archives of Psychiatry and Clinical Neuroscience* 253: 248–51.

Latkin CA, Curry AD (2003) Stressful neighborhoods and depression: a prospective study of the impact of neighborhood disorder. *Journal of Health and Social Behavior*: 4: 34–44.

Leighton DC (1956) The distribution of symptoms in a small town, *American Journal of Psychiatry* 112: 716–23.

Mead M (1978) *Culture And Commitment: the New Relationships Between the Generations in the 1970s.* New York, NY: Columbia University Press.

Media Focus on Africa (2012) Media Focus on Africa. http://www.mediafocusonafrica.org (accessed July 2013).

Merrill Lynch (2000) The Knowledge Web. Merrill Lynch & Co.

Muñoz RF, Glish M, Soo-Hoo T, Robertson J (1982) The San Francisco mood survey project: preliminary work toward the prevention of depression. *American Journal of Community Psychology* 10: 317–29.

Muñoz RF, Lenert LL, Delucchi K, *et al.* (2005) Toward evidence-based internet interventions: a Spanish/English web site for international smoking cessation trials. *Nicotine and Tobacco Research* 8: 77–87.

Murray JP (2008) Media violence: the effects are both real and strong. *American Behavioral Scientist* 51: 1212–30.

Paykel ES, Tylee A, Wright A, *et al.* (1997) The Defeat Depression Campaign: psychiatry in the public arena. *American Journal of Psychiatry* **154**: 59–66.

Penn DL, Chamberlin C, Mueser KT (2003) The effects of a documentary film about schizophrenia on psychiatric stigma. *Schizophrenia Bulletin* **29**: 383–91.

PricewaterhouseCoopers (2011) *Global Entertainment and Media Outlook.* London: PwC. http://www.pwc.com/gx/en/global-entertainment-media-outlook/index.jhtml (accessed July 2013).

Raad voor Volksgezondheid en Zorg (2010) *Perspectief op Gezondheid 2020* Den Haag: RVZ.

Regier DA, Hirschfeld RMA, Goodwin FK, *et al.* (1988) The NIMH depression awareness, recognition, and treatment program: structure, aims, and scientific basis. *American Journal of Psychiatry* **145**: 1351–7.

Ritterfeld U, Jin SA (2006) Addressing media stigma for people experiencing mental illness using an entertainment-education strategy. *Journal of Health Psychology* **11**: 247–67.

Riva G, Baños R, Botella C, Wiederhold BK, Gaggioli A (2012) Positive technology: using interactive technologies to promote positive functioning. *Cyberpsychology, Behavior, and Social Networking* **15**: 69–77.

Rose G (2008) *Rose's Strategy of Preventive Medicine*, 2nd edn. Oxford: Oxford University Press.

Ruiter A, Abraham C, Kok G (2001) Scary warnings and rational precautions: a review of the psychology of fear appeals. *Psychology and Health* **16**: 613–30.

Sanders MR, Montgomery DT, Brechman-Toussaint ML (2000) The mass media and the prevention of child behavior problems: the evaluation of a television series to promote positive outcomes for parents and their children. *Journal*

of Child Psychology and Psychiatry and Allied Disciplines **41**: 939–48.

Sartorius N, Schulze H (2005) *Reducing the Stigma of Mental Illness.* Cambridge: Cambridge University Press.

Saugstad LF (1989) Age at puberty and mental illness: towards a neurodevelopmental aetiology of Kraepelin's endogenous psychoses. *British Journal of Psychiatry* **155**: 536–44.

Singhal A, Rogers EM (2004) The status of entertainment-education worldwide. In A Singhal, MJ Cody, EM Rogers, M Sabido, eds., *Entertainment-Education and Social Change: History, Research, and Practice.* Mahwah, NJ: Lawrence Erlbaum Associates; pp. 3–20.

Smit F, Cuijpers P, Oostenbrink J, *et al.* (2006) Costs of nine common mental disorders: implications for curative and preventive psychiatry. *Journal of Mental Health Policy and Economics* **9**: 193–200.

Stip E, Caron J, Mancini-Marie A (2006) General population perceptions and attitudes towards schizophrenia and bipolar disorder. *Primary Care and Community Psychiatry* **11**: 157–65.

Stuckler D, Basu S, Suhrcke M, Coutts A, McKee M (2009) The public health effect of economic crises and alternative policy responses in Europe: an empirical analysis. *Lancet* **374**: 315–23.

Substance Abuse and Mental Health Services Administration (2011) SAMHSA's social health hub. http://www.samhsa.gov/socialmedia/socialhealth.aspx (accessed July 2013).

Toffler A (1970) *Future Shock.* New York, NY: Random House.

Tully M (2010) An analysis of the Fist to Five for Change Strategy: impact of the program, mobile screenings, and facilitated workshops. Internal report, Media Focus on Africa, Nairobi, Kenya.

Tully M, Ekdale B (2010) Beyond "soap opera for social change": an analysis

of Kenya's *The Team*. Paper presented at the Association for Education in Journalism and Mass Communication Annual Convention Denver, Colorado August 4–8, 2010.

Twardzicki M (2008) Challenging stigma around mental illness and promoting social inclusion using the performing arts. *Journal of the Royal Society for the Promotion of Health* **128**: 68–72.

Usdin S, Singhal A, Shongwe T, Goldstein S, Shabalala A (2004) No short cuts in entertainment-education: designing Soul City step-by-step. In A Singhal, MJ Cody, EM Rogers, M Sabido, eds., *Entertainment-Education and Social Change: History, Research, and Practice.* Mahwah, NJ: Lawrence Erlbaum Associates; pp. 153–75.

Voelker R (1996) Depression awareness. *JAMA* **276**: 936.

Wahl OF (1992) Mass media images of mental illness: review of the literature. *Journal of Community Psychology* **20**: 343–52.

Warner R (2005) Local projects of the World Psychiatric Association Programme to Reduce Stigma and Discrimination. *Psychiatric Services* **56**: 570–5.

Whitehorn K (1989) The use of media in the promotion of mental health. *International Journal of Mental Health* **18**: 40–6.

World Health Organization (2008a) *Closing the gap in a generation: health equity through action on the social determinants of health. Final Report of the Commission on Social Determinants of Health.* Geneva: WHO.

World Health Organization (2008b) *mhGAP: Mental Health Gap Action Programme. Scaling up Care for Mental, Neurological, and Substance Use Disorders.* Geneva: WHO.

WSIS (2010) *World Summit on the Information Society*: WSIS Forum 2010. Document 2010. Geneva: WHO.

Chapter

Suicide and depression

38

Diego De Leo and Lay San Too

Introduction

Suicide is a complex and multicausal phenomenon. It has a strong association with mental disorders, particularly major depressive disorder. Suicidal behaviors (both fatal and non-fatal) in patients with mood disorders are determined by their severity. Suicidal acts likely occur during depressive episodes, less often during mixed states, and very rarely in hypomania. However, the prevalence of suicidal behaviors in depressive disorders might be over-represented as a result of the misdiagnosis of normal sadness as a psychiatric disorder. There is a large amount of evidence showing that antidepressants are effective in preventing suicidal behaviors in mood disorders, but their effect remains controversial in young patients. The reduction in suicide is more prominent when combining pharmacotherapy and psychotherapy, rather than either therapy alone. This chapter reports on the epidemiology of suicidal behaviors in each type of mood disorder, discusses the boundaries between sadness and depressive disorders in relation to suicide, and highlights possible prevention strategies for suicide in patients with mood disorders.

Mood disorders

Mood disorders are a leading public health problem worldwide. They are not only enormously detrimental to society and the economy and have negative consequences on personal and interpersonal circumstances (Richards 2011), but are also related to the fatal outcome of suicide. A meta-analysis of psychological autopsy studies published between 1990 and 2007 indicated that mood disorders are strongly predictive of suicide risk, particularly in women (OR = 12.95, 95% CI 3.06–54.83) but also in men (OR = 6.56, 95% CI 2.65–16.28) (Yoshimasu et al. 2008). Other reviews

demonstrated that mood disorders are the most life-threatening of psychiatric illnesses: approximately 90% of suicide cases are diagnosed with a psychiatric disorder, and almost half of these with a diagnosis of mood disorder (Bertolote et al. 2004; Arsenault-Lapierre et al. 2004). Nevertheless, there are still many individuals with a mood disorder who have never completed or attempted suicide. In 1970, Guze and Robins performed a review of studies on the suicide mortality of inpatients diagnosed with mood disorders, which indicated that, in general, an average of 15% of depressed patients complete suicide. However, Bostwick and Pankratz (2000) reassessed the lifetime prevalence of suicide in patients with mood disorders. They showed that the lifetime risk of suicide was 8.6% for hospitalized patients with suicidality, 4.0% for hospitalized patients without suicidality, 2.2% for mixed inpatients/outpatients, and 0.5% for non-depressed people. In terms of non-fatal outcomes, a cross-national analysis of mental disorders and suicidal behavior carried out in 21 countries with a total sample of 108 664 reported that major depressive disorder (MDD), dysthymic disorder (DD), and bipolar disorder (BD) each significantly contributed to the potential onset of a suicide attempt. The odd ratios ranged from 5.1 (DD), 5.8 (MDD) to 7.1 (BD) in developed countries and from 5.1 (MDD), 6.7 (BD) to 7.1 (DD) in developing countries (Nock et al. 2009).

Unipolar disorders

Unipolar disorders primarily include major depressive disorder and dysthymic disorder. Based on the *Diagnostic and Statistical Manual of Mental Disorders Fourth Edition (Text Revision) (DSM-IV-TR)* (American Psychiatric Association 2000), major depressive

Essentials of Global Mental Health, ed. Samuel O. Okpaku. Published by Cambridge University Press. © Cambridge University Press 2014.

disorder is a diagnosis determined by the presence of a specified number of symptoms for a duration of at least two weeks. The individual must have experienced symptoms primarily of either depressed mood or loss of interest or pleasure, and at least three of the following symptoms: disturbance of appetite or sleep, psychomotor agitation or retardation, inability to think, feelings of worthlessness and guilt, and suicidal thoughts and ideation. Dysthymic disorder is characterized by symptoms that are less severe than those for major depressive disorder, but persist for at least two years. It includes symptoms of depressed mood and two or more of the following: problems with appetite or sleep, low energy, low self-esteem, poor concentration, and feelings of hopelessness. An individual is not diagnosed if he/she is symptom-free for at least two months. A systematic review of the literature published between 1980 and 2000 revealed a lifetime prevalence of 6.7 per 100 for major depressive disorder and 3.6 per 100 for dysthymic disorder in the general population (Waraich *et al.* 2004).

As indicated by Rihmer's review (2007), the most predictive clinical risk factors for suicide in depressive disorders are major depressive episodes, while minor depression and pure dysthymic disorder are relatively rare among subjects who die by suicide and among attempters. A five-year prospective study examining suicidal behavior in Finnish patients with major depressive disorder showed that the prevalence of suicide attempt varied markedly depending on the state of depression, being highest during major depressive episodes (OR = 7.74, 95% CI 3.40–17.6) and four times higher during partial remission (OR = 4.20, 95% CI 1.71–10.3) than in full remission (Holma *et al.* 2010). Another prospective study on suicide incidence between 1947 and 2006 was conducted in the south of Sweden, revealing that depression played a major role in contributing to suicide (44%). In particular, severe depression with psychotic and/or melancholic features was diagnosed in 66% (19/29) of all cases of depression. Twenty-nine per cent (19/66) of all suicide victims had major depression with severe features, while 15% (10/66) had depression without these features (Bradvik *et al.* 2010).

The importance of the severity of the illness in the risk of suicide in depression was further emphasized by a study on a sample of American outpatients (Witte *et al.* 2009). This was the first study to distinguish between the predictive powers of the different forms of depressive illness (dysthymic disorder, single

episode of major depression, recurrent major depressive disorder, and double depression). A cluster analysis showed that only recurrent major depressive disorder exclusively contributed to an increased risk of suicide (B = 1.27, SE B = 0.27, p < 0.0001). Individuals with recurrent major depressive disorder were about three times more likely to be in the higher risk rather than lower risk cluster, even after controlling for the number of comorbid Axis I and Axis II diagnoses. By contrast, none of the other depressive diagnoses was identified as a significant risk factor for suicide (Witte *et al.* 2009).

Bipolar disorders

Bipolar disorder is characterized by alternating episodes of mania and depression over the course of life. A diagnosis of bipolar I disorder requires at least one manic or mixed episode, while a diagnosis of bipolar II disorder requires neither of these but at least one each of hypomanic and depressive episodes (DSM-IV-TR). A cross-sectional World Mental Health Survey was conducted in 11 countries with a sample of 61 392 adults to measure the prevalence of bipolar disorders using DSM-IV classifications (Merikangas *et al.* 2011). The findings demonstrated that the lifetime prevalence of bipolar I disorder, bipolar II disorder, and subthreshold bipolar disorder were 0.6%, 0.4%, and 1.4% respectively, while the 12-month prevalence was 0.4%, 0.3%, and 0.8% respectively. In total, the lifetime and 12-month prevalence of bipolar disorders was 2.4% and 1.5%, respectively (Merikangas *et al.* 2011).

Initial reports estimated that between 4% and 19% of patients with bipolar disorder would complete suicide, and between 25% and 60% would attempt suicide, at least once in their lifetimes (Goodwin & Jamison 1990). However, a more recent review concluded that incidence of both non-fatal and fatal suicidal behaviors in bipolar disorders (especially bipolar II disorders) is overestimated (Rihmer 2005). This was further highlighted in a 35-year (1965–99) longitudinal study on the suicide mortality of British patients with bipolar disorder (Dutta *et al.* 2007). The analyses showed that, compared to the general population, the standardized mortality ratio (SMR) for suicide was 9.77 (95% CI 4.22–19.24), higher than all other causes of death (SMR = 1.03, 95% CI 0.71–1.44). In particular, the suicide ratio for males was 12 times higher (SMR = 12.76, 95%

CI 5.13–26.29) and for females was four times higher (SMR = 4.27, 95% CI 0.11–23.78) than in the general population. Overall, only 2.5% of those with bipolar disorder eventually completed suicide, an incidence lower than commonly cited (Dutta *et al.* 2007). In 2010, Novick and colleagues performed a comprehensive meta-analytic review on suicide attempts in both bipolar I and bipolar II disorders. For bipolar II individuals, retrospective, prospective, and descriptive studies reported a lifetime history of suicide attempt in 32.4%, 19.8%, and 20.5%, of individuals, respectively. The difference in the prevalence of attempted suicide in bipolar II (32.4%) and bipolar I (36.3%) cases was not significant (OR = 1.21, 95% CI 0.98–1.48, $p = 0.07$).

Moreover, a prospective 18-month study examined the incidence of suicide attempts in different phases of bipolar disorder in Finnish inpatients and outpatients (Valtonen *et al.* 2008). In comparing the phases of the illness, the findings indicated that the incidence of suicide attempt was 37 times higher (95% CI 11.8–120.3) during combined mixed and depressive mixed states, and 18 times higher (95% CI 6.5–50.8) during major depressive phases. Both phases were independent predictors of suicide attempt. It was suggested that the overall risk for suicide attempt among bipolar disorder patients is likely to be determined by the amount of time in high-risk illness phases (Valtonen *et al.* 2008).

Sadness and suicidal behaviors

While suicidal behaviors are convincingly predicted by clinical depression, as indicated above, their association with "normal" sadness has been neglected and never properly examined. This is likely the result of the confusion between normal sadness and depressive disorders among contemporary psychiatrists and researchers. In 2007, Horwitz and Wakefield discussed this issue extensively and stressed that the increasing occurrence of major depressive disorder is not the consequence of a genuine rise in the prevalence of mental illnesses, but the result of a process of the medicalization of sadness in recent decades. This means that individuals with fluctuations in mood due to sadness as a physiological reaction to a life event would easily fulfill the symptomatic requirements for major depressive disorder in the DSM, and would then be misdiagnosed as mental disorder sufferers. Other consequences of this phenomenon include a

dramatic increase in the number of patients receiving treatment for depression, an increase in the prescription and sale of antidepressants, and an inflated estimate of the social and economic costs of depression (Horwitz & Wakefield 2007).

Horwitz and Wakefield (2007) hypothesize that normality and abnormality exist along a continuum: it is difficult to distinguish between them without knowing the internal mechanisms of response to loss. Nonetheless, normal sadness is mainly different from depression by the existence of a cause or context, such as negative life events. That is, normal sadness is context-specific, and reasonably proportional to the nature of the loss, and it either ends when the circumstances become better or when the individual adjusts to the new circumstances, or endures if the circumstances persist. On the other hand, clinical depression tends to be unnatural, dysfunctional, recurrent, chronic, and disproportionate to the loss, rather than context-specific and time-restricted.

The DSM excludes the bereavement of a loved one from the diagnosis of a major depressive disorder. However, apart from this type of loss, individuals encountering other life stressors (e.g., the ending of a romantic relationship, losing a valued job, or being diagnosed with a severe physical illness) similarly tend to experience symptoms such as depressed mood, sleep problems, a lack of interest in usual activities, an inability to concentrate, and reduced appetite that might naturally persist for a period of at least two weeks (American Psychiatric Association 2000). These symptoms easily meet the DSM criteria for a diagnosis of major depressive disorder, but they are neither abnormal nor inappropriate in light of the situation. Horwitz and Wakefield (2007, p. 14) highlighted that the fundamental flaw of the DSM concept of MDD is that it "fails to take into account the context of the symptoms and thus fails to exclude from the disorder category intense sadness, other than in reaction to the death of a loved one, that arises from the way human beings naturally respond to major losses."

Recently, a study investigated whether individuals were able to distinguish between normal sadness and clinical depression (Holzinger *et al.* 2011). People in Vienna were presented a vignette depicting a case of depression fulfilling the DSM-IV criteria. The vignette was provided either with or without information about preceding life stressors. It was found that, as opposed to the conceptualization in the DSM, people were less likely to perceive depressive symptoms caused from losses as an indication of a major depressive disorder, and less likely to recommend professional help in such circumstances. This seems to confirm that the DSM has mistakenly considered normal responses to loss as a mental disorder.

The partially flawed understanding of depression in the DSM and its use by contemporary clinicians deserves further attention, as it has important social, clinical, and scientific implications. Importantly, given that clinicians and scientists might fail to differentiate sadness from depression, the available literature on the prevalence of suicidal behaviors associated with depression may depict the relationship in a biased manner. While stressful life events may place an individual at risk of suicide (Logan *et al.* 2011), the normal response of sadness that can be "physiologically" tied to these stressors is likely associated with suicide. Therefore, it is possible that suicide rates attributed to depression are in fact inflated by the inclusion of non-pathological sadness in the diagnosis of depressive disorder. This highlights the significance of the need to distinguish between normal and abnormal human behavior in order to capture a more accurate picture and enable relevant organizations to develop effective suicide prevention initiatives. Similarly, particular attention should also be paid to the recent controversy over the pathologizing of "suicidal behavior," as there is insufficient scientific evidence available to support this, as discussed by De Leo (2011).

Suicide prevention for patients with mood disorders

It is challenging to prevent suicide in individuals diagnosed with mood disorders. As suicide is strongly associated with mood disorders, particularly major depressive episodes, the hypothesis that suicide could be prevented by the treatment of depression is certainly not implausible. In recent years, a growing amount of research has examined the effect of antidepressants on suicidal behaviors. As presented by Isacsson *et al.* (2010), ecological studies showed that the use of antidepressants was inversely associated with suicide rates in 40 countries (Australia, Sweden, Denmark, Finland, Great Britain, Hungary, Israel, Italy, Japan, New Zealand, Norway, Slovenia, the USA, and 27 other countries, with the exception of Iceland). Similarly, a 27-year observational study

conducted at five US academic medical centers found that the risk of suicidal behaviors was reduced by 20% among depressed patients who were prescribed antidepressants (OR = 0.80, 95% CI 0.68–0.95, $z = -2.54$, $p = 0.11$) (Leon *et al.* 2011). Other long-term observational studies revealed the degree of risk reduction to be more than 50% (Baldessarini *et al.* 2006, Guzzetta *et al.* 2007).

Nevertheless, a systematic review of 702 randomized controlled trials showed that, compared to other active treatments or a placebo, individuals prescribed with antidepressants were at double the risk of both fatal and non-fatal suicidal behaviors (Fergusson *et al.* 2005). This was particularly prominent in depressed adolescents. The opposite effect was found in depressed adults, especially those aged 65 or above (Barbui *et al.* 2009). The adverse effect of antidepressants in young people was further evidenced by a meta-analytic review indicating that the use of antidepressants such as paroxetine, sertraline, citalopram, and venlafaxine, but not fluoxetine, increased the risk of suicidal behaviors in children and adolescents with depression (Whittington *et al.* 2004). Further, selective serotonin reuptake inhibitors (SSRIs) were found not to significantly increase suicidality in individuals under 19 years of age (Isacsson *et al.* 2005). Similarly, a non-significant increase in the rate of suicide associated with SSRIs was found among Danish youths (Søndergård *et al.* 2006). Recently, a comprehensive review analyzed 130 studies (including ecological, cohort, case–control, and randomized controlled) on antidepressants and suicide risk published during the period 1965–2010 (Pompili *et al.* 2010). It emphasized that antidepressants generally contributed to a decrease in the risk of suicide in adults with major affective disorders, but that the controversy surrounding the potential suicidal risk caused by antidepressants in younger patients remains. Pompili *et al.* (2010) further explained that the latter phenomenon might be due to the possible presence of many unrecognized "pseudo-unipolar mixed states" in younger patients that could contribute to suicidality.

Different types of antidepressants/mood stabilizers seem to have different effects on suicidal behaviors in depressed patients (Pompili *et al.* 2010). In 2011, Moncrieff and Goldsmith investigated the psychoactive and physical effects of two commonly used antidepressants: fluoxetine and venlafaxine. They indicated that these antidepressants were rarely associated with suicidal thoughts, but that they were correlated with unpleasant emotional effects, which may account for increased suicidal impulses in some users. Another study comparing suicidal risk in adults taking venlafaxine, citalopram, fluoxetine, and dothiepin showed that patients taking venlafaxine were prone to a higher risk of suicide compared to those taking citalopram, fluoxetine, and dothiepin. However, adjustment for possible confounders substantially minimized the excess risks of venlafaxine (Rubino et al. 2007). Further, a review article on the effect of lithium treatment among patients with major affective disorders found an approximately 80% lower risk of suicidal behaviors during lithium treatment (for an average of 18 months), in both randomized and open clinical trials (Baldessarini et al. 2006). The favorable impact of lithium on suicide has also been observed in the general population, as found in an epidemiologic study that revealed a significant negative relationship between lithium levels in tap water in 18 Japanese municipalities and the suicide rate in each municipality for 2002–06 (Ohgami et al. 2009). A similar finding was found in a study across 99 Austrian districts, further demonstrating an inverse association between suicide and lithium levels in drinking water (Kapusta et al. 2011).

In 2001, O'Leary et al. reviewed 75 follow-up studies concerning the impacts of electroconvulsive therapy (ECT) and antidepressants on the rates of suicide in patients with mood disorders. It was found that the average suicide rate was 6.3 per 1000 for the pre-treatment era, 5.7 per 1000 for the ECT treatment era (1940–59), and 3.3 per 1000 for the antidepressant treatment era (from 1960 onward). This implies that the utilization of treatment – particularly antidepressants – helps in preventing suicide in depressed patients. Further, a review of controlled studies on the enhancement of treatment adherence among bipolar patients showed that interpersonal group therapy, cognitive behavioral therapy, group sessions for partners of bipolar patients, and psycho-education were effective in improving the compliance of patients and may indirectly reduce the rates of suicides (Sajatovic et al. 2004). This suggests that the decline in suicide rates in depressed patients was likely also the result of psychological interventions, rather than the increased use of antidepressants alone.

The advantages of combined pharmacotherapy and psychotherapy appear to be greater than those offered from either therapy alone. This was supported by an investigation on the impact of psychotherapies on suicide mortality between 1991 and 2005 in Austria, revealing an association between a fivefold increase in antidepressant sales and a twofold increase in the density of psychotherapists on the one hand and a decrease in overall suicide rates on the other (Kapusta et al. 2009). Rucci et al. (2002) examined the effects of adjunctive psychotherapy and long-term lithium therapy on suicidal behavior in bipolar patients, showing that bipolar patients who received both lithium and psychotherapy had a 17.5-fold decline in lifetime suicidal rate compared to the average rate for bipolar sufferers. However, no difference between specific psychotherapy and intensive clinical management (involving regular visits with empathetic clinicians) on patients receiving lithium was found, which may indicate that any of the psychosocial interventions is beneficial in reducing suicide rates.

Conclusions

Although mood disorders are a strong predictor of suicidal behaviors, most individuals diagnosed with these disorders have never attempted or completed suicide. Studies show that suicidal behaviors in patients with mood disorders are state-severity dependent, and are most likely to occur during major depressive episodes. However, the rate of suicidal behaviors in depressive disorders is possibly inflated by the misdiagnosis of normal sadness as a psychiatric disorder. This counters the suggestion that mood disorders are likely underdiagnosed and undertreated in the general population. It is important to clearly distinguish normal sadness and clinical depressive disorders, because inaccurate identification, and thus wrongly prescribed antidepressants, may bring short- or long-term undesired effects, including increased suicidal risk. The DSM needs to take into account cause and context in the criteria used to diagnose major depressive disorder.

There is ample evidence that antidepressants are generally effective in reducing suicidal behaviors in adults with major affective disorders, but the question of the risk of suicide caused by antidepressants in younger patients remains. This indicates that high-quality mental health care is of paramount importance in monitoring suicidality in young individuals prescribed with antidepressants. Nevertheless, the decline in suicide rates in recent years is not the result of pharmacotherapy alone, but likely also an indirect effect of psychotherapy. The effect is more evident in the combination of these therapies, as medicines may ease distress, making patients more receptive and compliant to psychosocial therapies in the long term.

Continued efforts to improve early detection and assessment, as well as pharmacotherapy and psychotherapy, are required to sustain the decline in self-destructive behaviors.

References

American Psychiatric Association (2000) *Diagnostic and Statistical Manual of Mental Disorders, Fourth Edition Revised (DSM-IV-TR)*. Washington, DC: APA.

Arsenault-Lapierre G, Kim C, Turecki G (2004) Psychiatric diagnoses in 3275 suicides: a meta-analysis. *BMC Psychiatry* **4**: 37.

Baldessarini RJ, Tondo L, Davis P, *et al.* (2006) Decreased risk of suicides and attempts during long-term lithium treatment: a meta-analytic review. *Bipolar Disorders* **8**: 625–39.

Barbui C, Esposito E, Cipriani A (2009) Selective serotonin reuptake inhibitors and risk of suicide: a systematic review of observational studies. *Canadian Medical Association Journal* **180**: 291–7.

Bertolote JM, Fleischmann A, De Leo D, *et al.* (2004) Psychiatric diagnoses and suicide: revisiting the evidence. *Crisis* **25**: 147–55.

Bostwick JM, Pankratz VS (2000) Affective disorders and suicide risk: a reexamination. *American Journal of Psychiatry* **157**: 1925–32.

Bradvik L, Mattisson C, Bogren M, *et al.* (2010) Mental disorders in suicide and undetermined death in the lundby study. The contribution of severe depression and alcohol dependence. *Archives of Suicide Research* **14**: 266–75.

De Leo D (2011) DSM-V and the future of suicidology. *Crisis* **32**: 233–9.

Dutta R, Boydell J, Kennedy N, *et al.* (2007) Suicide and other causes of mortality in bipolar disorder: a longitudinal study. *Psychological Medicine* **37**: 839–47.

Fergusson D, Doucette S, Cranley K, *et al.* (2005) Association between suicide attempts and selective serotonin reuptake inhibitors: systematic review of randomised controlled trials. *BMJ* **330**: 396–9.

Goodwin FK, Jamison KR (1990) Suicide. In *Manic-Depressive Illness*. NewYork, NY: Oxford University Press; pp. 227–44.

Guze SB, Robins E (1970) Suicide and primary affective of major affective disorder. *British Journal of Psychiatry* **117**: 437–8.

Guzzetta F, Tondo L, Centorrino F, *et al.* (2007) Lithium treatment reduces suicide risk in recurrent major depressive disorder. *Journal of Clinical Psychiatry* **68**: 380–3.

Holma KM, Melartin TK, Haukka J, *et al.* (2010) Incidence and predictors of suicide attempts in dsm-iv major depressive disorder: a five-year prospective study. *American Journal of Psychiatry* **167**: 801–8.

Holzinger A, Matschinger H, Schomerus G, *et al.* (2011) The loss of sadness: the public's view. *Acta Psychiatrica Scandinavica* **123**: 307–13.

Horwitz A and Wakefield J (2007) *The Loss of Sadness: How Psychiatry Transformed Normal Sorrow Into Depressive Disorder*. New York, NY: Oxford University Press.

Isacsson G, Holmgren P, Ahlner J (2005) Selective serotonin reuptake inhibitor antidepressants and the risk of suicide: a controlled forensic database study of 14,857 suicides. *Acta Psychiatrica Scandinavica* **111**: 286–90.

Isacsson G, Rich CL, Jureidini J, *et al.* (2010) The increased use of antidepressants has contributed to the worldwide reduction in suicide rates. *British Journal of Psychiatry* **196**: 429–33.

Kapusta ND, Niederkrotenthaler T, Etzersdorfer E, *et al.* (2009) Influence of psychotherapist density and antidepressant sales on suicide rates. *Acta Psychiatrica Scandinavica* **119**: 236–42.

Kapusta ND, Mossaheb N, Etzersdorfer E, *et al.* (2011) Lithium in drinking water and suicide mortality. *British Journal of Psychiatry* **198**: 346–50.

Leon AC, Solomon DA, Li CS, *et al.* (2011) Antidepressants and risks of suicide and suicide attempts: a 27-year observational study. *Journal of Clinical Psychiatry* **72**: 580–6.

Logan J, Hall J, Karch D (2011) Suicide categories by patterns of known risk factors a latent class analysis. *Archives of General Psychiatry* **68**: 935–41.

Ohgami H, Terao T, Shiotsuki I, *et al.* (2009) Lithium levels in drinking water and risk of suicide. *British Journal of Psychiatry* **194**: 464–5.

O'Leary D, Paykel E, Todd C, *et al.* (2001) Suicide in primary affective disorders revisited: A systematic review by treatment era. *Journal of Clinical Psychiatry* **62**: 804–11.

Merikangas KR Jin R, He JP, *et al.* (2011) Prevalence and correlates of bipolar spectrum disorder in the world mental health survey initiative. *Archives of General Psychiatry* **68**: 241–51.

Moncrieff J, Goldsmith L (2011) The psychoactive effects of antidepressants and their association with suicidality. *Current Drug Safety* **6**: 115–21.

Nock MK, Hwang I, Sampson N, *et al.* (2009) Cross-national analysis of the associations among mental disorders and suicidal behavior: findings from the who world mental health surveys. *Plos Medicine* **6** (8): e1000123.

Novick DM, Swartz HA, Frank E (2010) Suicide attempts in bipolar i and bipolar ii disorder: A review and meta-analysis of the evidence. *Bipolar Disorders* **12**: 1–9.

Pompili M, Serafini G, Innamorati M, *et al.* (2010) Antidepressants and suicide risk: a comprehensive overview. *Pharmaceuticals* **3**: 2861–83.

Richards D (2011) Prevalence and clinical course of depression: A review. *Clinical Psychology Review* **31**, 1117–1125.

Rihmer Z (2005) Prediction and prevention of suicide in bipolar disorders. *Clinical Neuropsychiatry* **2**: 48–54.

Rihmer Z (2007) Suicide risk in mood disorders. *Current Opinion in Psychiatry* **20**: 17–22.

Rubino A, Roskell N, Tennis P, *et al.* (2007) Risk of suicide during treatment with venlafaxine, citalopram, fluoxetine, and dothiepin: Retrospective cohort study. *BMJ* **334**: 242–5.

Rucci P, Frank E, Kostelnik B, *et al.* (2002) Suicide attempts in patients with bipolar i disorder during acute and maintenance phases of intensive treatment with pharmacotherapy and adjunctive psychotherapy. *American Journal of Psychiatry* **159**: 1160–4.

Sajatovic M, Davies M, Hrouda DR (2004) Enhancement of treatment adherence among patients with bipolar disorder. *Psychiatric Services* **55**: 264–9.

Søndergård L, Kvist K, Andersen PK, *et al.* (2006) Do antidepressants precipitate youth suicide? *European Child and Adolescent Psychiatry* **15**: 232–40.

Valtonen HM, Suominen K, Haukka J, *et al.* (2008) Differences in incidence of suicide attempts during phases of bipolar i and ii disorders. *Bipolar Disorders* **10**: 588–96.

Waraich P, Goldner EM, Somers JM, *et al.* (2004) Prevalence and incidence studies of mood disorders: a systematic review of the literature. *Canadian Journal of Psychiatry* **49**: 124–38.

Witte TK, Timmons KA, Fink E, *et al.* (2009) Do major depressive disorder and dysthymic disorder confer differential risk for suicide? *Journal of Affective Disorders* **115**: 69–78.

Whittington CJ, Kendall T, Fonagy P, *et al.* (2004) Selective serotonin reuptake inhibitors in childhood depression: Systematic review of published versus unpublished data. *Lancet* **363**: 1341–5.

Yoshimasu K, Kiyohara C, Miyashita K (2008) Suicidal risk factors and completed suicide: Meta-analyses based on psychological autopsy studies. *Environmental Health and Preventive Medicine* **13**: 243–56.

Chapter

39

Violence as a public health problem

Claire van der Westhuizen, Katherine Sorsdahl, Gail Wyatt, and Dan J. Stein

Introduction

Violence and its consequences have a profound impact on global health. More than 1.6 million people die annually due to violence, with 90% of these deaths occurring in low- and middle-income countries (LMICs) (World Health Organization 2008), where health systems are less equipped to cope with the burden of injuries. Violence affects millions of people globally by contributing significantly to mental and physical disability throughout the lifespan. The effect of violence on mental health is enormous, and the role of poor mental health in the perpetuation of violence in society is a much-debated topic (Arseneault et al. 2000, Elbogen & Johnson 2009). A public health approach offers a vital solution insofar as it focuses on preventing violence, promoting mental health, and mitigating the impact of the existing disease burden.

Mental health professionals have a vital role to play in preventing violence and responding to the existing disease burden, although this role is not often recognized. In the past, violence has predominantly been relegated to the jurisdiction of the criminal justice system. If we are to make any progress in preventing violence and reducing its consequences, a number of sectors (including the health sector) must be mobilized in order to produce a coordinated, effective solution. This chapter will focus on providing an overview of violence in its different forms, its impact, and opportunities for preventing violence, but with a particular emphasis on the role of the mental health practitioner.

We will begin by describing a theoretical framework that views violence as a preventable public health problem. Then we review the literature on the prevalence and implications of violence, followed by a description of risk and protective factors. Thereafter, the literature available on effective evidence-based interventions will be discussed.

Theoretical framework

From a public health viewpoint, violence is regarded as a preventable problem that can potentially be solved by a joint effort from a number of disciplines, with leadership from the health sector. The World Health Organization (WHO) offers a useful definition of violence:

> The intentional use of physical force or power, threatened or actual, against oneself, another person, or against a group or community, that either results in or has a high likelihood of resulting in injury, death, psychological harm, maldevelopment or deprivation.
>
> (WHO Global Consultation on Violence and Health 1996)

Four public health steps have been used successfully to tackle a number of health threats, and these are equally applicable to violence (Mercy et al. 1993):

- defining the problem (data collection and surveillance)
- identifying causes and risk factors
- developing and testing interventions
- implementing and monitoring interventions

Public health aims to make a population-wide impact on a health problem. The ecological model (Figure 39.1) has been utilized effectively by WHO to categorize risk and protective factors and plan interventions for health issues, including violence prevention.

Essentials of Global Mental Health, ed. Samuel O. Okpaku. Published by Cambridge University Press. © Cambridge University Press 2014.

Risk factors for violent behavior are not confined to any one age group or context. Thus, different life-stage categories are often combined with the ecological model when mapping risk factors and intervention opportunities. For example, nurse-led home visiting impacts parent–child relationships, influencing young children at the relationship level, while social marketing campaigns promoting gender equality target an adult audience at a society level (World Health Organization 2010). Within the ecological levels of impact various types of violence may be targeted.

The WHO typology of violence (Figure 39.2) distinguishes between different types of violence using the context and type of relationship between the victim and the perpetrator. Within these categories

various "methods" of violence may be identified. While such a typology provides a useful approach to the broad issue of violence, it must be stressed that the types of violence are not mutually exclusive, and often share common risk factors and consequences. Additionally, despite vast cultural differences across the globe, some risk and protective factors for violence may be identified in many different settings (for example, poverty) (Lund *et al.* 2010), while some factors are confined to certain cultures or communities (for example, the practice of female genital mutilation) (UNICEF 2005).

Prevalence of violence

Violence is a global phenomenon, yet there are vast differences in prevalence rates across geographical regions, income per capita groupings of countries, gender and age groups. The WHO African and Eastern Mediterranean regions appear to experience the highest rates of overall violence, with LMICs reporting a greater burden of violence than high-income countries (HICs). For every one death due to violence in an HIC, nine people die in an LMIC (World Health Organization 2008).

Globally, men are considerably more affected by violence, with 32.9 violent deaths per 100 000 males, compared to 11.8 per 100 000 females (World Health Organization 2011b). With the exception of the 0–4-year age group, the gap in mortality rates

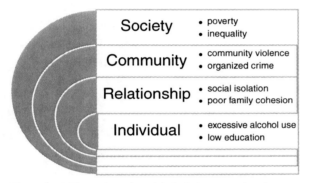

Figure 39.1 The ecological model, displaying examples of cross-cutting risk factors for violence and poor mental health.

A typology of violence

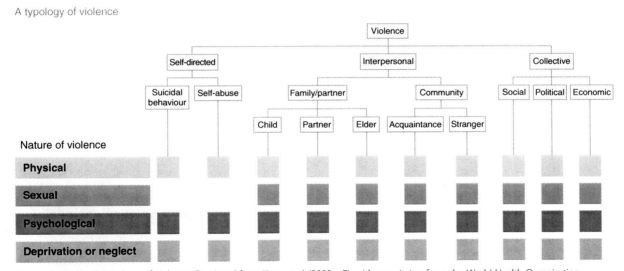

Figure 39.2 WHO typology of violence. Reprinted from Krug *et al.* (2002 p.7), with permission from the World Health Organization.

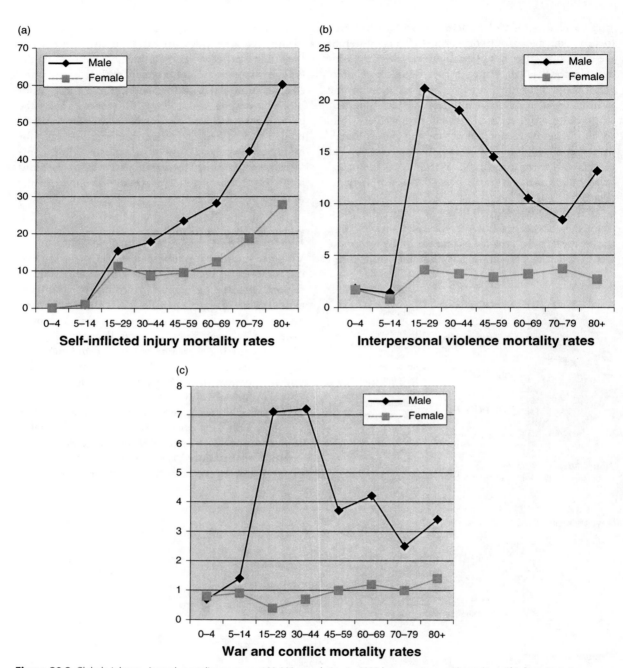

Figure 39.3 Global violence. Annual mortality rates per 100 000 population in 2008 by age group and gender: self-inflicted injuries, interpersonal violence injuries, and injuries due to war and conflict. Compiled using WHO data (World Health Organization 2011a).

between males and females is substantial. Young people are most at risk for all types of violence, especially in the 15–44-year age group, although there is a peak in self-directed violence after the age of 60 (Figure 39.3).

Burden of disease and implications of violence

Mortality rates and absolute numbers of deaths are often used to indicate the severity of a public health issue, yet these figures only partially illuminate the problem. It has been estimated that for every death due to interpersonal violence, there are approximately 28 serious injuries requiring medical care (World Health Organization 2008). Yet non-fatal injury data are often difficult to find, since many countries do not have injury surveillance systems in place (Krug *et al.* 2002). Data on non-fatal injuries, and particularly on various violence types such as self-inflicted injuries, child abuse, elder abuse, and sexual violence, are particularly scarce. There are a number of reasons for this lack of accurate data, including stigma (resulting in under-reporting) (Krug *et al.* 2002), the acceptance of violence as a cultural norm (for example, "honor killings") (Korteweg & Yurdakul 2009), and elder abuse victims being "misdiagnosed" as suffering from a physical illness (Lachs & Pillemer 2004). Data on non-fatal injuries due to war or conflict are also often incomplete due to the chaotic nature of the conflict environment. This involves the breakdown of public services, including two sectors often involved in mortality and injury data collection: health care and policing. Lack of accurate data is a barrier to an effective response to this public health problem.

Disability-adjusted life years (DALYs) attempt to depict the impact of a disease process or injury type on a population by quantifying the number of healthy life years lost to a certain cause. Globally, the list of DALYS is dominated by infectious and non-communicable diseases, with interpersonal violence ranked 18th, accounting for 1.4% of total DALYs (World Health Organization 2008). The impact of the combined violence figures (interpersonal violence, self-inflicted injuries, and war and conflict) would bring the ranking up to sixth, just behind HIV/AIDS. Thus, violence makes a considerable impact on global health, and in addition there are many "hidden" implications of injuries due to violence.

Physical disability, death, and economic implications have been investigated previously, but many sequelae of violence are not so easily quantified. A group of injury prevention researchers developed the LOAD framework to address this gap in the injury prevention literature (Lyons *et al.* 2010). In this framework (Figure 39.4), the ecological approach helps to frame the consequences of injury by using the society, family, and individual categories, while the community category is not included.

Violence in a society ("society" in the Figure 39.4) impacts many members of the society, even those who were not victims or witnesses. International terrorism provides such an example. Research in the United States a few days after the 9/11 terrorist attacks in 2001 showed significant emotional distress present in 44% of American individuals contacted for the study, with 90% reporting at least low levels of stress related to the attacks (Schuster *et al.* 2001). Major incidents, such as the 9/11 terrorist attacks, as well as more localized ongoing violence, have a profound impact on society and on communities.

The community level is absent from the framework shown in Figure 39.4, but community violence may considerably affect community health and economic behaviors. Studies have suggested that violence (and fear of violence) in a community may be associated with increased risky health behaviors, such as smoking and excessive drinking (Vermeiren *et al.* 2003), as well as decreasing beneficial health behaviors, such as exercising outdoors and traveling further to access healthy food (Harrison *et al.* 2007). In turn, these behaviors lead to an increased risk for a number of non-communicable diseases, such as diabetes mellitus and ischemic heart disease. Community violence impacts the health of communities in various ways, and inevitably infiltrates the home. Family and close friends of a violence victim may be exposed to stressors related to the injury scenario, recovery, and disability of the victim.

Children ("family" in the figure) exposed to inter-parental violence in the home, even in the absence of child abuse, appear to be vulnerable to developing psychological problems later in life. These problems include depression, alcohol dependence, perpetration of family violence, or vulnerability to victimization due to family violence (Roustit *et al.* 2009).

For the victim of violence ("individual" in the figure), psychological consequences of the injury scenario, pain, and other factors may result in serious functional impairment, which may be identified throughout the lifespan. In the US National Comorbidity Survey Replication, childhood adversities (specifically "maladaptive family functioning" adversities) were associated with 44.6% of all childhood-onset disorders and 25.9–32.0% of disorders with onset after childhood (Green *et al.* 2010). Maladaptive family functioning adversities were identified by the researchers as: parental mental disorder, substance use disorder, and criminality; physical abuse; sexual abuse; neglect and family violence. In particular, child sexual abuse (CSA) has been found to be associated

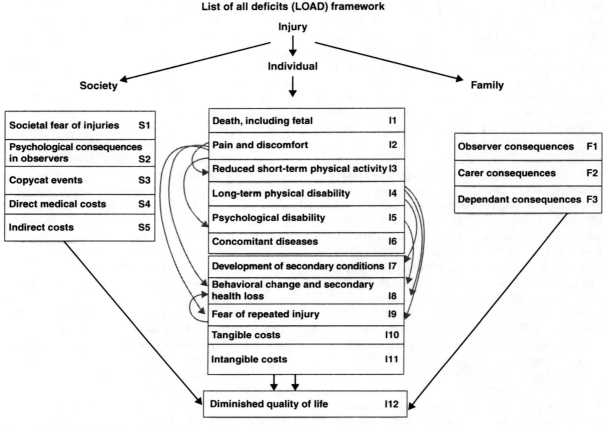

Figure 39.4 List of all deficits (LOAD) framework, reproduced from Lyons *et al.* (2010).

with long-term, serious health outcomes in both female and male victims (Dube *et al.* 2005). These outcomes include psychiatric disorders, substance abuse, sexual dysfunction, and vulnerability to repeat sexual victimization (Molnar *et al.* 2001, Paolucci *et al.* 2001, Loeb *et al.* 2002, Classen *et al.* 2005). The World Health Report of 2002 estimated that CSA accounted for 33% of post-traumatic stress disorder (PTSD) in females and 21% of PTSD in males. CSA was also estimated to play a significant role in the development of panic disorders, suicidality, mood disorders, and substance abuse (World Health Organization 2002).

Whether or not victims of CSA will experience these negative outcomes, and to what extent they experience them, may depend on the severity of CSA and the relationship proximity of the perpetrator to the victim. More severe forms of CSA involve attempted or actual penetration by an object, digit, or penis;

repeated incidents; and the perpetrator being a family member (Beitchman *et al.* 1992, Merrill *et al.* 2003). In a study involving ethnic-minority women in the USA, for example, Glover *et al.* (2010) found that more severe CSA predicted higher levels of post-traumatic stress symptoms. Negative reactions to disclosure of the abuse may also be associated with an increase in PTSD symptom severity. Using the ecological model, the impact of violence can be identified at many levels. The consequences of violence at these levels then place individuals at risk of violent experiences.

Risk and protective factors

Violence is "endemic" in society and has far-reaching implications. The public health approach maintains that violence is preventable, and that in seeking to understand violence one must understand the factors which place individuals or groups at risk for violence victimization or perpetration. Yet individuals or groups exposed to similar risk factors do not all react in the same way. Recently, the idea of protective factors for violence has attracted much attention, with research being published on topics such as violence, mental health, and social capital (McIlwaine & Moser 2001, Harpham *et al.* 2004). This section will focus on individual, relationship, community, and societal factors.

Individual factors

In the violence prevention arena, much research focuses on opportunities within the individual level of the ecological model, such as excessive use of alcohol by victims and perpetrators in various violence scenarios (Collins & Messerschmidt 1993), and demographic factors such as education and income levels. More recently, biological factors have been implicated in predicting or contributing to the development of aggressive behavior. These factors include hormone levels and function (Carré *et al.* 2011), brain executive function (Moffitt & Henry 1989), and genotypes or gene–environment interactions (Widom & Brzustowicz 2006).

The link between individual risk factors and aggressive behavior is often mediated through an individual's mental health. For example, an individual exposed to a neurological insult such as birth trauma (Kandel & Mednick 1991) may suffer neurocognitive deficits placing him or her at risk for future aggressive behavior (Chiodo *et al.* 2004). Gene–environment interactions have been studied for various genes linked to delinquency and aggression: for example, the monoamine oxidase A (MAOA) gene (Kim-Cohen *et al.* 2006). An individual carrying a polymorphism of a certain gene who is exposed to abuse in childhood could be at risk for impulsivity, placing the person at risk for developing aggressive behavior.

Previous exposure to violence is a risk factor not only for poor mental health, but also for future violence victimization or perpetration. Studies conducted internationally have found that sexual violence in children was strongly associated with later suicidal ideation (Beitchman *et al.* 1992, Brown *et al.* 2009). Individuals with a history of violent behavior, particularly those with a mental disorder such as schizophrenia or a personality disorder, have been found to be more at risk for future violence perpetration (Arseneault *et al.* 2000). Links have been reported between perpetration of intimate partner violence

(IPV) and mood disorders (among others) in the perpetrator, as well as between IPV and psychosis or antisocial personality disorder (Kessler *et al.* 2001). IPV not only affects the protagonists, but may have a profound impact on other members of the household, ultimately conferring violence risk on those members.

Relationship factors

Relationships have been shown to confer risk or protection for an individual's later exposure to violence. The presence and quality of relationships in an individual's life may be protective or damaging. For example, a young person's interaction with delinquent peers may have deleterious consequences.

Limited interpersonal relationships and living alone contribute to an individual's suicide risk in the presence of other factors, most notably mental disorders (Cheng *et al.* 2000). In the elderly, a lack of (or few) interpersonal relationships constitutes a risk factor for elder abuse in these vulnerable individuals; although in some studies living alone has been found to be a protective factor, as potential perpetrators have limited access to the individual (Lachs *et al.* 1997). Individuals exposed to other family members' unhealthy or violent interpersonal relationships are also placed at risk. Male children who witness IPV against their mothers have an increased risk for perpetrating IPV later in life (Abrahams *et al.* 2004).

The recent surge of interest in protective factors and resilience has led to research into family factors such as family functioning and parental support of youth as protective factors in youth violence. Even in violent communities, family factors may confer some protection on youth regarding reducing exposure to violence in the community, and mitigating the effects of exposure to community violence (Gorman-Smith *et al.* 2004). Factors from the different levels of the ecological level interact to modify the risk profile of individuals and groups of individuals.

Community factors

An individual's environment has a profound effect on his or her development and daily functioning. Positive social capital in a community appears to mitigate risk factors for both poor mental health and violent behavior (Harpham *et al.* 2004). Social capital has been described as "the stock of investments, resources and networks that produce social cohesion, trust and a willingness to engage in community activities"

(Lynch & Kaplan 1997). These "investments, resources and networks" appear to mitigate the effects of negative life events and stressors (including violence) on the mental health of an individual and a community (Harpham *et al.* 2002), although it seems that not all types of social capital are positive.

Some researchers studying violence and social capital in South America have commented on the occurrence of "perverse social capital" in the form of organized crime and gangs. These groups often perpetrate violence in a community, contributing to fear and distrust and thereby eroding the "productive social capital" (Rubio 1997). For many young people in such a community the benefits of this perverse social capital include survival and social inclusion (McIlwaine & Moser 2001). Increased exposure to community violence, such as gang violence, acts as a risk factor for violent behavior, violent victimization, and poor mental health (Fowler *et al.* 2009). These factors then contribute to further decreasing social capital and fueling violence in a community. Various socioeconomic factors such as rapid urbanization, social disorganization, and income inequality have also been implicated in the escalation of individual and collective community violence (Krug *et al.* 2002).

Economic factors feature prominently in the mental health and violence prevention literature. Previously, poverty alone has been cited as an important driver of these issues, but it appears that income inequality in a community or geographical area has a stronger association with poor mental health and violence outcomes (Lund *et al.* 2010). Many of the socioeconomic stressors affecting communities are directly linked to broader socioeconomic issues affecting societies globally.

Societal factors

The effects of social norms, and economic and political trends, may be seen globally and in the lives of individuals, even affecting violent behavior. For example, women are more at risk for IPV victimization in societies where they occupy a subservient position in the family, community, and society (Taft *et al.* 2009, Uthman *et al.* 2009). The role of economics is illustrated by the far-reaching effects of the recent economic crisis. Researchers in Greece reported an increase in suicidal behavior associated with high economic distress (Economou *et al.* 2011). In the United Kingdom, the government's response to the prevailing

economic climate played a role in sparking the 2011 riots (Baker 2011). An international organization such as the WHO, a government, or an individual politician may be instrumental in shaping a policy approach to a particular problem. National policies and strategies are vital in tackling any large-scale public health issue. The treatment gap in global mental health is a symptom of a paucity of national mental health policies and strategies (Eaton *et al.* 2011). Without the integration of mental health services into primary health care, health services will remain suboptimal, and a vital part of the violence prevention approach will be missing. Public opinion can also shape the politics of a nation or region, and has recently played a role in the conflict in the Middle East and North Africa.

The so-called "Arab Spring" has swept across these regions since its inception in Tunisia in December 2010. In these conflicts and in the United Kingdom riots, opinions expressed on social media platforms did much to fuel the actions of groups of people. The instant mobilization of numerous young individuals (online and geographically) brought a new dimension to collective action. Other factors in societies, such as attitudes and norms, influence various behaviors including firearm carrying, positive and negative interactions between spouses, and alcohol consumption (World Health Organization 2010).

Understanding the risk and protective factors associated with violence provides valuable insight into developing targeted interventions for at-risk groups. The next section will describe evidence-based interventions for reducing violence, with the exception of interventions preventing self-inflicted injuries (see Chapter 38), and mental health interventions during war and conflict (see Chapter 32), as these are beyond the scope of this chapter.

Evidence-based interventions to reduce violence

Although a multitude of interventions for violence prevention have been proposed, and in some cases implemented, a lack of evidence still remains. Particularly in resource-limited developing countries, it is vital that only interventions with the highest chance of success be implemented, and that existing interventions be monitored to ensure fidelity to the intervention and ongoing effectiveness.

A recent WHO publication outlined evidence-based interventions for interpersonal violence spread across the different levels of the ecological model and the different life stages (World Health Organization 2010). Many of the interventions necessitate a mental health approach, with the majority showing positive mental health outcomes for the intervention participants or recipients.

The seven proposed violence prevention strategies are:

- developing safe, stable and nurturing relationships between children and their parents and caregivers
- developing life skills in children and adolescents
- reducing the availability and harmful use of alcohol
- reducing access to guns, knives, and pesticides
- promoting gender equality to prevent violence against women
- changing cultural and social norms that support violence
- victim identification, care and support programs

Mental health professionals must play a leading role in the last group of interventions, namely those involved in "victim identification, care and support programs." The other intervention strategies focus on the primary prevention of violence, while the last strategy comes into play after the violent incident. Thus the violence prevention role of these interventions appears limited; yet the appropriate and effective management of these victims and their families is instrumental in limiting the impact of violence and preventing future violent events.

Functions of mental health professionals in the post-injury context include screening for mental disorders, psychiatric treatment, psychotherapy, etc. Mental health professionals can provide invaluable training and support for primary healthcare staff in screening for, and basic treatment of, mental disorders. After the violent incident, there are also numerous opportunities for involving other disciplines in patient care and violence prevention. Primary healthcare professionals should be trained to recognize and screen for various types of violence, such as IPV and elder abuse. Liaison with local schools in the management of bullying or vulnerable youths may be

beneficial. Social problems will benefit from the involvement of a social worker (World Health Organization 2010). Anonymized data from the primary healthcare unit can be used to alert local crime prevention officials to "hot spots" where increased security is needed (Florence et al. 2011). Members of the medical community can be involved in advocacy for violence prevention and improved mental health services. A medical perspective is an effective tool in communicating with the public and policy makers on these issues. The gaps in scope of practice, data, and research hamper the development of policies and interventions, and patient care.

Conclusion

In many countries, especially LMICs, injury data are scarce. Within countries, mortality data collection is patchy and non-fatal injury figures are even more difficult to find. Data collection seems to be the most efficient and accurate where various data sources are combined. Injury surveillance is a vital part of any health system (Krug et al. 2002).

Further research is needed in many different areas of violence and in many geographical regions. "Male-on-male" violence has been neglected in many countries, despite the overwhelming numbers of young men being injured in violent incidents. Other violence types, such as elder absue, are under-researched. Injury and mental health research in developing countries is lagging behind the developed world, with the bulk of resources devoted to research being allocated to infectious diseases (Hofman et al. 2005). The monitoring and evaluation of interventions is also lacking in many areas, and novel methodologies are required.

We have argued here that the mental health community must be an integral part of the public health approach to violence prevention in order to provide effective solutions. Success in the violence prevention arena will have a positive impact on the mental health of a population, and improved mental health service delivery can greatly benefit the field of violence prevention.

References

Abrahams N, Jewkes R, Hoffman M, et al. (2004) Sexual violence against intimate partners in Cape Town: prevalence and risk factors reported

by men. *Bulletin of the World Health Organization* 82: 330–7.

Arseneault L, Moffitt TE, Caspi A, et al. (2000) Mental disorders and violence in a total birth cohort:

results from the Dunedin study. *Archives of General Psychiatry* 57: 979–86.

Baker SA (2011) The mediated crowd: new social media and new forms of rioting. *Sociological Research Online* **16**: 21.

Beitchman JH, Zucker KJ, Hood JE, *et al.* (1992) A review of the long-term effects of child sexual abuse. *Child Abuse and Neglect* **16**: 101–18.

Brown DW, Riley L, Butchart A, *et al.* (2009) Exposure to physical and sexual violence and adverse health behaviours in African children: results from the Global School-based Student Health Survey. *Bulletin of the World Health Organization* **87**: 447–55.

Carré JM, McCormick CM, Hariri AR (2011) The social neuroendocrinology of human aggression. *Psychoneuroendocrinology* **36**: 935–44.

Cheng ATA, Chen THH, Chen C, *et al.* (2000) Psychosocial and psychiatric risk factors for suicide. *British Journal of Psychiatry* **177**: 360–5.

Chiodo LM, Jacobson SW, Jacobson JL (2004) Neurodevelopmental effects of postnatal lead exposure at very low levels. *Neurotoxicology and Teratology* **26**: 359–71.

Classen CC, Palesh OG, Aggarwal R (2005) Sexual revictimization: a review of the empirical literature. *Trauma, Violence, and Abuse* **6**: 103–29.

Collins JJ, Messerschmidt PM (1993) Epidemiology of alcohol-related violence. *Alcohol Health and Research World* **17**: 93–100.

Dube SR, Anda RF, Whitfield CL, *et al.* (2005) Long-term consequences of childhood sexual abuse by gender of victim. *American Journal of Preventive Medicine* **28**: 430–8.

Eaton J, McCay L, Semrau M, *et al.* (2011) Scale up of services for mental health in low-income and middle-income countries. *Lancet* **278**: 1592–603.

Economou M, Madianos M, Theleritis C, *et al.* (2011) Increased suicidality amid economic crisis in Greece. *Lancet* **378**: 1459.

Elbogen EB, Johnson SC (2009) The intricate link between violence and mental disorder: results from the National Epidemiologic Survey on Alcohol and Related Conditions. *Archives of General Psychiatry* **66**: 152–61.

Florence C, Shepherd J, Brennan I, *et al.* (2011) Effectiveness of anonymised information sharing and use in health service, police, and local government partnership for preventing violence related injury: experimental study and time series analysis. *BMJ* **342**: d3313.

Fowler PJ, Tompsett CJ, Braciszewski JM, *et al.* (2009) Community violence: a meta-analysis on the effect of exposure and mental health outcomes of children and adolescents. *Development and Psychopathology* **21**: 227–59.

Glover DA, Loeb TB, Carmona JV, *et al.* (2010) Childhood sexual abuse severity and disclosure predict posttraumatic stress symptoms and biomarkers in ethnic minority women. *Journal of Trauma and Dissociation* **11**: 152–73.

Gorman-Smith D, Henry DB, Tolan PH (2004) Exposure to community violence and violence perpetration: the protective effects of family functioning. *Journal of Clinical Child and Adolescent Psychology* **33**: 439–49.

Green JG, McLaughlin KA, Berglund PA, *et al.* (2010) Childhood adversities and adult psychiatric disorders in the National Comorbidity Survey Replication I: associations with first onset of DSM-IV disorders. *Archives of General Psychiatry* **67**: 113–23.

Harpham T, Grant E, Thomas E (2002) Measuring social capital within health surveys: key issues. *Health Policy and Planning* **17**: 106–11.

Harpham T, Grant E, Rodriguez C (2004) Mental health and social capital in Cali, Colombia. *Social Science and Medicine* **58**, 2267–77.

Harrison RA, Gemmell I, Heller RF (2007) The population effect of crime and neighbourhood on physical activity: an analysis of 15 461 adults. *Journal of Epidemiology and Community Health* **61**: 34–9.

Hofman K, Primack A, Keusch G, *et al.* (2005) Addressing the growing burden of trauma and injury in low- and middle-income countries. *American Journal of Public Health* **95**: 13–17.

Kandel E, Mednick SA (1991) Perinatal complications predict violent offending. *Criminology* **29**: 519–29.

Kessler RC, Molnar BE, Feurer ID, *et al.* (2001) Patterns and mental health predictors of domestic violence in the United States: results from the National Comorbidity Survey. *International Journal of Law and Psychiatry* **24**: 487–508.

Kim-Cohen J, Caspi A, Taylor A, *et al.* (2006) MAOA, maltreatment, and gene–environment interaction predicting children's mental health: new evidence and a meta-analysis. *Molecular Psychiatry* **11**: 903–13.

Korteweg A, Yurdakul G (2009) Islam, gender, and immigrant integration: boundary drawing in discourses on honour killing in the Netherlands and Germany. *Ethnic and Racial Studies* **32**: 218–38.

Krug EG, Dahlberg LL, Mercy JA, Zwi AB, Lozano R, eds. (2002) *World Report on Violence and Health.* Geneva: World Health Organization.

Lachs MS and Pillemer K (2004) Elder abuse. *Lancet* **364**: 1263–72.

Lachs MS, Williams C, O'Brien S, *et al.* (1997) Risk factors for reported elder abuse and neglect: a nine-year observational cohort study. *Gerontologist* **37**: 469–74.

Loeb TB, Williams JK, Carmona JV, *et al.* (2002) Child sexual abuse: associations with sexual functioning of adolescents and adults. *Annual Review of Sex Research* **13**: 307–45.

Lund C, Breen A, Flisher AJ, *et al.* (2010) Poverty and common mental disorders in low and middle income countries: a systematic review.

Social Science and Medicine **71**: 517–28.

Lynch JW, Kaplan GA (1997) Understanding how inequality in the distribution of income affects health. *Journal of Health Psychology* **2**: 297–314.

Lyons RA, Finch CF, McClure R, *et al.* (2010) The injury List Of All Deficits (LOAD) framework: conceptualising the full range of deficits and adverse outcomes following injury and violence. *International Journal of Injury Control and Safety Promotion* **17**: 145–59.

Mercy JA, Rosenberg ML, Powell KE, *et al.* (1993) Public health policy for preventing violence. *Health Affairs* **12**: 7–29.

McIlwaine C, Moser CON (2001) Violence and social capital in urban poor communities: perspectives from Colombia and Guatemala. *Journal of International Development* **13**: 965–84.

Merrill LL, Guimond JM, Thomsen CJ, *et al.* (2003) Child sexual abuse and number of sexual partners in young women: the role of abuse severity, coping style, and sexual functioning. *Journal of Consulting and Clinical Psychology* **71**: 987–96.

Moffitt TE, Henry B (1989) Neuropsychological assessment of executive functions in self-reported delinquents. *Development and Psychopathology* **1**: 105–18.

Molnar BE, Buka SL, Kessler RC (2001) Child sexual abuse and subsequent psychopathology: results from the national comorbidity survey. *American Journal of Public Health* **91**: 753–60.

Paolucci EO, Genius ML, Violato C (2001) A meta-analysis of the published research on the effects of child sexual abuse. *Journal of Psychology* **135**: 17–36.

Roustit C, Renahy E, Guernec G, *et al.* (2009) Exposure to interparental violence and psychosocial maladjustment in the adult life course: advocacy for early prevention. *Journal of Epidemiology and Community Health* **63**: 563–8.

Rubio M (1997) Perverse social capital: some evidence from Colombia. *Journal of Economic Issues* **31**: 805–16.

Schuster MA, Stein BD, Jaycox LH, *et al.* (2001) A national survey of stress reactions after the September 11, 2001, terrorist attacks. *New England Journal of Medicine* **345**: 1507–12.

Taft CT, Bryant-Davis T, Woodward HE, *et al.* (2009) Intimate partner violence against African American women: an examination of the socio-cultural context. *Aggression and Violent Behavior* **14**: 50–8.

Unicef (2005) *Female Genital Mutilation/Cutting: a Statistical Analysis.* New York: Unicef.

Uthman OA, Lawoko S, Moradi T (2009) Factors associated with attitudes towards intimate partner violence against women: a comparative analysis of 17 sub-Saharan countries. *BMC International Health and Human Rights* **9**: 14.

Vermeiren R, Schwab-Stone M, Deboutte D, *et al.* (2003) Violence exposure and substance use in adolescents: findings from three countries. *Pediatrics* **111**: 535–40.

WHO Global Consultation on Violence and Health (1996) *Violence: a Public Health Priority.* Geneva: World Health Organization.

Widom CS, Brzustowicz LM (2006) MAOA and the "cycle of violence:" childhood abuse and neglect, MAOA genotype, and risk for violent and antisocial behavior. *Biological Psychiatry* **60**: 684–9.

World Health Organization (2002) *The World Health Report 2002. Reducing Risks, Promoting Healthy Life.* Geneva: WHO.

World Health Organization (2008) *The Global Burden of Disease: 2004 Update.* Geneva: WHO.

World Health Organization (2010) *Violence Prevention: the Evidence.* Geneva: WHO.

World Health Organization (2011a) *Cause-Specific Mortality: Regional Estimates for 2008, by World Bank Income Groups.* Geneva: WHO.

World Health Organization (2011b) *Deaths by Age, Sex and Cause for the Year 2008.* Geneva: WHO.

Chapter

40

The war on drugs in the USA, Mexico, and Central America: Plan Colombia and the Mérida Initiative

Samuel O. Okpaku and Jayanthi Karunaratne

Introduction

Drug trafficking, drug consumption, and their concomitants are major public health and international health problems. From a public health perspective, it would not be an exaggeration to suggest that drug trafficking and consumption are a pandemic – spreading all over the world. From a global mental health and foreign policy point of view, it represents, par excellence, the principal issues involved in framing international health in relation to foreign policy.

For example, Labonté and Gagnon (2010) found that various governments use certain frames in making their foreign policy statements more prominent in global health in terms of health and society, health and development, health and global public goods, health as a human right, health and trade, and human rights and ethical/moral arguments for global health assistance. Drug trafficking contributes to violence, the spread of diseases, and increased morbidity. In this study, Labonté and Gagnon reviewed major English-language health and foreign policy statements made by various governments between 2005 and 2009. They also reviewed academic literature that was pertinent to the different frames against a background of their actual or potential effects.

The processes of drug trafficking, drug consumption, and their effects have a high relevance for positioning the international drug problem as a health and foreign policy issue. The ramifications are protean and include violence, human trafficking and prostitution, the contribution to the spread of HIV/AIDS, and the direct mortality and morbidity associated with drug use. The problems related to illicit drug consumption and trafficking are borderless.

Drug use: a global phenomenon

The United Nations Office on Drugs and Crime (UNODC) estimates that of the current global population of 7 billion people, about 230 million use an illegal drug at least once annually. This figure equals to approximately 1 in 20 persons in the age group 15–64. In this category about 1 in 40 people regularly use drugs at least once a month, and under 1 in 160 use drugs that put them at risk of serious health problems (UNODC 2012). Cannabis is the most frequently used illicit drug, with about 170 million people using it at least once a year. This is about 3.8% of the world's adult population. The corresponding numbers for the other major drugs are as follows: amphetamine type drugs, 30 million users; "ecstasy" (MDMA), 20 million; opiates, 17 million; cocaine, 16 million.

North America has the highest rate of illicit drug use. The regions with the rates of highest production of illicit drugs are as follows: cannabis, Africa and North America; opiates, Asia; cocaine, South America and Europe; synthetic drugs, Asia and North America (Figure 40.1)

Cannabis use is highest in Oceania, North America, and Africa; opiate use is highest in the Middle East, Central Asia, Europe; and the use of synthetic drugs is highest in Oceania, East and Southeast Asia, and Europe. UNODC goes on to report that drug use remains a youth phenomenon that peaks at the ages 18–25. Data from the USA indicate that in terms of current drug use, females use drugs 40% less than males. The figure is higher for other developed countries and higher for developing countries for which data are available. School surveys carried out in Europe and the USA show smaller gender gaps. The UNODC report (2012) also gives economic figures as follows: the total retail market for opiates and cocaine

Essentials of Global Mental Health, ed. Samuel O. Okpaku. Published by Cambridge University Press. © Cambridge University Press 2014.

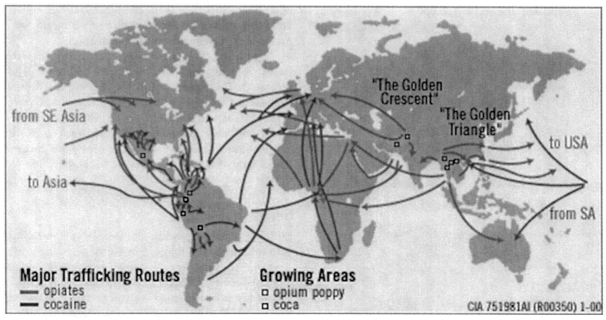

Figure 40.1 Major drug trafficking routes. US Federal Government image, in the public domain.

(2009 figures) were US$68 billion and US$85 billion respectively. The total contribution to the global GDP in 2003 was 0.9%, i.e., US$320 billion. The largest markets in rank order for 2005 were North America (44%) and Europe (33%), followed by Asia, Oceania, Africa, and South America. Trading drugs ranks as number 1 in illicit activities.

US presidents and the war on drugs

Since Eisenhower, every US president has attempted to curtail the spread of illicit drugs, and each one has built on his predecessor's plans.

Richard Nixon

The modern "war on drugs" is usually attributed to Richard Nixon. On June 17, 1971, Nixon declared that drug addiction was "public enemy number one" and asserted that drug addiction had "assumed the dimensions of a national emergency" (Nixon 1971). Throughout Nixon's term as president, he tied drug addiction to national crime, and according to his Oval Office tapes, he asked for US$84 million to initiate the fight on all fronts. The year after Nixon's declaration of the "war on drugs," marijuana arrests jumped by nearly 100 000 people. Historical records indicate that Nixon was driven by his personal prejudices rather

than reliable information in his approach to the marijuana problem. The following are few of Nixon's comments on marijuana:

- Jews and marijuana: "I see another thing in the news summary this morning about it. That's a funny thing, every one of the bastards that are out for legalizing marijuana is Jewish. What the Christ is the matter with the Jews, Bob, what is the matter with them? I suppose it's because most of them are psychiatrists . . ."
- Marijuana and the culture wars: "You see, homosexuality, dope, immorality in general. These are the enemies of strong societies. That's why the Communists and the left-wingers are pushing the stuff, they're trying to destroy us."
- Marijuana compared to alcohol: marijuana consumers smoke "to get high" while "a person drinks to have fun." Nixon also saw marijuana leading to loss of motivation and discipline but claimed, "At least with liquor I don't lose motivation."
- Marijuana and political dissent: "radical demonstrators that were here . . . two weeks ago . . . They're all on drugs, virtually all."
- Drug education: "Enforce the law, you've got to scare them." (Common Sense for Drug Policy 2002).

385

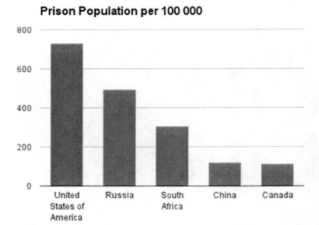

Figure 40.2 Prison population worldwide. Data from World Prison Brief, International Centre for Prison Studies.

Jimmy Carter

The Carter administration did not make drug policy a priority. In place of the law-and-order approach of Nixon, Carter's campaign for the US presidency had a major policy platform on the decriminalization of marijuana and the removal of federal criminal penalties for possession of less than 1 oz. of marijuana (Valelly 2010).

When he was president, he warned against filling US prisons with "young people who were no threat to society." President Carter had expressed the view that "penalties against possession of a drug should not be more damaging to an individual than the use of the drug itself." In a recent *New York Times* opinion piece, he quoted the statistic that before he left office in 1980, 500 000 people were incarcerated in America; by the end of 2009 the number had risen to about 2.3 million. For every 100 000 Americans, 743 are in prison (Figure 40.2). This figure is seven times greater than the equivalent figures for Europe (Carter 2011).

Ronald Reagan

In 1982 Reagan tied drug addiction to national security. It is believed that some of the strictest drug control legislation in American history was passed during Reagan's Presidency. In 1986 and 1988 anti-drug abuse acts were passed by Congress and the "zero tolerance" policy was announced (Keesings Worldwide 1998). The mandatory minimum drug sentencing guidelines were approved, causing judges to lose their sentencing discretion and turning it over to prosecutors. In addition, factors such as the character of the defendant and the impact of the incarceration on his family were no longer to be considered in sentencing.

Meanwhile, the prison population continued to climb as drug enforcement efforts and sentencing increased. The Anti-Drug Abuse Act increased punishment for selling the cheap new cocaine derivative, "crack." This was criticized for causing racial disparities in the prison population between crack users and cocaine users, as crack users were mostly low-income blacks or Hispanics and cocaine users were mainly middle-class whites (Valelly 2010).

George H. W. Bush

Bush built on the foundation of Reagan's war on drugs with substantial funding. Under Bush Sr., as vice president and as president, the federal antidrug budget increased from US$1.5 billion to US$12.3 billion, 70% of which was to go to law enforcement, including jails, and 30% to prevention, education, and treatment approaches. His plan put considerable pressure on the states and municipal authorities to fight the war because of the federal government's limited resources. As president, Bush increased the role of the military in fighting drugs. There were more efforts toward drug interdiction and campaigns to stop production, particularly of cocaine in South America (Valelly 2010).

Bill Clinton

Clinton's administration devoted less attention to federal drug control, but did not cut back on the stringent drug policies he inherited from Reagan and Bush. He expanded the drug eradication and interdiction initiatives such as the Plan Colombia enacted in 2000. These included seizure of property and a growth in the prison system. When he came into office the national prison population was 1.3 million and when he left the number was 2 million – reflecting the highest rate in a democratic society worldwide. Due to overcrowded prison and budget pressures, his drug policy did shift towards increasing treatment efforts (Valelly 2010).

George W. Bush

President G. W. Bush equated his "war on drugs" to a "war on terrorism." He linked the events of 9/11 to heroin production in Afghanistan. According to reports, nearly 70% of the world's heroin supply comes from Afghanistan. Bush linked his domestic agenda to foreign policy, remarking that the drug trade provided "a significant amount of money to the people that were harboring and feeding and hiding those who attacked and killed thousands of innocent Americans." He also emphasized the demand side of drug trafficking and called for greater federal involvement in the fight against drug traffickers on the US–Mexican border. His drug policy also established the social and moral effects on societal stability. He supported a more aggressive approach to drug education, treatment, and prevention. In addition, he promoted faith-based programs for reducing drug addiction (Zeleny 2002).

Barack Obama

There are conflicting predictions as to the direction of Obama's "war on drugs." His drug czar is quoted as having said that "war on drugs" was a misnomer, and some of his aides have been quoted as suggesting that the president will reform the current war on drugs. Some policy changes include emphasizing the public health aspects of drug use and lifting the practice that denies a drug convict an opportunity to gain fruitful rehabilitation. However, there have been some mixed signals. While campaigning for his first term, he had promised a more flexible and lenient approach to the medical use of marijuana, yet under his administration a significant number of interagency cannabis crackdowns and swat-style raids were carried out, predominantly in medical marijuana states (Walther 2012).

Plan Colombia and the Mérida Initiative

Plan Colombia and the Mérida Initiative are two major treaties that attempt to control and restrict drug trafficking in the USA, Mexico, and Central America.

In the late 1990s, it was estimated that 90% of the cocaine coming into the USA originated from Colombia. During that time, Colombia faced growing political instability, with terrorism and conflicts between government troops, paramilitary organizations, and terrorist paramilitary groups. Colombia was close to being a failed state. The opposition paramilitary groups seized upon the poverty in the rural areas to entice poor farmers to cultivate coca leaves and poppy seeds. In an attempt to bring some stability to his country, President Pastrana developed Plan Colombia. Originally, the plan was to involve a number of

partners including the USA. President Clinton embraced Pastrana's plan and committed the United States to fund the project. The USA contributed US$1.3 billion to fund the plan. Some of the original donors were either eclipsed or decided to play a minor role in the project. This was because of opposition to the then prominent military aspect of the plan. The plan entailed the provision of military hardware including helicopters and airplanes, and their servicing, training, and support by US forces and contractors. In addition, there were alternative measures to improve human rights conditions and provide an improved judiciary system. Also the equipment provided was to be used in spraying coca leaves, as well as destroying poppy fields. Supporters of the plan believed that it was successful. Critics disagreed with this. They felt that greater recognition should have been given to the plight of poor farmers in achieving economic security other than by cultivation of coca or poppy seeds. The aerial spraying had mixed results in discouraging cultivation of coca. No sooner was a field sprayed than planting started at another front (popularly known as the balloon effect). The use of herbicides that sometimes polluted rivers and caused health risks and other damage was also cited (Sipress 2001). President George W. Bush continued the Clinton policy and continued funding Plan Colombia.

The Mérida Initiative is basically an international treaty primarily between the USA and Mexico to combat drug trafficking problems and improve the US–Mexico border conditions. The treaty was signed by Mexican President Felipe Calderón and US President George W. Bush. Although the bulk of the funding went to Mexico, other Central American states including Haiti and the Dominican Republic were also funded.

This initiative was signed into law on June 30, 2008. It is estimated that annually the drug traffickers earned in cash above US$12–15 billion and that the Mexican cartels earned more than US$23 billion a year. The Mexican authorities believe that the demand for drugs by Americans was a prime factor for the cultivation and production of illicit drugs in Mexico and the Central American states (Seelke & Finklea 2013). The programs and activities of the Mérida Initiative have been summarized as follows:

- The United States is supporting Mexico's implementation of comprehensive justice-sector reforms through the training of personnel including police, prosecutors, and defenders, correction systems development, judicial exchanges, and partnerships between Mexican and US law schools.

- The US Agency for international Development (USAID) is partnering with the government of Mexico and civil society to promote the rule of law and build strong and resilient communities by supporting the implementation of Mexico's new justice system, increasing knowledge of and respect for human rights, strengthening social networks and community cohesion, addressing the needs of vulnerable populations (young and victims of crime) and increasing community and governmental cooperation.

- Air mobility has been increased through the delivery of eight Bell helicopters to the Mexican Army/Air Force, three UH-60M Black Hawk helicopters to the Federal Police and three UH-60M Black Hawk helicopters to provide for rapid transport of personnel for counter-narcotics and other security operations.

- The US government has provided scanners, x-ray machines, and other non-intrusive inspection equipment to enhance the Mexican authorities' ability to detect illicit goods at key checkpoints of land and air ports of entry.

- The Mexican government has established a corrections academy to train Mexican federal correctional staff at Xalapa in Mexico's Veracruz state (US Department of State 2012).

The major objectives of the initiative are (US Department of State 2012, Seelke & Finklea 2013):

(1) disrupt organized criminal groups
(2) strengthen institutions
(3) build a twenty-first-century border
(4) build strong and resilient communities

This program was funded by US$1.6 billion.

Recently, Ambassador Brownfield, in a visit to the border town of Juarez in Mexico, stated that he is the US official responsible for the Mérida Initiative. He emphasized a shift in the policy to expand the collaboration beyond the federal level and to include states and municipalities. He also sounded optimistic about the Mérida Initiative, as he had been in a news conference about 15 years previously, when he spoke about the Colombia Plan.

Some of the criticisms leveled at Plan Colombia were also made with respect to the Mérida Initiative. Two major criticisms concern the lack of adequate attention to the demand side of drug trafficking and the over-militaristic approach. During Calderón's presidency of six years the drug death toll was nearly 47 500 (Shoichet 2012).

The experiences from these two plans have no doubt contributed to the current movement even by past Central American presidents urging for a newer approach to drug trafficking.

Assessing the war on drugs

The war on drugs "philosophy" has been seriously challenged from many sides.

Some of the consequences of the harsh prohibitive philosophy and practice of the war on drugs have been greater availability of drugs, cheaper drugs, bloodbaths and gory crimes in Mexico and Central America. It has also led to a high prison rate in the United States. Hundreds and thousands of young people have been imprisoned in the USA and Central America for drug offences. These consequences have fallen disproportionately upon minorities – African-Americans and Hispanics.

There is now a push to decriminalize marijuana use as a first step and then to carry out further studies to explore how best to reduce the use of hard drugs such as cocaine and amphetamine. For a variety of reasons the current policies are being seen as a failure.

The Economist on March 5, 2009, published the following commentary:

> The war on drugs has been a disaster, creating failed states in the developing world even as addiction has flourished in the rich world. By any sensible measure, this 100-year struggle has been illiberal, murderous and pointless. That is why *The Economist* continues to believe that the least bad policy is to legalise drugs. Legalisation would not only drive away the gangsters; it would transform drugs from a law-and-order problem into a public-health problem, which is how they ought to be treated. Governments would tax and regulate the drug trade, and use the funds raised (and the billions saved on law-enforcement) to educate the public about the risks of drug-taking and to treat addiction.
>
> (*Economist* 2009)

The *Wall Street Journal* on February 23, 2009, also published an article on the failure of the "war on drugs," carrying the central message of a report commissioned by the Latin American Commission on

Drugs and Democracy and authored by Fernando Henrique Cardoso, former president of Brazil, César Gaviria, former president of Colombia, and Ernesto Zedillo, former president of Mexico:

> The war on drugs has failed. And it's high time to replace an ineffective strategy with more humane and efficient drug policies ... The revision of US inspired drug policies is urgent in light of the rising levels of violence and corruption associated with narcotics. The alarming power of the drug cartels is leading to a criminalization of politics and a politicization of crime. And the corruption of the judicial and political system is undermining the foundations of democracy in several Latin American countries.
>
> (Cardoso *et al.* 2009)

The move to decriminalize marijuana has gained an impetus by the recent ballot approved in Colorado and Washington (USA). Some observers have suggested that such a move could in fact encourage greater trafficking of marijuana to these states. Others argue that the resources being spent on interdiction can be better applied to the demand side, i.e., education, treatment, and rehabilitation. They argue that the traffickers will be discouraged by the fall in their business. Meanwhile, UNODC has asked the US Federal Government to discourage the states of Colorado and Washington from implementing the result of the votes for decriminalization. It should be noted that at this time of writing two bills have been introduced in Congress. The bills are aimed at allowing states to regulate marijuana as they deem fit and to seek a framework for taxation of the drug. This is not the first time that such bills have been introduced to the US Congress. It is generally believed that they stand no chance, but there is increasing support for legalization of marijuana use in the USA.

This chapter would be incomplete if mention were not made of the initiatives been taken by individual Central American and some South American countries in formulating their own drug policies. For example, in 2009 the Mexican legislature passed a law to decriminalize all drugs. Soon after, the Argentine Supreme Court struck down the law criminalizing drugs. Colombia similarly passed a law to decriminalize small amounts of drug.

Other countries, such as Guatemala and Ecuador, have passed or are about to pass similar laws (Gamarra 2005), and President Otto Pérez Molina of Guatemala has considered legalizing the use and transport of illicit drugs (Associated Press 2012).

Uruguay has passed contentious legislation whose objective is to separate the two components of the market, i.e., to separate users from traffickers and marijuana from other drugs such as cocaine. The Uruguayan officials have created a monopoly for marijuana and other substances prohibited by the 1961 UN single convention on narcotic drugs. The legislatures of Argentina and Brazil share similar views. They believe that separation between drug users and traffickers will allow the authorities to focus on traffickers instead of others. In addition to these shifts in legislature, these countries have requested a high-level UN meeting to discuss the future of drug policies and how best to deal with the problem (Gamarra 2005).

Conclusion

From the above, it can be seen that drug trafficking and consumption pose severe regional and international economic, social, political, and health problems. It has created considerable public health and other health-related problems in the USA, Mexico, and elsewhere in Central America. These activities are interconnected in a web-like fashion. These phenomena in the USA and neighboring Central American countries constitute a study in global mental health and diplomacy. The war on drugs in this hub has led to a dispersion of drugs to Canada and Europe. As the drug cartels are confronted in one area, they search for alternative transits. This results in the spread of cocaine and opiate use, for example, to poor West African countries who are ill-equipped to begin to deal with the associated problems of drug use and trafficking. The potential for fearful consequences is great. The war on drugs in the Southern hemisphere is now undoubtedly a failure. There does not appear to be any easy solution in attempting to control a major regional problem which appears intractable.

The consequences spill over globally. So it is truly a global health issue requiring a collective international effort to manage and control.

The current state of events poses challenges for the Obama administration in many ways. First, because of the hegemony of the USA, the pro-prohibition stance is reported to be largely due to US influence. A complete reversal of US policy is unlikely, as it is not realistic or pragmatic. It will jettison the whole philosophical basis of the current UNODC approaches. There are also implications for the countries of Central America and Mexico who have relied on US funding in obtaining equipment and alternative approaches. These approaches include institutional building and development as well as spraying of coca leaves. These alternatives also include greater emphasis on treatment, education, prevention, and rehabilitation.

Attention has to be paid to the consequences of the incarceration of young people for marijuana misdemeanors. The imprisonment of young individuals alongside violent and hardened criminals serves no purpose but to expose them to the possibilities of crime as a career.

References

Associated Press (2012) Guatemala president mulls drug legalization, blames U.S. failure to combat trafficking. *CBC News*. http://www.cbc.ca/news/world/story/2012/02/14/guatemala-drug-cartel.html (accessed July 2013).

Cardoso FH, Gaviria C, Zedillo E (2009) The war on drugs is a failure. *Wall Street Journal*, February 23, 2009. http://online.wsj.com/article/SB123535114271444981.html (accessed July 2013).

Carter J (2011) Call off the global drug war. *New York Times: The Opinion Pages*, June 11, 2011. http://www.nytimes.com/2011/06/17/opinion/17carter.html?_r=0 (accessed July 2013).

Economist (2009) How to stop the drug wars. *The Economist* March 5, 2009. http://www.economist.com/node/13237193 (accessed July 2013).

Common Sense for Drug Policy (2002) Nixon tapes show roots of marijuana prohibition: misinformation, culture wars and prejudice. *CSDP Research Report*. http://www.csdp.org/research/shafernixon.pdf (accessed July 2013).

Gamarra EA (2005) State, drug policy, and democracy in the Andes. *Andean: Inter-American Dialogue Working Paper*.

Keesing's Worldwide (1998) Measures to combat illegal drug use: mandatory drug testing of federal employees, arrest of drug traffickers, human rights. *Keesing's Record of World Events* **34**: 36089.

Labonté R, Gagnon ML (2010) Framing health and foreign policy: lessons for global health diplomacy. *Globalization and Health* **6** (14): 1–19.

Nixon R (1971) Remarks about an intensified program for drug abuse prevention and control, June 17, 1971. Online by Gerhard Peters and John T. Woolley, *The American Presidency Project*. http://www.presidency.ucsb.edu/ws/?pid=3047 (accessed July 2013).

Seelke CR, Finklea KM (2013) *U.S.-Mexican Security Cooperation: the Mérida Initiative and Beyond*. CRS Report for Congress 7-5700 R41349. Washington, DC: Congressional Research Service. http://www.fas.org/sgp/crs/row/R41349.pdf (accessed July 2013).

Shoichet CE (2012) Outgoing Mexican president defends legacy in wake of drug war. CNN. http://edition.cnn.com/2012/11/29/world/americas/mexico-president/index.html?hpt=hp_bn2 (accessed July 2013).

Sipress A (2001) U.S. reassesses Colombia Aid: anti-drug efforts studied as Powell visits Bogota *Washington Post*, September 10, 2001. http://www.latinamericanstudies.org/colombia/efforts.htm (accessed July 2013).

United Nations Office on Drugs and Crime (UNODC) (2012) *World Drug Report 2012*. New York, NY: UN.

US Department of State (2012) Merida Initiative. http://www.state.gov/j/inl/merida (accessed July 2013).

Valelly RM, ed. (2010) Drug policy (1976 to present). *Encyclopedia of U.S. Political History*, Vol. 7. Washington, DC: CQ Press.

Walther MF (2012) *Insanity: Four Decades of U.S. Counterdrug Strategy*. Carlisle Paper. Carlisle, PA: Strategic Studies Institute. http://www.strategicstudiesinstitute.army.mil/pdffiles/PUB1143.pdf (accessed July 2013).

Zeleny J (2002) Bush's drug policy highlights terror link. *Chicago Tribune*, February 13, 2002. Available from articles.chicagotribune.com.

Chapter

41

Medical education and global mental health

Clare Pain and Atalay Alem

Introduction

The prevalence of mental disorders has been found to be similar in countries of similar income levels. It is the gap between the number of trained mental health workers and the burden of mental disorders which is the most pressing problem for low-income countries (LICs). This human resources lack is reported to be the most significant limiting factor to the provision of appropriate, evidence-informed psychiatric care and services (Saxena *et al.* 2007).

In this chapter we will briefly identify issues related to the problem of the gap between mental health needs and services. Following this, two examples of educational partnerships will illustrate how high-income countries (HICs), in this case Sweden and Canada, were able to collaborate with a LIC, Ethiopia, and specifically how they addressed training needs by increasing the number of mental health specialists and their access to PhD training. These partnerships are between the Departments of Psychiatry at the University of Toronto (UofT) in Canada and Addis Ababa University (AAU) in Ethiopia, known as the Toronto Addis Ababa Psychiatry Project (TAAPP) (Alem *et al.* 2010); and between Umeå University in Sweden and the Department of Psychiatry, AAU.

In 2003, the TAAPP educational partnership began to develop specialist mental health capacity by assisting the three Ethiopian psychiatry faculty in the Department of Psychiatry at AAU. UofT supplemented local teaching by providing on-the-ground core teaching and supervision for three months a year for the first psychiatry residency training program in the country. Psychiatrists could now train locally, and the faculty enlarged as new graduates were recruited, establishing the department's educational capacity

and sustainability. This strategy also reduced the risk of the out-migration of potential residents seeking training in the west.

Prior to and concurrent with TAAPP, the Department of Psychiatry at AAU established a collaboration with Umeå University to assist with PhD training. This fertile association enabled Ethiopian psychiatrists to gain their PhDs in a well-designed "sandwich" program, where the Ethiopian candidate spent brief focused visits in Umeå and the majority of time in Ethiopia. This arrangement provided excellent postgraduate training, boosting the research capacity of the Department of Psychiatry at AAU with the same reduction of "brain drain" risk. These two collaborations (Umeå University and TAAPP) have been successful in enhancing clinical, educational, research, and leadership capacity for Ethiopian psychiatrists, and have been key components in the emergence of the Department of Psychiatry at AAU as the fastest-growing research department on the continent. This has a significant bearing on the enhancement of mental health services in the country (Alem & Pain 2010).

Prevalence of mental disorders

The contribution of mental disorders to the burden of disease in the world is high, accounting for 14% of the overall burden of disease as measured with disability-adjusted life years (DALYs), and 28% of the non-communicable burden of disease (World Health Organization 2001).

A third of the years lived with disability (YLD) are attributable to mental disorders in adults worldwide, and five mental disorders make up 10 of the leading causes of disability globally (WHO 2008). Depression was the fourth largest contributor to the disease

Essentials of Global Mental Health, ed. Samuel O. Okpaku. Published by Cambridge University Press. © Cambridge University Press 2014.

burden in 1990 and is expected to be the second largest after ischemic heart disease by 2020 (WHO 2001).

Although suicide accounts for about 800 000 deaths a year globally, there is significant non-suicide mortality associated with mental illness, particularly in LICs. For instance, if a child born to an impoverished mother dies as a result of her mother being too depressed to ensure she drinks clean water or is vaccinated, the death is not linked statistically to the depression of her mother. In addition, much of the disability and mortality of mental illness is strongly associated with physical illness; mental illness increases the risk of physical illness and vice versa (Sartorius 2007).

In emphasizing the importance of health in an LIC the World Health Organization (2012) wrote in a statement following the Rio+20 conference that health is a "precondition for, an outcome of, and an indicator of sustainable development." And mental health emerges as a key determinant of overall health. As noted by the Institute of Medicine (2001):

> The evidence is clear: mental health is fundamentally linked to physical health outcomes. Mental health status is a key consideration in changing the health status of a community. Health and behavior are influenced by factors at multiple levels, including biological, psychological and social. Interventions that involve only the individual are unlikely to change long-term behavior unless family, work and broader social factors are aligned to support a change.

Of note, one of the important impacts of the two partnerships is that the Ethiopian psychiatrists successfully lobbied the government of Ethiopia to work towards full integration of mental health services into the primary to tertiary healthcare system. This constitutes an essential move away from a custodial or asylum model of mental health service delivery, and addresses the false division of mental and physical illness. Integration of services begins to be possible as the number of psychiatrists trained locally increases, and with a high proportion of psychiatrists gaining a PhD, clinical, educational, and enhanced leadership can be expected.

Disparity of mental health resources

There is a massive disparity in health human resources, namely trained mental health professionals (psychiatrists, psychologists, psychiatric nurses, social workers, and occupational therapists) for people suffering from mental disorders in low- and middle-income countries (LMICs). In HICs the median number of psychiatrists is 172 times higher than in LMICs (Kakuma et al. 2011). Importantly Kakuma reports that this situation is not improving; between 2005 and 2011 the median number of psychiatrists rose by 0.65 per 100 000 population in HICs and fell by 0.01 per 100 000 population in LICs. There is an overall shortage of mental health workers in LICs (WHO 2011), and Kakuma et al. note that "all LICs and about two-thirds of middle-income countries (MICs) had far fewer mental health workers to deliver a core set of mental health interventions than were needed."

In addition, the availability of local postgraduate training in mental health is very limited in LICs. To become a psychiatrist, psychologist, or social worker, overseas training is required and the return rate is very low. To quote Dr. Lee Jong-Wook, former Director-General of the World Health Organization:

> People are a vital ingredient in the strengthening of health systems . . . Countries need their skilled workforce to stay so that their professional expertise can benefit their populations. When health workers leave to work elsewhere, there is a loss of hope and a loss of years of investment. The solution is not straightforward, and there is no consensus on how to proceed.
>
> (World Health Organization 2006)

Certainly the "brain drain" or attrition of specialized medical professionals is a central issue of concern for many sub-Saharan countries including Ethiopia. In 1965, the doctor-to-population ratio in Ethiopia was 1:85 000; by 2006 it had worsened to 1:118 000. This shows a 74.1% deficit according to WHO's minimum doctor-to-population ratio (Berhan 2008), made more worrying by the fact that HICs stand to gain from this migration of physicians out of LICs. In a recent article, Mills et al. (2011) calculated the cost to nine sub-Saharan African countries of a medical doctor's education. They then estimated the overall loss of returns from investment for all doctors trained in LICs and currently working in the USA, UK, Canada, and Australia to be US$2.17 billion, with costs for each country ranging from US$2.16 million to US$1.41 billion. For Ethiopia it was US$24.63 million. The benefit to destination countries of doctors trained in LICs was largest for the United Kingdom (US$2.7 billion) and the United States (US$846 million), with Canada benefiting by US$384 million. Mills and colleagues concluded that "destination countries should consider investing in measurable training for source countries and strengthening of their health systems."

It is important to note that non-governmental organizations (NGOs) and other similar operations within an LIC can precipitate an "internal brain drain." They attract local health professionals and employ them in high-salaried jobs, thereby preventing these government-trained doctors and nurses from contributing to their healthcare systems (Southall *et al.* 2010).

Strategies to help

There is an increasing awareness of the problem, and a consensus that HICs must address the huge disparity between mental disorders and the lack of mental health workers and services in LICs (Frenk *et al.* 2010). In considering strategies, a number of suggestions have been made. One idea is to task-shift, or, as Vikram Patel prefers as a less autocratic term, task-share. This refers to the scaling up of training to enable non-specialist health workers to do some of the tasks that in HICs are usually performed by more specialized healthcare workers. Another suggestion is to pay sustained attention to stigma, which, among other things, can be a barrier to the recruitment of mental health professionals. Thirdly, it is necessary to address the attrition due to the emigration of mental health professionals out of LMICs; and fourthly, Fricchione and colleagues (2012) suggest the growth of effective local leadership. The development of university partnerships between HICs and LMICs is an idea that is increasingly mentioned as a strategy to address the gap (Kakuma *et al.* 2011, 2012). In the two examples in this chapter, the twinning has been on a smaller scale than the ideal proposed by Fricchione *et al.*, restricted to partnering between departments rather than university to university. However, with the benefit of time they have been able to grow and develop farther than was initially imagined.

Psychiatry in Ethiopia: background

TAAPP was founded primarily in order to address the request by Ethiopian colleagues for teaching assistance in the first psychiatry residency training program opened by the Department of Psychiatry, Faculty of Medicine, AAU, and located at Amanuel and St. Paul's Hospitals. When the residency program opened in 2003, there were only three psychiatrists on faculty, and they had trained in the UK and in the Netherlands; the total number of Ethiopian psychiatrists in the country was 11, two of whom had retired and were in private practice. This resulted in a psychiatrist-to-population ratio of about 1 to 6 million. Very few of those who had been sent abroad for psychiatry training had returned.

TAAPP and the partnership with Umeå University followed a number of developments in the growth of psychiatry in Ethiopia. The following paragraphs will contextualize both partnerships more thoroughly.

The formal Western history of psychiatry began in 1966 with the creation, by Professor Robert Giel from the University of Groningen in the Netherlands, of the Department of Psychiatry as a unit in the Department of Internal Medicine at Addis Ababa University. At that time, AAU, known then as the Haile Selassie I University, was the only university in the country. By 1973, the psychiatry unit had become a fully fledged department with one Ethiopian psychiatrist, Dr. Fikre Workneh, who had returned after his training abroad in the USA.

Amanuel Hospital, the only civilian inpatient facility, had been built by the Italians during the 1936–41 occupation. After the Italians left, and because of its location (at that time) on the outskirts of the capital, it was deemed an appropriate institution for psychiatric patients. In 1987 the first psychiatric nurses graduated with a diploma in psychiatric nursing thanks to the National Mental Health Action Group (NMHAG) chaired by the then vice minister of health, who established a one-year psychiatric training program for nurses (Alem *et al.* 1996). These nurses were employed at Amanuel Hospital and in several regional psychiatric units and general hospitals throughout the country. In conjunction with this progress, in the late 1980s Drs. Atalay Alem and Mesfin Araya returned from their psychiatry residency trainings abroad (in the UK and the Netherlands, respectively) and continued the reorganization of Amanuel Hospital, from a long-stay custodial institution to a psychiatric hospital, which they had started before they went abroad for training. This prepared the way for the first psychiatry residency training, which was formally identified as a need in 1992.

Two HIC–LIC educational partnerships

In 1994, nine years prior to the start of TAAPP, the important partnership between the Departments of Psychiatry of AAU and Umeå University, Sweden, was initiated through a research collaboration by Dr. Atalay Alem when he started his PhD training at Umeå University. Through this partnership eight other Ethiopian psychiatrists have obtained their PhDs.

In Ethiopia the main research site for collaborative research has been Butajira, a predominantly rural district situated 130 km south of Addis Ababa. A demographic surveillance site (DSS) was established in Butajira District by the Department of Community Health, AAU, and the Department of Epidemiology and Public Health, Umeå University, in 1986. This DSS was named the Butajira Rural Health Program (BRHP). Ten sub-districts were randomly selected to establish the DSS or the study base in the district. An initial census was taken in order to determine the baseline population and establish a system of demographic surveillance with continuous registration of vital and migratory events (birth, death, marriage, new household, out-migration, in-migration, and internal movement). The information gathered through monthly household interviews has been used for numerous studies, including ones concerned with reproductive health and both childhood- and later-onset diseases.

It was through using this population in Butajira, and the infrastructure established by the BRHP, that the Departments of Psychiatry at Umeå and AAU started conducting mental health research. Since the collaboration between the two departments began, a number of epidemiological studies of common and severe mental disorders have been conducted in Ethiopia (Alem *et al.* 1999, Kebede & Alem 1999, Beyero *et al.* 2004, Fekadu *et al.* 2004, Shibre *et al.* 2010). Most of these studies were linked to PhD studentships. Since there was no PhD program in related fields in Ethiopia at the time, candidates had to register at Umeå University. All of the candidates were required to conduct their studies in Ethiopia, but took requisite courses at Umeå and other European universities. Through this collaboration, it has been possible to conduct the largest community-based epidemiological study in the world for schizophrenia and bipolar disorders, in which 68 378 adults in Butajira aged 15 to 49 were screened for these disorders through a door-to-door survey and close to 900 cases were identified (Kebede *et al.* 2004). These cases have been under follow-up for the last 14 years, and longitudinal data are being generated to describe the course and outcome of these disorders, and published in international peer reviewed journals (Alem *et al.* 2009, Teferra *et al.* 2011, 2012). Free psychotropic drugs are made available for study participants and non-participants who come to the hospital for treatment. This care is now being successfully transferred from the research project to the local government. Of note, this is the only community-based schizophrenia and bipolar cohort on the African continent.

Because of the achievements demonstrated through this collaboration, other higher learning institutions such as the Institute of Psychiatry (IoP) at King's College London, Nottingham University, and the Harvard School of Medicine have become involved in research collaborations and teaching in the Department of Psychiatry at AAU. Through these collaborations significant capacity building has been achieved among Ethiopian psychiatrists and public health specialists. So far, 13 Ethiopians have obtained their PhDs: eight psychiatrists and one epidemiologist from Umeå University, Sweden; a public health specialist, a psychiatrist, and a biostatistician from the King's College London; and one natural scientist from Nottingham University, UK. In addition, seven public health students have obtained their Masters degrees using data generated from these mental health projects.

Since these collaborations started, 33 different mental health studies have been conducted in Butajira and other districts of the country, and close to 100 scientific papers have been published in local and international scientific journals. Through these research projects millions of dollars have come to the country from funding agencies, mental health services have been initiated in the districts where mental health research has been conducted, and employment opportunities have been created for the local people.

One of the important outcomes of the research capacity built through these collaborations, in particular the Umeå University partnership, is that in 2011 the Department of Psychiatry at AAU opened a PhD program in mental health epidemiology. This is the only program of its kind in the country, and the Department of Psychiatry is the only clinical department at AAU to start a PhD program. It has 15 PhD candidates; seven have completed their first year of training, and eight began their training in 2012.

The Toronto Addis Ababa Psychiatry Project (TAAPP)

TAAPP is now 10 years old; this section will use some of the details of this partnership to illustrate the deliverables, outcomes, and impacts that are associated with it.

An invitation was sent for partnership consideration from Drs. Araya and Alem, who were the Head of the Department of Psychiatry and Chief of the Postgraduate program in Ethiopia at the time, to Dr. Don Wasylenki, the Chair of the Department of Psychiatry, UofT. Dr. Wasylenki suggested a one-week exploratory visit to AAU. As a result, a three-year letter of intent was signed agreeing to three teaching trips a year from UofT, each consisting of two UofT faculty psychiatrists and a psychiatry resident, starting in the fall of 2003. This first three-year period, called TAAPP Phase I, resulted in the graduation of the first six locally trained Ethiopian psychiatrists. The agreement is reviewed and reconsidered every three years. In TAAPP Phase II, 2006–08, teaching trips were reduced to two a year, and one Ethiopian faculty fellowship was offered annually at UofT. TAAPP Phase III replicated the previous three years and, with the aid of a DelPHI grant from the British Council, additional trips by UofT psychiatry faculty to the four new decentralized psychiatric departments were possible. Also, TAAPP assisted with the initiation of continuing medical education (CME) for all psychiatrists in the country. In TAAPP Phase IV the number of teaching trips has been increased to three a year, and CME development continues, as does the provision of an annual fellowship at UofT. In this phase we have also added one one-month trip a year of occupational therapy rehabilitation training into Amanuel hospital.

The main deliverables that TAAPP has partnered to provide are 26 on-site teaching months, delivering core content based on the Ethiopian curriculum. During these teaching months the formal didactic and seminar teaching occurs on three afternoons a week. During the remainder of the week, the UofT teachers spend one-on-one time clinically supervising the residents on site. This is very popular and highly valued by the Ethiopian residents because, despite the inconvenience it causes them (clinical teaching slows clinics and results in the residents having to work longer to get through their list), with a small overstretched faculty individual supervision is a luxury.

The partnership has considered the question of both cumulative and formative evaluation, and has developed a formative evaluation tool (FEDR) in the form of EthioMEDS (Alem *et al.* 2010). This single-sheet evaluation tool is of particular assistance to the UofT faculty, enabling quick feedback to residents based on their one-to-one clinical supervision on site during the TAAPP teaching months. TAAPP also co-prepares annual written examinations for all three years of residents to ensure they reflect the TAAPP teaching as well as the important findings of the Ethiopian mental health research.

As a result of a number of conversations between UofT and AAU colleagues, it was decided to incorporate five core competencies into the Ethiopian residency curriculum, adapted from CanMEDS (Royal College of Physicians and Surgeons of Canada 2013) to EthioMEDS. The roles are Clinical Expert, Leader, Educator, Scholar, and Advocate. In fact, all of the seven CanMED roles are included into the five EthioMED roles, which actually increase the number of roles by two: leader and educator. These were felt to be especially important and necessary for Ethiopian psychiatrists, given their particular context.

Perhaps the most relevant outcome of TAAPP is that since the program started 40 Ethiopian psychiatrists have graduated in-country. The current number of Ethiopian psychiatrists is 51 for a growing population estimated at 90 million. Of great interest is that the in-country retention rate is 95%, in contrast to the postulated 80% "brain drain." We hypothesize a critical mass effect together with the strong stabilizing effect of the senior Ethiopian psychiatrists' commitment to the expansion of mental health education and services, and their leadership mentoring effect.

Contingent on the increased number of psychiatrists in the country there have been several significant developments, two of the most important of which are addressed here. As noted earlier, mental health services are now moving towards becoming integrated into general health care, which necessitates training in aspects of psychiatry for all levels of healthcare professionals. Prior to this training, general healthcare workers would not have felt qualified to identify or assist patients who had mental disorders, with or without concurrent medical problems. The need for large-scale mental health education links up with the EthioMEDS role of educator. All new Ethiopian psychiatrists are grounded in the several skills of the educator role. Moving to train non-specialists is in line with task-shifting/sharing as mentioned earlier, and the *World Health Report* of 2006.

The second associated development of note is that one-third of the new graduates in psychiatry are employed regionally, and have opened the first five departments of psychiatry in their local university hospitals. TAAPP obtained a small DelPHI grant in Phase III and was able to send UofT psychiatrists for two-week stints to provide support and encouragement to these newly graduated heads of psychiatry departments over three years. The establishment of peripheral departments of psychiatry is a proud achievement. With devolution, the possibility of decentralized training can occur, and the development of locally tiered community-to-hospital services becomes far more likely. It sets the way for an evidence-supported optimum community psychiatry model for accessible, cost-efficient psychiatric care with improved outcomes. Through this model primary care workers are able to identify and provide local treatment for people with mental disorders (Desjarlais *et al.* 1995, Wiley-Exley 2007, World Health Organization 2001, 2003).

Patel (2009) suggests that as task-sharing is developed, the psychiatrist's role needs to shift accordingly to support a responsive system where the majority of mental health care is provided by primary health workers. For instance, the new regional departments of psychiatry in Ethiopia will become "hubs," with the psychiatrists in roles that promote community service development and assist in supporting primary care workers. Primary care workers also require training, supervision, and assistance to access psychiatric inpatient beds for patients in need of acute psychiatric care in a general hospital setting. The psychiatrist's roles will include attention to the forensic needs of the region, and overseeing the ordering of psychiatric medications and the development of integrated psychiatric care into a general hospital – including the future development of psychiatric residency programs.

On the UofT side of the partnership, over 40 faculty psychiatrists have traveled to AAU as volunteer teachers and supervisors for a month, and several have been there more than once. They are accompanied by a UofT resident who competes to go on this one-month educational elective. One of the impacts of TAAPP in the Department of Psychiatry at UofT has been the revision and doubling of the curriculum in the transcultural psychiatry core training for UofT

residents. The partnership has won five national and international awards. Perhaps most notably, TAAPP has produced a workable, effective model for accelerating the creation of medical specialists in Ethiopia, which in 2008 was embraced as a model collaboration for AAU and other Western university educational partnerships in general. In the same year, the government of Ethiopia mandated an increase in the number of universities from 13 to 31 and medical schools from 3 to 12. The number of medical student intakes has been increased from under 100 to 400 a year per school. In the 10 years between 2008 and 2018 the government requires 5000 PhD and 10 000 Masters students to graduate. With this massive focus on university postgraduate education, UofT and AAU have increased their number of departmental educational partnerships. TAAPP was the first, but there are now 16 such partnerships, out of five faculties at UofT, including the Faculties of Engineering and Arts and Science. The umbrella collaboration under which TAAPP and the other partnerships fall is now known as the Toronto Addis Ababa Academic Collaboration (TAAAC).

Conclusions

The two partnerships described in this chapter were established to address the gap in Ethiopia, a low-income country, between mental health services and care delivery personnel and systems. In concluding this summary, there are many considerations and questions that arise. We have emphasized five impacts of the educational partnerships that were set up between Addis Ababa University (AAU) and the University of Toronto, and between AAU and Umeå University: (1) the increase in research capacity and academic productivity; (2) the development of local psychiatric training capacity; (3) the progress that has been made in Ethiopia in the integration of mental health into the health system at all levels; (4) the regionalization of access and training for mental health in community systems; and (5) task-sharing. We believe the longevity of both partnerships has been an important asset enabling the AAU Department of Psychiatry to achieve capacity and sustainability in mental health education, which, as has been noted, impacts the system as a whole in a variety of ways. However, this longevity exceeds the life of any grant. In order therefore to provide such long-term partnering, systemic structures including reliable funding within both the HIC and LIC universities is needed to enable similar possibilities in future.

Finally, the question of the effect of America-centric psychiatric training on trainees and on local paradigms of mental distress and traditional healing has been raised frequently by global mental health experts (Fernando & Weerackody 2009), and this is a concern that we share. In 2012 TAAPP was a recipient of the Grand Challenges Canada grant which focused on tiered training to task-share mental health services centrally and in the regional hubs. This scaling-up opportunity offers a chance for feedback and a refined understanding of local explanatory models of mental health and wellness and local traditions of healing. We end this chapter by hoping that partnerships between HICs and LICs in mental health education will act to foster research into, and development of, culturally appropriate models of education.

References

Alem A, Pain C (2010) North–south collaboration for training psychiatrists: a template for Africa? Presented at the 36th Annual Harvey Stancer Research Day, Department of Psychiatry, University of Toronto.

Alem A, Jakobssen L, Argaw MD (1996) Traditional perceptions and treatment of mental disorders in central Ethiopia. In M Winkelman, W Andritzky, eds., *Yearbook of Cross-Cultural Medicine and Psychotherapy*. Berlin: Veerland & Vertrieb; pp. 105–19.

Alem D, Kebede G, Woldesemiat L, *et al.* (1999) The prevalence and socio-demographic correlates of mental distress in Butajira, Ethiopia. *Acta Psychiatrica Scandinavica* **100**: 48–55.

Alem A, Kebede D, Fekadu A, *et al.* (2009) Clinical course and outcome of schizophrenia in a predominantly treatment-naive cohort in rural Ethiopia. *Schizophrenia Bulletin* **35**: 646–654.

Alem A, Pain C, Araya M, *et al.* (2010) Co-creating a psychiatric resident program with Ethiopians, for Ethiopians, in Ethiopia: the Toronto Addis Ababa Psychiatry Project (TAAPP). *Academic Psychiatry* **34**: 424–32.

Berhan Y (2008) Medical doctor's profile in Ethiopia: production, attrition and retention. *Ethiopian Medical Journal* **46**: 23–4.

Beyero T, Alem A, Kebede D, *et al.* (2004) Mental disorders among the Borana semi-nomadic community in southern Ethiopia. *World Psychiatry* **3**: 110–14.

Desjarlais R, Eisenberg L, Good B, Kleinman A, eds. (1995) *World Mental Health: Problems and Priorities in Low-Income Countries*. New York, NY: Oxford University Press.

Fekadu A, Shibre T, Alem A, *et al.* (2004) Bipolar disorder among an isolated island community in Ethiopia. *Journal of Affective Disorders* **80**: 1–10.

Fernando S, Weerackody C (2009) Challenges in developing community mental health services in Sri Lanka. *Journal of Health Management* **11**: 195–208.

Frenk J, Chen L, Bhutta ZA, *et al.* (2010) Health professionals for a new century: transforming education to strengthen health systems in an interdependent world. *Lancet* **376**: 1923–58.

Fricchione G, Borba C, Alem A, *et al.* (2012) Capacity building in global mental health: professional training. *Harvard Review of Psychiatry* **20**: 47–57. http://www.royalcollege.ca/portal/page/portal/rc/canmeds (accessed July 2013).

Institute of Medicine (2001) *Health and Behavior: the Interplay of Biological, Behavioral, and Societal Influences*. Washington, DC: National Academies Press.

Kakuma R, Minas H, van Ginneken N, *et al.* (2011) Human resources for mental healthcare: current situation and strategies for action. *Lancet* **378**: 1654–63.

Kebede D, Alem A (1999) The prevalence and socio-demographic correlates of mental distress in Addis Ababa, Ethiopia. *Acta Psychiatrica Scandinavica* **100**: 5–10.

Kebede D, Alem A, Shibre T, *et al.* (2004) The sociodemographic correlates of schizophrenia in Butajira, rural Ethiopia. *Schizophrenia Research* **69**: 133– 141.

Mills EJ, Kanters S, Hagopian A, *et al.* (2011) The financial cost of doctors emigrating from sub-Saharan Africa: human capital analysis. *BMJ* **343**: 1–13.

Patel V (2009) The future of psychiatry in low- and middle-income countries. *Psychological Medicine* **39**: 1759–62.

Royal College of Physicians and Surgeons of Canada. (2013) CanMEDS. http://www.royalcollege.ca/portal/page/portal/rc/canmeds (accessed July 2013).

Sartorius N (2007) Physical illness in people with mental disorders. *World Psychiatry* **6**: 3–4.

Saxena S, Thornicroft G, Knapp M, *et al.* (2007) Resources for mental health: scarcity, inequity, and inefficiency. *Lancet* **370**: 878–89.

Shibre T, Tefera S Morgan C, Alem A (2010) Exploring the apparent absence of psychosis amongst pastoralist community of southern Ethiopia: a mixed method follow-up study. *World Psychiatry* **9**: 98–102.

Southall D, Cham M, Sey O (2010) Health workers lost to international

bodies in poor countries. *Lancet*
376: 498–9.

Teferra S, Shibre T, Fekadu A, *et al*
(2011) Five-year mortality in a
cohort of people with schizophrenia
in Ethiopia. *BMC Psychiatry* **11**:
165.

Teferra S, Shibre T, Fekadu A, *et al.*
(2012) Five-year clinical course and
outcome of schizophrenia in
Ethiopia. *Schizophrenia Research*
136: 137–42.

Wiley-Exley E (2007) Evaluations of
community mental healthcare in

low-and-middle-income countries:
a 10-year review of the literature.
Social Science and Medicine **46**:
1231–41.

World Health Organization (2001) *The
World Health Report 2001. Mental
Health: New Understanding, New
Hope.* Geneva: WHO.

World Health Organization (2003)
*Organization of Services for Mental
Health.* Geneva: WHO.

World Health Organization (2006) *The
World Health Report 2006. Working
Together for Health.* Geneva: WHO.

World Health Organization (2008) *The
Global Burden of Disease: 2004
Update.* Geneva: WHO.

World Health Organization (2011)
Mental Health Atlas 2011. Geneva:
WHO.

World Health Organization (2012) Rio
+20 declares health key to
sustainable development World
Health Organization. WHO news
statement, June 22, 2012. http://
www.who.int/mediacentre/news/
statements/2012/rio20_20120622/
en (accessed July 2013).

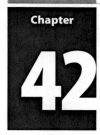

Chapter 42

Research priorities for mental health in low- and middle-income countries

Samuel O. Okpaku and Grace A. Herbert

Introduction and background

The field of medicine is no longer purely an art, as contemporary practice brings science and research to the forefront. With more emphasis on evidence and the need to understand the contributions of genetics and biology as well as the psychosocial factors that determine health outcomes, there is a priority for research in mental health. Why research? Research in medicine plays a vital role for a variety of reasons. It promotes discipline and critical examination of what we do rather than just relying on anecdotes, intuitions, and clinical myths. It provides greater knowledge and data for decision making, planning, and administrative rationales. It also impacts prestige and helps to satisfy curiosity.

The scientific validity of the knowledge base of global mental health itself has been questioned (Summerfield 2008). It becomes important, therefore, to take seriously the idea of research in global mental health. However, before undertaking such a project, it helps any research endeavor to have a foundation and a philosophical basis for that line of research. Global health is predicated on a value system. This system incorporates the following – access to care, equity in care, a focus on poor individuals and poor countries, country ownership, transparency, accountability, human dignity, and human rights. As we are talking about limited resources, the issue of effectiveness becomes a central value. Such a value system should serve as a core for mental health research and priority-setting exercises.

A major area of concern in global health is the disparity in research between developing nations and high-income countries. The concept "10/90" has become a slogan, referring to the research gap between low-income and high-income countries

(Patel 2007). It is estimated that both public and private funding sources contribute about US$56 billion a year to health research. Of this amount, less than 10% is devoted to diseases that account for about 90% of the global disease burden. A variant of the "10/90" concept is the limited contribution to prestigious journals by researchers from developing countries (Ad Hoc Committee 1996). There is a desire to close this research gap, a desire that is expressed by several agencies including the World Health Organization (WHO), major governments and their agencies, foundations such as the Bill and Melinda Gates Foundation, the Wellcome Trust, the Council on Health Research for Development (COHRED), the Global Forum for Health Research, and the pharmaceutical industry.

Several factors have led to the current interest. In 1990 a report by COHRED (1990) recommended that each country should have a national and international research agenda. In 1996 a report was published by the WHO Ad Hoc Committee on Health Research relating to future intervention options, and COHRED assisted a number of countries in setting up health research and health systems research agendas (Ad Hoc Committee 1996). Regrettably, many such plans did not translate into demonstrable action.

In response to the Ad Hoc Committee report, the Global Forum for Health Research was founded in 1998. The goal of this organization is to reduce the research gap between the developing world and the developed world (Independent Evaluation Group 2009). Another influence is the availability of funds from the US government (PEPFAR) for the fight against HIV/AIDS. The US government has contributed over US$37 billion to date in bilateral funding and over US$7 billion to the Global Fund to Fight

Essentials of Global Mental Health, ed. Samuel O. Okpaku. Published by Cambridge University Press. © Cambridge University Press 2014.

AIDS, Tuberculosis and Malaria (US Department of State 2012). There have been many positive results from this. In accordance with the recommendations from the Global Forum for Health Research, HIV/AIDS studies have been buttressed by a developing evidence base.

Another significant driving force is the perceived potential of research for health and development. This is then a matter of diplomacy. Global health research is fully embraced by the US government, as indicated by an international conference held in Rockville, Maryland, on January 6, 2000. The conference was attended by 60 leading experts including heads of major US agencies and representatives from foundations, pharmaceutical companies, industries, and overseas countries.

Several of the US speakers referred to a win–win situation, and described research funding activity as "soft and smart" diplomacy (National Institutes of Health 2010).

It is important to note that the NIH conference focused mostly on the big three diseases (HIV/AIDS, tuberculosis, and malaria) and non-communicable disorders. Attention was drawn to neglected tropical diseases. Mention was made of mental illness as a non-communicable disorder. In the recommendations at the end of the conference, the behavioral aspects of interventions were suggested. The major recommendations were suggestions to the NIH to be more relevant and active in global health (National Institutes of Health 2010). Also, the USA is by far the major donor of foreign aid. Therefore its leadership role is pivotal. Its vision and mission can be a useful template for all major donor countries.

Identifying barriers, challenges, and opportunities

Surveys of research priorities for mental health

In the last decade, there have been surveys, conferences, and commentaries to showcase the dearth of research activities and priorities in low- and middle-income countries (LMICs). Prominent amongst these were the surveys carried out by the Global Forum for Research, the WHO Department of Mental Health and Substance Abuse, the US National Institute of Mental Health (NIMH), the conference held by the

British Academy of Medical Sciences, and the *Lancet* Global Mental Health series.

Global Forum and WHO

In 2007, the Global Forum and WHO published the results of a mapping project named *Research Capacity for Mental Health in Low- and Middle-Income Countries* (Sharan *et al.* 2007). The participants in the study were two teams each from Africa, Asia, Latin America, and the Caribbean. The study respondents, or mapping actors, were individuals working in the field of mental health. These respondents were researchers, decision makers, university administrators, and association officers engaged in the field of mental health. The research team was able to glean information on the current research agendas in the various regions and to identify the priorities for mental health research. They gained insight into the dissemination of results of such research along with their impact on mental health policy and practice in the areas that were studied.

The major findings were significant disparities between and within regions in terms of research activities and mental health research. The respondents placed the highest priorities on epidemiological studies, health systems, and social science research. Depression/anxiety, substance abuse disorders, and psychosis were ranked as having the highest priority. The highest-ranked populations were children, adolescents women, and individuals at risk for violence and trauma. The study results underscored a gap between researchers and policy makers, which may account for the limited impact of research findings on policy. Other factors that contributed to the disparities included a lack of baseline studies and the absence of a critical mass of researchers and administrators. Together, these have consequences for communication across disciplines. Some of the major recommendations from the study included promoting the importance of mental health, setting up networks with the health research system, and increasing funding and investment in mental health research capacity (Sharan *et al.* 2007).

In a commentary on this study, Araya (2009) remarked that while the establishment of mental health research priorities may be desirable, there are many reasons why it may not be an easy task. He argued that the inequalities between LMICs point to the fact that the behavior of high-income countries, who make up 10% of the world population, may not be responsible for the inequalities. He questioned the allocation of resources for mental health research, vis-a-vis treatment, in the face of limited funding and when policy decisions are not necessarily based on research findings. He cited some strengths of the study:

- the inclusion of researchers and stakeholders from a variety of countries
- the concordance between responses from researchers and stakeholders

According to Araya, some weaknesses of the study included:

- lack of representativeness of the sample
- the exclusion of clinicians and users/survivors (this was a major omission)

I believe Araya (2009) was wrong in his opinion about the competition between clinical work and research activities. In our opinion research is an integral part of clinical services. Clinical services provide considerable opportunities for a variety of psychological, psychosocial, and biological studies, at the level of basic data collection and cross-sectional studies.

The *Lancet* series

The *Lancet* Global Mental Health series (2007) has contributed to the priority-setting exercises. The series pointed to deficits in evidence-based approaches to the major psychiatric disorders, alcohol and substance abuse, and mental health issues in childhood and adolescence. The list of priorities from the *Lancet* group included the need for mental health systems research on the cost-efficacy of interventions and epidemiological studies on childhood disorders and substance abuse disorders (*Lancet* 2007).

One of the major critisms of the *Lancet* series is the idea that a pattern of "one size fits all" is unacceptable. Some of the comments are in opposition to the continuation of previous colonial practices. They discuss strategies of targeting multilateral agencies, multinational interentions, and diverse settings.

The Academy of Medical Sciences

In 2008 the British Academy of Medical Sciences held a one-day symposium on challenges and priorities for global mental health research in LMICs. The symposium focused on three areas:

(1) highlighting the latest research activities in global mental health

(2) promoting awareness of the burden of mental illness in LMICs

(3) identifying priority areas for action

The participants included national and international experts as well as key funders of global mental health research. The discussions covered funding issues, low human capacity, lack of adequate infrastructure, and the burden on researchers because of service and administrative needs. The report also mentioned the lack of a research-oriented culture and weak peer networks and collaborations. The recommendations from the symposium included the need to scale up mental health services capacity, increase resources and funding for cost-effective interventions, achieve greater dissemination of research findings, and promote further understanding of task shifting. Additional recommendations included the need for greater attention to chronic mental disorders, increased knowledge of health systems, and more epidemiological studies in LMICs that cut across a variety of socioeconomic, ethnic, and community groups. Lastly, the report urged more communication between researchers and donors in the area of stigma, more studies in fragile states and areas of conflict, and greater support and training for researchers in LMICs (Academy of Medical Sciences 2008).

The Grand Challenges in Global Mental Health

On July 7, 2011, the journal *Nature* carried an article on the "grand challenges in global mental health" (Collins *et al.* 2011). This was the result of an initiative sponsored by NIMH, the Global Alliance for Chronic Diseases, the Wellness Trust, the McLaughlin Rotman Center for Global Health, and the London School of Hygiene and Tropical Medicine. Other contributors from the US National Institutes of Health included the Fogarty International Center; the National Heart, Lung and Blood Institute; and the National Institute of Neurological Disorders and Stroke (NINDS). The goal of the study was to identify the top 40 barriers to improving mental health globally. The participants included 422 experts from neuroscience, epidemiology, and mental health services research. There were representatives from more than 60 countries. The methodology used was the Delphi method, a strategy that was previously used by the Grand Challenges. The representatives were initially asked to suggest challenges to mental health care and services. The initial test consisted of 1565 challenges. The list was pruned down to 154 and ultimately to 40.

The highest-ranked challenges and needs were an emphasis on (1) evidence-based approaches, (2) the development of culturally informed methods to deal with stigma and associated behaviors, (3) task-shifting integration of mental health into screening in primary settings, (4) capacity building by creating regional hubs for training, education, and research, and (5) a deeper understanding of the consequences of poverty, violence, civil conflict, and migration on mental illness (Collins *et al.* 2011).

The above report met with outcry in some quarters. This was the case especially amongst the members of the transcultural psychiatry community. The researchers were accused of showing little sensitivity to cultural factors and local conditions in mental illness. In addition, powerful stakeholders and pharmaceutical companies were implicated in the study. Others have expressed the view that *The Lancet* and *Nature* should take the responsibility for fuelling the contentiousness.

A group of individuals including a user/survivor wrote a response to the *Nature* article – A reply to "Grand Challenges in the Mental Health" to the somatosphere. They criticized the study as being not representative and having too much of a focus on biomedical medicine. The response also questioned the premise that there is a norm in mental health (Timmi 2011).

The authors recommended that (1) mental health service delivery should reflect local realities and needs, (2) the frameworks should have, as their core, the protection of human rights, (3) the services should be "interactive" and not "imposed" from outside, (4) if the US NIMH is truly interested in improving the mental health of individuals in LMICs, then there should be direct discussions with a representative sample of the communities involved. The sample should not represent solely a selection of Western experts and "social and psychiatric elites" from LMICs (Timmi 2011).

Overall, the above surveys, conference reports, and the *Lancet* series have been derived essentially from the global burden of disease. While this is useful, it is deficient in that it does not take a contextual and ecological approach to the issue. The disease-burden approach implies a "one-size-fits-all" approach, while the contextual approach takes into account the variables and factors that have

been addressed as the social determinants of health – levels of poverty, the policies, the economy – all of which may have an impact on the research priorities. Labonté and Spiegel (2003) make a strong case for this latter perspective.

Editorial and research productivity

One measure of research productivity is the publication of papers in prestigious journals. Several groups have explored this area.

Keiser *et al.* (2004) published a report on the "representation of authors and editors from countries with different human development indexes in the leading literature of tropical medicine." The results obtained from their survey were as follows:

(1) About 71% of the editorial and advisory board members of the 12 referenced tropical medicine journals were from countries with a high human development index, with only 5.1% from countries with a low human development index.

(2) Of the 2384 articles published in 2000–02 in the six highest-ranking tropical medicine journals, 48.1% were from authors affiliated with high human development index countries, 13.7% from those affiliated with low human development index countries.

(3) There is significant collaboration between authors from high human development index and those from countries with a low or medium index.

The authors suggested that the current collaborations should be transferred into research partnerships to promote mutual learning and enhance capacity building in developing countries (Keiser *et al.* 2004).

Patel and Kim (2004) surveyed the contribution of LMICs to leading general psychiatric journals by reviewing the original research articles published between 2002 and 2004 in six of the highest-impact general psychiatric journals. They found out that although 60% of the global population is in LMICs only 3.7% of published materials were from developing countries. The European journals had higher representation than the American journals. About half of the research studies from LMICs were led by individuals from developing countries. Submission of articles from LMICs was very low and a high percentage of articles were rejected. They concluded that strengthening the research capacity of LMICs, as well as a revision of the editorial policies of major psychiatric journals, may enhance the contribution of LMICs to psychiatric research (Patel & Kim 2004).

The World Psychiatric Association (WPA) project in collaboration with representatives from the Global Mental Health Movement took on an initiative (1) to enhance support for a selected group of journal editors from LMICs, and (2) to assist the editors of LMIC mental health journals to improve the quality and standards of their publications by meeting the requirements for full indexation (de Jesus Mari *et al.* 2009).

In 2003, the WHO Department of Mental Health and Substance Abuse convened a conference of 25 editors representing journals in the field of mental health. Topics discussed included (1) the responsibilities of scientific journals towards international mental health, (2) the task of supporting mental health researchers from LMICs, (3) the task of supporting mental health journals from LMICs, and (4) the need to enhance dissemination of mental health research publications and opportunities for LMICs to access and disseminate research knowledge (Saxena *et al.* 2004). Practical suggestions for supporting and encouraging researchers from developing countries to gain access to the highly prestigious journals were made during the meeting.

Monitoring progress: the US and Canadian government efforts

It is worth commenting on some of the progress and follow-up to the above recommendations. In this regard, two major institutions have made some strides in providing funding to enhance research. Since 2010, the US NIMH has been active in pursuing goals to meet its global mental health objectives, and has organized workshops and conferences to promote opportunities in global mental health research and training. In addition, it has provided funds to set up regional research hubs. The Grand Challenges of Canada has also contributed 20 million Canadian dollars to innovative research in number of developing countries.

Observations and discussion

From the above survey results and conference recommendations some central themes emerge. These themes overlap, but for heuristic reasons they will be discussed separately.

Need for evidence-based approaches

It does not take a scientific mind to be aware of the disparities that exist within and between regions in terms of research activities, productivity, and resources. However, what is important, in the spirit of evidence-based approaches, is the ability to document the observations. Evidence-based approaches have an impact on policy, practice, and administration.

Cultural context

Every human engagement exists within a cultural context. Foreign aid is no exception. During the NIH conference several speakers made references to health research as diplomacy for health and development. For those speakers, research in global health is seen as a win–win situation, but this may have different meanings and implications in a variety of cultural settings.

Many decades ago I had a discussion with a prominent anthropologist. I do not remember what the antecedent was but we came to a point in our conversation at which we discussed the simple etiquette of opening the door for someone else. According to him, if an individual A opens the door for an individual B, there is the understanding that at some time in the future, B will open the door for A. I disagreed. I illustrated my point with the following examples. The first example is an elderly person who has limited funds. She is trying to decide what to buy in the grocery. If one were to give her a $5 bill, I do not believe that the donor expects anything back. Another example might be an eight-year-old child in a grocery. She is upset and has big beads of tears rolling down her cheeks. If one intervenes to inquire what the matter is, one is not expecting a reward.

This matter is not sufficiently discussed in diplomacy; however, it has been raised with reference to the Association of South East Asian Nations (ASEAN). The diplomatic approach of the leaders of that organization has been described as "a process of regional interactions and cooperation based on discussions, informality, consensus building, and non-confrontational bargaining styles" as opposed to the adversarial posturing, majority vote, and other legalistic decision-making procedures in Western multilateral organizations. A dictum in American social policy is "conflict and compromise." In all fairness, each system has its strengths and weaknesses. The tension between altruism and profit motive is real, which is indeed a problem in global research goals.

A good example is suspicion regarding the sincerity of the pharmaceutical industry.

Another aspect of the cultural dimensions of global health has to do with the cultural familiarity that occurs in exchange programs. It is true that sometimes aid workers may experience severe cultural shock, but there are instances where exchange programs have led eventually to health diplomatic activities. A good example is the recent Peace Corps award of excellence given to Dr. Mohamud Sheikh Nurein Said of Kenya. As a youngster, he was taught science under very rural and poor circumstances by a young American Peace Corps worker. The American aid worker had to teach theories of magnetism in extremely deprived circumstances where candles burned in place of electric lights. Dr. Said later went to Russia to study medicine and then returned to his homeland. He served as president of the International Rehabilitation Council for Torture Victims (*US Africa Journal* 2013).

There are many such examples of friendships developed in international exchanges that provide the human background to diplomatic engagements. A major consideration in global health and mental health is for projects, research, and intervention to be locally and culturally relevant and sensitive.

Culture of research

One should not fail to mention the need for a culture of research. This is critical for research productivity. A multidisciplinary approach with social scientists, anthropologists, economists, and statisticians can greatly benefit the research agenda. An important cultural component is the attitude that individuals, institutions, policy makers, and administrators have towards research. For the individual clinician, he/she should be asking himself/herself questions such as, what am I doing; what results do I expect; what outcomes am I getting; and why is some treatment approach better than others? Similarly, policy makers and administrators can gain useful insights by asking questions parallel to the above questions. One is reminded of the discovery of the causative pathogen in cholera by John Snow, the discovery of the usefulness of lithium carbonate in the treatment of manic depressive illness, and other serendipities in the history of medicine.

The culture of research should begin early in life. It is beneficial for young boys and girls to learn critical skills from their time in primary schools, through high school and college. Cross-cultural academic collaboration between schools is helpful in this endeavor. In the developed world, there are government-run and industry-led programs that stimulate young people's interest in science, mathematics, and engineering. Such strategies are also valuable to young students from the developing world.

Resources

A major barrier to research in developing countries is the lack of resources. This has implications for infrastructure and capacity building. Many agencies advocate increased investment in developing countries by the developed countries. Qualified personnel tend to be handicapped by administrative and clinical commitments. Undeniably, funding is critical. However, this should not be overemphasized or overrated. There are opportunities for non-funded research. While funding is not to be discouraged, the limited resources can be a driver in their own right – necessity is the mother of invention. At a 1986 conference in Nairobi, Kenya, organized by the African Psychiatric Association, the Black Psychiatrists of America, and the American Psychiatric Association, I had the privilege to hear some lamentations from our African colleagues as to the limited resources that were available to them. A colleague once mentioned that even in the busy schedule of physicians there are weekends. Another insinuated that what one needs is a good idea, a pencil, and some paper – to which I said it is the attitude and orientation of the individual. This is not to excuse the paucity of resources.

Education, training, exchange programs, and mentorships

The recommendation of COHRED is that each nation should have a national research agenda as well as an international agenda. There are multiple opportunities for institutions and experts from developed countries to participate in assisting institutions from developing countries in this area. Fellowships at different levels have been suggested. Scientists from major institutes may gain first-hand knowledge of the recipient institutions by exchange agreements. Talented students from developing countries may be trained abroad – and here there is the sensitive topic of "brain drain." It is believed that by making research more attractive in students' home countries, the temptation to study and stay abroad may be reduced.

Information technology

Lastly, the potential use of modern information technology (IT) was touched upon at the NIH conference. A frequently suggested goal is for greater epidemiological studies with cohorts and multiple-site involvement. IT is useful in this regard. The opportunities for "e-mobile health" and "e-education" are to be further experienced. Data sharing, access to large databanks, multimedia presentations, as well as multiple scientific presentations and conferences, can have considerable application in bridging the research gap between the developing countries and the developed world.

Promotion and advocacy

A frequent recommendation for global mental health is to make civil society policy and decision makers more aware of mental health issues. A good example is the deleterious effect of stigma and discrimination on mentally ill individuals and their families.

Innovative and creative partnerships

The need for innovative partnerships is gaining momentum. New south–south and north–south private and public partnerships have been encouraged. Entrepreneurship also has a role in setting up innovative consortiums among stakeholders, including academia, pharma, start-up companies, and foundations.

Conclusions

In conclusion, there is an urgent need to enhance mental health research in LMICs. Such research will help to address the unmet needs of those countries. The results can shape policy. Developed countries also benefit from this research, as they contribute to understanding the contextual nature of interventions and the variability of outcomes.

Evidence-based research is a priority, and all stakeholders should be more aware of the need for research. The prestigious mental health research journals can contribute to the effort of promoting and disseminating the work of researchers from LMICs. Partnerships and mentorships should be encouraged between researchers from LMICs and those from high-income countries. Usage of advances in IT and other technologies is a priority. Attempts should be made for early transfer of technological advances to LMICs, so as not to cause delays in knowledge transfer in a rapidly changing world.

References

Academy of Medical Sciences (2008) *Challenges and Priorities for Global Mental Health Research in Low- and Middle-Income Countries. Symposium Report, December 2008.* London: The Academy.

Ad Hoc Committee on Health Relating to Future Intervention Options (1996) *Investing in Health Research and Development.* Document TDR/Gen/96.1. Geneva: WHO.

Araya R (2009) Invited commentary on . . . Mental health research priorities in low- and middle-income countries. *British Journal of Psychiatry* **195**: 364–5.

Collins PY, Patel V, Joestl SS, *et al.* (2011) Grand challenges in global mental health. *Nature* **475**: 27–30.

Commission On Health Research for Development (COHRED) (1990) *Health Research Essential Link to Equity in Development.* New York, NY: Oxford University Press.

de Jesus Mari J, Patel V, Kieling C, *et al.* (2009) The 5/95 gap on the dissemination of mental health research: the World Psychiatric Association (WPA) task force report on project with editors of low and middle income (LAMI) countries. *African Journal of Psychiatry* **12**: 33–9.

Independent Evaluation Group (2009) *The Global Forum for Health Research.* Global Program Review, Vol 3 Issue 3. Washington, DC: World Bank Group. http://siteresources.worldbank.org/EXTGLOREGPARPROG/

Resources/gfhr.pdf (accessed July 2013).

International Consortium on Mental Health Policy and Services (2000) First Meeting of the Africa Region Meeting, Lusaka, Zambia 27–29 November 2000: report. http://www.mental-neurological-health.net/media/documents/A2-RegionalMeetings_Regional-Lusaka.pdf (accessed July 2013).

Keiser J, Utzinger J, Tanner M, Singer BH (2004) Representation of authors and editors from countries with different human development indexes in the leading literature on tropical medicine: survey of current evidence. *BMJ* **328**: 1229–32.

Labonté R, Spiegel J (2003) Setting global health research priorities. *BMJ* **326**: 722–3.

Lancet (2007) Global mental health: executive summary. *Lancet*, September 3, 2007. http://www.thelancet.com/series/global-mental-health (accessed July 2013).

National Institutes of Health (2010) Global Health Research Meeting, January 6, 2010, in Rockville, Maryland. http://commonfund.nih.gov/pdf/Global%20Health%20Research%20Meeting.pdf (accessed July 2013).

Patel V (2007) Closing the 10/90 divide in global mental health research. *Acta Psychiatrica Scandinavia* 115: 257–9.

Patel V, Kim YR (2007) Contribution of low- and middle-income countries to research published in leading general psychiatry journals, 2002–2004. *British Journal of Psychiatry* 190: 77–8.

Saxena S, Sharan P, Saraceno B (2004) Research for change: the role of scientific journals publishing mental health research. *World Psychiatry* 3 (2): 66–72.

Sharan P, Levav I, Olifson S, de Francisco A, Saxena S, eds. (2007) *Research Capacity for Mental Health in Low- and Middle-Income Countries: Results of a Mapping Project.* Geneva: WHO & Global Forum for Health Research.

Summerfield D (2008) How scientifically valid is the knowledge base of global mental health? *BMJ* 336: 992–4.

Timimi S (2011) A reply to "Grand Challenges in Mental Health". *Somatosphere*, October 11, 2011. http://somatosphere.net/2011/10/a-reply-to-grand-challenges-in-mental-health.html (accessed July 2013).

US Africa Journal (2013) Kenyan doctor receives Peace Corps Alumni's Global Citizen Award. *US Africa Journal*, June 2013. http://www.usafricajournal.com/2013/06/25 (accessed July 2013).

US Department of State (2012) The President's Emergency Plan for AIDS Relief (PEPFAR) Blueprint: creating an AIDS-free generation. Fact sheet. http://www.state.gov/r/pa/prs/ps/2012/11/201195.htm (accessed July 2013).

Chapter

43

Research infrastructure

Athula Sumathipala

Definition

The *Oxford English Dictionary* (OED) definition of *infrastructure* is "basic structural foundations of a society or enterprise." Therefore research infrastructure can best be defined as the "basic structural foundations of a research enterprise."

Research infrastructure is an indispensible component of research enterprise. "If the history of science teaches us anything, it is that an infrastructure is an indispensable adjunct to the efforts of individual researchers" (National Research Council 1998).

Therefore, it is worth examining right at the outset the working definition of research infrastructure used by the scientific community globally. However, this is not a comprehensive systematic review of literature, because such an exercise is beyond the scope of a short chapter in this book.

For the project on Mapping of the European Research Infrastructure Landscape (MERIL), the European Commission and the European Strategy Forum on Research Infrastructures (ESFRI) use the following definition: "a European Research Infrastructure is a facility or (virtual) platform that provides the scientific community with resources and services to conduct top-level research in their respective fields. These research infrastructures can be single-sited or distributed or an e-infrastructure, and can be part of a national or international network of facilities, or of interconnected scientific instrument networks" (European Science Foundation 2013). This definition appears to be a fairly broad one, and considers not only resources but also services and virtual facilities.

The European Commission Work Programme for 2010, under research infrastructure, has also included radiation sources, data banks in genomics and in social science, observatories for environmental sciences, systems of imaging or clean rooms for the study and development of new materials or nano-electronics, computing and communication-based e-infrastructures also as part of the infrastructure.

According to the definition used by the National Research Infrastructure Council of the Australian Department of Innovation and Industry, Science and Research, "research infrastructure comprises the assets, facilities and services which support research across the innovation system and which maintain the capacity of researchers to undertake excellent research and deliver innovation outcomes" (National Research Infrastructure Council 2011).

The University of South Australia's Research Infrastructure Working Party (RIWP) has adopted a working definition of research infrastructure as "equipment, facilities and 'soft' infrastructure such as software, subscriptions, digital archives, databases which enable the process of research and support the generation of research outcomes of high impact and quality" (National Research Infrastructure Council 2011). The RIWP definition is consistent with the Australian Research Council definition of research infrastructure (http://www.arc.gov.au).

The Research Infrastructure Task Force (RITF) of the University of Minnesota felt that a workable definition of "research infrastructure" must be sufficiently broad to encompass the support needed for all scholarly activities not directly related to teaching. The RITF therefore adopted the definition of infrastructure as "the facilities (e.g., laboratories, studios, clinics) and services (e.g., libraries, computing services, grants management systems, research safety and subject protection organizations, and secretarial services) needed to produce novel and influential

Essentials of Global Mental Health, ed. Samuel O. Okpaku. Published by Cambridge University Press. © Cambridge University Press 2014.

scholarly output (e.g., publications, exhibits, performances)" (University of Minnesota Research Infrastructure Task Force 2006).

The German Federal Ministry of Education and Research (2011) includes scientific collections too as a significant part of research infrastructure: "Scientific collections and objects form an essential basis for research in numerous scientific disciplines; many disciplines came into existence only as a result of collections, particularly in research fields such as evolution, the environment, biodiversity, ethnology and archaeology, art and culture, the history of science and engineering."

The PAERIP (Promoting African European Research Infrastructure Partnership) definition of research infrastructure includes "facilities, resources and services used by the scientific community for conducting cutting edge research for the generation, exchange and preservation of knowledge. It includes associated human resources, major facilities, equipment or sets of instruments, collaborative networks and knowledge-containing resources such as collections, archives and data- and bio banks too" (Botha & Gruenewaldt 2012).

New knowledge and innovation depends on high-quality and accessible infrastructure. Research infrastructures are therefore at the center of the knowledge triangle of research, education, and innovation, producing knowledge through research, diffusing it through education, and applying it through innovation.

A search for a Chinese definition of research infrastructure did not yield any specific results. However, there was evidence that the European Economic Council was working closely with the Chinese on this. Similarly, a search for a definition from another growing economy, India, did not yield any results either. Therefore it is difficult to compare the conceptualizations of Chinese and Indian definitions of research infrastructure.

This raises a fundamental question. Should the conceptual definition of research infrastructure be the same across different cultures and countries?

Types of research infrastructures

In summary, the above review suggests that the term *research infrastructure*, according to the Western definition, is very broad and refers to facilities, resources, and related services used by the scientific community

to conduct research, ranging from the social sciences to genomics and nanotechnologies. Examples include singular large-scale research installations, collections, special facilities, libraries, databases, biological archives, clean rooms, integrated arrays of small research installations, high-capacity/high-speed communication networks, research vessels, satellite and aircraft observation facilities, coastal observatories, telescopes, synchrotrons and accelerators, networks of computing facilities, as well as infrastructure centers and hubs which provide a service for the wider research community based on an assembly of techniques and know-how.

However, it is notable that people, salaries, and buildings have been considered outside the definition of research infrastructure.

Despite infrastructure being widely cited as a core component of research capacity building, it has been restricted to a narrow category of physical or administrative inputs. The terms *research infrastructure*, *capacity*, and *culture*, which are overlapping components, have been artificially separated and used in inconsistent ways, dissociating their relationships with associated concepts (Coen *et al.* 2010). Coen *et al.* strongly argued for "an expanded conceptualization of research infrastructure; one that moves beyond conventional 'hardware' notions." Drawing on a case analysis of NEXUS, a multidisciplinary health research center/hub based at the University of British Columbia, Canada, they have proposed a conceptual framework to integrate the tangible and intangible structures that interactively underlie research center functioning, and they envision infrastructure as a relational construct comprised of multiple and interactive parts.

In their conceptual framework, "infrastructure consists of various structures that interactively create a composite greater than the sum of its parts." They characterize the framework as "relational" because "it is the relationships between these elements that define the whole, not simply the ingredients called for in the recipe."

Elaborating on interrelationships, "particular features of research centers take form as a result of an iterative, interactive process, and this form is not necessarily tangible." Instead, Coen *et al.* (2010) comment that "abstruse collective structures, such as internal knowledge, culture, or identity (that may not be quantifiable) are nevertheless significant factors in centre success."

One of the core assertions of this framework is that features of research environments such as culture or identity are in effect resources upon which center members can draw in advancing the work. Therefore these aspects form part of the underlying structures (albeit social) that support research. Hence infrastructures are not necessarily material.

Research infrastructures play a crucial role in the advancement of knowledge and technology. They are an essential tool in science. They are key to bringing together a wide diversity of stakeholders. Research infrastructures may be "single-sited" (a single resource at a single location), "distributed" (a network of distributed resources), or "virtual" (the service is provided electronically).

Proxy indicators of research infrastructure and capacity in health services research

Even though at a conceptual level the West is propagating a global attitude, does the reality reflect that agenda in an equitable manner?

Less than 10% of research funds are spent on the diseases that account for 90% of the global disease burden. Although 93% of the world's burden of preventable mortality occurs in developing countries, too little research funding is dedicated to health problems in developing countries (Global Forum for Health Research 2000). There is also a significant publication divide in medical as well as in mental health research (Patel & Sumathipala 2001, Sumathipala et al. 2004), which could be indirect evidence of poor research capacity, whatever the reasons may be.

Mapping mental health research capacity and resources in low- and middle-income countries (LMICs) has provided evidence for scarcity and unequal distribution of mental health research capacity in LMICs. A global survey mapped research and researchers from 114 LMIC countries around the world and found that researchers and publications were concentrated in 10% of the countries surveyed (Razzouk et al. 2010). This paper, based on a project of the Global Forum for Health Research, found, among other things, that Asian researchers were more likely to be based in private institutions than their colleagues from other continents. This finding poses the question whether the situation demands research infrastructure beyond traditional and conventional institutions such as universities.

The paper further concludes that low publication rates from LMICs are due to a lack of human resources, and it cites access to journals and databases, research fellowships, and funding as main resources that are lacking in LMICs (Razzouk et al. 2010).

In a survey carried out by Sumathipala et al. (2004), the average contribution of countries outside Europe, North America, and Australia (rest of the world, RoW) to overall research literature in five high-impact medical journals was 6.5%. An analysis of the authorship of 151 articles from RoW showed that 104 (68.9%) had co-authors from Europe, North America, or Australia. This study adds to a previous study reveaing that over 90% of psychiatric research articles published in six leading journals originated from European and American societies (Patel & Sumathipala 2001).

Therefore, can equal capacity or output, in a significantly divided world, ever be a reality?

Mental health researchers in LMICs have little access to resources, such as research networks, fellowships, technical support or well-resourced libraries. Global surveys of mental health researchers in LMICs indicate that major challenges facing researchers are perceived to be a lack of funding, shortage of trained staff, and difficulties in the provision of training owing to poor institutional infrastructure. The absence of a strong research "culture" is reflected through constraints on researchers' time owing to service delivery and teaching commitment, weak peer networks and collaborations. Partnerships between, institutions or researchers in the South and/or North (South–South or North–South partnerships) can provide important support and guidance.

In December 2002 the World Health Organization (WHO) organized a meeting in Cape Town, South Africa, on "Research for Change" to discuss mental health research in LMICs. Participants at this meeting included researchers from developing and developed countries, WHO Collaborating Centers, national research institutes and research councils, international research organizations, editors of scientific journals, policy advisors and program planners, as well as representatives of funding agencies and donors. The meeting clearly brought out the paucity of mental health research activities and the inadequacy of infrastructure to support such research in these countries. The need for concerted actions for supporting research was recognized, and many steps have been taken. One of these was the Atlas Research Project, which aims to obtain information about mental health-related research (research amount and quality) and mental health research infrastructure.

Research infrastructure funding schemes

It is encouraging to see that international research funding agencies and governments have recognized the need to support capacity building in LMICs. There is an increasing trend globally to recognize the need to support research infrastructure.

- The Swiss National Science Foundation (SNSF) provides direct funding on a discretionary basis for research infrastructure.
- The Unicef/UNDP/World Bank/WHO Special Programme for Research and Training in Tropical Diseases (TDR) also supports Research Capacity Strengthening (RCS) activities.
- The EU Framework Programme is a cross-border research support system. It now expands the scope of its network worldwide beyond the 27 EU member states.
- Japan also has established the Human Frontier Science Program (HFSP) as a global research support system at the end of the 1980s. Recently, it launched a system to support research and human resource development in developing countries as a joint project between the Japan Science and Technology Agency (JST) and the Japan International Cooperation Agency (JICA), and is receiving high praise.
- Grand Challenges Canada is another initiative dedicated to supporting bold ideas with big impact in global health. It is funded by the Government of Canada to support innovators in low- and middle-income countries and Canada.
- The Australian government and state and territory governments contribute significant funding for research infrastructure. This includes funding to universities and funding to mission-oriented publicly funded research agencies such as CSIRO and DSTO. The Australian government also provides support to national, international, regional, institutional, and thematic groups' strategies and priorities.
- The Consortium for Advanced Research Training in Africa (CARTA) brings together a network of nine academic and four research institutions from west, east, central, and southern Africa, and selected northern universities and training institutes. CARTA's program of activities comprises two primary, interrelated, and mutually reinforcing objectives: to strengthen research infrastructure and capacity at African universities, and to support doctoral training through the creation of a collaborative doctoral training program in population and public health. The ultimate goal of CARTA is to build local research capacity to understand the determinants of population health and effectively intervene to improve health outcomes and health systems.

- The Wellcome Trust in the UK, which is the world's second-largest research charity, had been offering extensive funding and support to enhance research capacity in the LMICs for a long time well in advance of the campaign to increase research capacity in LMICs. It supports over 3000 researchers in more than 50 different countries and offers around £720 million per year, including around £100 million for international activities, especially international networks and partnerships focused on the problems of resource-poor countries. There are major overseas programs (centers) in Vietnam, Thailand, Kenya, and Central Africa.
- The National Institute of Mental Health (NIMH) offered funding to establish regional research hubs to increase the evidence base for mental health interventions in World-Bank-designated LMICs. Each regional hub is to conduct research and provide capacity-building opportunities in one of six geographical regions (East Asia and the Pacific, Europe and Central Asia, Latin America and the Caribbean, Middle East and North Africa, South Asia, sub-Saharan Africa). As a group, awardees will constitute a collaborative network for mental health research in LMICs with capabilities for answering research questions (within and across regions) aimed at improving mental health outcomes for men, women, and children.
- The SHARE initiative – SHARE is the South Asian Hub for Advocacy, Research and Education on mental health. It is one of the five Collaborative Hubs for International Research on Mental Health funded by the US National Institute of Mental Health (NIMH). It is a five-year program, starting in 2012, that focuses on research, research

capacity building, and shared research. It is a collaboration between the London School of Hygiene and Tropical Medicine, the University of Liverpool, the Public Health Foundation of India, Sangath, the Institute of Psychiatry (Pakistan), the Human Development Research Foundation (Pakistan), the Institute of Psychiatry (UK), the Johns Hopkins School of Public Health (USA), and a network of about a dozen research institutions in India, Afghanistan, Nepal, Bangladesh, and Sri Lanka. The Institute for Research and Development (IRD) is the Sri Lankan collaborative partner of this initiative. The goal of SHARE is to establish a collaborative network of institutions in South Asia, to carry out and to utilize research that answers policy-relevant questions related to reducing the treatment gap for mental disorders in the region.

The above is not an exhaustive list, but some selected examples of existing work taking place to address the gap.

All these funding efforts should be lauded and appreciated. However, the big question is: Can funding alone deliver? Also, is the commitment sustainable and adequate?

Infrastructure and capacity development

A good methodologist with a sound research question and a protocol, along with generous funding, alone will not succeed in carrying out high-quality research. There are many other factors such as team building and leaderships that matters. North–South and South–South collaboration are also necessary to produce high-quality research. Research infrastructures can facilitate good-quality research. Expatriates also have a significant role to play in this regard.

Research in developing countries at present is mostly influenced by a semi-colonial model (Costello & Zumla 2000): "postal research," where developing countries courier biological samples to the West, or "parachute research," where Western researchers travel to developing countries and take back data or biological samples without much benefit back to the host countries. However, "annexed sites research" led and managed by expatriate staff can produce influential and innovative research.

One of the potential threats is when the Western partner's motives could be driven purely by a need to conduct research cheaply on developing-country populations. This is why local infrastructure and capacity building should be an essential component of the project.

The collaboration between the Institute for Research and Development (www.ird.lk) in Sri Lanka and the Institute of Psychiatry, King's College London, in the UK (www.kcl.ac.uk/iop) was a "partnership model," a model which can produce high-quality research. In this model local academic leaders manage the research, and expatriates having active links to both worlds playing a significant leadership role with significant inputs from the Western partners.

The Sangath Foundation of India is another organization that materialized through North–South partnership, and which has achieved much in mental health and public health in India (www.sangath.com). It is doing valuable work in capacity building and mental health research in India.

How can LMIC research contribute to global knowledge?

High-quality collaborative research conducted in developing countries can provide evidence of relevance and value to the developed world. For example, the use of anticonvulsants in the management of eclampsia has been the subject of controversy over 70 years, until a large clinical trial (1687 patients) conducted in South America, Africa, and India, coordinated by the Oxford Eclampsia Trial Collaborative Group (ETCG) from Britain, demonstrated that magnesium sulphate was the drug of choice." The results of this trial have been widely accepted by the international obstetric community, with the Royal College of Obstetricians and Gynaecologists (London), for example, incorporating this evidence into its practice guidelines (Mari *et al.* 1997).

Another good example is provided by a large population-based study of vaginal discharge (Patel *et al.* 2005, 2006). WHO had previously recommended syndromic management, in which women complaining of vaginal discharge are treated for some or all of the five common reproductive tract infections (RTIs): *Chlamydia trachomatis* infection, gonorrhea, and trichomoniasis, which are sexually transmitted infections (STIs), and bacterial vaginosis (BV) and candidiasis, which result from disturbances in the normal bacterial flora of the vagina (World Health

Organization 1994). This approach had significant social and marital implications for women and families, especially as it implied that vaginal discharge was indicative of STI. In the population-based cohort study in Goa, India, Patel *et al.* (2005, 2006) revealed that the vaginal discharge had a strong association with bacterial vaginosis, but not with sexually transmitted infection. Vaginal discharge also had association with psychosocial stressors and common mental disorders. This study was the first population-based cohort study investigating the etiology of one of the most common, and disabling, reproductive and sexual symptoms affecting women in developing countries. In terms of impact, the practice has changed to the extent that the syndromic approach is now not considered foolproof, and diagnostic tests for STI are considered before antibiotics – even though these are not available in most places in rural India, and mental health issues are not quite addressed as they should be. However, the policy shift at least has been initiated.

Another good example is a randomized controlled trial of a community-based complex intervention delivered by community health workers for maternal depression and child development in Pakistan (Rahman *et al.* 2008). Commenting on the paper, Patel & Kirkwood (2008) noted that these trials have implications for both the developing and the developed world. The study demonstrated that suitably modified cognitive behavioral therapy can be given by community health workers who had not completed high school, if sufficiently trained and supervised.

Sri Lankan experience

In this section, the author's Sri Lankan experience is revisited to present an option for capacity building, including research infrastructure development, in the form of a case study from an LMIC.

Traditionally most research, particularly individual-led research, is focused on one or a few subject areas of research interest. If a particular researcher is interested or involved in too many fields that is considered, at least by some, as lack of focus. Giving leadership to research capacity in resource-poor settings cannot be artificially narrowed or "focused." This is one of the major issues I faced during some of my grant applications. For historical reasons, my research interests are centered on interconnected disciplines. They are seemingly diverse but very

much interconnected. For example, epidemiology of chronic non-communicable diseases; evaluation and implementation of complex interventions; and ethics related to research in the context of international collaborations, including disaster-related research and ethics. All these are grounded through real-life experience in conducting research in a developing country. But for some this was seen as a lack of focus.

I consider my greatest contribution throughout my academic and research career to have been the establishment of the Institute for Research and Development (IRD) in Sri Lanka (www.ird.lk). Being a researcher from a developing country, where the infrastructure for research is not well established, I founded the IRD in an effort to overcome systematic barriers in an LMIC. The IRD is a research organization independent of government, industry, and universities. The institute has been a vehicle for developing a series of large-scale local and international research projects. Working with senior colleagues at the Institute of Psychiatry (IoP) at King's College London and in Sri Lanka, the resource has been extended to establish a state-of-the-art genetic laboratory and a bio-bank. This infrastructure now complements my efforts by promoting capacity building through a cadre of high-caliber junior academics.

Sri Lankan experience: the wider context

Sri Lanka is classified by the World Bank as an LMIC. By 2004 Sri Lanka had only around 25 specialist psychiatrists for a population of over 20 million (Sumathipala & Siribaddana 2005). Mental health services were based on institutional care and lacked public health, primary care, and multidisciplinary perspectives (World Health Organization 2005). Nationwide epidemiological data were not available to quantify the burden of disease, death, and disability due to mental disorders in Sri Lanka (World Health Organization 2005). The IRD was later commissioned in 2007 by the Ministry of Health and the World Health Organization (WHO) to conduct the first national mental health survey to be conducted in Sri Lanka.

A survey revealed that over a period of five years, only 47 indexed and 32 non-indexed articles had been published on mental health in Sri Lanka (Sharan *et al.* 2009). Apart from that, opportunities for full-time (mental) health research at local universities are almost non-existent in Sri Lanka (Konradsen & Munk-Jorgensen 2007). Research is not a popular career option for mental health professionals.

The Institute for Research and Development (IRD)

This brief account about the Institute for Research and Development in Sri Lanka is presented here to show an example of a successful private research institution based in an LMIC, and a showcase of a successful North–South partnership for capacity building. A comprehensive account of the work carried out by the IoP and IRD partnership since 1997 has been published elsewhere (Siriwardhana et al. 2011).

The IRD is a not-for-profit research institution. Its academic members include epidemiologists, psychiatrists, physicians, geneticists, veterinarians, public health specialists and others who are not employed full-time by the institution. It now has over 20 full-time research staff, and many other associates involved at various levels while employed in other academic institutions. The IRD was initiated following a Wellcome Trust project grant awarded to the author in 1997. There had to be immense individual commitments and personal sacrifices on the part of those who initiate such endeavors in the developing world. A sound research question and a protocol along with generous funding were necessary, but were not sufficient to develop research infrastructure or build capacity. Experiences from Sri Lanka (and other developing countries) suggest that there are many other factors that contribute and play a decisive role. Examples include the ability to conduct teamwork and establish networks, negotiating skills, and supervising and training others.

The IRD was commissioned in 2007 by the Ministry of Health and the WHO to conduct the first national mental health survey, using a population-based adult sample of 6000 and a school-based child sample of 4000. The institute was also commissioned by the International Organization on Migration to carry out a study on the impact of spouse migration on the family left behind.

The IRD has already addressed the Global Health Forum survey team's call to meet challenges in mental health research in LMICs (Razzouk et al. 2010) by investing in capacity building. It stands as a model for successful North–South partnerships in

mental health research and other research areas. It also stands as a perfect example of how Northern financial support can be successfully utilized to improve Southern research resources, capacity, and output.

However, international funding agencies, academics, and other bodies need to address the issue of sustaining such initiatives as a priority, in order to reduce scarcity and inequity in mental health research in developing countries.

The Sri Lankan Twin Registry

The Sri Lankan Twin Registry (SLTR), which is part of IRD, was also established through a strategic North–South collaboration, a multidisciplinary partnership between the IRD and IoP, with generous but competitive charitable funding from the West leading to influential research and publications in high impact journals.

The SLTR was proposed by the author and founded in 1997 (Sumathipala et al. 2000, 2002, Siribaddana et al. 2006). It is a unique resource for twin and genetic research in an LMIC (Boomsma et al. 2002). It comprises of a volunteer cohort with 14 130 twins (7065 pairs) and a population-based cohort of 19 040 twins (9520 pairs) (Sumathipala et al. 2013). Several studies have been conducted using this registry, including a twin and singleton study which explored the prevalence and heritability of a range of psychiatric disorders as well as gene–environment interplay. The establishment of a state-of-the-art genetic laboratory was also a major accomplishment. A full account of the SLTR has been published elsewhere (Boomsma et al. 2002), and only an outline is presented here.

Twin research helps to determine the degree to which traits and disorders are heritable within specific populations. Most such studies use volunteer registers of twins, and most are in North America, Europe, and Australasia. Population-based registers are rare even in the West. The uniqueness of the SLTR lies in the fact that it is the first in the developing world. It is still one of the few large-scale functioning population based registries in the developing world (Boomsma et al. 2002).

Currently a follow-up study of the same cohort is under way, looking at the prevalence and interrelationship of key cardiovascular and metabolic risk markers ("metabolic syndrome"). A significant advance in the follow-up study is the establishment of a bio-bank (DNA and serum/plasma), which is considered an important research infrastructure (Sumathipala *et al.* 2013). This will open up opportunities for epigenetic, genome-wide association (GWA), and candidate-gene studies.

A specific research project, the Colombo Twin and Singleton Study (CoTaSS 1), was successfully completed. A number of papers have been published using data from CoTaSS 1 (Siribaddana *et al.* 2008, Ball *et al.* 2010a, 2010b, 2010c, 2010d, Zavos *et al.* 2012), and a follow-up study aims to estimate the prevalence of the component phenotypes which make up the "metabolic syndrome" in Sri Lanka. A secondary study aims to investigate the genetic architecture of metabolic syndrome phenotypes, and estimate the extent to which phenotypic correlations are explained by shared genetic or environmental effects. A third study aims to determine whether there is a significant etiological overlap between depression and the component phenotypes of metabolic syndrome. A sub-study within the follow-up phase aims to evaluate the contribution of sleep and activity levels

to the prevalence of metabolic syndrome and depression in Sri Lanka, using self-report and actigraphy funded by the Australian Research Council. It will be the first study to determine population-based estimates of validated sleep parameters in a developing country (Sumathipala *et al.* 2013).

In the context of scarcity of research capacity in LMICs, which is well established, the SLTR and the wider IRD initiatives have showcased how successful North–South partnerships can overcome barriers to minimize the 10/90 divide (Konradsen & Munk-Jorgensen 2007). In this perfect example of North–South collaboration, support and expertise came from colleagues at Kings College, London to establish SLTR and ensure its sustenance.

Conclusion

In this chapter, an attempt has been made to explore the various definitions of research infrastructure. Examples were also given of major funding and successful projects. Lastly, successful North–South collaborations were cited.

References

Ball H, Glozier N, Kovas Y, *et al.* (2010a) The aetiology of fatigue in Sri Lanka and its overlap with depression *British Journal of Psychiatry* **197**: 106–13.

Ball H, Glozier N, Kovas Y, *et al.* (2010b) Epidemiology and symptomatology of depression in Sri Lanka: a cross-sectional population-based survey in Colombo District. *Journal of Affective Disorders* **123**: 188–96.

Ball H, Glozier N, Kovas Y, *et al.* (2010c) Genetic and environmental contributions to the overlap between psychological, fatigue and somatic symptoms: a twin study in Sri Lanka. *Twin Research and Human Genetics* **14**: 53–63.

Ball HA, Siribaddana SH, Sumathipala A, *et al.* (2010d) Environmental exposures and their genetic or environmental contribution to depression and fatigue: a twin study in Sri Lanka. *BMC Psychiatry* **2**: 13.

Boomsma DI, Busjahn A, Peltonen L (2002) Classical twin studies and beyond. *Nature Reviews Genetics* **11**: 872–82.

Botha PA, Gruenewaldt G (2012) Promoting African European Research Infrastructure Partnership (PAERIP). TechnoScience PVT Ltd South Africa.

Coen SE, Bottorff JL, Johnson JL, Ratner PA (2010) A relational conceptual framework for multidisciplinary health research centre infrastructure, *Health Research Policy and Systems* **8**: 29 http://www.health-policy-systems. com/content/8/1/29 (accessed July 2013).

Costello A, Zumla A (2000) Moving to research partnerships in developing countries. *BMJ* **321**: 827–9.

European Science Foundation (2013) MERIL: Mapping of the European Research Infrastructure Landscape. http://www.esf.org/serving-science/ ec-contracts-coordination/meril-mapping-of-the-european-research-

infrastructure-landscape.html (accessed July 2013).

German Federal Ministry of Education and Research (2011) Recommendations on Scientific Collections as Research Infrastructures http://www. wissenschaftsrat.de/download/ archiv/10464-11-11_engl.pdf (accessed July 2013).

Global Forum for Health Research (2000) *The 10/90 Report on Health Research*. Geneva: Global Forum for Health Research.

Konradsen J, Munk-Jorgensen A (2007) The destinies of the low and middle-income country submissions. *Acta Psychiatrica Scandinavica* **115**: 331–4.

Mari JJ, Lozano JM, Duley L (1997) Erasing the global divide in health research: collaborations provide answers to developing and developed countries. *BMJ* **314**: 390.

National Research Council (1998) *Investing in Research Infrastructure in the Behavioral and Social*

Sciences. Wasington, DC: National Academies Press.

National Research Infrastructure Council (2011) Strategic framework for research infrastructure investment. http://www.innovation.gov.au/Science/ResearchInfrastructure/Documents/StrategicFrameworkforResearchInfrastructureInvestment.pdf (accessed July 2013).

Patel V, Kirkwood B (2008) Perinatal depression treated by community health workers. *Lancet* **372**: 868–9.

Patel V, Sumathipala A (2001) International representation in psychiatric literature: survey of six leading journals. *British Journal of Psychiatry* **178**: 406–9.

Patel V, Pednekar S, Weiss H, *et al.* (2005) Why do women complain of vaginal discharge? A population survey of infectious and psychosocial risk factors in a South Asian community. *International Journal of Epidemiology* **34**: 853–62.

Patel V, Weiss HA, Kirkwood BR, *et al.* (2006) Common genital complaints in women: the contribution of psychosocial and infectious factors in a population-based cohort study in Goa, India. *International Journal of Epidemiology* **35**: 1478–85.

Rahman A, Malik A, Sikander S, Roberts C, Creed F (2008) Cognitive behaviour therapy-based intervention by community health workers for mothers with depression and their infants in rural Pakistan: a cluster-randomised controlled trial. *Lancet* **372**: 902–9.

Razzouk D, Sharan P, Gallo C, *et al.* (2010) Scarcity and inequity of mental health research resources in low-and-middle income countries: a global survey. *Health Policy* **94**: 211–20.

Sharan P, Gallo C, Gureje O, *et al.* (2009) Mental health research priorities in low- and middle-income countries of Africa, Asia, Latin America and the Caribbean. *British Journal of Psychiatry* **195**: 354–63.

Siribaddana S, Hewege S, Siriwardena D, *et al.* (2006) Update from Sri Lankan twin registry: establishment of population based register and ongoing project on common mental illness, alcohol and suicidal ideations. *Twin Research and Human Genetics* **9**: 868–74.

Siribaddana S, Ball H, Hewage S, *et al.* (2008) Colombo Twin and Singleton Study (CoTASS): a description of a population-based twin study of mental disorders in Sri Lanka *BMC Psychiatry* **8**: 49.

Siriwardhana C, Sumathipala A, Siribaddana S, *et al.* (2011) Working to minimize the 10/90 divide in global mental health research: a case study from Sri Lanka on successful North–South, South–South collaborations. *International Review of Psychiatry* **23**: 77–83.

Sumathipala A, Siribaddana S (2005) Research and clinical ethics after the tsunami: Sri Lanka. *Lancet* **366**: 1418–20.

Sumathipala A, Fernando DJS, Siribaddana SH, *et al.* (2000) Establishing a twin register in Sri Lanka. *Twin Research* **3**; 202–4.

Sumathipala A, Siribaddana SH, De Silva N, *et al.* (2002) Sri Lankan Twin Registry. *Twin Research* **5**: 424–6.

Sumathipala A, Siribaddana A, Patel V (2004) Under-representation of developing countries in the research literature: ethical issues arising from a survey of five leading medical journals. *BMC Medical Ethics* **5**: E5.

Sumathipala A, Siribaddana S, Hotopf M, *et al.* (2013) The Sri Lankan Twin Registry: 2012 update. *Twin Research and Human Genetics* **16**: 307–12.

University of Minnesota Research Infrastructure Task Force (2006) Transforming the university: recommendations of the Task Force on Research Infrastructure. http://www1.umn.edu/systemwide/strategic_positioning/tf_final_reports_060512/res_infra_final.pdf (accessed July 2013).

World Health Organization (1994) *Management of Sexually Transmitted Diseases*. Geneva: WHO.

World Health Organization (2005) *Psychosocial Care of Tsunami-Affected Populations Manual for Community-Level Workers*. New Delhi: WHO Regional Office for South-East Asia.

Zavos HMS, Kovas Y, Ball HA, *et al.* (2012) Genetic and environmental etiology of nicotine use in Sri Lankan male twins. *Behavior Genetics* **42**: 798–807.

Chapter

44

Monitoring the progress of countries

Jorge Rodríguez and Víctor Aparicio

Introduction

Mental disorders represent 22% of the total burden of disease in Latin America and the Caribbean. An efficient mental health system is fundamental for reducing this high burden, which translates into morbidity, mortality, and disability, as well as for closing the large gap in terms of affected patients who are not receiving any kind of treatment (Kohn *et al.* 2005, PAHO 2007, 2009a, Rodríguez *et al.* 2009).

Although it is important to have valid and reliable information, more than 24% of countries across the world lack a system to collect and analyze basic mental health information, while in other countries the information systems are weak or inappropriate (World Health Organization 2005a, 2008). Lack of information generates problems such as deficiency in planning, lack of accountability, lack of evaluation and monitoring of ongoing processes, and the possibility of developing solutions before appropriately understanding the situation.

The current situation of mental health in Central America is complex and is associated with a long history of suffering caused by the onslaught of frequent natural disasters, in addition to bloody armed conflicts and other forms of violence (e.g., social violence or violence linked to drug and human trafficking) that for decades have affected these countries, leaving important psychosocial sequels; all this in a context of high levels of poverty and chronic socially excluded population groups, such as indigenous peoples. The last internal armed conflicts ended in the 1990s, and this opened the way for peace building and for strengthening the respect for human rights (Rodríguez *et al.* 2007, PAHO 2009b).

Notwithstanding the aforementioned situation, mental health systems in almost all Central American countries are unable to respond appropriately to the needs of the population. There still exists the asylum-type psychiatric hospital, which absorbs a sizeable proportion of mental health resources, while the participation of primary care in the provision of mental health services is limited. In addition, primary care workers are poorly prepared for handling psychosocial problems effectively. The Pan American Health Organization/Organización Panamericana de la Salud (PAHO/OPS) has increased its technical support to reform processes in the region, as evidenced by the Caracas Declaration (PAHO 1990) and PAHO Directing Council Resolutions (PAHO 1997, 2001). The regional "Strategy and plan of action on mental health" was approved for the PAHO Directing Council in 2009 (PAHO 2009a).

This chapter presents a set of indicators on the status of mental health systems in six Central American countries and the Dominican Republic. The results should help to promote changes and serve as a baseline for monitoring the process.

Methodology for the assessment of mental health systems

The World Health Organization Assessment Instrument for Mental Health Systems (WHO-AIMS) consists of a tool and methodology developed by the World Health Organization (WHO) for collecting essential data about the mental health programs and services of a country (WHO 2005b). WHO-AIMS is being used in most Latin American and Caribbean countries with the technical cooperation of PAHO.

This instrument and methodology is a tool for the comprehensive evaluation of mental health plans and services especially designed for low- and middle-income countries (LMICs). The second version, WHO-AIMS 2.2 (WHO 2005b), has six sections: (1) policy and legislative framework; (2) mental health services; (3) mental health in primary care; (4) human resources; (5) health education and the relation with other sectors; and (6) evaluation and research. This instrument, which comprises 28 sections and 155 items, provides essential information on mental health policies, plans, and services, and facilitates the monitoring of the implementation of service reform and restructuring, with emphasis on the community, as well as the involvement of users, families, and other actors in actions of promotion, prevention, treatment, and rehabilitation in mental health.

WHO-AIMS facilitates the evaluation of weaknesses in the mental health system and clarifies how to make the needed reforms. The evaluation process can promote reflection among decision makers and government officials.

The countries assessed between 2006 and 2009 were Nicaragua, El Salvador, Guatemala, Honduras, Costa Rica, Panama, and the Dominican Republic (PAHO 2009b). In each country, data collection was performed by a consultant, who received appropriate training. Technical support was provided by each country's ministry of health and their mental health programs or offices, and by PAHO/WHO representation in the country. The information was initially reviewed by the PAHO/WHO Mental Health Subregional Advisor for Central America and the Caribbean, and in the second phase by a team from the WHO Department of Mental Health and Substance Abuse in Geneva, Switzerland. Upon completion of

the review and validation of the data, national teams drafted a final report.

The next step was to present the final report and its findings to mental health workers, to national authorities and to other institutions and stakeholders involved (e.g. users and/or family associations, members of the judicial and educational systems, and representatives of traditional medicine, among others) to design an operational plan reflecting the priorities that required intervention in the short, medium, and long term.

Sociodemographic country framework

Among the countries studied, Guatemala has the lowest percentage of literate population (69.1%) and an average life expectancy of 70 years, which is also the lowest. It should be noted that Guatemala is the country with the largest number of inhabitants (about 13 million), representing over a quarter of the population of the countries where the study was conducted. It is estimated that about half of its population is indigenous, one of the most vulnerable sectors of society.

At the other end is Costa Rica, with one of the highest life expectancy rates in the Americas (78.8 years) and a literate population of almost 95%, closely followed by Panama, which has the oldest population in Central America. These two countries have the smallest populations. Costa Rica, Panama, and the Dominican Republic have the highest per capita income (US$9680, US$7310, and US$7150, respectively), and Honduras and Nicaragua the lowest (US$2900 and US$3650) (Table 44.1).

Table 44.1 Sociodemographic data, Central America and the Dominican Republic.

Country	Population (2007)	Life expectancy at birth (years) (2007)	Literate population (> 15 years) (%)a	Per capita income 2005 (US$) purchasing power parity
Costa Rica	4 468 000	78.8	94.9	9680
El Salvador	6 857 000	71.9	80.6	5120
Guatemala	13 354 000	70.3	69.1	4410
Honduras	7 106 000	70.2	80.0	2900
Nicaragua	5 603 000	72.9	76.7	3650
Panama	3 343 000	75.5	93.1	7310
Dominican Republic	9 760 000	72.2	87.0	7150

Source: Report on mental health systems in Central America and the Dominican Republic (2005–2007) using the WHO-AIMS (PAHO 2009b).
[a] Data from national surveys between 1999 and 2005.

Results of the evaluation of mental health systems

Policies, plans, and legislative framework

It was noted that all countries had begun or completed the formulation or revision of their national mental health plans after 2003, except for Guatemala, which had carried it out in 1997. However, after this assessment, Guatemala developed a new version of its mental health plan. Four countries (El Salvador, Guatemala, Nicaragua, and Panama) had no explicit policy on mental health, and in three countries (El Salvador, Guatemala, and Nicaragua) there was no defined legislative framework on the subject (Table 44.2). After the evaluation, Guatemala began preparing a document outlining its mental health policy, and El Salvador is in the process of doing so.

At the legislative level, although there were no mental health laws as such, most countries had many pieces of legislation related to the topic, scattered in different legal instruments, but they needed to be revised and updated in line with current international standards.

In summary, all countries have been more likely to generate operational frameworks (plans) than strategic or legal-normative frameworks (policies and laws). However, the WHO-AIMS analysis has enabled them to start the process for the improvement of their policies and laws.

Human rights

Some weaknesses were noted regarding the protection of patients' human rights. Five countries (Costa Rica, El Salvador, Guatemala, Nicaragua, and Panama) mentioned the existence of an institution generally called *Procuraduría de los Derechos Humanos* (in Spanish) or Ombudsman. They are governmental human rights review bodies, although their resolutions are not legally mandatory in nature, but moral.

Costa Rica, Guatemala, Nicaragua, and Panama reported inspections of mental health services by external human rights review bodies, although generally they were not carried out systematically and regularly, or through a predetermined program or agreement. Costa Rica and Guatemala reported having received an annual inspection in their psychiatric hospitals.

The control of involuntary admissions and the application of measures of physical restraint or

Table 44.2 Policy and legislative framework, Central America and the Dominican Republic

Country	Year of last version		
	Policy	Plan	Law
Costa Rica	2006	2004	1999
El Salvador	No	2005	No
Guatemala	No	1997	No
Honduras	2001	2007	1999
Nicaragua	No	2004	No
Panama	No	2003	2003
Dominican Republic	2006	2006	2006

Source: Report on mental health systems in Central America and the Dominican Republic (2005–07) using the WHO-AIMS (PAHO 2009b).

isolation to people with mental disorders in hospitals are directly related to healthcare quality and human rights protection, and, in general, there were no clear and precise regulations this regard. In practice, no country systematically collected data on the implementation of such measures. Only El Salvador and Panama provided information on the proportion of involuntary admissions to psychiatric beds, which was collected under the framework of this study.

In general, we observe that there are not programs for regular reviews of human rights protection of patients in psychiatric hospitals, and there is no provision of systematic training in the field of human rights for workers in mental health services.

Financing of mental health services

The ministries of health mental health budget, measured in relation to the total health budget, was 3% in Costa Rica and Panama; in most of the other countries it was around 1%, and in the Dominican Republic it was less than 1%.

The structure of mental health expenditures varied by country. In Panama and the Dominican Republic 50% or less of the mental health budget was allocated to the funding of psychiatric hospitals. Costa Rica was in an intermediate position, with 67.0%; while Guatemala, El Salvador, Honduras, and Nicaragua spent more than 88% of the budget on mental hospitals. On average, the seven countries devoted 1.6% of the health budget to mental health,

Table 44.3 Mental health financing, Central America and the Dominican Republic

Country	Percentage of health budget devoted to mental health	Percentage of mental health budget devoted to psychiatric hospitals
Costa Rica	2.9	67
El Salvador	1.1	92
Guatemala	1.4	90
Honduras	1.6	88
Nicaragua	0.8	91
Panama	2.9	44
Dominican Republic	0.4	50
Average	1.6	75

Source: Report on mental health systems in Central America and the Dominican Republic (2005–07) using the WHO-AIMS (PAHO 2009b).

Table 44.4 Number of beds per 100 000 population in general and psychiatric hospitals, Central America and the Dominican Republic

Country	General hospitals	Psychiatric hospitals
Costa Rica	1.97	22.1
El Salvador	0.0	6.3
Guatemala	0.02	2.64
Honduras	0.0	5.14
Nicaragua	0.33	2.98
Panama	3.93	11.3
Dominican Republic	0.9	1.75

Source: Report on mental health systems in Central America and the Dominican Republic (2005–07) using the WHO-AIMS (PAHO 2009b).

of which 75% went to psychiatric hospitals (Table 44.3). This structure of health spending has a negative impact on the development of a community health care model.

In Costa Rica, El Salvador, Guatemala, Honduras, and Panama, social security public institutions covered the costs of care for mental disorders; but only in Costa Rica and Panama did they offer significant coverage extending to most of the population.

Psychotropic medicines are practically inaccessible to people with low income levels. For example, the proportion of a minimum wage that a user should spend on purchasing the necessary daily dose of an antipsychotic or an antidepressant (the least expensive generic medicines) in El Salvador would be 46% and 28%, respectively; in Guatemala, 29% and 17%; and in Nicaragua, 5% and 4%.

Mental health services

The mental health care model is still predominantly institutional, centered on psychiatric or mental hospitals, but with nuances and exceptions. In El Salvador and Honduras there were no inpatient psychiatric units in general hospitals, and in Guatemala only two, with little functionality. In Costa Rica and Panama

there had been a certain development of psychiatric hospitalization in general hospitals (Table 44.4). The highest number of beds in general hospitals was in Panama (3.93 per 100 000 population), followed by Costa Rica (1.97 per 100 000). The latter was the country with the largest number of psychiatric units in general hospitals, a total of 26 (Table 44.5).

Psychiatric hospitals are usually located in capital cities and concentrate almost all the psychiatric beds in these countries. To a large extent, care models still follow the pattern of old psychiatric institutions – asylums – with poor living conditions for hospitalized persons and some problems regarding the protection of human rights. Often, the average stay remains high; for example, over 40% of patients admitted to the Psychiatric Hospital of Managua had remained there for over 10 years. These hospitals usually do not respond to the growing mental health needs of the population. Costa Rica had the highest rate of beds in psychiatric hospitals (22.1 per 100 000 populations), and the Dominican Republic the lowest (1.75 per 100 000) (Table 44.4).

In Panama, there had been a significant reduction in psychiatric hospital beds (63%) in the five years preceding the study. In the Dominican Republic the reduction was 25%; in El Salvador, 7%; and in Costa Rica, 6%. The rest of the countries showed no change in the number of beds in these institutions.

Community residential facilities for patients with long-standing mental disorders were almost

Table 44.5 Mental health facilities, Central America and the Dominican Republic

Country	General hospitals with psychiatric beds	Psychiatric hospitals	Outpatient mental health services	Outpatient services (children only)	Day hospitals	Residential community services
Costa Rica	26	2	38	1	2	35
El Salvador	0	2	49	1	0	0
Guatemala	2	2	32	1	2	0
Honduras	0	2	31	3	1	0
Nicaragua	3	1	34	3	5	31
Panama	8	1	103	2	3	0
Dominican Republic	9	1	56	3	1	1
Total	48	11	343	14	14	67

Source: Report on mental health systems in Central America and the Dominican Republic (2005–07) using the WHO-AIMS (PAHO 2009b).

non-existent. Basically this category includes asylum-type centers, privately owned, for the elderly or for people with intellectual disabilities; some of them are dedicated to treating substance abuse disorders.

All countries had a network of outpatient mental health services, with varying levels of development. Panama had the highest number of such services (103), while Honduras, Guatemala, and Nicaragua had the fewest (31, 32, and 34, respectively) (Table 44.5). The main problem lies in the fact that outpatient services were concentrated in the capital or major urban centers, while there were large areas, mostly rural, without coverage. Most outpatient services essentially provided clinical care; psychosocial and prevention–promotion interventions were very limited and community support was not offered routinely. Only Nicaragua reported that 50% of its health facilities provided community support.

A total of 389 262 users were treated in outpatient mental health services in the seven countries (annual basis), with an average of 55 608 users per country. This represents a rate of 803.95 per 100 000 users treated in a period of one year. Table 44.6 shows the performance of this indicator in each country. Sixty percent of people served by these mental health facilities were female, and 6% of users were children or adolescents (17 years old or younger). According to data from six of the seven countries surveyed, the average of contacts per user was 3.43 (annual basis). Partial hospitalization facilities are scarce. In El Salvador there were none, while Nicaragua had the best

Table 44.6 Users treated in outpatient facilities, Central America and the Dominican Republic

Country	Number of users per 100 000 general population
Costa Rica	1916.31
El Salvador	627.28
Guatemala	781.55
Honduras	1579.97
Nicaragua	145.06
Panama	587.83
Dominican Republic	265.53

Source: Report on mental health systems in Central America and the Dominican Republic (2005–07) using the WHO-AIMS (PAHO 2009b).

network of this type of service (five "day hospitals" in the country) (Table 44.5).

Given the very high percentages of young population (over 40%), mental health services dedicated to children and adolescents were scarce or limited (1–3 per nation) (Table 44.5).

In general, all countries reported evident rates of inequality:

- Psychiatric beds and human and financial resources were concentrated in the capitals, particularly in hospitals.

Table 44.7 Number of mental health professionals per 100 000 population, Central America and the Dominican Republic

Country	Psychiatrists	Psychologists	Nursing staff
Costa Rica	3.06	1.88	4.13
El Salvador	1.39	1.68	2.11
Guatemala	0.57	0.35	1.28
Honduras	0.81	0.77	2.58
Nicaragua	0.90	2.11	1.7
Panama	3.46	2.99	4.38
Dominican Republic	2.07	3.17	1.61

Source: Report on mental health systems in Central America and the Dominican Republic (2005–07) using the WHO-AIMS (PAHO 2009b).

Table 44.8 Percentage of doctors and nurses in primary health care with at least two days of refresher training in psychiatry/mental health in the last year, Central America and the Dominican Republic

Country	Doctors (%)	Nursing staff (%)
Costa Rica	3	—[a]
El Salvador	16	13
Guatemala	—[a]	—[a]
Honduras	4	2
Nicaragua	4	0
Panama	7	—[a]
Dominican Republic	12	0

Source: Report on mental health systems in Central America and the Dominican Republic (2005–07) using the WHO-AIMS (PAHO 2009b).
[a] No data available at the national level.

- Users of rural areas, indigenous groups, and other ethnic and linguistic minorities were significantly under-represented in the use of outpatient mental health services.
- There were no formal strategies to ensure equitable access to mental health services for indigenous groups and other ethnic minorities.

Costa Rica was the only country in the study where over 50% of the centers had protocols or procedures manuals for the care of key mental conditions in primary care. A relationship with traditional medicine was almost non-existent; only Panama and Nicaragua had information about a limited relationship between primary health care workers and traditional healers.

Human resources

Despite being the country with the largest population in Central America, Guatemala had the lowest number of professionals in the field of mental health (0.57 psychiatrists per 100 000 population), compared with 3.06 in Costa Rica and 3.46 in Panama. The Dominican Republic and Panama had the highest rates of psychologists (3.17 and 2.99 per 100 000, respectively); Guatemala and Honduras, the lowest (0.35 and 0.77 per 100 000). The number of nursing staff trained in the specialty was limited, despite being an important resource for those countries that need to develop their mental health systems. Panama and

Costa Rica were the exception, with a rate of more than four mental health nurses per 100 000 population. In general, there was a better situation in terms of human resources in Costa Rica and Panama (Table 44.7).

The countries with the highest concentration of human resources were Honduras and Nicaragua. Those with greater decentralization of psychiatrists were Costa Rica and the Dominican Republic, and in the case of nurses, El Salvador and Panama.

The percentage of time devoted to mental health issues in medical schools varied from country to country (from 1% in Guatemala to 7% in El Salvador). The percentage of time devoted to mental health issues in nursing schools varied from 3% in Guatemala to 12% in Panama. Training on mental health issues for physicians and nurses in primary care is very limited. In El Salvador, only 16% of primary care doctors had a minimum standard of training in mental health, and in the Dominican Republic, 12%. Costa Rica had the lowest level (3%), and in Guatemala the data could not be identified (Table 44.8).

In all countries there are programs for training specialists in the field of psychiatry (residential) for a period of three or four years. The number of teaching units for the training of specialists varies, and most of them are located in psychiatric hospitals, which is a contradiction if we want professionals to work in a

Table 44.9 Number of graduates, specialists in psychiatry, in the year preceding the study, Central America and the Dominican Republic

Country	Graduate specialists in psychiatry
Costa Rica	5
El Salvador	6
Guatemala	5
Honduras	4
Nicaragua	1
Panama	5
Dominican Republic	6

Source: Report on mental health systems in Central America and the Dominican Republic (2005–07) using the WHO-AIMS (PAHO 2009b).

community mental health model. In all countries, psychiatric specialists graduate annually; the figures of the last year assessed range from one in Nicaragua to six in the Dominican Republic and El Salvador (Table 44.9).

The migration to other countries registered in the first five years after reaching the specialty was zero in Honduras and El Salvador. In the other countries, emigration ranged from 1% to 20%.

The associations of users of mental health services and of families of people with mental disorders still lack strength. In all the seven participating countries, there was a total of 747 users who were members of consumer associations, and another 292 individuals who were involved in family organizations. In general, the public sector does not provide financial or any other form of support to users' associations. There were seven such organizations in Costa Rica and 12 in Nicaragua; the associative movement was almost non-existent in Honduras, El Salvador, and Guatemala.

Mental health links with other sectors

Honduras and Nicaragua reported having some mechanism or institutional body to coordinate mental health promotion activities aimed at the population.

Costa Rica, the Dominican Republic, El Salvador, Nicaragua, and Panama had legislative provisions concerning the obligation of employers to hire a percentage of employees with disabilities. However, Costa Rica was the only country that effectively enforced those provisions and where mental health facilities provided or managed outside employment for people with severe mental disorders.

In assessing the number of primary and secondary schools employing a mental health worker (technical or professional) on full time or part time basis, the study showed that the rate was generally very low (from 0.5% in El Salvador up to 16% in the Dominican Republic). This is an important index, because it will largely determine the ability to develop programs to promote and protect mental health in the educational context.

In El Salvador and Costa Rica, prisons provided mental health services to inmates. Very few prisons in the Dominican Republic, Guatemala, Honduras, and Panama provided mental health care.

Research and information systems

With the exception of Guatemala, all mental health offices and services in the countries assessed collected data. Psychiatric hospitals were the ones that provided more information, based on the number of beds, admissions, length of stay, and diagnosis. No country collected data on involuntary admissions, or about persons suffering physical restraint or isolation in hospitals. The Dominican Republic was the only country that delivered an annual report analyzing the data.

An analysis of national reports concluded that there were limitations and weaknesses in the information systems: not all mental health services reported to the ministries of health; the data collected were insufficient for proper analysis; there was underreporting or poor quality in the primary record; there were no data available from the private sector; there were no publications or annual reports on mental health; and there were no epidemiological surveillance systems. The lack of research is, undoubtedly, another weakness of the countries evaluated. Costa Rica appeared to be the strongest in mental health research, because it had a greater number of mental health professionals formally committed to the topic. However, Nicaragua and Costa Rica had a higher percentage of mental health publications over the country's total health publications registered in PubMed (24% and 20%, respectively).

Conclusions

There have been advances in the development of mental health systems in the Central American countries and the Dominican Republic, but it is evident that important work remains to be done. The priorities identified for the coming years should include (Rodriguez *et al.* 2007, PAHO 2009b):

- Strengthening the implementation of mental health national policies and plans at the country level.
- Improving funding of mental health programs and services. Modify the current structure of expenses (centralized in mental hospitals) so that more resources can be devoted to mental health outpatient services, primary health care, and community-based services.
- Developing more extensive, decentralized mental health services in the community including outpatient facilities, day hospitals, inpatient units in general hospitals, residential services, and others.
- Re-structuring existing mental hospitals. It is necessary to reduce the number of severe psychiatric patients treated in mental hospitals and reduce their lengths of stay in these facilities; many of these patients have lived there for long periods of time.
- Admission of people with mental disorders, when necessary, to mental health units in general hospitals.

- Increasing the availability of psychotropic medications in primary care facilities.
- Strengthening the human resources in mental health including pre- and postgraduate training for mental health professionals and technicians. Increasing the mental health training for primary care providers.
- Supporting consumers and family members associations by strengthening their direct participation in the design and implementation of mental health plans.
- Continuing to work in human rights protections for people with mental disorders by increasing the oversight of mental health services.
- Improving information collection and dissemination systems.

An important conclusion is that mental health systems, in most of these countries, do not satisfactorily respond to the population needs. Mental hospitals continue to be the core of mental health care, absorbing a considerable amount of available resources. The development of the mental health component in primary health care is still limited, and health workers at this level do not have the problem-solving capacity to address this kind of problem. However there are positive experiences in Central America that may be used as examples to follow in this field.

References

Kohn R, Levav I, Caldas de Almeida JM, *et al.* (2005) Los trastornos mentales en América Latina y el Caribe: asunto prioritario para la salud pública. *Revista Panamerica de Salud Pública* **18**: 229–40. http://www.scielosp.org/pdf/rpsp/v18n4-5/28084.pdf (accessed July 2013).

Pan American Health Organization (1990) *The Caracas Declaration.* http://new.paho.org/hq/dmdocuments/2008/DECLARATIONOFCARACAS.pdf (accessed July 2013).

Pan American Health Organization (1997) Resolution CD40.R19. Washington, DC: PAHO. http://www.paho.org/English/gov/cd/ftcd_40.htm#R19 (accessed July 2013).

Pan American Health Organization (2001) 43rd Directing Council, Document CD43/15. Mental health in the Americas. New challenges in a new millennium. Washington, DC: PAHO. http://www.paho.org/english/gov/cd/cd43_15-e.pdf (accessed July 2013).

Pan American Health Organization (2007) *Salud en las Américas.* Publicación Científica y Técnica No. 622. Washington, DC: PAHO.

Pan American Health Organization (2009a) *Strategy and Plan of Action on Mental Health.* Resolution CD49.R17. Washington, DC: PAHO. http://www2.paho.org/hq/dmdocuments/2009/MENTAL_HEALTH.pdf (accessed July 2013).

Pan American Health Organization (2009b) *Report on the Mental Health Systems in Central America and Dominican Republic.* Panama: PAHO. http://www.who.int/mental_health/evidence/report_on_mental_health_systems_2009_ENG.pdf (accessed July 2013).

Rodríguez J, Barret T, Narvaez S, *et al.* (2007) Sistemas de salud mental en El Salvador, Guatemala y Nicaragua. Resultados de una evaluación mediante el WHO-AIMS. *Revista Panamerica de Salud Pública* **22**: 348–57. http://www.scielosp.org/pdf/rpsp/v22n5/a08v22n5.pdf (accessed July 2013).

Rodríguez J, Kohn R, Aguilar-Gaxiola S, eds. (2009) *Epidemiología de los Trastornos Mentales en America*

Latina y el Caribe. Publicación Cinetífica y Técnica No. 632 / OPS. Washington, DC: PAHO/OPS.

World Health Organization (2005a) *Mental Health Atlas 2005.* Geneva: WHO.

World Health Organization (2005b) *Assessment Instrument for Mental Health Systems (WHO-AIMS, Version 2.2).* Geneva: WHO. http://www.who.int/mental_health/evidence/AIMS_WHO_2_2.pdf (accessed July 2013).

World Health Organization (2008) *mhGAP: Mental Health Gap Action Programme. Scaling up Care for Mental, Neurological, and Substance Use Disorders.* Geneva: WHO.

Epilogue

The synthesis of public health and international health approaches constitute the core of global mental health. The burden of mental health and neuropsychiatric disorders is great, as it constitutes about 13% of the global disability burden. The treatment gaps are enormous, irrespective of what studies are being quoted. As outlined by Robert Kohn in Chapter 3, the range in 2004 was from 32.2% for schizophrenia to 78.1% for alcohol abuse and dependence. There is also great variation in service utilization. All in all, there is a great discrepancy between service needs and service utilization. The situation for children and adolescents is even worse. The figures frequently cited, however, omit any discussion of cultural definitions of health and variation in mental health policies. Many countries still do not have any specific policy on mental health service delivery, in spite of WHO efforts in this area.

The impact of the multiple determinants of health has also gained some currency. Traditional health approaches are no longer sufficient, rather policy makers and practitioners have to consider the broader portfolio of mental health determinants to include the economic, transportation, education and employment, and site of treatment factors for individuals and communities. More emphasis needs to be placed on community-level approaches. In this regard mention should be made of a study that showed that the availability of transportation can be a predictor of compliance with psychotherapy. Needless to say that higher socioeconomic status correlates with higher health status.

All the above implies that to promote mental health and provide for adequate treatment requires a broad range of services, policies, capacity, and sustainability programs. At present, no society can boast of having enough psychiatrists or formally trained mental health workers. This implies the need for greater research and application of findings in the prevention of mental disorders and the promotion of mental health as suggested by the Grand Challenges in Global Mental Health. There is a need for task shifting and the provision of reliable public health information.

Humanitarianism and equity are driving factors in global health. Poverty and material handicaps are prime factors in health determinants.

The Millennium Development Goals (MDG) has amongst its goals two objectives – the eradication of poverty and the availability of basic education to all. Globalization is one mechanism that can contribute to this. Two issues have become apparent. One is the fact that some nations that have committed themselves to the stated objectives of the MDG only pay lip service to their commitments. A major handicap of UN declarations and treaties is that they often do not have any binding force. The other factor is that globalization has not been a perfect model, and a by-product of globalization is the deterioration of the economic situation of some poor countries.

The major international agencies such as the World Trade Organization (WTO) and the International Monetary Fund (IMF), by their insistence on structural adjustments, have made the plight of many low-income countries even worse. Some of these countries are being excluded from the global economy as they see their traditional export products lose economic and competitive value in the global market. This is aggravated by the high-income countries that heavily subsidize their farmers.

Globalization has not been a panacea, the playing field has not been equal, and – as articulated by the former Prime Minister of Norway, Kjell Magne Bondevik:

The soccer players are fortunate to play on a level field, by the same rules, with referees to ensure their

even-handed application. The development field is far less level. The rules are less clear, and more unevenly applied. Some refuse to play at fields not of their liking. The poor are mostly excluded from every field. There are no generally recognized referees. This is the challenge that the poor face.
(http://www.dpmf.org/images/OccasionalPaper12.pdf, p. 7)

It is important that the developing countries be not left behind with respect to modern technology. It will be more desirable for the developed countries to accelerate the modernization of technology in developing countries. The developing countries should not be made to go through the same trajectories that have led to improved information technologies and sciences in the developed world. Therefore, attention has to be paid to greater acceleration of innovative strategies in this area. In this regard, developing countries should strive more in seeking assistance. Health policy in developing countries should collaborate more intensely with their educational authorities for a head start in training young scientists. Practitioners from developing countries should adopt a more research-oriented attitude. Every clinical situation presents an opportunity for research. This will encourage them to pursue locally relevant questions which may have application in developed countries. By so doing, they can gain more respect and contribute to the global field. Similarly, practitioners and policy makers have to emphasize the idea of country ownership of their problems. Although this has been done mostly in the field of HIV/AIDS, global mental health is also likely to benefit from this. This hopefully will reduce the tendency to foreign-aid dependency.

The above, therefore, requires multiple-level models of intervention involving multisectoral and multiprofessional groups.

Keenly aware of the colonization experiences of the not too distant past, some advocates are very vocal in their suspicion as to the extent that global health, and by implication global mental health, can provide any real relief in the suffering of the individuals in low- and middle-income countries plagued by mental disorders.

As high-income countries frame their foreign policies with a component of health policy, the low- and middle-income countries should do likewise in order to fully participate in donor–recipient relations and not leave that area unattended.

"Smart" diplomacy rather than "muscle" diplomacy has become the order of the day. Admittedly, it is hoped that this is being driven by humanitarianism and equity. However, if it is diplomacy, it implies an attempt to also win friends in the international arena. We have to recognize that there may be real or good motives for the actions of donors. For example, I heard a recent radio commentary on human trafficking in Southeast Asia. A US representative emphasized the US interest in reducing human trafficking in that area. However, the US government was more concerned about the consequences of the use of cheap labor, provided by human "slaves" in over-fishing in that area. So recipients have to be aware of the "donors" when they bring gifts. There is a need to be watchful for backdoor opportunities for recolonization. Hence, the contentious debate about the "grand challenges" in global mental health. This is besides the fact that one size suits all cannot be applied to the field of mental health services. In spite of the homogenizing effects of globalization and our interconnectedness, there remain distinct cultural patterns in different parts of the globe. Even within the same country and region there may be different institutional traditions and trajectories of service delivery. Countries may vary as to their modernization and priorities. As previously indicated, there is a need for local ownership of problems as well as autonomy in approaching local problems.

Furthermore, the process of globalization in the area of mental health can benefit from efforts toward mutuality between donor and recipient countries. There are opportunities for the high-income countries to benefit from demonstration projects and interventions carried out in low- and middle-income countries. This is particularly relevant in those highly diverse high-income countries where the interaction of genetic and environmental determinants of health can be studied. The US National Institute of Mental Health funding of regional hubs of research is a good example in this area. An assistant asked me recently, what is the evidence for the impact of global mental health, in view of all the money being expended in this area? That is the million-dollar question. Such a question frequently refers to the need for good governance, accountability, and transparency. Mention should be made of the Swiss foreign policy which is imbedded in that country's health policy. While not providing more financial assistance, it emphasizes greater efficiency.

Finally, this project has been very instructive to me in terms of the need for a greater recognition of the issues of stigma, violence to women and girls, and the various frameworks of foreign policy and global health.

I would encourage any student or practitioner of global mental health to appraise themselves of some fundamentals of foreign policy. In so doing, our work and contribution become more interesting and more relevant as we search for a common ground and purpose in the arena of global mental health.

Index

Locators in **bold** refer to figures and tables.

445

CPSIA information can be obtained
at www.ICGtesting.com
Printed in the USA
LVOW09*1311230418
574521LV00012B/93/P